OBJECTIVE BIOLOGY

for

NEET

(National Eligibility Cum Entrance Test)

and Other Medical Entrance Examinations

Dr Rajiv Vijay, MBBS

Government Medical College, Kota

Pearson

Editor–Acquisitions: Abhilash Ayyappan
Editor–Production: Sakshi Kansal

ISBN 978-93-325-7535-6

First Impression, 2016
Second Impression, 2017

Published by Pearson India Education Services Pvt Ltd, CIN: U72200TN2005PTC057128, formerly known as TutorVista Global Pvt Ltd, licensee of Pearson Education in South Asia.

Head Office: 7th Floor, Knowledge Boulevard, A-8(A), Sector 62, Noida 201 309 U.P., India.

Registered Office: 4th floor, Software Block, Elnet Software City,
TS 140 Block 2 & 9, Rajiv Gandhi Salai, Taramani, Chennai - 600 113.
Fax: 080-30461003, Phone: 080-30461060
www.pearson.co.in, Email: companysecretary.india@pearson.com

Compositor: SRS Technologies, Puducherry
Printed in India by Rahul Print O Pack.

Contents

Preface v
Acknowledgments vi
About the Author vii
Trend Analysis of Biology From 2010–2016 ix
NEET Phase I, 2016 xi

Unit I Diversity in the Living World
1. Living World 1.1–1.12
2. Biological Classification 2.1–2.18
3. Plant Kingdom 3.1–3.26
4. Animal Classification 4.1–4.26

Unit II Structural Organization in Plants and Animals
5. Plant Morphology 5.1–5.22
6. Anatomy of Flowering Plants 6.1–6.20
7. Structural Organization in Animals 7.1–7.14

Unit III Cell: Structures and Functions
8. Cell: The Unit of Life 8.1–8.24
9. Biomolecules 9.1–9.20
10. Cell Cycle and Cell Division 10.1–10.14

Unit IV Plant Physiology
11. Transport in Plants 11.1–11.20
12. Mineral Nutrition 12.1–12.14
13. Photosynthesis in Higher Plants 13.1–13.18
14. Respiration in Plants 14.1–14.12
15. Plant Growth and Development 15.1–15.16

Unit V Human Physiology
16. Digestion and Absorption 16.1–16.18
17. Breathing and Exchange of Gases 17.1–17.18
18. Body Fluids and Circulation 18.1–18.20
19. Excretory Products and Their Elimination 19.1–19.22

	20. Locomotion and Movement	20.1–20.18
	21. Neural Control and Co-ordination	21.1–21.18
	22. Chemical Co-ordination and Integration	22.1–22.16
Unit VI	**Reproduction**	
	23. Reproduction in Organisms	23.1–23.20
	24. Sexual Reproduction in Flowering Plant	24.1–24.34
	25. Human Reproduction	25.1–25.30
	26. Reproductive Health	26.1–26.14
Unit VII	**Genetics and Evolution**	
	27. Principles of Inheritance and Variation	27.1–27.36
	28. Molecular Basis of Inheritance	28.1–28.28
	29. Evolution	29.1–29.28
Unit VIII	**Biology in Human Welfare**	
	30. Human Health and Disease	30.1–30.30
	31. Strategies for Enhancement in Food Production	31.1–31.16
	32. Microbes in Human Welfare	32.1–32.18
Unit IX	**Biotechnology**	
	33. Biotechnology Principles and Processes	33.1–33.20
	34. Biotechnology and Its Application	34.1–34.14
Unit X	**Ecology**	
	35. Organisms and Populations	35.1–35.26
	36. Ecosystem	36.1–36.20
	37. Biodiversity and Conservation	37.1–37.16
	38. Environmental Issues	38.1–38.16
	Mock Test 1	*M1.1–M1.6*
	Mock Test 2	*M2.1–M2.10*
	Mock Test 3	*M3.1–M3.8*
	Sample Paper-I	*S1.1–S1.7*
	Sample Paper-II	*S2.1–S2.8*
	Sample Paper-III	*S3.1–S3.7*

Preface

Objective Biology for NEET and other Medical Entrance Examinations is a complete study package of biology questionnaire with their answers for the students who dream of becoming medical professionals and desire to get admission in prestigious medical colleges. The content of this book will familiarize the students with the latest trends of questions and theory asked in the medical entrance examinations. This book can be used as an add on for your Board preparations also, right from the start of class XI, as this book closely adheres to the NCERT syllabus.

Some unique features of this book are:

1. Written in accordance with the class XI and XII syllabus as directed by NCERT.
2. Provides a sound revision plan for maximizing your biology score in the medical entrance examinations.
3. Plenty of Assertion and Reason questions are given to help students prepare for exams like AIIMS.
4. Previous years question from 2010 are included.
5. NEET Phase I, 2016 question paper is also included before the start of the chapters.
6. Few Mock tests and Sample papers are provided at the end of the book for student's self-practice.

As an experienced teacher, I would suggest that before starting any chapter of this book, a student should minutely scan the theory and diagrams of the NCERT Textbook and minimum three reading of its chapters is a must. In my opinion, the book will prove to be an asset and will serve to fulfill the requirement of the medical aspirants.

Rajiv Vijay

Acknowledgments

This book is a result of the enormous effort and support given by my team members who were always there to support me. I believe that the blessings of my parents (Late Gopallal Vijay and Late Suryakanta Vijay) and my grandparents have always played a prime role in making me more focused and determinant towards my goal. My wife Shubha Vijay, brother Jeetu Vijay and all other family members inspired me throughout the preparation of this book.

My sincere thanks to the team of Pearson Education for providing me the platform to serve students and I appreciate their efforts in bringing out this book in such an excellent manner.

Once again special thanks to my wife Shubha Vijay for always being there with me and helping me in proof reading of this book.

Careful attempts have been made in making the book error free; however, errors can always creep in. Suggestions, queries, criticism will always be welcomed from one and all to improve the quality of this book.

Rajiv Vijay

About the Author

Dr Rajiv Vijay has completed his schooling from JNV HURDA, Bhilwara, Rajasthan and qualified for MBBS through PMT in 1997. After completing MBBS in 2003 from Government Medical College, Kota, he established his Medical and Engineering Entrance Coaching Institute in Vadodara (Gujarat) which is today known as RJ VISION Pvt. Ltd.

In his career of 14 years, he has taught a lot of students and most of them are extremely successful in various reputed pre-medical entrance examinations. In 2011, he was selected as the head of the pre-medical division of Resonance, Kota. As the head of pre-medical division and HOD of biology he nurtured, developed, installed and supervised the pre-medical division at Kota and all centers across India.

One of his students secured AFMC ALL INDIA RANK 1 in NEET-UG, 2013 and ALL INDIA RANKING 35 in NEET and is presently studying in MAMC, New Delhi. He also helps his students by providing free lectures on his youtube channel www.youtube.com/c/drrajivvijay.

Trend Analysis of Biology From 2010-2016

Ch. No	Chapter Name	Number of Question(s) in						
		2010	2011	2012	2013	2014	2015	2016
1	The Living World	0	1	0	1	0	0	1
2	Biological Classification	3	8	4	1	6	2	5
3	Plant Kingdom	3	1	3	4	4	4	2
4	Animal Kingdom	4	3	1	4	4	3	3
5	Morphology of Flowering Plants	3	4	4	2	5	5	5
6	Anatomy of Flowering Plants	3	4	5	3	2	4	1
7	Structural Organisations in Animals	1	3	2	1	2	2	2
8	Cell: The Unit of Life	4	4	5	3	4	4	5
9	Biomolecules	1	2	3	4	2	1	3
10	Cell Cycle and Cell Division	2	1	2	2	3	2	3
11	Transport in Plants	0	0	0	1	0	1	2
12	Mineral Nutrition	3	4	3	1	1	2	1
13	Photosynthesis	3	2	2	1	1	2	3
14	Respiration in Plants	1	0	0	2	1	0	0
15	Plant Growth and Development	2	0	0	2	4	2	1
16	Digestion and Absorption	2	2	1	1	2	2	2
17	Breathing and Exchange of Gases	2	0	1	2	1	2	2
18	Body Fluids and Circulation	3	5	0	1	2	3	1
19	Excretory Products and their Elimination	3	5	1	1	1	2	1
20	Locomotion and Movement	0	0	1	3	1	2	1
21	Neural Control and Coordination	1	2	3	2	3	2	1
22	Chemical Coordination and Regulation	4	2	3	3	2	1	3
23	Reproduction in Organisms	0	1	1	3	0	0	1
24	Sexual Reproduction in Flowering Plants	4	5	3	6	3	4	5
25	Human Reproduction	13	3	4	3	3	3	2

Ch. No	Chapter Name	Number of Question(s) in						
		2010	**2011**	**2012**	**2013**	**2014**	**2015**	**2016**
26	Reproductive Health	1	2	2	3	3	1	2
27	Principles of Inheritance and Variations	5	4	2	4	4	3	7
28	Molecular Basis of Inheritance	4	1	4	2	4	6	3
29	Evolution	1	1	4	4	2	1	3
30	Human Health and Disease	3	5	6	2	2	6	4
31	Strategies for Enhancement in Food Production	2	3	2	1	1	2	1
32	Microbes in Human Welfare	3	2	7	2	1	0	1
33	Biotechnology: Principles and processes	5	2	5	2	3	0	3
34	Biotechnology and its Applications	3	3	1	1	2	3	2
35	Organisms and Environment	2	4	0	2	4	2	3
36	Ecosystem	2	2	6	3	1	6	2
37	Biodiversity and its Conservation	1	3	2	1	4	2	2
38	Environmental Issues	4	4	3	3	2	3	3
	Total Questions	**100**	**100**	**100**	**90**	**90**	**90**	**90**

NEET Phase I, 2016

The Living World

1. Nomenclature is governed by certain universal rules. Which one of the following is contrary to the rules of nomenclature?
   (a) Biological names can be written in any language
   (b) The first word in a biological name represents the genus name, and the second is a specific epithet
   (c) The names are written in Latin and are italicized
   (d) When written by hand, the names are to be underlined

Biological Classification

2. Which of the following statements is wrong for viroids?
   (a) They lack a protein coat
   (b) They causes infections
   (c) They are smaller than viruses
   (d) Their RNA is of high molecular weight
3. Which of the following statements is wrong?
   (a) Cyanobacteria are also called blue-green algae.
   (b) Golden algae are also called desmids.
   (c) Eubacteria are also called false bacteria.
   (d) Phycomycetes are also called algal fungi.
4. Which of the following would appear as the pioneer organisms on bare rocks?
   (a) Lichens
   (b) Mosses
   (c) Liverworts
   (d) Green algae
5. Chrysophytes, Euglenoids, Dinoflagellates and Slime moulds are included in the kingdom:
   (a) Monera
   (b) Fungi
   (b) Protista
   (d) Animalia
6. The primitive prokaryotes responsible for the production of biogas from the dung of ruminant animals, include the:
   (a) Halophiles
   (b) Thermoacidophiles
   (c) Methanogens
   (d) Eubacteria

Plant Kingdom

7. Select the correct statement:
   (a) Gymnosperms are both homosporous and heterosporous
   (b) *Salvinia*, *ginkgo* and *Pinus* all are gymnosperms
   (c) *Sequoia* is one of the tallest trees
   (d) The leaves of gymnosperms are not well adapted to extremes of climate

Animal Kingdom

8. Which of the following features is not present in the Phylum – Arthropoda?
   (a) Chitinous exoskeleton
   (b) Metameric segmentation
   (c) Parapodia
   (d) Jointed appendages

9. Which of the following characteristic features always holds true for the corresponding group of animals?

(a) Cartilaginous endoskeleton – Chondrichthyes
(b) Viviparous – Mammalia
(c) Possess a mouth with an upper and a lower jaw – Chordata
(d) 3-chambered heart with one incompletely divided ventricle. – Reptilia

10. Which one of the following characteristics is not shared by birds and mammals?
(a) Ossified endoskeleton
(b) Breathing using lungs
(c) Viviparity
(d) Warm blooded nature

Morphology of Flowering Plants

11. The standard petal of a papilionaceous corolla is also called:
(a) Carina
(b) Pappus
(c) Vexillum
(d) Corona

12. Tricarpellary, syncarpous gynoecium is found in flowers of:
(a) Liliaceae
(b) Solanaceae
(c) Fabaceae
(d) Poaceae

13. Which of the following is not a stem modification?
(a) Pitcher of Nepenthes
(b) Thorns of citrus
(c) Tendrils of cucumber
(d) Flattened structures of Opuntia

14. Cotyledon of maize grain is called:
(a) plumule
(b) coleorhiza
(c) coleoptile
(d) scutellum

15. Stems modified into flat green organs performing the functions of leaves are known as:
(a) Cladodes
(b) Phyllodes
(c) Phylloclade's
(d) Scales

Anatomy of Flowering Plants

16. Specialized epidermal cells surrounding the guard cells are called:
(a) Complementary cells
(b) Subsidiary cells
(c) Bulliform cells
(d) Lenticels

Structural Organisation in Animals

17. Which of the following features is not present in *Periplaneta americana*?
(a) Schizocoelom as body cavity
(b) Indeterminate and radial cleavage during embryonic development
(c) Exoskeleton composed of N – acetyl glucosamine
(d) Metamerically segmented body

18. Which type of tissue correctly matches with its location?

	Tissue	Location
(a)	Smooth muscle	Wall of intestine
(b)	Areolar tissue	Tendons
(c)	Transitional epithelium	Tip of nose
(d)	Cuboidal epithelium	Lining of stomach

Cell: The Unit of Life

19. Mitochondria and chloroplast are:
(i) Semi-autonomous organelles.
(ii) Formed by division of pre-existing organelles and they contain DNA but lack protein synthesizing machinery.
Which one of the following options is correct?
(a) Both (i) and (ii) are correct
(b) (ii) is true and (i) is false
(c) (i) is true and (ii) is false
(d) Both (i) and (ii) are false

20. Microtubules are the constituents of:
(a) Cilia, Flagella and Peroxisomes
(b) Spindle fibres, Centrioles and Cilia
(c) Centrioles, Spindle fibres and Chromatin
(d) Centrosome, Nucleosome and Centrioles

21. A complex of ribosome attached to a single strand of RNA is known as:
(a) Polysome
(b) Polymer
(c) Polypeptide
(d) Okazaki fragment

22. Which one of the following cell organelles is enclosed by a single membrane?
(a) Mitochondria
(b) Chloroplasts
(c) Lysosomes
(d) Nuclei

23. Water soluble pigments found in plant cell vacuoles are:
(a) Xanthophylls
(b) Chlorophylls
(c) Carotenoids
(d) Anthocyanins

Biomolecules

24. One of the major components of cell wall of most fungi is:
(a) Chitin
(b) Peptidoglacan
(c) Cellulose
(d) Hemicellulose

25. Which one of the following statements is wrong?
(a) Sucrose is a disaccharide
(b) Cellulose is a polysaccharide
(c) Uracil is a pyrimidine
(d) Glycine is a sulphur containing amino acid

26. A typical molecule is made up of:
(a) Three glycerol molecules and one fatty acid molecule
(b) One glycerol and three fatty acid molecules
(c) One glycerol and one fatty acid molecule
(d) Three glycerol and three fatty acid molecules

Cell Cycle and Cell Division

27. Spindle fibres attach on to:
(a) Telomere of the chromosome
(b) Kinetochore of the chromosome
(c) Centromere of the chromosome
(d) Kinetosome of the chromosome

28. In meiosis crossing over is initiated at:
(a) Pachytene
(b) Leptotene
(c) Zygotene
(d) Diplotene

29. Which of the following is not characteristic feature during mitosis in somatic cells?
(a) Spindle fibres
(b) Disappearance of nucleolus
(c) Chromosome movement
(d) Synapsis

Transport in Plants

30. Water vapour comes out from the plant leaf through the stomatal opening. Through the same stomatal opening carbon dioxide diffuses into the plant during photosynthesis. Reason out the above statements using one of following options:
(a) Both processes cannot happen simultaneously
(b) Both processes can happen together because the diffusion coefficient of Water and CO_2 is different
(c) The above processes happen only during night time
(d) One process occurs during time and the other at night

Mineral Nutrition

31. In which of the following all three are macronutrients?
(a) Boron, zinc, manganese
(b) Iron, copper, molybdenum
(c) Molybdenum, magnesium, manganese
(d) Nitrogen, nickel, phosphorus

Photosynthesis in Higher Plants

32. Emerson's enhancement effect and Red drop have been instrumental in the discovery of:
(a) Photophosphorylation and non-cyclic electron transport
(b) Two photosystems operating simultaneously
(c) Photophosphorylation and cyclic electron transport
(d) Oxidative phosphorylation

33. In a chloroplast the highest number of protons is found in:
(a) Stoma
(b) Lumen of thylakoids
(c) Inter membrane space
(d) Antennae complex

34. A plant in your garden avoids photorespiratory losses, has improved water use efficiency shows high rates of photosynthesis at high temperatures and has improved efficiency of nitrogen utilization. In which of the following physiological groups would you assign this plant?
(a) C_3
(b) C_4
(c) CAM
(d) Nitrogen

Plant Growth and Development

35. The Avena curvature is used for bioassay of:
(a) ABA
(b) GA_3
(c) IAA
(d) Ethylene

Digestion and Absorption

36. In the stomach, gastric acid is secreted by the:
(a) gastrin secreting cells
(b) parietal cells
(c) peptic cells
(d) acidic cells

37. Which of the following guards the opening of hepatopancreatic duct into the duodenum?
(a) Semilunar valve
(b) Ileocaecal valve
(c) Pyloric sphincter
(d) Sphincter of Oddi

Breathing and Exchange of Gases

38. Name the chronic respiratory disorder caused mainly by cigarette smoking:
(a) Emphysema
(b) Asthma
(c) Respiratory acidosis
(d) Respiratory alkalosis

39. Reduction in pH of blood will:
(a) Reduce the rate of heart beat
(b) Reduce the blood supply to the brain
(c) Decrease the affinity of hemoglobin with oxygen
(d) None of these

Body Fluids and Circulation

40. Blood pressure in the pulmonary artery is:
(a) same as that in the aorta
(b) more than that in the carotid
(c) more than that in the pulmonary vein
(d) less than that in the vena cavae

Excretory Products and Their Elimination

41. In mammals, which blood vessel would normally carry largest amount of urea?
(a) Renal Vein
(b) Dorsal Aorta
(c) Hepatic Vein
(d) Hepatic Portal Vein

Locomotion and Movement

42. Lack of relaxation between successive stimuli in sustained muscle contraction is known as:
(a) Spasm
(b) Fatigue
(c) Tetanus
(d) Tonus

Neural Control and Coordination

43. Photosensitive compound in human eye is made up of:
(a) Guanosine and Retinol
(b) Opsin and Retinal
(c) Opsin and Retinol
(d) Transducin and Retinene

Chemical Coordination and Integration

44. Which of the following pairs of hormones are not antagonistic (having opposite effects) to each other?
(a) Parathormone–Calcitonin
(b) Insulin–Glucagon
(c) Aldosterone–Atrial Natriuretic Factor
(d) Relaxin–Inhibin

45. Changes in GnRH pulse frequency in females is controlled by circulating levels of:
(a) Estrogen and progesterone
(b) Estrogen and inhibin
(c) Progesterone only
(d) Progesterone and inhibin

46. Identify the correct statement on 'inhibin':
(a) Inhibits the secretion of LH, FSH and Prolactin
(b) Is produced by granulose cells in ovary and inhibits the secretion of FSH
(c) Is produced by granulose cells in ovary and inhibits the secretion of LH
(d) Is produced by nurse cells in testes and inhibits the secretion of LH

Reproduction in Organisms

47. In bryophytes and pteridophytes, transport of male gametes requires:
(a) Wind
(b) Insects
(c) Birds
(d) Water

Sexual Reproduction in Flowering Plants

48. The correct water from tender coconut represents:
(a) Endocarp
(b) Fleshy mesocarp
(c) Free nuclear proembryo
(d) Free nuclear endosperm

49. Proximal end of the filament of stamen is attached to the:
(a) Anther
(b) Connective
(c) Placenta
(d) Thalamus or petal

50. Which one of the following statements is not true?
(a) Tapetum helps in the dehiscence of anther
(b) Exine of pollen grains is made up of sporopollenin
(c) Pollen grains of many species cause severe allergies
(d) Stored pollen in liquid nitrogen can be used in the crop breeding programmes

51. Seed formation without fertilization in flowering plants involves the process of:
(a) Sporulation
(b) Budding
(c) Somatic hybridization
(d) Apomixis

52. Which of the following statements is not correct?
(a) Pollen grains of many species can germinate on the stigma of a flower, but only one pollen tube of the same species grows into the style
(b) Insects that consume pollen or nectar without bringing about pollination are called pollen nectar robbers
(c) Pollen germination and pollen tube growth are regulated by chemical components of pollen interacting with those of the pistil
(d) Some reptiles have also been reported as pollinators in some plant species

Human Reproduction

53. Fertilization in humans is practically feasible only if
(a) The sperms are transported into vagina just after the release of ovum in fallopian tube.
(b) The ovum and sperms are transported simultaneously to ampullary–isthmic junction of the fallopian tube.
(c) The ovum and sperms are transported simultaneously to ampullary–isthmic junction of the cervix.
(d) The sperms are transported into cervix within 48 hrs of release of ovum in uterus.

54. Select the incorrect statement:
(a) FSH stimulates the sertoli cells which help in spermiogenesis
(b) LH triggers ovulation in ovary
(c) LH and FSH decrease gradually during the follicular phase
(d) LH triggers secretion of androgens from the Leydig cells

Reproductive Health

55. In context of Amniocentesis, which of the following statements is incorrect?
(a) It is usually done when a woman is between 14–16 weeks pregnant
(b) It is used for prenatal sex determination
(c) It can be used for detection of Down syndrome
(d) It can be used for detection of Cleft palate

56. Which of the following approaches does not give the defined action of contraceptive?

(a) Barrier methods	Prevent fertilization
(b) Intra uterine devices	Increases phagocytosis of sperms suppress sperm motility and fertilizing capacity of sperms
(c) Hormonal contraceptives	Prevent retard entry of sperms, prevent ovulation and fertilization
(d) Vasectomy	Prevents spermatogenesis

Principles of Inheritance and Variation

57. Which of the following most appropriately describes haemophilia?
(a) Recessive gene disorder
(b) X–linked recessive gene disorder
(c) Chromosomal disorder
(d) Dominant gene disorder

58. A tall true breeding garden pea plant is crossed with a dwarf true breeding garden pea plant. When the F1 plants were selfed the resulting genotypes were in the ratio of:
(a) 1:2:1: Tall homozygous: Tall heterozygous : Dwarf
(b) 1:2:1: Tall heterozygous: Tall homozygous: Dwarf
(c) 3 : 1 : : Tall Dwarf
(d) 3 : 1 : : Dwarf : Tall

59. Match the terms in Column I with their description in Column II and choose the correct option:

Column I	Column II
(a) Dominance	(i) Many genes govern a single character
(b) Codominance	(ii) In a heterozygous organism only one allele expresses itself.
(c) Pleiotropy	(iii) In a heterozygous organisms both alleles express themselves fully
(d) Polygenic inheritance	(iv) A single gene influences many characters

Code:

	(a)	(b)	(c)	(d)
(a)	ii	i	iv	iii
(b)	ii	iii	iv	i
(c)	iv	i	ii	iii
(d)	iv	iii	i	ii

60. Pick out the correct statements:
(A) Haemophilia is a sex-linked recessive disease.
(B) Down's syndrome is due to aneuploiday.
(C) Phenyllketonuria is an autosomal recessive gene disorder.
(D) Sickle cell anaemia is an X-linked recessive gene disorder.
(a) A and D are correct (b) B and D are correct
(c) A, C and D are correct (d) A, B and C are correct

61. The amino acid Tryptophan is the precursor for the synthesis of:
(a) Melatonin and Serotonin (b) Thyroxine and Triiodothyronine
(c) Estrogen and Progesterone (d) Cortisol and Cortisone

62. In a testcross involving F1 dihybrid flies, more parental-type offspring were produced the recombinant-type offspring. This indicates:
(a) The two genes are located on two different chromosomes
(b) Chromosomes failed to separate during meiosis
(c) The two genes are linked and present on the same chromosome
(d) Both of the characters are controlled by more than one gene

63. A cell at telophase stage is observed by a student in a plant brought from the field. He tells his teacher that this cell is not like other cells at telophase stage. There is no formation of cell plate and thus the cell is containing more number of chromosomes as compared to other, dividing cells. This would result in:
(a) Aneuploidy (b) Polyploidy
(c) Somaclonal variation (d) Polyteny

Molecular Basis of Inheritance

64. Which of the following is required as inducer(s) for the expression of Lac operon?
(a) Glucose (b) Galactose
(c) Lactose (d) Lactose and galactose

65. Which of the following is not required for any of the techniques of DNA fingerprinting available at present?
(a) Polymerase chain reaction (b) Zinc figure analysis
(c) Restriction enzymes (d) DNA – DNA hybridization

66. Which one of the following is the starter codon?
(a) AUG (b) UGA
(c) UAA (d) UAG

Evolution

67. Which of the following structures is homologues to the wing of a birds?
(a) Dorsal fin of a Shark (b) Wing of a Moth
(c) Hind limb of Rabbit (d) Flipper of Whale

68. Following are the two statements regarding the origin of life:
(A) The earliest organisms that appeared on the earth were non-green and presumably anaerobes.
(B) The first autotrophic organisms were the chemoautotroph that never released oxygen.
Of the above statements which one of the following options is correct?
(a) (A) is correct but (B) is false (b) (B) is correct but (A) is false
(c) Both (A) and (B) are correct (d) Both (A) and (B) are false

69. Analogous structures are a result of:
(a) Divergent evolution
(b) Convergent evolution
(c) Shared ancestry
(d) Stabilizing selection

Human Health and Disease

70. Asthma may be attributed by:
(a) Bacterial infection of the lungs
(b) Allergic reaction of the mast cells in the lungs
(c) Inflammation of the trachea
(d) Accumulation of fluid in the lungs

71. In higher vertebrates, the immune system can distinguish self-cells and non-self. If this property is lost due to genetic abnormality and it attacks self-cells, then it leads to:
(a) Allergic response
(b) Graft rejection
(c) Auto-immune disease
(d) Active immunity

72. Antivenom injection contains preformed antibodies while polio drops that are administered into the body contain
(a) Activate pathogens
(b) Harvested antibodies
(c) Gamma globulin
(d) Attenuated pathogens

73. Which of the following statements is not true for cancer cells in relation to mutations.
(a) Mutations in proto-oncogenes accelerate the cell cycle
(b) Mutations destroy telomerase inhibitor
(c) Mutations inactivate the cell control
(d) Mutations inhibit production of telomerase

Strategies for Enhancement in Food Production

74. A system of rotating crops with legume or grass pasture to improve soil structure and fertility is called:
(a) Ley farming
(b) Contour farming
(c) Strip farming
(d) Shifting agriculture

Microbes in Human Welfare

75. Which of the following is wrongly matched in the given table?

	Microbe	Product	Application
(a)	Trichoderma polysporum	Cyclosporin A	Immunosuppressive drug
(b)	Monascus purpureus	Statins	Lowering of blood cholesterol
(c)	Streptococcus	Streptockinase	Removal of clot from blood vessel
(d)	Clostridium butylicum	Lipase	Removal of oil stains

Biotechnology: Principles and Processes

76. Which of the following is not a feature of the plasmids?
(a) Independent replication
(b) Circular structure
(c) Transferable
(d) Single-stranded

77. The taq polymerase enzyme is obtained from:
(a) Thermus aquaticus
(b) Thiobacillus ferroxidans
(c) Bacillus subtilis
(d) Pseudomonas putida

78. Which of the following is a restriction endonuclease?
(a) Hind II
(b) Protease
(c) DNase I
(d) RNase

Biotechnology and Its Applications

79. The two polypeptides of human insulin are linked together by:
(a) Hydrogen bonds
(b) Phosphodiester bond
(c) Covalent bond
(d) Disulphide bridges

80. Which part of the tobacco plant is infected by *Meloidogyne incognita*?
(a) Flower
(b) Leaf
(c) Stem
(d) Root

Organisms and Populations

81. Gause's principle of competitive exclusion states that:
(a) More abundant species will exclude the less abundant species through competition
(b) Competition for the same resources excludes species having different food preferences
(c) No two species can occupy the same niche indefinitely for the same limiting resources
(d) Larger organisms exclude smaller ones through competition

82. When does the growth rate of a population following the logistic model equal zero? The logistic model is given as $dN/dt = rN(1\text{-}N/K)$:
(a) When N/K is exactly one
(b) When N nears the carrying capacity of the habitat
(c) When N/K equals zero
(d) When dearth rate is greater than birth rate

83. It is much easier for a small animal to run uphill than for animal, because:
(a) It is easier to carry a small body weight
(b) Smaller animals have a higher metabolic rate
(c) Small animals have a lower O_2 requirement
(d) The efficiency of muscles in large animals is less than in the small animals

Ecosystem

84. Which of the following is a characteristic feature of cropland ecosystem?
(a) Absence of soil organisms
(b) Least genetic diversity
(c) Absence of weeds
(d) Ecological succession

85. The term ecosystem was coined by:
(a) E. P. Odum
(b) A.G. Tansley
(c) E. Haeckel
(d) E. Warming

Biodiversity and Conservation

86. Which of the National Aquatic Animal of India?
(a) Gangetic shark
(b) River dolphin
(c) Blue whale
(d) Sea-horse

87. Which of the following is the most important cause of animals and plants being driven to extinction?
(a) Over-exploitation
(b) Alien species invasion
(c) Habitat loss and fragmentation
(d) Co-extinctions

Environmental Issues

88. Joint Forest Management Concept was introduced in India during:
(a) 1960s (b) 1970s
(c) 1980s (d) 1990s

89. Depletion of which gas in the atmosphere can lead to an increased incidence of skin cancers:
(a) Nitrous oxide (b) Ozone
(c) Ammonia (d) Methane

90. A river with an inflow of domestic sewage rich in organic waste may result in:
(a) Drying of the river very soon due to algal bloom
(b) Increased population of aquatic food web organisms
(c) An increased production of fish due to biodegradable nutrients
(d) Death of fish due to lack of oxygen

Answer Keys

1. (a)	2. (d)	3. (c)	4. (a)	5. (b)	6. (c)	7. (c)	8. (c)	9. (a)	10. (c)
11. (c)	12. (a)	13. (a)	14. (d)	15. (c)	16. (b)	17. (b)	18. (a)	19. (c)	20. (b)
21. (a)	22. (c)	23. (d)	24. (a)	25. (d)	26. (b)	27. (b)	28. (a)	29. (d)	30. (b)
31. (b)	32. (b)	33. (b)	34. (b)	35. (c)	36. (b)	37. (d)	38. (a)	39. (c)	40. (c)
41. (c)	42. (c)	43. (b)	44. (d)	45. (b)	46. (d)	47. (d)	48. (d)	49. (d)	50. (a)
51. (d)	52. (a)	53. (b)	54. (c)	55. (d)	56. (d)	57. (b)	58. (a)	59. (b)	60. (d)
61. (a)	62. (c)	63. (b)	64. (c)	65. (b)	66. (a)	67. (d)	68. (c)	69. (b)	70. (b)
71. (c)	72. (d)	73. (d)	74. (a)	75. (d)	76. (d)	77. (a)	78. (a)	79. (d)	80. (d)
81. (c)	82. (a)	83. (b)	84. (b)	85. (b)	86. (b)	87. (c)	88. (c)	89. (b)	90. (d)

Unit

I

Diversity in The Living World

Unit I is one of the most important units from the examples point of view. As this unit contains animal and plant classifications which require some extra input, so prepare these two chapters in some more detail. Do not deviate so much from textbook. By solving questions you can learn all the examples. Also nowadays, a question may be asked from Chapter 1, i.e. 'Living World'. Since all diagrams are important, you need to analyze each diagram because questions can be asked in any format. Unit I contributes 8–10 questions in AIPMT. Employ the process of *mnemonic* to increase the efficiency of memory. To elaborate, for examples coming under Echinodermates given in textbook, you can employ the following:

[**A, B, C, D, E**]: **A** for **A**sterias (star fish) **B** for **B**rittle star (ohpiura) **C** for **C**ucumaria (sea cucumber) **D** for ante**D**on(sea lily) and **E** for **E**chinus (sea urchin)].

CHAPTER

1

Living World

1. Who is known as 'the Darwin of the 20th century'?
   (a) Lamarck (b) Ernst Mayr
   (c) Carolus Linneaus (d) Robert May
2. The number of species that are known and described range between
   (a) 1.3–1.4 million (b) 1.4–1.5 million
   (c) 1.7–1.8 million (d) 1.9–2.2 million
3. Twin characteristics of growth are
   (a) increase in mass (b) increase in number
   (c) both of the above (d) none of the above
4. Growth in living organism
   (a) is from outside (b) is from inside
   (c) both (a) and (b) (d) does not take place
5. Which of the following does not grow?
   (a) Amoeba (b) Yeast (c) Dead body (d) Planaria
6. Growth cannot be taken as a defining property of living organisms because
   (a) all living organism do not show growth
   (b) non-living thing also grow from inside
   (c) non-living things also grow
   (d) some living organism not showing process of reproduction
7. Select the total number from the following organism that multiply by budding
   Hydra, Sponges, yeast, earthworm, Planaria, honey bee
   (a) 2 (b) 3 (c) 4 (d) 5
8. For which organism, growth is synonymous with reproduction?
   (a) Unicellular algae (b) Amoeba (c) Bacteria (d) All
9. Which of the following multiply through fragmentation?
   (a) Fungi (b) Filamentous algae (c) Planaria (d) All of these
10. Mark the correct statement.
    (a) The growth in living organisms is from inside
    (b) Plants grow only up to a certain age
    (c) Only living organisms grow
    (d) All of these
11. The growth and reproduction are mutually exclusive events in
    (a) plants only (b) animals only
    (c) higher animal and plants (d) lower organisms

12. Reproduction cannot be an all-inclusive defining characteristic of living organisms because
(a) all living organism do not show growth
(b) many organism do not reproduce
(c) non-living things show reproduction
(d) all living organism show small period of reproductive phase in their life
13. Living organism shows
(a) self-replication (b) evolution
(c) self-regulation and response to external stimuli (d) all
14. The sum total of chemical reactions occurring in our body is called
(a) metabolism (b) homeostasis (c) catabolism (d) anabolism
15. Select the incorrect statement from the following
(A) NBRI is situated at Lucknow.
(B) Plant families like Convolvulaceae and Solanaceae are included in the order polymoniales mainly based on the floral characters.
(C) All living organisms – present, past and future, are linked to one another by the sharing of the common genetic material but to varying degree.
(D) Order Solanum, Datura and Petunia are placed in family Solanaceae.
(a) A only (b) B and D only
(c) D only (d) B and C only
16. Which of the following statement is incorrect?
(a) All plants, animals, fungi and microbes exhibit metabolism
(b) Interactions among the molecular components of the organelles result into the properties of cell organelles
(c) Properties of cellular organelles are present in the molecular constituents of the organelles
(d) Celluar organisation of the body is the defining feature of life forms
17. Properties of organs are
(a) present in the constituent cells
(b) due to different cells in them
(c) due to their similar origin
(d) a result of interactions among the constituent tissues
18. Which two points are known as the twin characteristics of growth?
(1) Increase in mass (2) Metabolism
(3) Increase in number of individuals (4) Sense of environment
(a) (1) and (2) (b) (1) and (4) (c) (2) and (3) (d) (1) and (3)
19. Growth by cell division occurs ______________ in plants and ______________ in animals
(a) Continuously, only up to a certain age
(b) Only up to a certain age, continuously
(c) Continuously, never
(d) Continuously, continuously
20. Which of the following matching is incorrect?

	Common name	Genus	Order	Class
(a)	Man	Homo	Primata	Mammalia
(b)	Mango	Mangifera	Sapindales	Dicotyledonae
(c)	Housefly	Musca	Coelopetra	Insecta
(d)	Wheat	Tritium	Poales	Monocotyledonae

21. Which set of organisms multiply through fragmentation?
(a) Planaria, hydra, yeast
(b) Echinoderms, fungi, bacteria
(c) Fungi, filamentous algae, protonema of mosses
(d) Amoeba, hydra, virus

22. Which of the following organism does not reproduce?
(a) Mules (b) Sterile worker bees
(c) Sterile human couple (d) All

23. Which one of the following aspects is an exclusive characteristic of living things?
(a) Isolated metabolic reactions occur in vitro
(b) Increase in mass from inside only
(c) Perception of events happening in the environment and their memory
(d) Increase in mass by accumulation of material both on surface as well as internally

24. Which of the following is self-conscious?
(a) Human being (b) Tiger (c) Lion (d) Frog

25. Metabolic reactions take place
(a) Invitro (b) Invivo
(c) both (a) and (b) (d) only in unicellular organisms

26. Organisms that can sense and respond to environmental cues
(a) eukaryotes only
(b) prokaryotes only
(c) both (a) and (b)
(d) those with a well-developed neuroendocrine system

27. Growth, development and functioning of living body is due to
(a) a decrease in entropy (b) an increase in Gibbs free energy
(c) metabolism (d) adaptations

28. A living organism can be exceptionally differentiated from a non-living thing on the basis of its ability for
(a) reproduction and excretion
(b) growth and movement
(c) responsiveness to touch and temperature
(d) interaction with environment and progressive evolution

29. Two components of binomial nomenclature are
(a) generic name (b) specific epithet (c) both (a) and (b) (d) subspecies

30. In *Mangifera indica Linn*, Linn stands for
(a) Latin (b) lower organism (c) Linnaeus (d) Lamarck

31. Alsatian is a breed of
(a) dog (b) cat (c) cow (d) horse

32. Modern taxonomy studies require
(a) knowledge of external and internal structure
(b) knowledge of structure of cell
(c) knowledge development process and ecological information of organisms
(d) all

33. Which of the following term include all other terms?
(a) Classification (b) Nomenclature (c) Taxonomy (d) Systematics

34. Linnaeus evolved a system of nomenclature called
(a) trinomial (b) vernacular (c) binomial (d) polynomial

35. Binomial nomenclature seems to be difficult because a scientific name is derived from
(a) Hindi (b) Sanskrit (c) Latin (d) Arabic

36. A group of plants or animals with similar traits of any rank is
(a) species (b) order (c) genus (d) taxon

37. Binomial nomenclature means
(a) two names: one given by zoologist, other by botanist
(b) one scientific name consisting of a generic name and a specific epithet
(c) two names: one latinized, other french
(d) two names: one scientific, other local

38. Basic unit of taxonomic hierarchy is
(a) species (b) kingdom (c) class (d) phylum

39. Botanical name of mango is
(a) *Mangifera indica* (b) *Solanum tuberosum*
(c) *Solanum melongena* (d) *Panthera leo*

40. Botanical name of potato is
(a) *Mangifera indica* (b) *Solanum tuberosum*
(c) *Solanum melongena* (d) *Panthera leo*

41. Zoological name of lion is
(a) *Mangifera indica* (b) *Solanum tuberosum*
(c) *Solanum melongena* (d) *Panthera leo*

42. The branch connected with characterization, nomenclature, identification and classification is
(a) ecology (b) taxonomy (c) morphology (d) eugenics

43. The third name in trinomial nomenclature is
(a) species (b) subgenus (c) subspecies (d) holotype

44. In binomial nomenclature
(a) both genus and species are printed in italics
(b) genus and species may be of same name
(c) both the initial letters in genus and species is capital
(d) genus is written after the species

45. As we go higher from species to kingdom, the number of common characterstic goes on _______.
(a) increasing (b) decreasing (c) remains same (d) none of the above

46. The binomial nomenclature was given by
(a) Lamarck (b) Ernst Mayr (c) Carolus Linnaeus (d) Darwin

47. The term 'taxon' is used for
(a) the ranks of species and genus (b) the ranks up to phylum
(c) the species epithet only (d) any rank of taxonomic hierarchy

48. The taxonomic aid that provides information for the identification of names of species found in an area is
(a) monograph (b) manual (c) catalogue (d) periodical

49. The Indian Botanical Garden is located in
(a) Howrah (b) Lucknow (c) Mumbai (d) Mysore

50. The famous botanical garden 'Kew' is located in
(a) England (b) Lucknow (c) America (d) Australia

51. Identify the correct sequence of taxonomic categories.
(a) Species–order–kingdom–phylum
(b) Species–family–genus–class
(c) Genus–species–order–phylum
(d) Species–genus–order-phylum

52. Which biological name is wrongly written?
(a) *Apis indica*
(b) *Triticum aestivum*
(c) *Felis domesticus*
(d) *Mangifera Indica*

53. Descending arrangement of categories is called
(a) classification (b) taxonomy (c) hierarchy (d) key

54. Petunia is
(a) variety (b) subspecies (c) species (d) genus

55. Which one of the following is not a category?
(a) Species (b) Class (c) Phylum (d) Convolvulaceae

56. In hierarchy of classification, order is present between
(a) family and genus
(b) phylum and kingdom
(c) family and class
(d) family and species

57. Select the incorrect statement from the following
(a) Each statement in key is called lead
(b) Taxonomic keys are tools that help in identification based on characterstics
(c) ICZN stands for International Code of Zoological Nomenclature
(d) Ernst Mayr used *system a Nature* as the title of his publication

58. Place where we store dry plants for information purpose is called
(a) key (b) museum (c) monograph (d) herbarium

59. Which is not a part of taxonomic hierarchy?
(a) Genus and species
(b) Order and class
(c) Kingdom and class
(d) Catalogue and herbarium

60. Find out the incorrect statement from the following:
(a) Closely-related species differ in morphological features
(b) Genus comprises a group of related species
(c) Taxonomic studies are useful in agricultural, forestry and industries
(d) Notochord and ventral hollow neural system are common features of phylum chordata

61. ICBN is
(a) International Code for Biosphere Nomenclature
(b) International Code for Botanical Nomenclature
(c) International Class for Biological Nobel leurette
(d) International Committe for Biological Naming

62. Zoological name of tiger is
(a) *Mangifera indica*
(b) *Solanum tuberosum*
(c) *Solanum melongena*
(d) *Panthera tigris*

63. Zoological name of leopard is
(a) *Mangifera indica*
(b) *Solanum tuberosum*
(c) *Solanum melongena*
(d) *Panthera pardus*

64. Zoological name of house fly is
(a) *Mangifera indica*
(b) *Solanum tuberosum*
(c) *Solanum melongena*
(d) *Musca domestica*

65. Zoological name of man is
(a) *Mangifera indica*
(b) *Solanum tuberosum*
(c) *Solanum melongena*
(d) *Homo sapiens*

66. Botanical name of wheat is
(a) *Mangifera indica*
(b) *Solanum tuberosum*
(c) *Solanum melongena*
(d) *Triticum aestivum*

67. Zoological name of cat is
(a) *Mangifera indica*
(b) *Solanum tuberosum*
(c) *Solanum melongena*
(d) *Felis domesticus*

68. Botanical name of makoi is
(a) *Mangifera indica*
(b) *Solanum tuberosum*
(c) *Solanum melongena*
(d) *Solanum nigrum*

69. Potato and brinjal belongs to genus
(a) *Mangifera* (b) *Solanum* (c) *Allium* (d) *Brassica*

70. Genera Petunia and Datura belongs to family
(a) *Solanaceae* (b) *Fabaceae* (c) *Liliaceae* (d) any of the above

71. Select the total number of family from the following:
Felis, Felidae, Solanaceae, Liliaceae, Canidae, Hominidae, Poaceae, Muscidae, Insecta, Convolvulaceae,
(a) 5 (b) 6 (c) 7 (d) 8

72. Family *Solanaceae* and *Convolvulaceae* belongs to order
(a) *Poales* (b) *Polymoniales* (c) *Diptera* (d) *Dicot*

73. Common features of *Chordata* are
(a) presence of notochord in any stage of life
(b) dorsal hollow neural system
(c) paired pharyngeal gill slits
(d) all

74. Which of the following is a common feature of category 'insecta'?
(a) Presence of ostium
(b) Presence of coxal gland for excretion
(c) Three pair of jointed legs in thoracic region
(d) Exoskeleton of cutin

75. Which of the following represent the family of mango?
(a) *Sapindales* (b) *Anacardiaceae* (c) *Poales* (d) *Poaceae*

76. House fly belongs to order
(a) *Diptera* (b) *Carnivora* (c) *Primata* (d) *Insecta*

77. Which is not required for preservation of insect?
(a) Collecting (b) Killing (c) Pinning (d) Pressing

78. IBG is situated at
(a) Kew (b) Howrah (c) Lucknow (d) Jodhpur

79. A museum has a collection of
(a) preserved plants
(b) preserved animals
(c) skeleton of animals
(d) all

80. Which of the following animals usually stuffed and preserved?
(a) Large birds (b) Mammals (c) Small lizards (d) Both (a) and (b)

81. Zoological parks are places for
(a) wild animals (b) pet animals (c) wild plants (d) endangered crops

82. Zoological park is a place where
(a) wild animals are kept in protected environment under human care
(b) we can learn about wild animal's food habit
(c) we can learn about wild animal's behavior
(d) all

83. The keys are based on contrasting characters generally in pairs called
(a) duplex (b) couplet (c) dimer (d) all

84. Which of the following is incorrect about keys?
(a) Key is taxonomical aid used for identification of plants and animals based on the similarities and dissimilarities
(b) Separate taxonomic keys are required for each taxonomic category such as family, genusand species for identification purposes
(c) Keys are generally analytical in nature
(d) Key is another taxonomical aid used for nomenclature of plants and animals based on the similarities and dissimilarities

85. Which of the following is a mean of recording description?
(a) Flora and manuals (b) Monographs
(c) Catalogues (d) All

86. Flora contains information about habitat and distribution of
(a) Animals of a given area (b) Plants of a given area
(c) Some useful plants of a given area (d) Some useful animals of a given area

87. Monographs contains information of
(a) genus (b) species (c) family (d) any one taxon

88. Manuals contain information for
(a) habitat and distribution of animals of a given area
(b) habitat and distribution of plants of a given area
(c) identification of names of species found in an area
(d) habitat and distribution of some useful animals a given area

89. Organisms vary in
(a) size and colour (b) habitat
(c) physiological and morphological features (d) all

90. Live specimens of organisms are found in
(a) herbaria (b) museum
(c) zoological parks and botanical gardens (d) all

91. The name of a plant written on herbarium sheet is its
(a) English name (b) local name (c) botanical name (d) all

92. NBRI is situated in
(a) Kolkata (b) Lucknow (c) Delhi (d) Jodhpur

93. Which is the prime source of taxonomical studies?
(a) Collection of actual specimen (b) Nomenclature
(c) Characterization (d) Identification

94. Tiger, dog and cat are placed in order of

(a) insectivora (b) carnivora (c) primata (d) lagomorpha

95. Monkey, gorilla and gibbons belongs to which of the following order and class respectively

(a) primata and prototheria (b) primata and mammalia

(c) carnivora and eutheria (d) Carnivora and mammalia

96. In plants, families are characterized on the basis of

(a) vegetative structures (b) reproductive features

(c) both (d) none

97. Match the column:

Column I	Column II
A. Man	1. Order–Carnivora
B. Mango	2. Family–Poaceae
C. House fly	3. Genus–Musca
D. Tiger	4. Phylum–Chordata
E. Wheat	5. Family–Anacardiaceae

(a) A–1, B–5, C–3, D–4, E–2 (b) A–4, B–5, C–3, D–1 and 4, E–2

(c) A–4, B–2, C–3, D–1, E–5 (d) A–1, B–2, C–3, D–4, E–5

98. Select the incorrect combination:

(a) Fragmentation Fungi, Planaria, Protonema of moss

(b) Budding Yeast, hydra and sponges

(c) Order Mammalia, primata, diptera, poales, polymoniales, sapindales

(d) Genus *Homo*, *Triticum*, *Musca*, *Felis*, *Panthera*, *Datura*, *Petunia*, *Mangifera*, *Solanum*

99. Select the correct combination:

(a) Earliest classification based on – Uses of various organisms

(b) Reproduction is synonymous with growth – Primitive multicellular organism

(c) ICZN – International Code of Zoo Nomenclature

(d) NBRI – National Botanical Registered Institute

100. Single-horned Rhinoes are found in

(a) Ghana (b) Bastar of Madhya Pradesh

(c) Kaziranga National Park (d) Khasi in Meghalaya

101. Herbarium sheet provides information of

(a) collector's name (b) family of plant

(c) local, English and botanical name (d) all of the above

102. Select total number of correct statements from the following:

1. Photoperiod affects reproduction in seasonal breeders, both plants and animals
2. All organisms handle chemicals entering their bodies.
3. Metabolism is a characterstic feature of all living organisms.
4. In animals, growth is seen only up to a certain age.
5. Non-living object exhibits metabolism.
6. No non-living object is capable of reproducing or replicating by itself

(a) 2 (b) 3 (c) 4 (d) 6

103. All plants, animals, fungi and microbes exhibit

(a) reproduction (b) growth by increase in mass only

(c) metabolism (d) self consciousness

*Read the **assertion** and **reason** carefully to mark the correct option out of the options given below:*

(a) If both the assertion and the reason are true and the reason is a correct explanation of the assertion
(b) If both the assertion and reason are true but the reason is not a correct explanation of the assertion
(c) If the assertion is true but the reason is false
(d) If both the assertion and reason are false

104. Assertion: Systematics is an important branch of biology.
Reason: Systematics name the organisms and divides them into groups and subgroups according to set rules to make their study easy.

105. Assertion: Members of a species breed only with others of the same species.
Reason: In some cases, members of different species may also breed, producing sterile or fertile offspring.

106. Assertion: No non living object exhibit metabolism.
Reason: Cellular organisation is absent non living organism.

107. Assertion: Metabolic reactions can be demonstrated outside the body in cell free systems.
Reason: An isolated metabolic rection performed in test tube is neither living nor non living.

108. Assertion: Conservative characters are more useful in classification.
Reason: These characters do not change during evolution. Therefore, their similarities show relationships among organisms.

109. Assertion: Linnaeus insisted that the scientific names should be Latinized.
Reason: This gives beauty to the names.

110. Assertion: There is no difference between the terms taxon and category.
Reason: Aves is a taxon that includes the category “birds”.

111. Assertion: Each rank or taxon represents a unit of classification.
Reason: Taxonomic categories are distinct biological entities and not merely morhpological aggregates.

112. Assertion: Human being has self- conciousness.
Reason: Human is organism who is aware of himself.

113. Assertion: In unicellular organism reproduction is synonymous with growth.
Reason: Increase in number of cell is also growth.

AIPMT PREVIOUS YEAR QUESTIONS

1. The Indian rhinoceros is a natural inhabitant of which one of the Indian states? [AIPMT MAINS 2010]

(a) Uttarakhand
(b) Uttar Pradesh
(c) Himachal Pradesh
(d) Assam

2. Which one of the following aspects is an exclusive characteristic of living things? [AIPMT MAINS 2011]
   (a) Isolated metabolic reactions occurs in vitro
   (b) Increase in mass from inside only
   (c) Perceptions of events happening in the environment and their memory
   (d) Increase in mass by accumulation of material both on surface as well as internally
3. Which one of the following is common to multicellular fungi, filamentous algae and protonema of mosses? [AIPMT PRE 2012]
   (a) Diplontic life cycle
   (b) Members of kingdom Planate
   (c) Mode of Nutrition
   (d) Multiplication by fragmentation
4. Which one of the following is not a correct statement? [AIPMT MAINS 2013]
   (a) Herbarium houses dried pressed and preserved plant specimens
   (b) Botanical gardens have collection of living plants for reference
   (c) A museum has collection of photographs of plants and animals
   (d) Key is a taxonomic aid for identification of specimens.

Answer Keys

1. (b)	2. (c)	3. (c)	4. (b)	5. (c)	6. (c)	7. (b)	8. (d)	9. (d)	10. (a)
11. (c)	12. (b)	13. (d)	14. (a)	15. (c)	16. (c)	17. (d)	18. (d)	19. (a)	20. (c)
21. (c)	22. (d)	23. (b)	24. (a)	25. (c)	26. (c)	27. (c)	28. (d)	29. (c)	30. (c)
31. (a)	32. (d)	33. (d)	34. (c)	35. (c)	36. (d)	37. (b)	38. (a)	39. (a)	40. (b)
41. (d)	42. (b)	43. (c)	44. (a)	45. (b)	46. (c)	47. (d)	48. (b)	49. (a)	50. (a)
51. (d)	52. (d)	53. (c)	54. (d)	55. (d)	56. (c)	57. (d)	58. (d)	59. (d)	60. (d)
61. (b)	62. (d)	63. (d)	64. (d)	65. (d)	66. (d)	67. (d)	68. (d)	69. (b)	70. (a)
71. (d)	72. (b)	73. (d)	74. (c)	75. (b)	76. (a)	77. (d)	78. (b)	79. (d)	80. (d)
81. (a)	82. (d)	83. (b)	84. (d)	85. (d)	86. (b)	87. (d)	88. (c)	89. (d)	90. (c)
91. (d)	92. (b)	93. (a)	94. (b)	95. (b)	96. (c)	97. (b)	98. (c)	99. (a)	100. (c)
101. (d)	102. (c)	103. (c)	104. (a)	105. (b)	106. (a)	107. (b)	108. (a)	109. (c)	110. (d)
111. (b)	112. (a)	113. (a)							

AIPMT Previous Year Questions

1. (d) 2. (b) 3. (d) 4. (c)

CHAPTER 2

Biological Classification

1. Who was the first to attempt a more scientific basis of classification?
(a) Linnaeus (b) Aristotle
(c) Whittaker (d) Bentham and Hooker
2. Aristotle classified plants in herbs, shrubs and trees on the basis of
(a) anatomical feature (b) morphological characters
(c) physiological characters (d) biochemical characters
3. In how many groups Aristotle divided animals on the basis of presence/absence of RBC?
(a) 1 (b) 2 (c) 3 (d) 4
4. Two kingdom classification does not distinguish between
(a) eukaryote and prokaryote
(b) unicellular and multi cellular organism
(c) photosynthetic (green algae) and non-photosynthetic (fungi) organism
(d) all
5. In which year Whittaker proposed five kingdom classification?
(a) 1960 (b) 1959 (c) 1969 (d) 1979
6. Whittaker's kingdom are
(a) *Plantae* and *Animalia* (b) *Monera and Protista*
(c) *Fungi* (d) All
7. How many main criteria were used by Whittaker for classification?
(a) 1 (b) 3 (c) 4 (d) 5
8. What is the criteria used by Whittaker for classification?
(1). Cell structure (2). Thallus organization
(3). Mode of nutrition (4). Reproduction
(5). Phylogenetic relationship (6). Biochemical difference
(7). Physiological character
(a) All except (5) and (6) (b) All except (5) and (7)
(c) All except (6) and (7) (d) All except (3) and (4)
9. In earlier classification (like two kingdoms), the following are included in plant
(1). Bacteria, blue green algae, fungus (2). Mosses and fern
(3). Gymnosperms and angiosperm
(a) (1) only (b) (2) and (3) only (c) (3) only (d) all
10. What is common to bacteria, mosses and fungus?
(a) It is mode of nutrition (b) Presence of cell wall
(c) Autotrophic (d) Body organization
11. All prokaryotic groups are put under ——— kingdom
(a) monera (b) plantae (c) fungi (d) protista

12. Kingdom protista contain
(a) blue green algae (b) fungi
(c) unicellular eukaryotes (d) all

13. Chlamydomonas, chlorella, paramecium and amoeba are placed in which kingdom of Whittaker's classification?
(a) Monera (b) Plantae (c) Fungi (d) Protista

14. Phylogeny refers to
(a) morphology (b) physiology
(c) reproduction (d) evolutionary relationship

15. Kingdom monera contain
(a) bacteria (b) dianoflagellate
(c) slime moulds (d) euglenoid

16. Most abundant micro organism are
(a) bacteria (b) virus (c) amoeba (d) paramecium

17. Which of the following is incorrect about bacteria?
(A) It is grouped under five categories on the basis of shape
(B) It can live in hot spring, deep ocean, snow and desert
(C) It can live as parasite
(D) It is composed of simple behavior and complex structure
(a) A and B only (b) A and D only (c) B and C only (d) C and D only

18. Most extensive metabolic diversity found in
(a) protozoans (b) amphibian (c) bacteria (d) fungi

19. Most of the bacteria are
(a) chemo-autotrophs (b) photo-autotrophs (c) heterotroph (d) holozoic

20. Match the column:

Column I	**Column II**
A. Salty area	1. Thermoacidophil
B. Hot spring	2. Methanogen
C. Marshy area	3. Halophiles

(a) A–3, B–1, C–2 (b) A–1, B–2, C–3
(c) A–2, B–1, C–3 (d) A–2, B–3, C–1

21. Archaebacteria can live in some of the most harsh habitats because of
(a) presence of mesosome (b) high power of multiplication
(c) special cell wall structure (d) all of the above

22. Following are present in gut of cows and buffaloes and responsible for production of methane from dung of these animals
(a) Methanogen (b) Thermoacidophiles
(c) Halophils (d) All

23. Motile bacteria possess
(a) cilia (b) flagella (c) both (d) none

24. Which of the following statements is true about cyanobacteria?
(a) It is found in fresh water only
(b) It may be unicellular, colonial or filamentous
(c) They often form bloom in non-polluted fresh water bodies
(d) Colonies are not surrounded by gelatinous sheath

25. Specialized cell of nostoc and anabaena fix nitrogen are known as
(a) cyst (b) heterocyst (c) oocyts (d) cholecyst

26. Find out the total number of false statements:

A. Cyanobacteria have chlorophyll 'a' like green plants

B. Bacteria which oxidizes various inorganic substance such as nitrates and ammonia and use the released energy for ATP production are chemosynthesis autotrophic bacteria

C. Heterotrophic bacteria are less in abundance in nature.

D. Majority of heterotrophic bacteria are decomposers.

E. Chemosynthetic autotrophic bacteria play important role in recycling of nutrients like nitrogen, phosphorus iron and sulphur

(a) 1 (b) 2 (c) 3 (d) 4

27. Heterotrophic bacteria help in

(a) curding of milk (b) production of antibiotic
(c) nitrogen fixation in leguminous plant (d) all

28. Select the total number of disease from the following caused by bacteria
Mumps, Smallpox, Citrus canker, Cholera, Typhoid, Tetanus, Sleeping sickness, Malaria

(a) 2 (b) 4 (c) 5 (d) 6

29. Which one is correct about reproduction in bacteria?

(a) Mainly by binary fission
(b) Spores are formed under unfavorable condition
(c) Sexual reproduction by transfer of DNA from one to another
(d) All

30. Following features belong to

A. complete lacking of cell wall
B. anaerobic
C. smallest living cell
D. many of them are pathogenic to plant and animals

(a) Chrysophytes (b) Prions (c) Viroids (d) Mycoplasma

31. Which of the following is incorrect about protista?

(a) All are single cell eukaryotes
(b) Some have flagella or cilia
(c) Sexually reproduce by cell fusion and zygote formation
(d) Members of protista are primarily terrestrial

32. Kingdom protista include

(a) chrysophyte (b) dianoflagellate (c) euglenoids (d) all

33. Which kingdom of Whittaker are not well-defined?

(a) monera (b) protista (c) fungi (d) animalia

34. Which of the following is correct about chrysophytes?

I. Found in fresh and marine water. II. Microscopic plankton
III. Cell walls are embedded with $CaCO_3$. IV. Most of them are photosynthetic

(a) I and III only (b) I, III and IV only (c) I, II and IV only (d) I and IV only

35. Chief producers in ocean are

(a) euglenoids (b) dianoflagellate (c) BGA (d) chrysophytes

36. Chrysophytes include

(a) diatoms (b) golden algae (c) desmids (d) all

37. Diatomaceous earth is used in

(a) polishing (b) filteration of oils
(c) filteration of syrups (d) all

38. In _______ cell wall forms two thin overlapping shells which fit together as in a soap box.
(a) dianoflagellates (b) diatoms (c) euglenoids (d) none
39. Mostly marine, photosynthetic and biflagellate organisms are
(a) diatoms (b) desmids (c) dianoflagellates (d) euglenoids
40. Following features belong to
I. Appear yellow, green, brown, blue and red depending on pigment in cell.
II. Stiff cellulose plate forms cell wall.
III. One longitudiual and one transverse flagella present.
IV. Photosynthetic.
(a) diatoms (b) desmids (c) dianoflagellates (d) euglenoids
41. Red tide is because of
(a) desmids (b) gonyaulax (c) euglena (d) red algae
42. Which of the following is true about gonyaulax?
(a) Release toxin (b) Slow multiplication causing red tide
(c) Heterotropic (d) All
43. Habitat of euglenoids is
(a) fresh river water (b) fresh stagnant water
(c) marine water (d) all
44. Mode of nutrition in euglenoids is
(a) autotropic (b) heterotropic (c) symbiotic (d) mixotropic
45. Characteristic feature of euglenoids are
A. Presence of cell wall B. Presence of two flagella
C. Photosynthetic in presence of sunlight D. Presence of pellicle on their cell
(a) A, D only (b) B, D only (c) B, C, D only (d) All
46. Euglenoids have flexible body because of
(a) cellulosic wall (b) protein rich pellicle
(c) lipoic wall (d) pectinic wall
47. Pigments of euglenoids are identical to
(a) bacteria (b) diatoms (c) dianoflagellates (d) higher plants
48. Euglena posses all except
(a) pellicle (b) two equal flagella
(c) two unequal flagella (d) mixotrophic nutrition
49. Character belongs to slime moulds
A. Saprophytes.
B. Forms plasmodium under favorable condition.
C. Spores posses true walls.
D. Spores are dispersed by water.
E. Body moves along decaying twings and leaves engulfing organic matter.
(a) All except E (b) All except D
(c) All except C and E (d) All except B
50. Which protist are believed to be the relatives of animals?
(a) Slime moulds (b) Dianoflagellates (c) Protozoans (d) Diatoms
51. Protozoans are
A. Hetrotrops.
B. Parasites or predators.
C. Protist.
D. Belived to be primitive relative of animals.
(a) A, B only (b) B, C only (c) D, A only (d) All

52. Amoeboid protozoans
(a) live in fresh water, sea water or moist soil
(b) capture prey by putting pseudopodia
(c) marine forms have shells on their surface
(d) all of the above

53. False feet is the characteristic of which protozoan?
(a) Sporozoan (b) Ciliated protozoan
(c) Flagellated protozoan (d) Amoeboid protozoans

54. Sleeping sickness caused by
(a) plasmodium (b) paramoecium (c) trypanosoma (d) entamoeba

55. The protist which possess flagella is
(a) paramoecium (b) plasmodium (c) trypanosoma (d) entamoeba

56. Ciliated protozoan possess
(a) thousands of cilia (b) gullet that opens outsides to cell
(c) coordinated movement of rows of cilia (d) all

57. Sporozoans possesss
(a) spore like stage in life cycle (b) are infectious
(c) are motile (d) both (a) and (b)

58. Select correct statement from the following for kingdom fungi
A. They are heterotrophic.
B. They show less diversity in morphology and habitat.
C. Yeast is an unicellular fungus.
D. They prefer to grow in warm and humid places.
(a) A and D only (b) C and D only (c) A, C and D only (d) A and B only

59. Following are example of fungus
(a) Toadstool (b) Puccinia (c) Yeast (d) All

60. Following pairs belongs to same kingdom
(a) Mycoplasma and Euglena (b) Golden algae and Green algae
(c) Toadstool and Albugo (d) Lichens and Alternaria

61. Refrigeration prevent food from spoilage by
(a) fungus (b) bacteria (c) both (d) none

62. Which is not a correct matching?
(a) Rust → Puccinia (b) Yeast → Bread and beer
(c) Chrysophyte → Diatomaceous earth (d) Penicillium → Red tide

63. Following features belongs to
A. Body consist of long, slender thread-like structures called hyphae.
B. Cell wall consist of chitin.
C. Cosmopolitan.
(a) ciliated protozoans (b) slime moulds
(c) fungi (d) euglenoids

64. If hyphae are continuous tube filled with multinucleated cytoplasm is known as
(a) septate hyphae (b) coenocytic hyphae
(c) mycelium (d) none

65. Select correct matching:
A. Fungi depend on dead substrate – Saprophytic
B. Fungi depend on living plant and animals – Parasite

C. Fungi as symbiont with algae – Lichens
D. Fungi as symbiont with root of higher plant – Mycorrhazia
(a) A and B only (b) B and C only (c) C and D only (d) All

66. Vegetative reproduction in fungus takes place by
(a) fragmentation (b) fission (c) budding (d) all

67. Asexual reproduction in fungus occurs by spores known as
(a) conidia (b) sporangiospores
(c) zoospores (d) any of the above

68. Sexual reproduction in fungus is by
(a) oospores (b) ascospores
(c) basidiospores (d) any of the above

69. Sexual reproduction in fungus occurs in following sequential event. Arrange them properly.
A. Fusion of two nuclei called karyogamy.
B. Fusion of protoplasm between two motile or non-motile gametes.
C. Meiosis in zygote resulting in haploid spores.
(a) $A \rightarrow B \rightarrow C$ (b) $B \rightarrow A \rightarrow C$ (c) $C \rightarrow B \rightarrow A$ (d) $C \rightarrow A \rightarrow B$

70. Dikaryon and dikaryophase is seen in case of
(a) ascomycetes (b) basidiomycetes (c) phycomycetes (d) both (a) and (b)

71. Kingdom fungi divided into various classes on the basis of
(a) morphology of mycelium (b) mode of spore formation
(c) type of fruiting bodies (d) all

72. During sexual reproduction in fungus
(a) hyphae of same class come together and fuse
(b) hyphae of same genus come together and fuse
(c) hyphae of closely related species come together and fuse
(d) hyphae of compatible mating type come together and fuse

73. Habitats of phycomycetes are
(a) aquatic (b) decaying wood in moist and damp place
(c) obligate parasite in plant (d) all

74. Endogenously produced spores are found in all except
(a) mushroom (b) mucor (c) albugo (d) rhizopus

75. Following features belong to class
A. Asexual reproduction by zoospores or aplanospores.
B. Fusion of gametes may be isogamous, anisogamous or oogamous.
C. Mycelium is aseptate and coenocytic.
D. Spores are endogenously produced in sporangium.
(a) ascomycetes (b) deuteromycetes (c) phycomycetes (d) basidiomycetes

76. Following fungus belongs to class ascomycetes (count total number).
Rhizopus, Penicillium, Yeast, Mucor, Agaricus, Puccinia, Albugo, Claviceps, Neurospora, Alternaria, Trichoderma, Aspergillus, Ustilago, Morels, Buffles, Colletotrichum, Toadstool
(a) 5 (b) 7 (c) 9 (d) 10

77. Ascomycetes are mostly
(a) acellular (b) unicellular (c) multicellular (d) all

78. Unicellular ascomycetes is
(a) penicillium (b) alternaria
(c) saccharomyces (yeast) (d) agaricus

79. Following features belongs to class
A. Mycelium branched and septate.
B. Asexual spores conidia produced exogenously.
C. Sexual spores produced endogenously.
D. Many members of this class are edible.
(a) ascomycetes (b) phycomycetes (c) basidiomycetes (d) deuteromycetes

80. Which of the following is extensively used in biochemical and genetic work?
(a) Aspergillus (b) Claviceps (c) Neurospora (d) Penicillium

81. Commonly known form of basidiomycetes are
(a) mushrooms (b) bracket fungi (c) puffballs (d) all

82. Following characteristics are of which of the given fungi?
A. Mycelium branched and Septate.
B. Asexual spores are generally not found.
C. Vegetative reproduction by fragmentation is common.
D. Sex organs are absent but plasmogamy is by fusion of two somatic cells of different strains or genotype.
(a) phycomycetes (b) basidiomycetes (c) deuteromycetes (d) ascomycetes

83. Karyogamy and meiosis occur in basidium produces ______ basidiospores
(a) 1 (b) 2 (c) 3 (d) 4

84. Basidiospores are produced on basidium
(a) endogenously (b) exogenously (c) both (d) none

85. Find out the correct matching:
(a) Ustilago–Smut (b) Puccinia–Rust
(c) Agaricus–Mushroom (d) All

86. Which of the following fungi only reproduce by asexual spores conidia?
(a) Alternaria (b) Colletotrichum (c) Trichoderma (d) All

87. Deuteromycetes known imperfect fungi because
(a) only sexual phase is found
(b) only asexual or vegetative phase are known
(c) both asexual and sexual phase are known
(d) reproduction in these fungi is absent

88. Many members of ______ class are decomposers of litter and help in mineral cycling.
(a) ascomycetes (b) deuteromycetes (c) basidiomycetes (d) phycomycetes

89. Following features belongs to
A. Mycelium septate and branched.
B. Some members are saprophytes or parasites.
C. Reproduce only by conidia.
(a) ascomycetes (b) deuteromycetes (c) basidiomycetes (d) phycomycetes

90. Following are example of insectivorous plants.
(a) Bladderwort (b) Venus fly trap (c) Cuscuta (d) Both (a) and (b)

91. Kingdom plantae include
(a) algae and bryophytes (b) pteridophytes and gymnosperms
(c) angiosperms (d) all

92. Plant cells have all except
(a) chloroplast (b) cellulosic cell wall
(c) large vacuole (d) centriole

93. Alternation of generation seen in all except
(a) fucus (b) sphagnum (c) equisetum (d) alternaria

94. Life cycle in plant has generally two distinct phase the ______ sporophytic and the ______ gametophytic that alternate with each other. This phenomenon is called as alternation of generation.
(a) diploid, diploid (b) diploid, haploid
(c) haploid, diploid (d) haploid, haploid

95. Select from the following the total number of features belonging to animal kingdom.
1. Multicellular, heterotrophic.
2. Most of them capable of locomotion.
3. Have definite shape and size.
4. Digestion of food in internal cavity.
5. Holozoic mode of nutrition.
6. Stored food reserve as glycogen or fat.
7. Higher forms shows sensory and neuromotor mechanism.
8. Some members are autotrophic.
9. Presence of cellulose cell wall.
10. Sexual reproduction generally by copulation of male and female.

(a) 6 (b) 7 (c) 8 (d) 10

96. In five kingdom classification of Whittaker, some acellular organisms are not included, they are
(a) virus (b) viroids (c) lichens (d) both (a) and (b)

97. Virus is
(a) completely non-living
(b) inert crystalline structure outside the living cell
(c) cellular organism
(d) one of Whittaker's classification

98. 'Virus' name means
(a) venom or poisonous fluid
(b) acellular form
(c) non-cellular form
(d) connecting link between living and non-living

99. 'Virus' name was given by
(a) Ivanowsky (b) Pasteur (c) Whittaker (d) Beijerinek

100. *Contagium vivum fluidum* (infections living fluid) name given to fluid extract from infected tobacco plant was given by
(a) Ivanowsky (b) Pasteur (c) Whittaker (d) Beijerinek

101. Viruses are
(a) inert outside their specific host cell (b) obligate parasite
(c) passes through bacteria proof filter (d) all above statements are correct

102. Who showed that virus can be crystallized out?
(a) Ivanowsky (b) Beijerinek (c) Stanley (d) Pasteur

103. Virus contains
(a) protein (b) DNA
(d) RNA (d) (a) and either (b) or (c)

104. Viruses infect plants generally have
(a) single standard DNA (b) double standard DNA
(c) double standard RNA (d) single standard RNA

105. Viruses which infect animals have
(a) single standard RNA
(b) double standard RNA
(c) double standard DNA
(d) any of the above

106. Bacteriophage generally have
(a) single standard RNA
(b) double standard RNA
(c) double standard DNA
(d) any of the above

107. Capsomeres may be arranged in
(a) helical (b) polyhedral (c) ellipsoid (d) either (a) or (b)

108. In virus infected plants following symptoms can be observed
(a) Mosaic formation and stunted growth
(b) Leaf rolling and curling
(c) Yellowing and vein clearing
(d) All

109. Select the total number of diseases from the following which can be caused by virus in plant or animals.
Mumps, Small pox, Rust, Smut, Herpes, Influenza, Potato spindle tuber, Red rot of sugar cane, Turnip mosaic, Black rot crucifier
(a) 4 (b) 5 (c) 7 (d) 8

110. Potato spindle tuber disease is caused by
(a) virus (b) viroids (c) lichens (d) fungi

111. 'Viroids' is discovered by
(a) Ivanowsky (b) T.O. Diener (c) Beijerinek (d) Stanley

112. Viroids are
(a) free protein (b) free RNA (c) free DNA (d) free saccharides

113. The molecular weight of RNA of viroid is
(a) high
(b) low
(c) very high
(d) any of the above

114. Lichen are symbiotic association between
(a) algae and bacteria
(b) bacteria and fungus
(c) algae and fungus
(d) fungus and Root of higher plant

115. In lichen algal component is called ______ and fungal component is called ______
(a) mycobiont, phycobiont
(b) phycobiont, mycobiont
(c) phycobiont, mycorrhazia
(d) mycorrhaiza, mycobiont

116. Which one heterotrophic in lichen?
(a) Fungus (b) Algae (c) Both (d) None

117. Lichens are
(a) pollution indicator
(b) symbiotic association between algae and fungus
(c) pioneer species in primary succession on rocks
(d) all of the above

118. Which of the following is incorrect about lichens?
(a) Algae part is autotrophic
(b) Fungus part absorb nutrient and minerals
(c) Fungus provide shelter to algae
(d) Algae provide shelter to fungus

119. Identify the A, B, C and D in this figure.

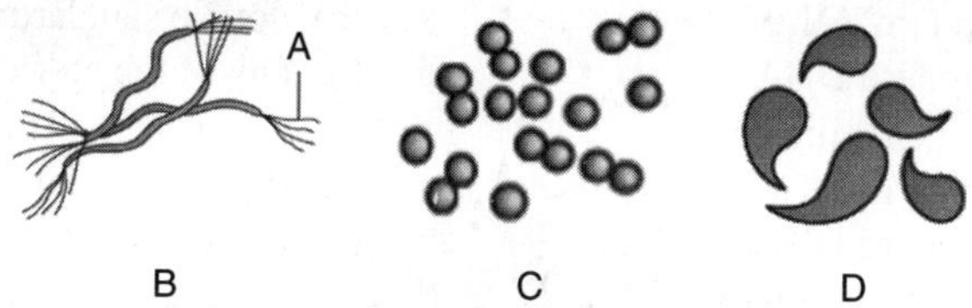

(a) A–Spirilla, B–Vibrio, C–Flagellum, D–Cocci
(b) A–Cocci, B–Flagellum, C–Spirilla, D–Vibrio
(c) A–Vibrio, B–Spirilla, C–Cocci, D–Flagellum
(d) A–Flagellum, B–Spirilla, C–Cocci, D–Vibrio

120. Identify around structure 'A' in this diagram

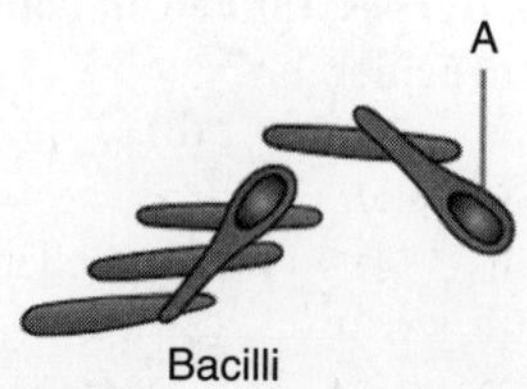

(a) ds DNA (b) Plasmid (c) Spore (d) Cosmid

121. What indicate A in this figure?

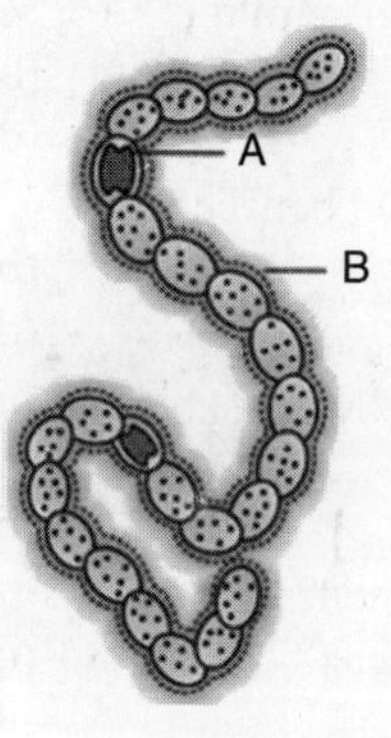

(a) Heterocyst (b) Mucilagenous sheath
(c) Cyanobacteria (d) ATP

122. Identify the A, B and C showing in this figure?

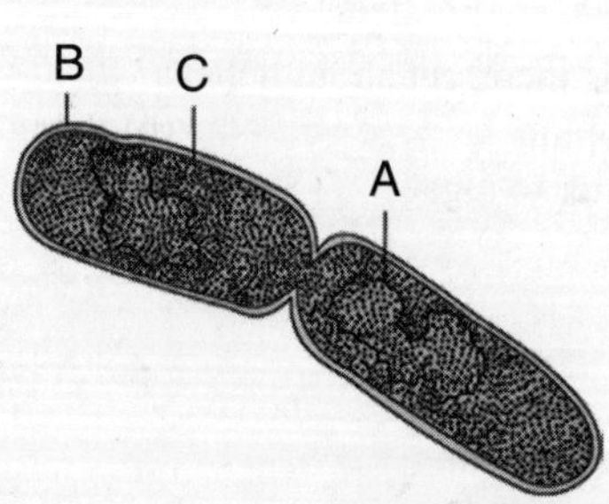

(a) A–Cell wall, B–DNA, C–Cell membrane
(b) A–DNA, B–Cell membrane, C–Cell wall
(c) A–Cell membrane, B–DNA, C–Cell wall
(d) A–DNA, B–Cell wall, C–Cell membrane

123. Identify organism given in this diagram and its feature?

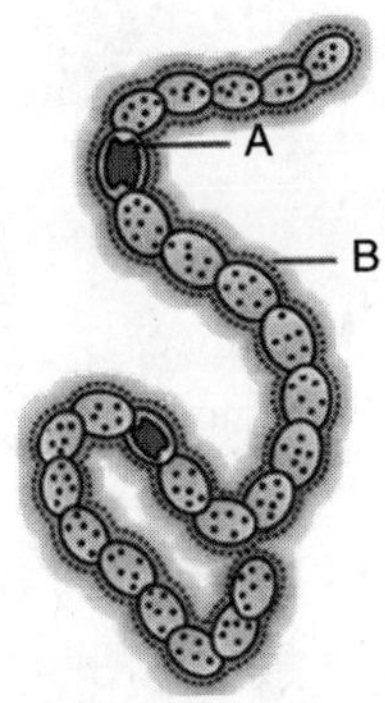

(a) Vibrio–Comma shape bacteria which causes cholera
(b) Fungi–Body organization is loose tissue level
(c) Blue green algae–Filamentous structure, help in nitrogen fixation
(d) Algae–Heterotrophic structure feeds on Nostoc

124. Select incorrect statement about organism given in this diagram

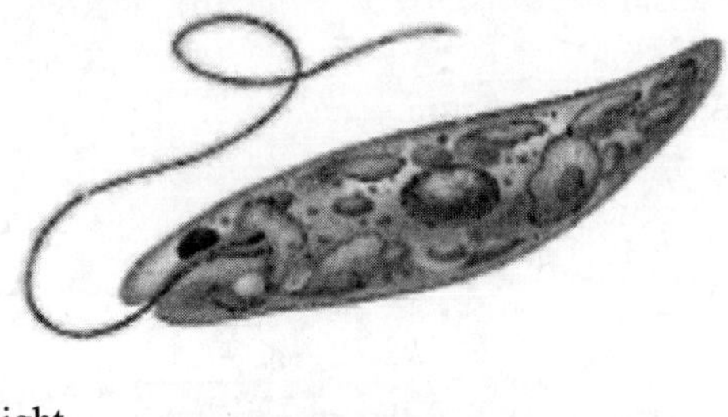

(a) Autotrophic in sunlight
(b) Heterotrophic in deprived sunlight
(c) Biflagellate
(d) They are surrounded by protein rich layer known as cell wall

125. Identify A, B, C in this diagram

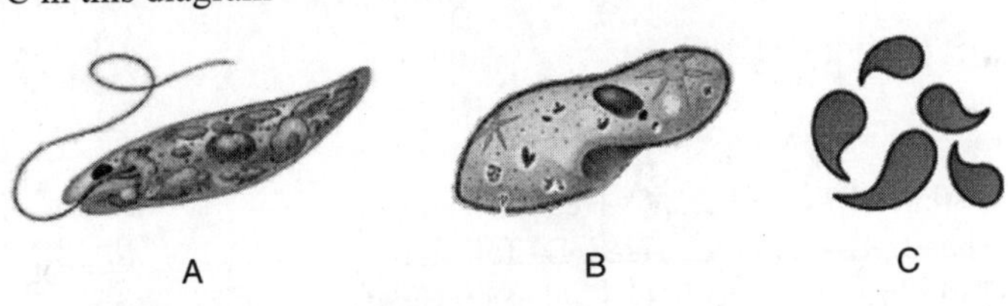

(a) A–Euglena, B–Paramoecium, C–Vibrio
(b) A–Paramoecium, B–Vibrio, C–Euglena
(c) A–Flagella, B–Paramoecium, C–Vibrio
(d) A–Paramoecium, B–Slipper animalcule, C–Vibrio

126. Identify the A, B and C in this figure.

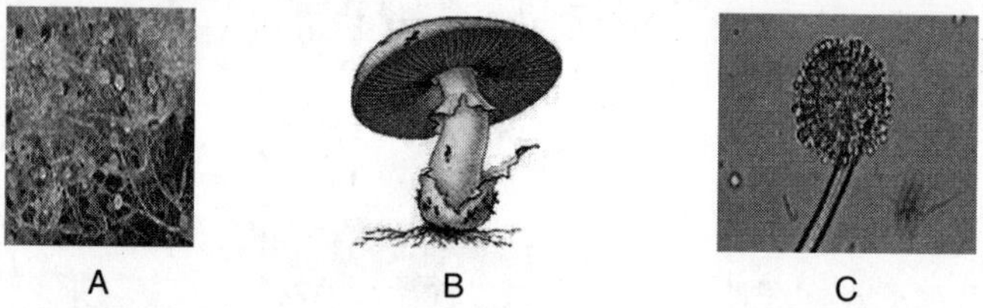

(a) A–Agaricus, B–Mucor, C–Aspergillus
(b) A–Mucor, B–Agaricus, C–Aspergillus
(c) A–Aspergillus, B–Mucor, C–Agaricus
(d) A–Agaricus, B–Aspergillus, D–Mucor

127. Identify the A and B shown in this figure.

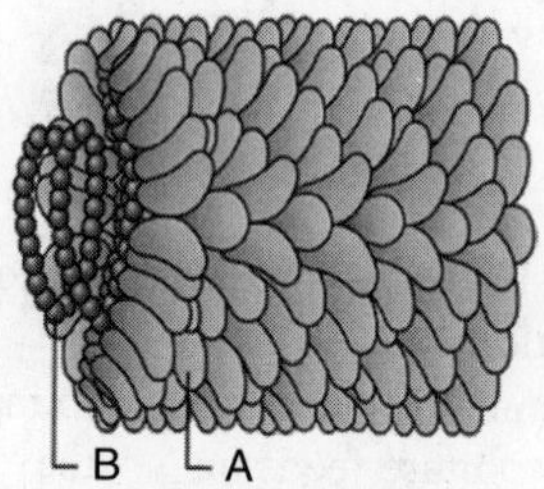

(a) A–DNA, B–Capsid
(b) A–RNA, B–DNA
(c) A–Capsid, B–RNA
(d) A–RNA, B–Capsid

128. What is indicate A to D in this figure.

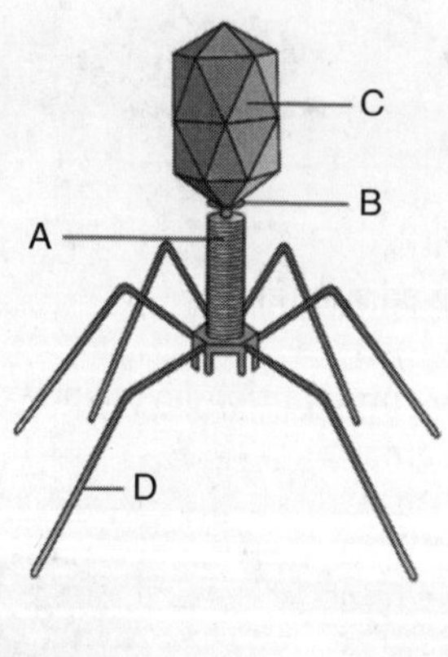

(a) A–Collar, B–Tail Fibres, C–Head, D–Sheath
(b) A–Sheath, B–Collar, C–Head, D–Tail fibres
(c) A–Tail fibres, B–Sheath, C–Collar, D–Head
(d) A–Tail fibres, B–Collar, C–Head, D–Sheath

*Read the **assertion** and **reason** carefully to mark the correct option out of the options given below:*

(a) If both the assertion and the reason are true and the reason is a correct explanation of the assertion

(b) If both the assertion and reason are true but the reason is not a correct explanation of the assertion

(c) If the assertion is true but the reason is false

(d) If both the assertion and reason are false

129. Assertion: Chemotaxonomy is classifying organisms at molecular level.
Reason: Cytotaxonomy is classifying organisms at cellular level.

130. Assertion: Bacteria are prokaryotic.
Reason: Bacteria do not possess true nucleus and membrane bound cell organelles.

131. Assertion: Bacteria are grouped under four categories based on their shapes.
Reason: Cocci and Bacilli may form clusters or chain of a definite length.

132. Assertion: Mycoplasma can survive with out oxygen.
Reason: They have no cell wall.

133. Assertion: Bacterial cell wall are not like the plant cell.
Reason: Bacterial cell wall is made up of cellulose.

134. Assertion: Bacteria do not always move with the help of flagella.
Reason: Flagellated bacteria employs rotary motion of flagellum when it moves.

135. Assertion: Amoeba contains a contractile vacuole.
Reason: It helps in both digestion and osmoregulation.

136. Assertion: Whittaker proposed a five kingdom classification.
Reason: The main criteria were cell structure, body organisation, mode of nutrition, reproduction and phylogenetic relationship.

137. Assertion: Paramecium is aquatic, actively moving organism.
Reason: Paramecium contains two nucleus.

138. Assertion: Fresh water protozoan possess contractile vacuoles.
Reason: The main function of the vacuole is contraction during digestion.

139. Assertion: Sexual reproduction in protozoan is not a frequent occurrence.
Reason: Sexual reproduction has no significance.

AIPMT PREVIOUS YEAR QUESTIONS

1. Give below is the diagram of a bacteriophage. In which one of the options all four parts A, B, C and D are correct?

[AIPMT MAINS 2010]

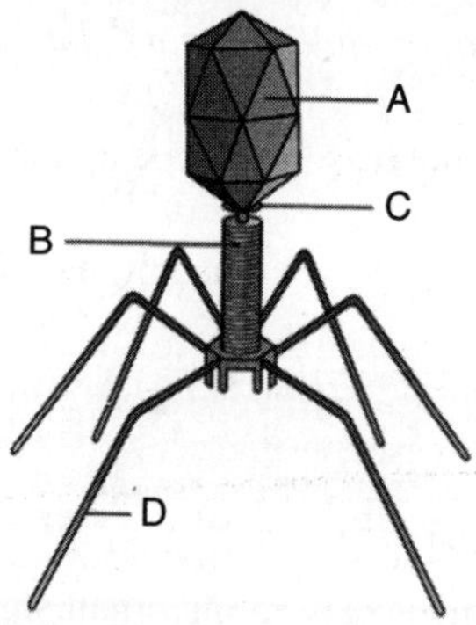

(a) A: Tail fibres, B: Head, C: Sheath, D: Collar
(b) A: Sheath, B: Collar, C: Head, D: Tail fibres
(c) A: Head, B: Sheath, C: Collar, D: Tail fibres
(d) A: Collar, B: Tail fibres, C: Head, D: Sheath

2. Select the correct combination of the statements (A-D) regarding the characteristics of certain organisms

[AIPMT MAINS 2010]

(A) Methanogens are archaebacteria which produce methane in marshy areas
(B) Nostoc is a filamentous blue –green alga which fixes atmospheric nitrogen
(C) Chemosynthetic autotrophic bacteria synthesize cellulose from glucose
(D) Mycoplasma lack a cell wall and can survive without oxygen

The correct statements are:

(a) (B) & (C)
(b) (A), (B) & (C)
(c) (B), (C) & (D)
(d) (A), (B) & (D)

3. Some hyperthermophilic organisms that grow in highly acidic (pH = 2) habitats belong to the two groups called

[AIPMT PRE 2010]

(a) Eubacteria and archaea
(b) Cyanobacteria and diatoms
(c) Protists and mosses
(d) liverworts and yeasts

4. Single-celled eukaryotes are included in:

[AIPMT PRE 2010]

(a) Protista
(b) Fungi
(c) Archaea
(d) Monera

5. Virus envelope is known as:

[AIPMT PRE 2010]

(a) Capsid
(b) Virion
(c) Nucleoprotein
(d) Core

6. Infectious proteins are present in:

[AIPMT PRE 2010]

(a) Gemini viruses
(b) Prions
(c) Viroids
(d) Satellite viruses

7. Organisms called Methanogens are most abundant in a

[AIPMT PRE 2011]

(a) Cattle yard
(b) Polluted stream
(c) Hot spring
(d) Sulphur rock

8. How many organisms in the list given below are autotrophs?
Lactobacillus, Nostoc, Chara, Nitrosomonas, Nitrobacter, Streptomyces, Saccharomyces, Trypanosoma, Porphyra, Wolffia

[AIPMT MAINS 2012]

(a) Five
(b) Six
(c) Three
(d) Four

9. The most abundant prokaryotes helpful to humans in making curd from milk and in production of antibiotics are ones categorised as:

[AIPMT PRE 2012]

(a) Cyanobacteria
(b) Archaebacteria
(c) Chemosynthetic autotrophs
(d) Heterotrophic bacteria

10. The cyanobacteria are also referred to as:

[AIPMT PRE 2012]

(a) Protists
(b) Golden algae
(c) Slime moulds
(d) Blue green algae

11. Which statement is wrong for viruses?

[AIPMT PRE 2012]

(a) All are parasites
(b) All of them have helical symmetry.
(c) They have ability to synthesize nucleic acids and proteins
(d) Antibiotics have no effect on them.

12. Which one single organism or the pair of organisms is correctly assigned to its or their named taxonomic group?

[AIPMT PRE 2012]

(a) Paramoecium and Plasmodium belong to the same kingdom as that of Penicillium
(b) Lichen is a composite organism formed from the symbiotic association an algae and a protozoan
(c) Yeast used in making bread and beer is a fungus
(d) Nostoc and Anabaena are examples of protista

13. Maximum nutritional diversity is found in the group:

[AIPMT PRE 2012]

(a) Fungi
(b) Animalia
(c) Monera
(d) Plantae

14. Pigment-containing membranous extensions in some cyanobacteria are:

[AIPMT PRE 2013]

(a) Heterocysts
(b) Basal bodies
(c) Pneumatophores
(d) Chromatophores

15. Five kingdom system of classification suggested by R.H. Whittaker is not based on:

[AIPMT PRE 2014]

(a) Presence or absence of a well defined nucleus
(b) Mode of reproduction
(c) Mode of nutrition
(d) Complexity of body organization

16. Which one of the following fungi contains hallucinogens?

[AIPMT PRE 2014]

(a) Morchella esculenta
(b) Amanita muscaria
(c) Neurospora sp.
(d) Ustilago sp.

17. Archaebacteria differ from eubacteria in: [AIPMT PRE 2014]

(a) Cell membrane structure
(b) Mode of nutrition
(c) Cell shape
(d) Mode of reproduction

18. Anoxygenic photosynthesis is characteristic of: [AIPMT PRE 2014]

(a) Rhodospirillum
(b) Spirogyra
(c) Chlamydomonas
(d) Ulva

19. Which of the following shows coiled RNA strand and capsomeres? [AIPMT PRE 2014]

(a) Polio virus
(b) Tobacco mosaic virus
(c) Measles virus
(d) Retrovirus

20. Viruses have: [AIPMT PRE 2014]

(a) DNA enclosed in a protein coat
(b) Prokaryotic nucleus
(c) Single chromosome
(d) Both DNA and RNA

21. A location with luxuriant growth of lichen on the trees indicated that the: [AIPMT PRE 2014]

(a) Tress are very healthy
(b) Trees are heavily infested
(c) Location is highly polluted
(d) Location is not polluted

22. Which of the matches is correct? [AIPMT 2015]

(a) Phytophthora → Aseptate mycelium → Basidiomycetes
(b) Alternania → Sexual reproduction absent → Deuteromycetes
(c) Mucor → Reproduction by conjugation → Ascomycetes
(d) Agaricus → Parasitic fungus → Basidiomycetes

23. The guts of cow and buffalo posses: [AIPMT 2015]

(a) Fucus spp
(b) Chlorella spp
(c) Methanogens
(d) Cyanobacteria

24. The imperfect fungi which are decomposers of litter and help in mineral cycling belong to [RE-AIPMT 2015]

(a) Basidiomycetes
(b) Phycomycetes
(c) Ascomycetes
(d) Deuteromycetes

25. Pick up the wrong statement: [RE-AIPMT 2015]

(a) Protista have photosynthetic and heterotrophic modes of nutrition
(b) Some fungi are edible
(c) Nuclear membrane is present in Monera
(d) Cell wall is absent in Animalia

26. Chromatophores take part in [RE-AIPMT 2015]

(a) Growth
(b) Movement
(c) Respiration
(d) Photosynthesis

27. Which of the following disease is caused by a protozoan? [RE-AIPMT 2015]

(a) Influenza (b) Babesiosis
(c) Blastomycosis (d) Syphilis

28. Select the wrong statement [RE-AIPMT 2015]

(a) W.M. Stanley showed that viruses could be crystallized
(b) The term 'contagium vivum fluidum' was coined by M.W. Beijerinek
(c) Mosaic disease in tobacco and AIDS in human being are caused by viruses
(d) The viroids were discovered by D.J. Ivanowsky

29. Cell wall is absent in [RE-AIPMT 2015]

(a) Funaria (b) Mycoplasma
(c) Nostoc (d) Aspergillus

30. In which group of organisms the cell walls from two thin overlapping shells which fit together? [RE-AIPMT 2015]

(a) Euglenoids (b) Dianoflagellates
(c) Slime moulds (d) Chrysophytes

31. Choose the wrong statement: [RE-AIPMT 2015]

(a) Neurospora is used in the study of biochemical genetics
(b) Morels and Buffles are poisonous mushrooms
(c) Yeast is unicellular and useful in fermentation
(d) Penicillium is multicellular and produces antibiotics

Answer Keys

1. (b)	2. (b)	3. (b)	4. (d)	5. (c)	6. (d)	7. (d)	8. (c)	9. (d)	10. (b)
11. (a)	12. (c)	13. (d)	14. (d)	15. (a)	16. (a)	17. (b)	18. (c)	19. (c)	20. (a)
21. (c)	22. (a)	23. (b)	24. (b)	25. (b)	26. (a)	27. (d)	28. (b)	29. (d)	30. (d)
31. (d)	32. (d)	33. (b)	34. (c)	35. (d)	36. (d)	37. (d)	38. (b)	39. (c)	40. (c)
41. (b)	42. (a)	43. (b)	44. (d)	45. (c)	46. (b)	47. (d)	48. (b)	49. (b)	50. (c)
51. (d)	52. (d)	53. (d)	54. (c)	55. (c)	56. (d)	57. (d)	58. (c)	59. (d)	60. (c)
61. (c)	62. (d)	63. (c)	64. (b)	65. (d)	66. (d)	67. (d)	68. (d)	69. (b)	70. (d)
71. (d)	72. (d)	73. (d)	74. (a)	75. (c)	76. (b)	77. (c)	78. (c)	79. (a)	80. (c)
81. (d)	82. (b)	83. (d)	84. (b)	85. (d)	86. (d)	87. (b)	88. (b)	89. (b)	90. (d)
91. (d)	92. (d)	93. (d)	94. (b)	95. (c)	96. (d)	97. (b)	98. (a)	99. (b)	100. (d)
101. (d)	102. (c)	103. (d)	104. (d)	105. (d)	106. (c)	107. (d)	108. (d)	109. (b)	110. (b)
111. (b)	112. (b)	113. (b)	114. (c)	115. (b)	116. (a)	117. (d)	118. (d)	119. (d)	120. (c)
121. (a)	122. (d)	123. (c)	124. (d)	125. (a)	126. (b)	127. (c)	128. (b)	129. (b)	130. (a)
131. (b)	132. (b)	133. (a)	134. (b)	135. (c)	136. (b)	137. (b)	138. (c)	139. (c)	

AIPMT Previous Year Questions

1. (c)	2. (d)	3. (a)	4. (a)	5. (a)	6. (b)	7. (a)	8. (b)	9. (d)	10. (d)
11. (b)	12. (c)	13. (c)	14. (d)	15. (a)	16. (b)	17. (a)	18. (a)	19. (b)	20. (a)
21. (d)	22. (b)	23. (c)	24. (d)	25. (c)	26. (d)	27. (b)	28. (d)	29. (b)	30. (d)
31. (b)									

CHAPTER

3

Plant Kingdom

1. Who suggested five kingdom classifications?
   (a) Robert Hooke (b) Joseph Dalton Hooker
   (c) Carolus Linnaeus (d) Whittaker
2. The earliest classification used only
   (a) physiological characters (b) gross anatomical characters
   (c) gross morphological characters (d) all
3. Artificial systems gave equal weightage to
   (a) morphological and anatomical characters
   (b) vegetative and sexual characters
   (c) vegetative and anatomical characters
   (d) morphological and sexual characters
4. _______ characters are easily affected by environment
   (a) Sexual (b) Somatic (c) Anatomical (d) All
5. Natural classification system developed were
   (a) natural affinities amongst organism (b) ultra structure and anatomy
   (c) embryology (d) all
6. The classification based on evolutionary history was
   (a) phylogenetic classification (b) artificial classification
   (c) numerical classification (d) none
7. Numbers and codes are assigned to the characters in
   (a) cytotaxonomy (b) chemotaxonomy
   (c) numerical taxonomy (d) none
8. Chemotaxonomy is based on
   (a) information are chromosome number, structure and behaviour
   (b) chemical constituents of plants
   (c) all observable characters
   (b) only sexual characters
9. According to phylogenetic classification organisms belonging to same taxa
   (a) are same in anatomy (b) have same genetic constituent
   (c) have a common ancestor (d) have all characteristics same
10. Characters used to classify organism when no fossil evidence is supportive is
    (a) numerical taxonomy (b) cytotaxonomy
    (c) chemotaxonomy (d) all
11. Chlorophyll bearing, thalloid, simply, autotropic, and mainly aquatic organisms are
    (a) bryophytes (b) protist (c) algae (d) all

12. Filamentous forms of algae are
(a) ulothrix (b) spirogyra (c) chlamydomonas (d) both (a) and (b)
13. Volvox is
(a) unicellular algae (b) filamentous algae
(c) colonial algae (d) symbiotic algae
14. Modes of reproduction found in algae are
(a) vegetative (b) asexual (c) sexual (d) all
15. Vegetative reproduction in algae is by
(a) binary fusion (b) fragmentation (c) budding (d) cyst formation
16. Spore formation in algae occur during
(a) vegetative reproduction (b) asexual reproduction
(c) sexual reproduction (d) during germination
17. Isogamy is seen in
(a) chlamydomonas (b) spirogyra (c) both (d) none
18. Algae possesing both isogamy and anisogamy is
(a) chlamydomonas (b) volvox (c) spirogyra (d) fucus
19. Male gamete is small and motile and female gamete is large and immotile in
(a) fucus (b) spirogyra (c) ulothrix (d) all
20. 50% CO_2 fixation on earth is carried out by
(a) protest (b) higher plants (c) algae (d) none
21. Marine algae used as food are
(a) laminaria (b) sargassum (c) porphyra (d) all
22. Hydrocolloids are secreted by
(a) all of the algae (b) only brown algae
(c) only red algae (d) both red and brown algae
23. Algin is secreted by:
(a) all of the algae (b) only brown algae
(c) only red algae (d) both red and brown algae
24. Carrageen is secreted by
(a) all the algae (b) only brown algae
(c) only red algae (d) both red and brown algae
25. Microbes used in preparation of ice-cream and jellies are grown on the product secreted by
(a) chlorella (b) spirullina
(c) gelidium and gracilaria (d) all
26. Algae rich in proteins and used as food by space travellers is
(a) chlorella (b) spirullina (c) both (d) laminaria
27. Agar is commercially obtained from
(a) gelidium and gracilaria (b) laminaria and spirullina
(c) chlorella and spirullina (d) chlamydomonas and spirogyra
28. Green algae are kept in
(a) phaeophyceae (b) xanthophylls (c) chlorophyceae (d) rhodophyceae
29. The organism which contain chlorophyll 'a' and 'b' cup-shaped chloroplast and is unicellular is
(a) spirogyra (b) chlamydomonas (c) volvox (d) ulothrix
30. Dominance of chlorophyll 'a' and 'b', pyrenoids and starch as stored food are found in
(a) members of chlorophyceae (b) members of rhodophyceae
(c) members of phaeophyceae (d) all

31. Chlorophyceae are grass green due to dominance of pigment
(a) chlorophyll a, c (b) chlorophyll b, a
(c) chlorophyll d, c (d) all
32. Pyrenoids are located in
(a) cytoplasm (b) mitochondria (c) chloroplast (d) nucleus
33. Pyrenoids store
(a) protein (b) starch (c) lipids (d) both (a) and (b)
34. Cell wall of green algae is made up of
(a) cellulose and pectose
(b) cellulose and pectin
(c) inner layer of pectose and outer layer of cellulose
(d) inner layers of cellulose and outer layer of pectose
35. Zoospores are formed during asexual reproduction of algae and formed in
(a) sporangia (b) zoosporangia (c) microsporangia (d) megasporangia
36. Sexual reproduction is of isogamous, anisogamous, and oogamous in
(a) chlorophyceae (b) rhodophyceae
(c) chlorophyceae and phaeophyceae (d) chlorophyceae and rhodophyceae
37. Algae which are primarily marine is
(a) red algae (b) brown algae (c) green algae (d) all
38. Filamentous brown algae is
(a) spirogyra (b) laminaria (c) ectocarpus (d) porphyra
39. Green algae perform _______ oogamous type sexual reproduction
(a) sphagnum (b) volvox (c) dictyota (d) spirogyra
40. Kelps represent the group of
(a) bryophytes (b) red algae (c) green algae (d) brown algae
41. Kelps may reach a height up to
(a) 120 m (b) 100 m (c) 1000 m (d) 10 m
42. The algae possess chlorophyll a, c, carotenoids and xanthophylls belong to
(a) green algae (b) brown algae (c) both (d) none
43. Brown algae vary in colour from _______ to various shades of _______ depending on the amount of _______ pigment and _______ present in them
(a) fucoxanthin, xanthophyll, blue, brown
(b) blue, brown, fucoxanthin, xanthophyll
(c) yellow, brown, fucoxanthin, xanthophyll
(d) olive green, brown, fucoxanthin, xanthophyll
44. Laminaria and mannitol are stored food of
(a) euglena (b) green algae (c) liverworts (d) brown algae
45. The plant body of algae divided in holdfast, stipe and fronds in
(a) chara (b) laminaria (c) porphyra (d) all
46. The plant body attached to substratum in brown algae by
(a) rhizoids (b) multicellular hair (c) holdfast (d) roots
47. The photosynthetic leaf like organ found in some of the algae are called
(a) sporophyll (b) fronds (c) leaves (d) scaly leaves
48. Zoospores of brown algae are
(a) uniflagellate (b) multiflagellate
(c) biflagellate (d) may be any of the above three

49. The arrangement of flagella in brown algae is
(a) one and equally arranged
(b) two unequal and laterally arranged
(c) many flagella arranged anywhere on the body
(d) depend from organism to organism

50. The biflagellate pear-shaped zoospores are characteristic of
(a) red algae (b) green algae (c) brown algae (d) all

51. Fertilization in brown algae occurs in
(a) water (b) within the oogonia (c) both (d) none

52. Sexual reproduction shown by members of brown algae is
(a) isogamous (b) anisogamous (c) oogamous (d) all

53. Pyriform gametes means
(a) pea-shaped gametes (b) pear shaped gametes
(c) gametes with one flagella (d) all

54. Dictyota belongs to
(a) bryophytes (b) green algae (c) brown algae (d) none

55. Red algae are red due to the presence of pigment
(a) phycoerythrin (b) r-phycocyanin (c) r-phycoerythrin (d) r-phepocyamin

56. Red algae are found in
(a) cold seas (b) seas with moderate temp
(c) warmer water (d) none

57. Algae found in the areas where no light penetrates is
(a) green algae (b) dinofalgellates (c) red algae (d) brown algae

58. Algae found in areas with abundant light as well as areas of great depths with no light is
(a) red algae (b) green algae (c) blue algae (d) brown algae

59. Red algae are mostly
(a) unicellular (b) multicellular
(c) may be multicellular and unicellular (d) none

60. Floridean starch is stored food found in
(a) some protist (b) some bryophytes (c) some algae (d) prokaryotes

61. Floridean starch is similar to
(a) amylopectin (b) glycogen (c) fructose (d) both (a) and (b)

62. The spores and gametes of red algae are
(a) motile and non motile (b) both are motile
(c) both non motile (d) motile spores and non motile gamete

63. Sexual reproduction of oogamous type is found in
(a) red algae (b) green algae (c) brown algae (d) all

64. Most reduced type of sexual reproduction is found in the members of
(a) red algae (b) green algae (c) brown algae (d) all

65. _______ reproduction shown by members of rhodophyceae
(a) Oogamous (b) Isogamous (c) Anisogamous (d) All

66. Fronds are found in which of the following algae?
I. Laminaria II. Fucus
III. Dictyota IV. Porphyra
(a) I, II, and III (b) I and II (c) II and III (d) All

67. Air bladders are shown by
(a) fucus (b) laminaria (c) dictyota (d) all

68. How many of the following algae belong to the category of red algae?
Polysiphonia, Gelidium, Laminaria, Spirogyra, Porphyra, Fucus, Chlamydomonas
(a) 2 (b) 3 (c) 4 (d) 5

69. Members of phaeophyceae are
(a) ectocarpus, dictyota, fucus and sargassum
(b) ectocarpus, dictyota, fucus and porphyra
(c) chlamydomonas, volvox, ulothrix
(d) gracilaria and gelidium

70. Poly sulphate esters are present in the cell wall of
(a) ectocarpus and dictyota (b) gelidium and gracilaria
(c) ectocarpus and sargassum (d) spirogyra and chara

71. Pear-shaped gametes are found in
(a) ectocarpus, dictyota and fucus
(b) ulothrix, spirogyra, and ectocarpus
(c) ectocarpus, gelidium and gracilaria
(d) none

72. Complex post fertilization events are seen in
(a) chlorella and spirullina (b) gracilaria and porphyra
(c) volvox and ulothrix (d) all

73. Organisms referred to as amphibians of plant kingdom are
(a) pteridophytes (b) bryophytes
(c) angiosperms (d) gymnosperms

74. Bryophytes are found in
(a) rocky places (b) hilly areas
(c) moist and shady places (d) aquatic areas

75. Organisms play import role in plant succession on base rocks are
(a) mosses (b) pteridophytes (c) protist (d) none

76. Bryophytes required _______ for fertilization
(a) nutrients (b) water (c) both (d) none

77. Which of the following statement is incorrect in respect to bryophytes?
(a) The plant body is thallus like, more differentiated than algae and attached to substratum by help of rhizoids
(b) The antherozoids are released in water for fertilization
(c) Zygote formed undergoes meiote division immediately
(d) They have leaf like, stem like and root like structures

78. The sporophyte of bryophytes develops after
(a) reduction division of zygote (b) multiplication in zygote
(c) before the formation of zygote (d) none

79. Sporophyte of bryophytes is
I. multicellular body.
II. parasite on gametophyte.
III. partially undergoes reduction division to form spores.
IV. derives the water from gametophytes.
(a) II and III (b) III and IV (c) Only I (d) All

80. _______ forms gametophyte of bryophytes
(a) Zygote (b) Sporophyte (c) Gametes (d) Spores
81. The organism having more differentiated plant body than algae
(a) protist (b) mosses (c) monera (d) none
82. The gametophyte possessing leaf like, root like and stem like structure is
(a) gymnosperm (b) chlorophyceae (c) slime molds (d) mosses
83. The male sex organ of bryophyte is called
(a) antherozoids (b) testes (c) globule (d) none
84. The sex organ in bryophytes are
(a) reduced to single celled stage (b) multicellular
(c) net cell developed (d) formed in sporophyte stage
85. The main plant body of bryophyte is
(a) haploid (b) diploid (c) polyploid (d) all
86. Female sex organ of bryophytes is
(a) oval in shape (b) irregular
(c) flask shaped (d) depends on the organism
87. Female sex organ of bryophyte is called
(a) nucule (b) ovary (c) oogonia (d) archegonium
88. Archegonium contains _______ egg cells in bryophytes
(a) more than one (b) two (c) four (d) one
89. Division in zygote results in formation of _______ in bryophytes
(a) gametophyte (b) sporophyte (c) antherozoids (d) archegonium
90. Gametophyte of bryophyte is
(a) free living and sporophyte (b) free living and autotrophic
(c) may be free living or autotropic (d) always pressure
91. Peat used in trans shipment is a product obtained by
(a) liverworts (b) phaeophyceae (c) mosses (d) none
92. Organisms which first colonize base rocks is
(a) mosses (b) mycorrhiza (c) lichens (d) both (a) and (c)
93. Mosses are ecologically important because
I. first organism to colonize base rocks.
II. decompose rocks making suitable for growth of higher plant.
III. forms dense mats on soil.
IV. reduce impact of falling rain and soil erosion.
(a) Only I (b) Only II (c) III and IV (d) All
94. Peat which is long used as fuel is a product obtained from
(a) gelidium (b) species of sphagnum
(c) all mosses (d) all liverworts
95. Organisms participating as pioneers in ecological succession belongs to
(a) lichens (b) mosses (c) liverworts (d) both (a) and (b)
96. Liverworts are found in
(a) moist shady places
(b) banks of steams, marshy ground
(c) damp soil, bard of trees and deep in the woods
(d) all of the above

97. The thallus of liverworts are
(a) sexual multiplication of the formation of sex organs called gemmae
(b) dorsiventral and appressed to substrate
(c) found in xeric habitats
(d) diploid

98. Asexual reproduction in liverworts means
(a) fragmentation of thalli
(b) formation of specialized structure called gemmae
(c) both of above
(d) none of above

99. Gemmae in liverworts are formed during
(a) sexual reproduction (b) asexual reproduction
(c) spore formation (d) adverse conduction

100. Marchantia is
(a) an algae (b) gymnosperm (c) fern (d) bryophyte

101. Sexual reproduction in liverworts takes place by
(a) formation of sex organs always on the same thallus
(b) formation of male and female sex organs on different thallus
(c) sexual reproduction is absent
(d) male and female sex organs may be present on same or different thalli

102. The sporophyte in liverworts
(a) is the dominant and main phase of the plant body
(b) is differentiated into foot, seta and capsule
(c) parasite on the gametophyte
(d) both (b) and (c)

103. Spore in bryophytes are formed
(a) on the gametophyte (b) on the sporophyte
(c) in the seta of sporophyte (d) in the capsule of sporophyte

104. The gametophyte of bryophyte develops from
(a) a haploid spore (b) a diploid spore (c) zygote (d) none

105. Zygote of bryophyte
(a) multiply and form gametophyte
(b) multiply and form the sporophyte
(c) undergoes reduction division just after formation
(d) all are correct

106. The dominant stage of gametophyte of mosses consist of
(a) protonema which develops from lateral bud
(b) a leafy stage developing from a spore
(c) both (a) and (b)
(d) a leafy stage developing form secondary protonema

107. Protonema is found in
(a) liverworts (b) selaginella (c) funaria (d) none

108. Which one is correct about protonema?
(a) It is a dominant stage mosses
(b) Develops from spore
(c) It is creeping, green, branched and frequently filamentous
(d) All are correct

109. Leafy stage in bryophytes
(a) Develops from secondary protonema
(b) Consist of upright, slender axis and bears consist of alternately arranged leaves
(c) Attached to the soil through unicellular and branched rhizoids
(d) All

110. Sex organs in mosses develops on
(a) secondary protonema (b) leafy stage
(c) on capsule of sporophyte (d) none

111. Vegetative reproduction in mosses takes place by
(a) fragmentation and budding in secondary protonema
(b) binary fission
(c) spore dispersal
(d) all

112. Sporophyte of mosses is more elaborated from
(a) ferns (b) pinus (c) polytrichum (d) marchantia

113. Spores in bryophytes are formed by
(a) mitosis (b) meiosis in gametophyte
(c) mitosis in zygote (d) meiosis in zygote

114. Elaborate mechanism of spore dispersal is found in
(a) ferns (b) mosses (c) liverworts (d) none

115. Sphagnum belongs to
(a) ferns (b) liverworts (c) mosses (d) none

116. The plants frequently grown as ornamentals and are used for medicinal purpose belong to
(a) angiosperms (b) pteridophytes (c) algae (d) some protist

117. The first terrestrial plants to posses vascular tissues are
(a) gymnosperms (b) bryophyte (c) pteridophytes (d) all

118. The main plant body of pteridophytes is
(a) gametophytes as well as sporophyte (b) sporophyte
(c) none (d) both

119. The plant body of pteridophyte is
(a) not well-developed (b) lacks vascular tissue
(c) is thalloid (d) posses true root, leaves and stem

120. Pteridophytes have only
(a) small microphyllous leaves
(b) large macrophyllous leaves
(c) both microphyllous as well as macrophyllous in some of the ferns
(d) all of above

121. Which one is false about pteridophyte?
(a) They flourish well moist and shady condition
(b) They are found in cool damp and shady place
(c) The xylem posses vessels
(d) None

122. Prothallus is the gametophyte of
(a) bryophytes (b) algae (c) pteridophyte (d) gymnosperm

123. The gametophyte of pteridophyte grows in damp, moist and shady places because
(a) they are limited and restricted to a narrow geographical region
(b) they need water for fertilization of gametes formed on the gametophyte
(c) water is required for gametogenesis
(d) egg cell swims in water to reach to the antheridia

124. Gametophyte of pteridophyte
(a) parasite on sporophyte (b) not a free living stage
(c) photosynthetical and free living (d) is unicellular

125. Vascular plants which do not bear seeds is
(a) angiosperms (b) pteridophytes (c) gymnosperms (d) none

126. Macrophylls leaves are characteristics of
(a) mosses (b) ferns (c) funaria (d) none

127. Pteridophyte having microphylls is
(a) ferns (b) psilotum (c) selaginella (d) all

128. The production of spores by the spore mother cells is the result of
(a) mitosis (b) meiosis
(c) mitosis and meiosis both (d) amitosis

129. The leaves bearing sporangia are called
(a) sporophylls (b) fronds (c) tropophylls (d) scaly leaves

130. Cones in pteridophytes are formed in
(a) salvinia (b) selaginella and lycopodium
(c) dryopteris (d) selaginella and Equisetum

131. Spores in pteridophytes give rise to
(a) sporophyte (b) parasite gametophyte
(c) free living gametophyte (d) free living sporophyte

132. Which of the following are correct about pteridophytes?
I. The sporophytes bear sporangia that are formed on the sporophylls.
II. They are frequently grown as ornamentals.
III. They are the first terrestrial plants to forms seeds.
IV. Vascular tissues are absent in pteridophytes.
V. some species flourish well in sandy soil conditions.
(a) V and IV (b) I, II and IV (c) III, IV and V (d) I and II

133. Sex organs in pteridophytes are formed on the
(a) multicellular well-developed sporophyte
(b) multicellular main gametophyte phase of the plant
(c) photosynthetic, free living gametophyte
(d) parasite gametophyte dependent on sporophyte

134. The male and female sex organs of pteridophyte are called
(a) globule and nucule respectively (b) antheridia and archegonia respectively
(c) spermatangia and oogonia respectively (d) tests and ovary respectively

135. Zygote of pteridophyte
(a) undergoes reduction division just often formation
(b) produces multicellular gametophyte
(c) produces multicellular sporophyte
(d) remains dormant

136. Maximum of pteridophytes are
I. homosporous and produce only one kind of spores.
II. aquatic in nature.
III. heterosporus and produce small and large spores.
IV. restricted to narrow geographical zone because of specific requirement of water.
(a) I and II (b) II and III (c) III and IV (d) IV and I

137. Heterosporous pteridophytes are
(a) dryopteris and pteris (b) selaginella and lycopodium
(c) selaginella and salvinia (d) equisetum and Adiantum

138. Heterosporous plants are
(a) plants producing one kind of spores
(b) plants producing large and small spores
(c) plants producing two type of spores which are similar in size
(d) none

139. Megaspore germinate into
(a) female gametophyte
(b) gametophyte having both male and female sex organs
(c) male gametophyte
(d) male sporophyte

140. The female gametophytes are retained on the parent sporophyte in
(a) homosporous species of pteridophytes
(b) heterosporous species of pteridophytes
(c) both are correct
(d) both are incorrect

141. Process similar to seed habit considerably observed in
(a) homosporous species of pteridophytes
(b) heterosporous species of pteridophyte
(c) all the members of pteridophytes
(d) net seen in pteridophyte

142. Vascular plants, with seeds but no fruits are
(a) bryophyte (b) angiosperms (c) gymnosperms (d) pteridophytes

143. In heterosporous pteridophyte
(a) zygote develops into young embryo in the female gametophyte
(b) zygote multiples and develop into the sporophyte in the soil
(c) all spores are similar
(d) none

144. Naked seed plants are
(a) algae (b) bryophyte (c) angiosperms (d) gymnosperms

145. Ovules are not enclosed by the ovaries in
(a) pteridophytes (b) angiosperms (c) gymnosperms (d) all

146. The tallest gymnosperms is
(a) sequoia (red wood tree) (b) pinus
(c) cycas (d) ginkgo

147. Coralloid roots having association with N_2 fixing bacteria are found in
(a) pinus (b) cedrus (c) sequoia (d) cycas

148. In gymnosperms mycorrhizal association are found in
(a) cycas (b) pinus (c) cedrus (d) all

149. Gymnosperms
(a) are naked seeds plants (b) have tap roots
(c) are heterosporous (d) all

150. Which of the following are correct for gymnosperms?
I. Have adventitious root system.
II. The leaves in gymnosperms can withstand extreme of temperature, humidity and wind.
III. Microspores are produced in microsporangia.
IV. They include medium or tall sized trees and shrubs.
(a) I and III (b) I, II and II (c) II, III and IV (d) I and IV

151. In cycas
(a) the stems are unbranched
(b) the pinnately compound leaves persist for years
(c) have symbiotic association with n_2 fixing cynobacteria
(d) all are correct

152. Which of the followings are correct for conifers?
I. Needle like leaves to reduce surface area.
II. Thick cuticle on leaves.
III. Sunken stomata to reduce water loss.
IV. The main plant body is gametophyte.
(a) II and III (b) IV only (c) I only (d) II, I and III

153. Which of the following are correct for gymnosperms?
I. They are heterosporous.
II. They are the first vascular plants.
III. Posses fruits.
IV. Require water for fertilization.
(a) I (b) I and II (c) II and III (d) I, II, III and IV

154. Which of the following sequence is correct?
(a) Strobili–Sporophylls→Sporangia→Spores
(b) Strobili–Sporangia→Sporophylls→Spores
(c) Sporophylls–Strobili→Sporangia→Spores
(d) Spores–Sporangia→Strobili→Cones

155. Male gametophyte which is highly reduced and confined to only limited numbers of cells is called
(a) autherozoid (b) spermatozoid
(c) pollen grain (d) all

156. Male and female cones are formed on the same tree of
(a) cycas (b) pinus (c) both (d) none

157. In gymnosperms
(a) pollen grains germinate inside the ovary
(b) the development of pollen grain takes place within the microsporangia
(c) the cones barring megasporophylls are called male cones or male strobili
(d) all are correct

158. Megaspore mother cell
(a) develops from one of the cell of nucleus (b) forms four megaspore after meiosis
(c) formed in the megasporangium (d) all

159. The female gametophyte of gymnosperms
(a) bear two archegonia
(b) retained within megasporangium
(c) is unicellular
(d) both (a) and (b)

160. In gymnosperms, male and female gametophyte
I. do not have independent free living existence.
II. remain within the sporangia retained on parent sporophyte.
III. may be born on same or different tree.
IV. perform meiosis to produce gametes.
(a) I and II
(b) II and III
(c) III and IV
(d) All

161. Pollination in gymnosperms take place by
(a) wind
(b) water
(c) only physical factors like wind and water
(d) all of the above

162. Angiosperms include
(a) vascular plants with naked seeds
(b) vascular plants with covered seeds
(c) few vascular plants with naked seeds
(d) few vascular plants with covered seeds

163. Microscopic angiosperm is
(a) sequoia
(b) eucalyptus
(c) wolfia
(d) never microscopic

164. Angiosperms include
(a) massive woody trees
(b) shrubs and herbs
(c) ranges from tiny microscopic plants to tall trees
(d) none

165. Height of eucalyptus tree is approximately
(a) 100 m
(b) 1000 m
(c) 10 m
(d) 10–20 m

166. Male sex organ in angiosperm is located in
(a) male cone
(b) sporophyll
(c) flower
(d) carpel

167. Male sex organ in flower is
(a) anthredia
(b) stamens
(c) spermatangia
(d) nucule

168. The female sex organ of flower is called
(a) archegonia
(b) nucule
(c) oogonia
(d) pistil

169. The pistil in flower encloses
(a) one ovule
(b) only two ovules
(c) three ovules
(d) one too many ovules

170. Embryo sacs in angiosperms is
(a) male gametophyte
(b) well-developed female gametophyte
(c) highly reduced female gametophyte
(d) well-developed female sporophyte

171. Embryo sac of angiosperms posses
(a) egg apparatus
(b) synergids
(c) antipodal
(d) all

172. Egg apparatus of angiosperms contain
(a) one egg cell
(b) two synergids
(c) both (a) and (b)
(d) two antipodals

173. The cells of embryo sac are
(a) diploid (b) haploid
(c) may be haploid or diploid (d) none

174. Diploid secondary nucleus in embryo sac of angiosperm is the product of
(a) fusion of two synergid cells (b) fusion of two antipodal cells
(c) fusion of two polar nuclei (d) fusion of egg cell and antipodal cell

175. The pistil in angiosperm is made up of
(a) ovary (b) stigma (c) style (d) all

176. Ovary is the characteristic feature of
(a) gymnosperms (b) angiosperm (c) pteridophyte (d) all

177. In double fertilization
(a) male gamete fuses with egg cell to form zygote
(b) male gamete fuses with diploid endosperm nucleus to produce triploid primary endosperm nucleus
(c) both (a) and (b)
(d) fertilization takes place in two plants simultaneously

178. Synergids and antipodals
(a) develop into new plans (b) are diploid
(c) degenerate after fertilization (d) are produced in male gametophyte

179. Fruit formation in angiosperm takes place by
(a) development of ovule after fertilization (b) development of ovary after fertilization
(c) axillary bud (d) terminal bud

180. Double fertilization is unique characters feature of
(a) angiosperm (b) gymnosperm
(c) pteridophyte (d) dicotyledons only

181. Zygote after multiplication in angiosperm develop in
(a) endosperm (n) (b) embryo (n) (c) endosperm (d) embryo (2n)

182. Endosperm in angiosperm is formed
(a) before fertilization (b) after fertilization
(c) vary from species to species (d) all

183. Meiosis in plants can take place in
(a) only haploid species
(b) only diploid species
(c) both in haploid as well as diploid species
(d) none

184. The haploid plant body produces _______ and is referred to as _______
(a) spores, sporophyte (b) gametes, gametophyte
(c) zoospores, zoosporangia (d) conidia, Conidiophores

185. Haploid spore divide by _______ to form haploid plant body
(a) mitosis (b) meiosis (c) amitosis (d) any of them

186. In haplontic life cycle, sporophytic generation is seen by
(a) well-developed multicellular sporophyte (b) zygote
(b) embryo (d) none

187. In haplontic life cycle zygote divides by
(a) mitosis (b) meiosis (c) any of them (d) amitosis

188. Volvox, spirogyra chlamydomonas come under
(a) haplodiplontic life cycle organism (b) diplohaplontic organism
(c) haplontic life cycle (d) diplontic life cycle

189. Sporophyte, dominant, photosynthetic and independent phase of plant represents
(a) haplontic (b) diplontic
(c) diplohaplontic life cycle (d) both (b) and (c)

190. Diplontic life cycle is seen in
(a) angiosperms and gymnosperms (b) spermatophytes
(c) both (d) pteridophyte

191. When both the phases of life cycle are multicellular i.e. haploid and diploid phases are more than one celled
(a) life cycles are called haplodiplontic
(b) they differ in the dominant phase
(c) they are in pteridophytes and bryophytes
(d) all

192. The bryophytes
(a) dominant diploid multicellular sporophyte alters dominant with multicellular gametophytes
(b) dominant haploid multicellular gametophyte alters with diploid sporophyte
(c) the plant body show diplontic life cycle
(d) the plant body show haplontic life cycle

193. Most of the alga show
(a) haplontic life cycle (b) diplontic life cycle
(c) haplodiplontic life cycle (d) none

194. Algae showing haplodiplontic life cycle are
(a) spirullina and spirogyra (b) ectocarpus and polysiphonia
(c) kelps (d) both (b) and (c)

195. Which alga shows diplontic life cycle?
(a) Chara (b) Fucus (c) Ectocarpus (d) Polysiphonia

196. How many organisms show haplodiplontic life cycle?
Sphagnum, Volvox, Ulothrix, Marchantia, Polytrichum, Selaginella, Pinus, Cedrus, Ectocarpus, Polysiphonia
(a) 8 (b) 6 (c) 7 (d) 9

197. How many organisms show diplontic life cycle?
Selaginella, Equisetum, Cycas, Cedrus, Ectocarpus, Fucus, Sequoia
(a) 7 (b) 5 (c) 4 (d) 6

198. Which of the organisms show haplontic life cycle?
(a) Chlamydomonas, volvox (b) Ectocarpus, polysiphonia
(c) Fucus (d) All

199. In diplontic life cycle gametogenesis takes place by
(a) mitosis (b) meiosis
(c) both (d) neither mitosis nor meiosis

200. Gametogenesis in organism showing haplontic life cycle takes place in
(a) mitosis (b) meiosis (c) both (d) amitosis

201. Identify a, b, c in diagram:

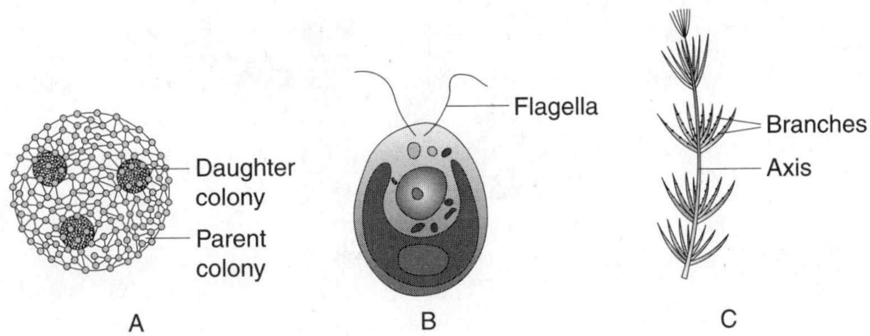

(a) A– Volvox, B–Chlamydomonas, C–Chara
(b) A–Chara, B–Volvox, C–Chlamydomonas
(c) A–Chlamydomonas, B–Chara, C–Volvox
(d) A–Chara, B–Chlamydomonas, C–Volvox

202. Identify a, b, c in diagram:

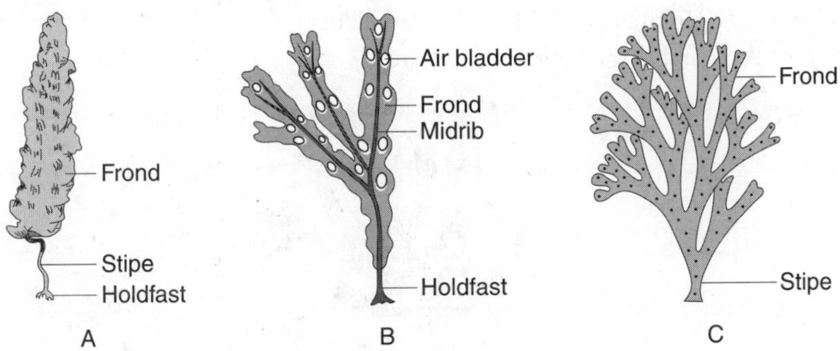

(a) A–Fucus, B–Laminaria, C–Dictyota
(b) A–Laminaria, B–Dictyota, C–Fucus
(c) A–Laminaria, B–Fucus, C–Dictyota
(d) A–Dictyota, B–Fucus, C–Laminaria

203. Identify A and B:

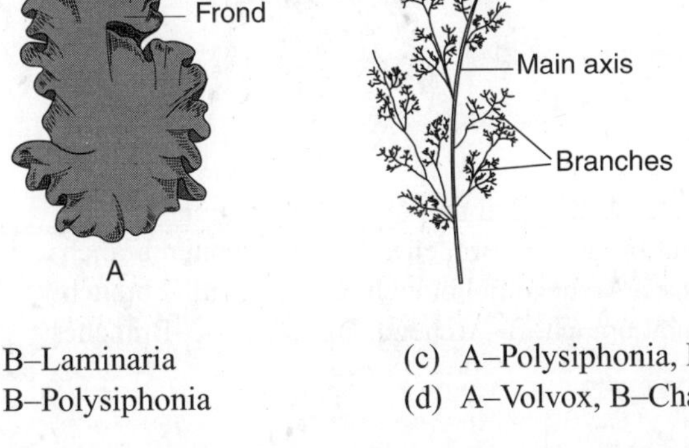

(a) A–Porphyra, B–Laminaria
(b) A–Porphyra, B–Polysiphonia
(c) A–Polysiphonia, B–Porphyra
(d) A–Volvox, B–Chara

204. Identify the A, B, C and D showing in this figure?

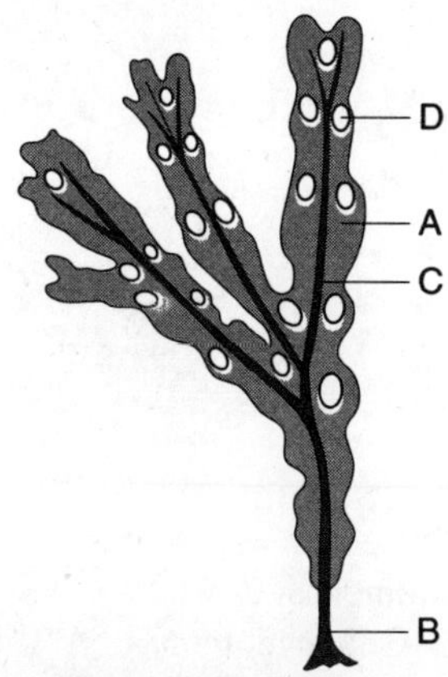

(a) A–Holdfast, B–Air bladder, C–Midrib, D–Frond
(b) A–Frond, B–Midrib, C–Air bladder, D–Holdfast
(c) A–Air bladder, B–Midrib, C–Holdfast, D–Frond
(d) A–Frond, B–Holdfast, C–Midrib, D–Air bladder

205. Identify the A, B and C showing in this figure?

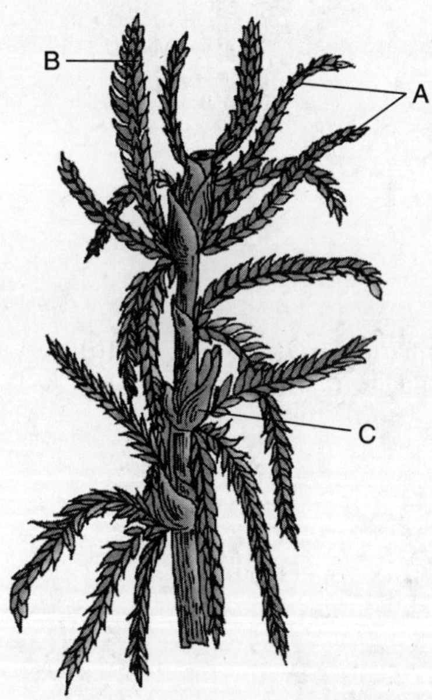

(a) A–Branches, B–Antheridial branch, C–Archegonial branch
(b) A–Antheridial branch, B–Branches, C–Archegonial branch
(c) A–Branches, B–Archegonial branch, C–Antheridial branch
(d) A–Archegonial branch, B–Archegonial branch, C–Branches

206. What indicate A to E in below figure.

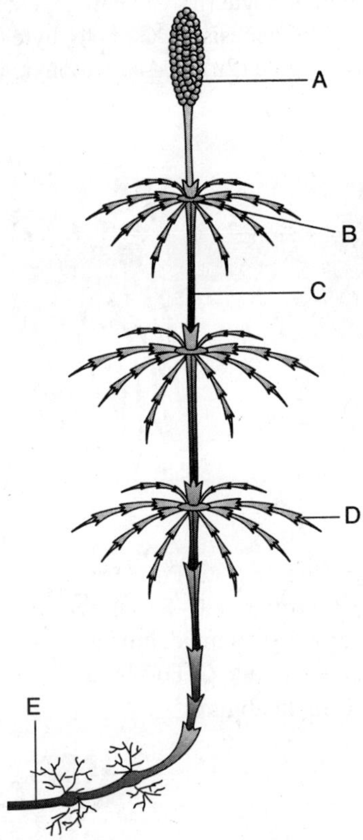

(a) A–Node, B–Rhizome, C–Internode, D–Strobilus, E–Branch
(b) A–Strobilus, B–Node, C–Internode, D–Branch, E–Rhizome
(c) A–Branch, B–Internode, C–Strobilus, D–Node, E–Rhizome
(d) A–Strobilus, B–Node, C–Branch, D–Internode, E–Rhizome

207. Identify the A, B and C showing in this figure?

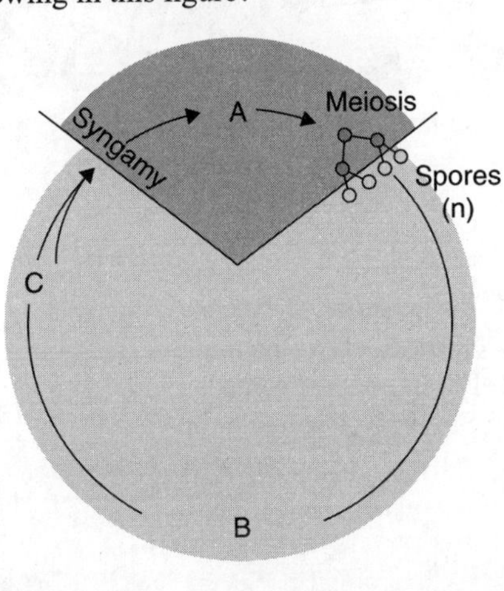

(a) A–Gametophyte (n), B–Zygote (2n), C–Gametogenesis
(b) A–Zygote (2n), B–Gametophyte (n), C–Gametogenesis
(c) A–Zygote (2n), B–Gametogenesis, C–Gametophyte (n)
(d) A–Gametogenesis, B–Zygote (2n), C–Gametophyte (n)

208. Identify the A, B and C.

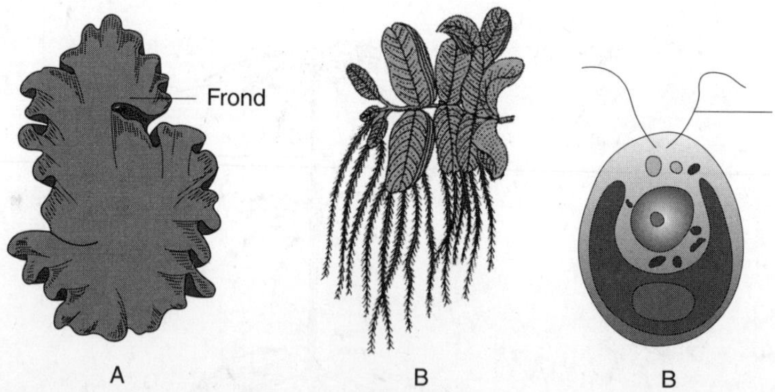

(a) A–Salvinia, B–Chlamydomonas, C–Porphyra
(b) A–Chlamydomonas, B–Porphyra, C–Salvinia
(c) A–Porphyra, B–Salvinia, C–Chlamydomonas
(d) A–Chlamydomonas, B–Salvinia, C–Porphyra

209. What indicates A, B and C in this figure.

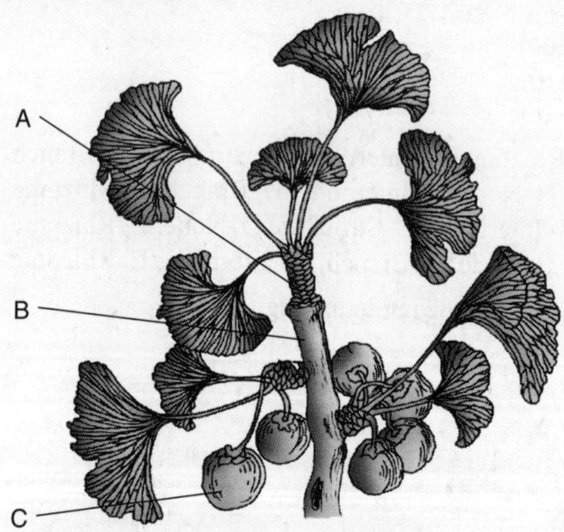

(a) A–Dwarf shoot, B–Long shoot, C–Seeds
(b) A–Long shoot, B–Seeds, C–Dwarf shoot
(c) A–Long shoot, B–Dwarf shoot, C–Seeds
(d) A–Seeds, B–Long Shoot, C–Dwarf Shoot

Read the **assertion** *and* **reason** *carefully to mark the correct option out of the options given below:*

(a) If both the assertion and the reason are true and the reason is a correct explanation of the assertion
(b) If both the assertion and reason are true but the reason is not a correct explanation of the assertion
(c) If the assertion is true but the reason is false
(d) If both the assertion and reason are false

210. Assertion: The earliest systems of classification used only superficial morphological characters.
Reason: Artificial system gave equal weightage to vegetative and sexual characterstics.

211. Assertion: Cytotaxonomy is based on cytological information like chromosome number, structure and behaviour.
Reason: Chemotaxonomy that uses the chemical constituents of the plants.

212. Assertion: In some species of Chlamydomonas the fusion of gamete is termed as anisogamous.
Reason: Because gametes which undergo fusion in these species are of dissimilar in size.

213. Assertion: Bryophytes are called amphibian of plant kingdom.
Reason: These plants live in soil but dependent on water for sexual reproduction.

214. Assertion: Mosses along with lichens are the first organisms to colonise rocks.
Reason: They decompose rocks by scereting acid substances.

215. Assertion: Pteridophytes are used for medicinal purposes and soil binders.
Reason: They are first terrestrial plants to possess vascular tissues.

216. Assertion: Only red algae are able to flourish at the great depth of sea.
Reason: Red algae has the pigments r phycoerythrin and r-phycocyanin.

217. Assertion: Gymnosperms are heterosporous.
Reason: They produce haploid microspores and megaspores.

218. Assertion: PEN is triploid in angiosperm.
Reason: PEN is formed by fusion of haploid male gamete with the dipoid secondary nucleus.

219. Assertion: The cells of highly reduced female gametophyte (embryo sac in angiosperm) is haploid.
Reason: The embryosac is formed by meiosis.

220. Assertion: In pinus coralloid roots are associated with nitrogen fixing cynobacteria.
Reason: In Cycas mycorrhiza is present.

AIPMT PREVIOUS YEAR QUESTIONS

1. Examine the figures A, B, C and D. In which one of the four options all the items A, B, C and D are correct?

[AIPMT MAINS 2010]

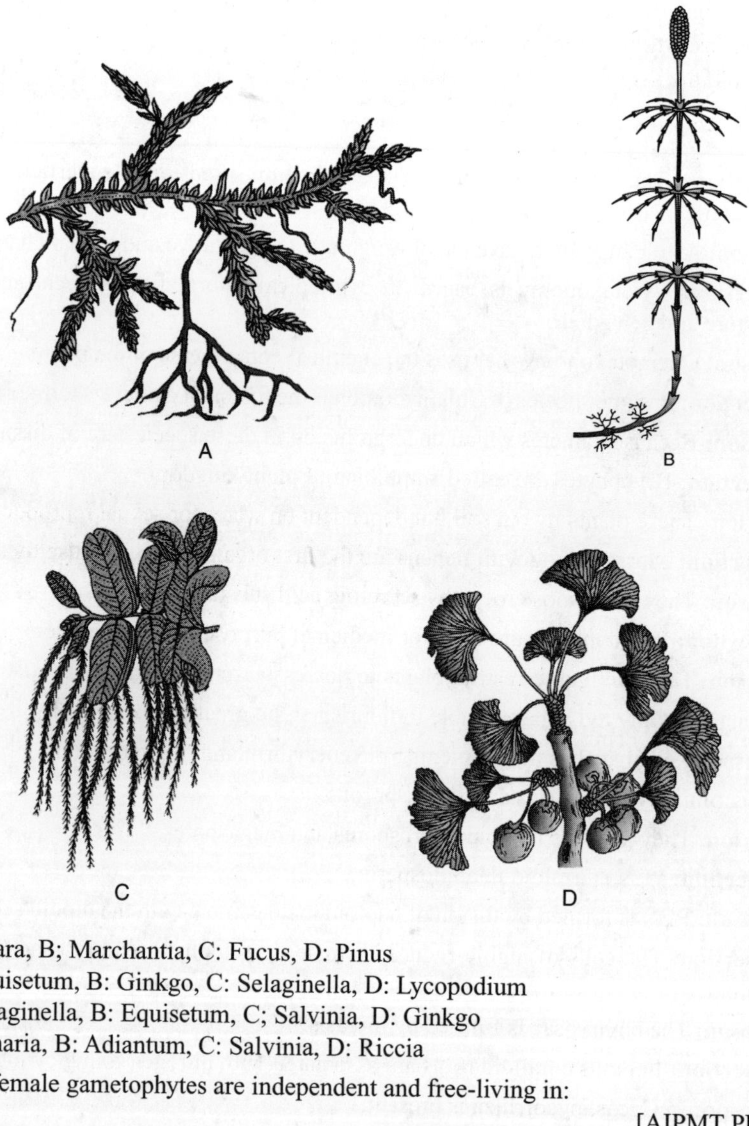

(a) A: Chara, B; Marchantia, C: Fucus, D: Pinus
(b) A: Equisetum, B: Ginkgo, C: Selaginella, D: Lycopodium
(c) A: Selaginella, B: Equisetum, C; Salvinia, D: Ginkgo
(d) A: Funaria, B: Adiantum, C: Salvinia, D: Riccia

2. Male and female gametophytes are independent and free-living in:

[AIPMT PRE 2010]

(a) Mustard
(b) Castor
(c) Pinus
(d) Sphagnum

3. Algae have cell wall made up of

[AIPMT PRE 2010]

(a) Cellulose, galactans and mannans
(b) Hemicellulose, pectins and proteins
(c) Pectins, cellulose and proteins
(d) Cellulose, hemicellulose and pectins

4. Consider the following four statements whether they are correct or wrong

[AIPMT MAINS 2011]

(A) The sporophyte in liverworts is more elaborate than that in mosses
(B) Salvinia in heterosporous
(C) The life-cycle in all seed-bearing plants is diplontic
(D) In Pinus male female cones are born on different trees

The two wrong statements together are

(a) A and C
(b) A and D
(c) B and C
(d) A and B

5. Selaginella and Salvinia are considered to represent a significant step toward evolution of seed habit because

[AIPMT MAINS 2011]

(a) Female gametophyte is free and gets dispersed like seeds
(b) Female gametophyte lacks archegonia
(c) Megaspores possess endosperm and embryo surrounded by seed coat
(d) Embryo develops in female gametophyte which is retained on parent sporophyte

6. Examine the figure given below and select the correct option giving all the four parts (A, B, C and D) rightly identified.

[AIPMT MAINS 2011]

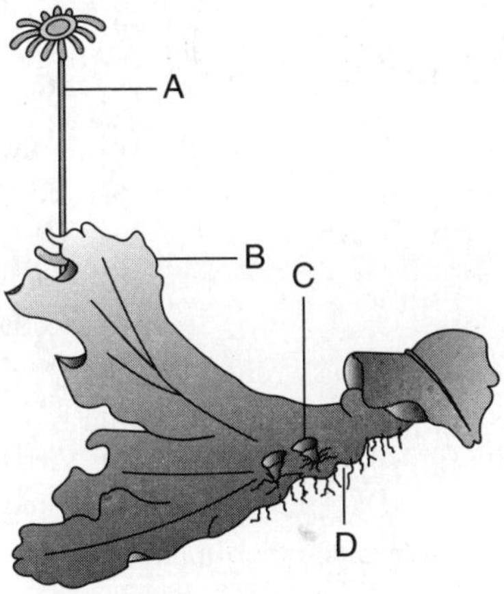

(a) A: Archegoniophore, B: Female thallus, C: Gemma cup, D: Rhizoids
(b) A: Archegoniophore, B: Female thallus, C: Bud, D: Food
(c) A: Seta, B: Sporophyte, C: Protonema, D: Rhizoids
(d) A: Antheridiophore, B: Male thallus, C: Globule, D: Roots

7. Compared with the gametophytes of the bryophytes, the gametophytes of vascular plants tends to be:

[AIPMT PRE 2011]

(a) Larger but to have smaller sex organs
(b) Larger and to have large sex organs
(c) Smaller and to have smaller sex organs
(d) Smaller but to have larger sex organs

8. The gametophyte is not an independent, free living generation in

[AIPMT PRE 2011]

(a) Adiantum (b) Marchantia
(c) Pinus (d) Polytrichum

9. Archegoniophore is present in

[AIPMT PRE 2011]

(a) Chara (b) Adiantum
(c) Funaria (d) Marchantia

10. A prokaryotic autotrophic nitrogen fixing symbiont is found in:

[AIPMT PRE 2011]

(a) Cycas (b) Cicer
(c) Pisum (d) Alnus

11. Read the following five statements (A - E) and answer as asked next to them.

[AIPMT MAINS 2012]

(A) In Equisetum the female gametophyte is retained on the parent sporophyte
(B) In Ginkgo male gametophyte is not independent
(C) The sporophyte in Riccia is more developed than that in Polytrichum
(D) Sexual reproduction in Volvox is isogamous
(E) The spores of slime moulds lack cell walls How many of the above statements are correct?

(a) Three (b) Four
(c) One (d) Two

12. In the five-kingdom classification, Chlamydomonas and Chlorella have been included in

[AIPMT MAINS 2012]

(a) Algae (b) Plantae
(c) Monera (d) Protista

13. Which one of the following pairs is wrongly matched?

[AIPMT MAINS 2012]

(a) Salvinia – Prothallus (b) Viroids – RNA
(c) Mustard-Synergids (d) Ginkgo-Archegonia

14. Cycas and Adiantum resemble each other in having

[AIPMT PRE 2012]

(a) Seeds (b) Motile Sperms
(c) Cambium (d) Vessels

15. Which one of the following is a correct statement?

[AIPMT PRE 2012]

(a) Pteridophyte gametophyte has a protonemal and leafy stage.
(b) In gymnosperms female gametophyte is free living

(c) Antheridiophores and archegoniophores are present in pteridophyte
(d) Origin of seed habit can be traced in pteridophytes.

16. Select the wrong statement: [AIPMT 2013]
(a) Isogametes are similar in structure, function and behaviour
(b) Anisogametes differ either in structure, function or behaviour
(c) In Oomycetes female gamete is smaller and motile, while male gamete is larger and non-motile
(d) Chlamydomonas exhibits both isogamy and anisogamy and Fucus shows oogamy

17. Isogamous condition with non-flagellated gametes is found in: [AIPMT 2013]
(a) Chlamydomonas (b) Spirogyra
(c) Volvox (d) Fucus

18. Besides paddy fields, cyanobacteria are also found inside vegetative part of: [AIPMT 2013]
(a) Pinus (b) Cycas
(c) Equisetum (d) Psilotum

19. Megasporangium is equivalent to: [AIPMT 2013]
(a) Embryosac (b) Fruit
(c) Nucellus (d) Ovule

20. Read the following statement (A-E) and answer the question which follows them.
(A) In liverworts, mosses, and ferns gametophytes are free-living
(B) Gymnosperms and some ferns are heterosporous
(C) Sexual reproduction in Fucus, Volvox and Albugo is oogamous
(D) The sporophyte in liverworts is more elaborate than that in mosses
(E) Both, Pinus and Marchantia are dioecious How many of the above statements are correct? [AIPMT 2013]
(a) One (b) Two
(c) Three (d) Four

21. Which one of the following shows isogamy with non-flagellated gametes? [AIPMT 2014]
(a) Sargassum (b) Ectocarpus
(c) Ulothrix (d) Spirogyra

22. Which one of the following is responsible for peat formation? [AIPMT 2014]
(a) Marchantia (b) Riccia
(c) Funaria (d) Sphagnum

23. Read the following give statements (A to E) and select the option with all correct statements:
(A) Mosses and Lichens are the first organisms [AIPMT 2015]
(B) *Selaginella* a homosporous pteridophyte.
(C) Coralloid roots in *Cycus* have VAM.
(D) Main plant body in bryophytes is gametophyte where as in pteridophytes it is saprophytic.
(E) In gymnosperms male and female gametophytes are present within sporangia located o sporophyte.

(a) (A), (C) and (D)
(b) (B), (C) and (D)
(c) (A), (D) and (E)
(d) (B), (C) and (E)

24. In which of the following gametophyte is not independent free living? [AIPMT 2015]

(a) Funaria
(b) Marchantia
(c) Pteris
(d) Pinus

25. Which one of the following statements is wrong? [AIPMT 2015]

(a) Algin and carrageen are product of algae
(b) Agar – agar is obtained from Gelidum and Gmeilaria
(c) Chlorella and Spirulina are used as space Food Mannitol is stored food in Rhodophyceae
(d) Mannitol is stored food in Rhodophyceae

26. Male gametes are flagellated in: [AIPMT 2015]

(a) Polysiphonia
(b) Anabena
(c) Ectocarpus
(d) Spirogyra

27. Which one is a wrong statement? [RE-AIPMT 2015]

(a) Mucor has biflagellate zoospores
(b) Haploid endosperm is typical feature of gymnosperms
(c) Brown algae have chlorophyll a and c, and fucoxanthin
(d) Archegonia are found in Bryophyta, Pteridophyta and Gymnosperms

Answer Keys

1. (d)	2. (c)	3. (b)	4. (b)	5. (d)	6. (a)	7. (c)	8. (b)	9. (c)	10. (d)
11. (c)	12. (d)	13. (c)	14. (d)	15. (b)	16. (b)	17. (c)	18. (a)	19. (a)	20. (c)
21. (d)	22. (d)	23. (b)	24. (c)	25. (c)	26. (c)	27. (a)	28. (c)	29. (b)	30. (a)
31. (b)	32. (c)	33. (d)	34. (d)	35. (b)	36. (c)	37. (b)	38. (c)	39. (b)	40. (d)
41. (b)	42. (b)	43. (d)	44. (d)	45. (b)	46. (c)	47. (b)	48. (c)	49. (b)	50. (c)
51. (c)	52. (d)	53. (b)	54. (c)	55. (c)	56. (c)	57. (c)	58. (a)	59. (b)	60. (c)
61. (d)	62. (c)	63. (d)	64. (a)	65. (a)	66. (d)	67. (a)	68. (b)	69. (a)	70. (b)
71. (a)	72. (b)	73. (b)	74. (c)	75. (a)	76. (b)	77. (c)	78. (b)	79. (d)	80. (d)
81. (b)	82. (d)	83. (a)	84. (b)	85. (a)	86. (c)	87. (d)	88. (d)	89. (b)	90. (b)
91. (c)	92. (d)	93. (d)	94. (b)	95. (d)	96. (d)	97. (b)	98. (c)	99. (b)	100. (d)
101. (d)	102. (d)	103. (d)	104. (a)	105. (c)	106. (d)	107. (c)	108. (d)	109. (a)	110. (b)
111. (a)	112. (d)	113. (d)	114. (b)	115. (c)	116. (b)	117. (c)	118. (b)	119. (d)	120. (c)
121. (c)	122. (c)	123. (b)	124. (c)	125. (b)	126. (b)	127. (c)	128. (b)	129. (a)	130. (d)
131. (c)	132. (b)	133. (c)	134. (c)	135. (c)	136. (d)	137. (c)	138. (b)	139. (a)	140. (b)
141. (b)	142. (c)	143. (a)	144. (d)	145. (c)	146. (a)	147. (d)	148. (b)	149. (d)	150. (c)
151. (d)	152. (d)	153. (a)	154. (a)	155. (c)	156. (b)	157. (b)	158. (d)	159. (d)	160. (d)
161. (a)	162. (b)	163. (c)	164. (c)	165. (a)	166. (c)	167. (b)	168. (d)	169. (d)	170. (c)
171. (d)	172. (c)	173. (b)	174. (c)	175. (d)	176. (b)	177. (c)	178. (c)	179. (b)	180. (a)
181. (d)	182. (b)	183. (b)	184. (b)	185. (a)	186. (b)	187. (a)	188. (c)	189. (b)	190. (c)
191. (d)	192. (b)	193. (a)	194. (d)	195. (b)	196. (b)	197. (c)	198. (a)	199. (b)	200. (a)

201. (a)	202. (c)	203. (c)	204. (d)	205. (a)	206. (b)	207. (b)	208. (c)	209. (a)	210. (b)
211. (b)	212. (a)	213. (a)	214. (a)	215. (b)	216. (a)	217. (a)	218. (a)	219. (a)	220. (d)

AIPMT Previous Year Questions

1. (c)	2. (d)	3. (a)	4. (b)	5. (d)	6. (a)	7. (c)	8. (c)	9. (d)	10. (a)
11. (c)	12. (d)	13. (a)	14. (b)	15. (d)	16. (c)	17. (b)	18. (b)	19. (d)	20. (c)
21. (d)	22. (d)	23. (c)	24. (d)	25. (d)	26. (c)	27. (a)			

CHAPTER 4

Animal Classification

1. Living organism differ in
   (a) shape (b) form (c) size and habit (d) all
2. Which is not a character of sponges?
   (a) Multicellular (b) Cells are functionally independent
   (c) Cellular level of organization (d) Tissue level of organization
3. Which phylum shows tissue level of organization?
   (a) protozoa (b) porifera (c) coelenterate (d) all
4. Organ system level of organization is not found in
   (a) annelida (b) arthropod (c) molluscs (d) platyhelminthes
5. Incomplete digestive tract (blind sac body plan) is found in
   (a) annelida (b) arthropod (c) molluscs (d) platyhelminthes
6. Closed type of circulatory system present in
   (a) annelida and arthropod (b) arthropod and mollusc
   (c) annelida and cephalopods (d) mollusc and echinodermates
7. In open type of circulatory system
   (a) blood flow in sinuses
   (b) blood pressure is low and irregular
   (c) it is found in arthropods and mollusc(except cephalopods)
   (d) all are true
8. Closed type of circulatory system is found in
   (a) annelida (b) cephalopods (c) vertebrate (d) all
9. What is false about closed circulatory system?
   (a) blood pressure is high and regular
   (b) amount of blood is limited
   (c) blood circulates through arteries, veins and capillaries
   (d) blood pressure is low and irregular
10. When body of animal can be divided into equal left and right halves by one plane symmetry. It is known as
    (a) bilateral (b) radial (c) biradial (d) asymmetric
11. Radial symmetry is shown by
    (a) coelenterate (b) platyhelminthes
    (c) adult echinodermates (d) both (a) and (c)
12. Most of the sponges are
    (a) bilateral (b) radial (c) biradial (d) asymmetric

13. First diploblastic animal is
(a) coelenterates (b) platyhelminthes (c) aschelminthes (d) annelida
14. First triploblastic animal is
(a) coelenterates (b) platyhelminthes (c) aschelminthe (d) annelida
15. Triploblastic animal contains
(a) ectoderm (b) mesoderm (c) endoderm (d) all
16. Aschelminthe are
(a) eucoelomate (b) pseudocoelomate (c) acoelomate (d) none
17. Following are acoelomate
(a) porifera (b) coelenterates (c) platyhelminthes (d) all
18. Metameric segmentation is found in
(a) annelida (b) arthropod (c) both (d) platyhelminthes
19. Notochord is derived from which layer?
(a) ectoderm (b) mesoderm (c) endoderm (d) all
20. Which of the following is correct about notochord?
(a) dorsally situated (b) mesodermal in origin
(c) rod like (d) all
21. Radial symmetry is shown by
(a) ctenophores (b) coelenterates
(c) adult echinodermates (d) all
22. Undifferentiated layer present between ectoderm and endoderm in coelenterate is
(a) mesophyll (b) gastral layer (c) archenteron (d) mesoglea
23. Which of the following is correct about metamerism (true segmentation)?
(a) every organ shows serial repetition
(b) body is divided externally as well as internally
(c) each segment not supplied with separate nerve and blood vessels
(d) all
24. In some animals, body cavity is not lined by mesoderm. Instead the mesoderm is present as scattered pouches in between the ectoderm and endoderm. Such a body cavity is called
(a) eucoelom (b) pseudocoelom (c) acoelom (d) any of the above
25. Following are coelomates except (true coelom)
(a) Annelida (b) platyhelminthes
(c) Mollusca (d) Chordata
26. Select total number of organism from the following which are sessile:
Amoeba, Euglena, Adamsia, Spongilla, Hydra, Jelly fish, Earthworm
(a) 1 (b) 2 (c) 3 (d) 4
27. Which of the following is incorrect about Porifera?
(a) It is solitary or colonial organism
(b) Majority live in sea and some live in fresh water
(c) Most of them are asymmetric
(d) All
28. Members of phylum Porifera are commonly known as
(a) flatworms (b) roundworms (c) sponges (d) corals
29. Water path in sponges is
(a) ostia $\rightarrow$ spongocoel $\rightarrow$ osculum (b) osculum $\rightarrow$ spongocoel $\rightarrow$ osculum
(c) ostia $\rightarrow$ spongocoel $\rightarrow$ ostia (d) spongocoel $\rightarrow$ ostia $\rightarrow$ osculum

30. Unique character of sponges is
(a) choanoctyes or collar cells line, the spongocoel and the canals
(b) that they are hermaphrodite
(c) that they live in marine water
(d) it reproduces by asexual means only

31. Character possessed by all sponges are
(a) that all are fresh water (b) all possess tissue level of organization
(c) external fertilisation (d) hermaphrodite

32. Select the total number of statements belonging to sponges:
(1) Cellular level of organization.
(2) Body is supported by endoskeleton made up of spicules or sponging fibres.
(3) Larva stage is morphologically different from adult.
(4) Pathway of water transport is helpful in gathering of food, respiratory exchange and removal of waste.
(5) Hermaphrodite organism.
(6) They show power of regeneration.
(a) 5 (b) 6 (c) 4 (d) 3

33. Select fresh water sponge from the following:
(a) Sycon (b) Euspongia (c) Spongilla (d) Haylonema

34. Another name of sycon is
(a) Scypha (b) Euspongia (c) Spongilla (d) Haylonema

35. Match the following:

Column I		Column II
A. Sycon	–	1. Bath sponge
B. Spongilla	–	2. Scypha
C. Euspongia	–	3. Fresh water sponge

(a) A–2, B–3, C–1 (b) A–1, B–2, C–3
(c) A–3, B–2, C–1 (d) A–3, B–1, C–2

36. Select total number of marine sponges from the following:
Leucosolenia, Euspongia, Spongilla, Sycon, Haylonema
(a) 3 (b) 4 (c) 5 (d) 2

37. Primitive multicellular animals having cellular level of organization are
(a) ctenophores (b) sponges (c) corals (d) crustacean

38. Water enters through minute pores in the body wall into central cavity in sponges. These minute pores are known as
(a) osculum (b) ostia (c) spongocoel (d) any of the above

39. In sponge, sperm and ova are produced by same individual. Such types of organisms are called
(a) asexual (b) unisexual (c) hermaphrodite (d) dioecious

40. Canal system and choanocytes are characteristic of
(a) ctenophora (b) coelenterates (c) platyhelminthes (d) porifera

41. In sponges commonly seen larva are
(a) Amphiblastula (b) Parenchymula (c) Planula (d) Both (a) and (b)

42. Digestion in sponges is
(a) intracellular (b) extracellular (c) both (d) none

43. Which of the following is correct about reproduction in sponges?
(a) the mode of asexual reproduction gemmule formation, budding and fragmentation
(b) fertilization is internal

(c) development is indirect
(d) all

44. Exogenous budding is seen in case of
(a) scypha (b) euspongia (c) spongilla (d) haylonema

45. Following characters are related to phylum:
(1) Aquatic, mostly marine. (2) Sessile or free swimming.
(3) Radially symmetrical animals. (4) They show polymorphism.
(a) Porifera (b) Ctenophora (c) Echinodermata (d) coelenterata

46. Cnidoblast is a characteristic feature of
(a) porifera (b) coelenterata (c) ctenophora (d) arthropoda

47. First diploblastic animal showing tissue level of organization is
(a) Sycon (b) Gorgonia (c) Taenia (d) Locust

48. Cnidoblast is used for
(a) anchorage (b) defense (c) capture of prey (d) all

49. Select the total number of organisms from the following which shows both intra and extra cellular digestion.
Physalia, Pleurobrachia, Taenia, Culex, Apis, Neries, Echinus, Salpa, Meandrina, Pennatula, Doliolum, Catla, Hyla, Adamsia, Gorgonia, Ctenoplana.
(a) 6 (b) 8 (c) 7 (d) 10

50. Select correct matching:
(a) Petromyzon – Hag fish
(b) Echinus – Brittle star
(c) Apis – Silkworm
(d) Pennatula – Sea pen

51. Select incorrect matching:
(a) Locusta – Locust
(b) Cucumaria – Sea cucumber
(c) Meandrina – Sea anemone
(d) Echinus – Sea urchin

52. Some cnidarians examples corals have a skeleton composed of
(a) spongin fibres (b) silica (c) calcium carbonate (d) any of the above

53. Metagensis is shown by
(a) hydra (b) adamsia (c) aurelia (d) obelia

54. Which of the following is not true fish?
(a) Exocoetus (b) Betta (c) Saw fish (d) Jelly fish

55. Umbrella shape and free swimming form of coelentrate reproduce by sexual reproduction is
(a) polyp (b) medusa (c) both (d) none

56. Sessile, cylindrical form of coelenterate reproduce by asexual reproduction is
(a) polyp (b) medusa (c) both (d) none

57. Polyp → Asexually → Medusa → Sexually → Polyp
The above cycle is shown by
(a) physalia (b) aurelia (c) obelia (d) hydra

58. Select from the following total number of organisms which contain the word 'sea' in their common names.
Physalia, Adamsia, Pennatula, Gorgonia, Meandrina, Hydra, Aurelia, Obelia
(a) 2 (b) 3 (c) 4 (d) 5

59. Following is known as Portuguese man-of-war
(a) gorgonia (b) aurelia (c) physalia (d) obelia

60. First phylum shows nerve net
(a) porifera (b) coelenterate (c) platyhelminthes (d) protozoa

61. Gastro-vascular cavity with single opening is found in
(a) porifera (b) coelenterate (c) aschelminthes (d) annelida

62. Coelenterates asexually reproduce by
(a) Budding (b) Gametes (c) Conidia (d) Gemmules

63. Larva stage shown by coelenterate is called
(a) Amphiblastula (b) Parenchymula (c) Planula (d) All

64. Match the following:

Column I		Column II
A. Physalia	–	1. Brain coral
B. Adamsia	–	2. Sea fan
C. Pennatula	–	3. Sea pen
D. Gorgonia	–	4. Sea anemone
E. Meandrina	–	5. Portuguese man-of-war
F. Aurelia	–	6. Jellyfish

(a) A–5, B–4, C–2, D–3, E–1, F–6
(b) A–5, B–4, C–3, D–2, E–1, F–6
(c) A–5, B–4, C–2, D–1, E–2, F–6
(d) A–5, B–3, C–4, D–2, E–1, F–6

65. Ctenophores are commonly known as
(a) Sea walnut (b) Comb jellies (c) Both (d) None

66. Following features belongs to which phylum?
(1) Exclusively marine. (2) Radial symmetry.
(3) Diploblastic. (4) Tissue level organization.
(a) Coelentrata (b) Porifera
(c) Ctenophora (d) platyhelminthes

67. Body bears eight external rows of ciliated comb plates present in phylum _____.
(a) Coelentrata (b) Porifera (c) Ctenophora (d) platyhelminthes

68. Ctenophores show
(a) Extra and intra cellular digestion (b) Sexual reproduction only
(c) Bio luminescence (d) All

69. Example of ctenophores is
(a) Pleurobrachia (b) Ctenoplana (c) Both (d) None

70. Following features belong to which phylum?
(1) Bilateral symmetry. (2) Triploblastic, Acoelomate.
(3) Organ level of organization. (4) Dorso-ventrally flattened body.
(a) Platyhelminthes (b) Aschelminthes (c) Annelida (d) Arthropoda

71. platyhelminthes called flat worms because
(a) They are triploblastic (b) They are without coelom
(c) They have organ level of organization (d) Their body is dorso-ventrally flattened

72. Following are characters present in platyhelminthes:
(1) Some absorb nutrients from the host directly through their body surface.

(2) Digestive system incomplete, branched and without anus.
(3) Flame cells/solenocyte protonephridia help in excretion and osmoregulation.
(4) Hooks and Suckers are present in parasitic form.
(5) Hermaphrodites.
(6) Fertilization internal.
(7) Indirect development through many larva stages.
(a) 1, 2, 3, 5, 6 (b) 2, 3, 4, 5, 7 (c) All except 1 (d) All

73. Which platyhelminthes posses high power of regeneration?
(a) Planaria/Dugesia (b) Taenia (c) Fasciola (d) Liver fluke

74. Flame cells helps in excretion and osmoregulation in
(a) earthworm (b) hookworm (c) roundworm (d) tapeworm

75. Internal fertilization is seen in
(a) pleurobrachia (b) fasciola (c) ctenoplana (d) all

76. (1) Fertilization ______.
(2) Development ______.
(3) Excretion and osmoregulation by ______.
Fill in the blanks for organism given in the figure.

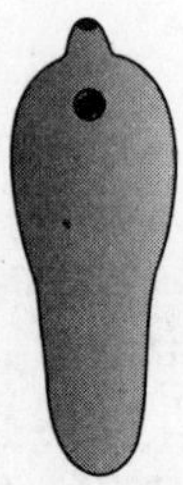

(a) Internal, direct, rennett cells
(b) Internal, indirect, flame cells
(c) External, direct, nephridia
(d) External, indirect, protonephridia

77. Phylum whose organism are mostly endoparasites is
(a) platyhelminthes (b) annelida (c) arthropoda (d) mollusca

78. Following are pseudocoelomate:
(a) Roundworm (b) Hookworm (c) Filarial worm (d) All

79. The body of the aschelminthes is circular in cross section. Hence it is named as
(a) tapeworm (b) earthworm (c) hookworm (d) roundworm

80. Roundworms/Nematodes are
(a) free living (b) aquatic or terrestrial
(c) parasitic on animals and plants (d) all

81. Select total number of organism shows internal fertilization.
Ascaris, Wuchereria, Ancylostoma, Taenia, Fasciola, Sycon, Euspongia, Spongilla, pleurobrachia, ctenoplana
(a) 6 (b) 7 (c) 8 (d) 5

82. Which character not belongs to phylum Aschelminthes?
(a) Excretory tube (branched ducts) remove body waste form the body cavity through excretory pore
(b) Usually sexes are separate (unisexual or dioecious)
(c) Development may be direct or indirect
(d) Alimentary canal is incomplete with a well-developed muscular pharynx

83. Match the following:

Column I		Column II
A. Ascaris	–	1. Intestinal Roundworm
B. Wuchereria	–	2. Filarialworm
C. Ancylostoma	–	3. Hookworm
D. Pheretima	–	4. Earthworm

(a) A–2, B–4, C–3, D–1
(b) A–1, B–2, C–3, D–4
(c) A–4, B–3, C–1, D–2
(d) A–2, B–1, C–4, D–3

84. Which of the following is correct about ascaris?
(a) females are smaller than males (b) posterior end of male curved dorsally
(c) females are longer than males (d) fertilization is external

85. Select total number of organism from the following contain well-developed muscular pharynx with complete alimentary canal.
Taenia, Fasciola, Planaria, Ascaris, Filarial worm, Hookworm
(a) 1 (b) 3 (c) 4 (d) 2

86. Metamerism is found in
(a) ascaris (b) leech (c) loligo (d) octopus

87. Nephridia help in excretion and osmoregulation in
(a) nereis (b) pheretima (c) hirudinaria (d) all

88. Closed circulatory system is present in
(a) nereis (b) pheretima (c) ascaris (d) both (a) and (b)

89. Animals having cylindrical body having organ system level of organization showing metamerism belong to phylum
(a) arthropoda (b) mollusca (c) annelida (d) platyhelminthes

90. Annelids may be
(a) aquatic (marine and fresh water), terrestrial
(b) free living
(c) parasite
(d) all

91. Neural system consists of paired ganglia connected by lateral nerve to a double ventral nerve cord present in
(a) fasciola (b) ancylostoma (c) nereis (d) taenia

92. Which of the following are monoecious?
Ascaris, Wuchereria, Ancylostoma, Neries, Pheretima, Hirudinaria
(a) 3 (b) 2 (c) 3 (d) 4

93. First true coelomates are
(a) nereis (b) centipede (c) crab (d) wuchereria

94. Following features belong to which of the following phylum?
(1) Triploblastic.
(2) Bilateral symmetry.
(3) Eucoelomate.
(4) Metamerism.
(a) Mollusca (b) Aschelminthe (c) Platyhelminthes (d) Annelida

95. Which of the following is correct about parapodia?
(a) they are longitudinal muscles which help in locomotion
(b) they are circular muscles which help in locomotion
(c) help in swimming
(d) it is dorsal appendages of nereis

96. Which of the following is largest phylum?
(a) Mollusca (b) Echinodermata (c) Arthropoda (d) Annelida

97. How many species named on earth is arthropoda?
(a) $\frac{1}{2}$ (b) $\frac{2}{3}$ (c) $\frac{1}{4}$ (d) $\frac{3}{4}$

98. In which of the following phylum body in generally divided in head, thorax and abdomen?
(a) Mollusca (b) Echinodermata (c) Arthropoda (d) Annelida

99. Which of the following phylum shows segmentation?
(a) Annelida (b) Arthropoda (c) Both (d) Platyhalmithes

100. Following features are of
(1) Exoskeleton of chitin.
(2) Malpighian tubules as excretory organ.
(3) Tracheal system for respiration.
(4) 3 pair of legs in thoracic region.
(a) limulus (b) prawn (c) spider (d) cockroach

101. Respiration occur through organs like gills, book gills, book lungs or tracheal system found in phylum
(a) mollusca (b) annelida (c) arthropoda (d) echinodermata

102. Which of the following are sensory organs in phylum Arthropoda?
(1) Simple or compound eye.
(2) Statocyst or balance organ.
(3) Malpighian tubules.
(4) Antennae.
(a) All except (4) (b) All except (1) (c) All except (3) (d) All except (2)

103. Which of the following is correct about reproduction in Arthropods?
(a) usually dioecious, mostly oviparous (b) internal fertilization
(c) some exhibit parthenogenesis (d) all

104. Ecdysis seen in case of
(a) nereis (b) pila
(c) sea urchin (d) cockroach

105. Exoskeleton of Arthropods are chitinous and it sheds at interval for growth and development process known as
(a) autotomy (b) metamerism
(c) ecdysis (moulting) (d) aestivation

106. Presence of joint appendages is speciality of phylum ______
(a) mollusca (b) echinodermata (c) arthropoda (d) annelidia

107. Bilaterally symmetrical, triploblastic, segmented, coelomate and covered by chitinous exoskeleton are features of
(a) anneldia (b) vertebrata (c) amphibia (d) arthropoda

108. Which of the following is true for Arthropoda?
(a) Development may be direct or indirect
(b) Open circulatory system
(c) Excretion takes place by green gland, coxal gland and Malpighian tubules
(d) All

109. Select from the following the total number of useful insects.
Apis, Bombyx, Laccifer, Anopheles, Culex, Aedes, Prawn, Scorpion, Locust, Limulus.
(a) 3 (b) 4 (c) 3 (d) 5

110. Select from the following the total number of organism that belongs to phylum arthropoda.
Locust, Butterfly, Scorpion, Prawn, Salpa, doliolums, Pila, Chiton, Antedon, Hyla, Myxine, Locust, Loligo, Culex, Cucumaria, Cuttle fish.
(a) 4 (b) 6 (c) 8 (d) 12

111. Select the living fossil from the following:
(a) culex (b) silkworm (c) lac insect (d) limulus

112. Following mosquitoes used as vector for various diseases:
(a) culex (b) anopheles (c) aedes (d) all

113. Other name of limulus is
(a) laccifer (b) locust (c) king crab (d) gregarious pest

114. Which of the following is a gregarious pest?
(a) Laccifer (b) Locusta (c) King crab (d) Both (a) and (b)

115. Match the following:

Column I		Column II
A. Locusta	–	1. Apis
B. Honey bee	–	2. Locust
C. Silkworm	–	3. Bombyx
D. Lac insect	–	4. Laccifer

(a) A–4, B–1, C–3, D–4 (b) A–2, B– 1, C–4, D–3
(c) A–2, B–1, C–3, D–4 (d) A–4, B–3, C–1, D–4

116. Which of the following belongs to arthropods?
(a) Peripatus and crab (b) Prawn and scorpion
(c) Centipede and cockroach (d) All

117. Animals with soft body, bilateral symmetry, triploblastic and unsegmented, usually protected by a shell made up of calcium carbonate belongs to phylum _____
(a) porifera (b) echinodermata (c) mollusca (d) arthropoda

118. The mouth contain file-like rasping organ for feeding called radula found in
(a) mollusca (b) hemichordata (c) echinodermata (d) arthropoda

119. The body of ___ is unsegmented with a distinct head, muscular foot and visceral mass
(a) asterias (b) ophiura (c) balanoglossus (d) devil fish

120. A. A soft and spongy layer of skin forms a _(i)_ over the visceral hump.
B. A _(ii)_ cavity contain _(iii)_ like gills.
C. A antenor head region has sensory _(iv)_.
Fill in the blanks in the above respective about mollusca.
(a) Mantle, Mantle, Comb, Papilla (b) Mantle, Mesoglea, Feather, Papilla
(c) Mantle, Mantle, Feather, Tentacles (d) Mantle, Mantle, Comb, Tentacles

121. Which of the following is true about reproduction in mollusca?
(1) Mostly dioecious. (2) Oviparous.
(3) Mainly indirect development. (4) Fertilization is external or internal.
(a) All except (4) (b) All except (3) (c) All except (2) (d) All

122. Which of the following is not a fish?
(a) Devil fish (b) Cuttle fish (c) Jelly fish (d) All

123. Match the following:

Column I		Column II
A. Pila	–	1. Tusk shell
B. Chiton	–	2. Apple snail

C. Dentalium – 3. Cuttle fish
D. Sepia – 4. Chaetopleura
(a) A–2, B–1, C–4, D–3
(b) A–2, B–4, C–1, D–3
(c) A–4, B–2, C–3, D–1
(d) A–4, B–3, C–2, D–1

124. Devil fish is called
(a) pearl oyster (b) tusk shell (c) sepia (d) octopus

125. Majority of mollusca are
(a) aquatic (b) terrestrial (c) aerial (d) any of the above

126. Select the total number of organism from the following which are mollusca:
Pila, Pinctada, Sepia, Loligo, Aplysia, Echinus, Antedon, Salpa, Bufo, Chelone, Neophron, Pteropus, Elephas, Pavo
(a) 7 (b) 6 (c) 5 (d) 9

127. Mantle cavity is a site of
(a) excretion (b) respiration (c) both (d) none

128. Shell in mollusc is
(a) external (b) internal (c) any of the above (d) shell absent

129. Unsegmented, triploblastic, eucoelomate is
(a) pheretima (b) laccifer (c) pila (d) all

130. Select incorrect matching:
(a) Aurelia – Jelly fish
(b) Sepia – Cuttle fish
(c) Octopus – Devil fish
(d) Loligo – Fighting fish

131. Select incorrect matching:
(a) Gorgonia – Sea fan
(b) Adamsia – Sea anemone
(c) Aplysia – Sea cucumber
(d) Antedon – Sea lily

132. Pinctada is a
(a) sea hare (b) cuttle fish (c) pearl oyster (d) apple snail

133. Common name of which organism contain 'sea' in their name?
(a) Chaetopleura (b) Dentalium (c) Sepia (d) Aplysia

134. Animals having calcareous endoskeleton with organ-system level of organization, completely marine are
(a) arthropoda (b) mollusca (c) hemichordates (d) echinodermates

135. In which phylum, larva is bilaterally symmetrical and adult have radial symmetry?
(a) Arthropoda (b) Mollusca (c) Hemichordata (d) Echinodermata

136. Most distinctive feature of echinoderm is
(a) gastro vascular cavity
(b) choanoctyes
(c) water vascular system/ambulacral system
(d) canal system

137. Water vascular system helps in
(a) locomotion (b) capture and transport of food
(c) respiration (d) all

138. Which of the following is true about reproduction in echinoderms?
(a) unisexuality
(b) usually external fertilization
(c) indirect development through free swimming larva
(d) all

139. Following are spiny-bodied animals:
Pila, Pinctada, Asterias, Echinus, Antedon, Cucumaria, Brittle star, Octopus
(a) 4 (b) 5 (c) 6 (d) 3

140. Select correct matching:
(a) Asterias – Sea urchin
(b) Pila – Pearl oyster
(c) Ophiura – Brittle star
(d) Loligo – Cuttle fish

141. Select incorrect matching:
(a) Asterias – Star fish
(b) Echinus – Sea urchin
(c) Antedon – Sea lily
(d) Cucumaria – Sea fan

142. Sea urchin belongs to phylum:
(a) echinodermata (b) hemichordata (c) ctenophora (d) mollusca

143. Another name of cucummaria is
(a) sea urchin (b) sea mouse (c) sea pen (d) sea cucumber

144. Which phylum shows regeneration of lost part?
(a) mollusca (b) annelida (c) arthropoda (d) echinodermata

145. Which phylum has the following features?
(1) Digestive track complete, straight or U shape
(2) Worm like, unsegmented marine animal
(3) Respiration by gills.
(4) Excretion by single proboscis gland
(5) Circulatory system open
(a) Arthropoda (b) Mollusca (c) Hemichordata (d) Urochordata

146. Which is a phylum?
(a) Hemichordata (b) Urochordata (c) Cephalochordata (d) All

147. Larva of hemichordate is
(a) Amphiblastula (b) Torneria (c) Ammocoet (d) Planula

148. Which of the following is correct about reproduction in hemichordata?
(a) Internal fertilization (b) Usually direct development
(c) Sexes are separate (d) Monoecious organism

149. The body is cylindrical and composed of anterior proboscis and a collar and a long trunk found in
(a) Ascidia (b) Salpa (c) Doliolum (d) Saccoglossus

150. Excretory organ proboscis gland is present in
(a) Ascidia (b) Salpa (c) Doliolum (d) Saccoglossus

151. Fundamental character of chordate is
(a) notochord (b) dorsal hollow nerve cord
(c) paired pharyngeal gill slits (d) all

152. Which is not a distiactive character of non-chordata?
(a) Notochoral absent (b) Ventral and double nerve cord
(c) Heart is ventral (d) Post-anal tail is absent

153. Following are the features of chordates:
(1) Notrchord present.
(2) CNS is dorsal, hollow and single.
(3) Pharynx perforated by gill slits.
(4) Heart ventral.
(5) A post-anal is present
(a) All except (4) (b) All except (2) (c) All (d) All except (5)

154. Animal belonging to phylum chordata shows
(a) bilateral symmetry, triploblastic and the coelom
(b) organ system level of organization
(c) closed circulatory system
(d) all

155. Urochordata and cephalochordate are referred as
(a) non chordates (b) vertebrates (c) protochordates (d) all

156. In which subphyla, notochord is present in tail of larva only?
(a) Hemichordata (b) Urochordata (c) Cephalochordata (d) All

157. Notochord is extended from head to tail region and persistent throughout their life in
(a) Hemichordata (b) Urochordata (c) Cephalochordata (d) All

158. How many of the following belongs to subphylum cephalochordate?
Ascidia, Salpa, Doliolum, Branchiostoma
(a) 1 (b) 2 (c) 3 (d) 4

159. Other name of Branchiostoma is
(a) amphioxus (b) lancelet (c) both (d) none

160. Select incorrect statement from the following:
(a) In vertebrates notochord is replaced by cartilaginous or bony vertebral column
(b) In cephalochordates, notochord extended from head to tail region and persistent throughout life
(c) Protochordates are exclusively marine
(d) Notochord is present in tail of adult in urochordata

161. Vertebrates have
(a) ventral muscular heart with 3, 2 or 4 chamber
(b) kidneys for excretion and osmoregulation
(c) paired appendages which may be fins or limbs
(d) all

162. Which of the following is exoskeleton in vertebrates?
(a) Scales (b) Feathers (c) Hair (d) Any of the above

163. All living members of which class is ectoparasite on fishes?
(a) Turbellaria (b) Chondrichthyes (c) Cephalopoda (d) Cyclostomata

164. Following are characters of cyclostomata:
(a) 6–15 pairs of gill slits for respiration (b) Sucking and circular mouth without jaws
(c) Body is devoid of scales and paired fins (d) All

165. Which of the following organism possess cartilaginous cranium, vertebral column, closed type of circulatory system, which helps them migrate to fresh water for spawning?
(a) Ascidia (b) Scoliodon (c) Petromyzon (d) All

166. Following are marine but migrate for spawning to fresh water. After spawning, within a few days, they die. Their larvae, after metamorphosis, return to ocean. Specify the correct one.
(a) Petromyzon (Lamprey) (b) Myxine (Hagfish)
(c) Scoliodon (d) Both (a) and (b)

167. Which of the following is correct about cyclostomes?
(a) Ectoparasite on fishes during their adult stage
(b) Skin with scales and contain unicellular mucous gland
(c) One kidney for excretion
(d) Heart is two chambered and possess 4 pair of gill slits for respiration

168. Class name 'cyclostomata' means
(a) Marine, but reproduction takes place in fresh water
(b) Mouth anterio ventral, suctorial and circular
(c) Ectoparasite of fishes
(d) Jaws are absent

169. Study of fishes is called
(a) Ichthyology (b) Serpentology (c) Saurology (d) Chonchology

170. (1) Marine with streamlined body
(2) Cartilaginous endoskeleton
(3) Mouth ventral
(4) Caudal fin in Heterocercal
(5) Notochord is persistent throughout life.
Above characters belong to which of the following organism (select total number)?
Dog fish, Saw fish, Flying fish, Fighting fish, Angle fish, Jelly fish, Star fish, Trygon, Torpedo, Rohu, Catla, Magur
(a) 3 (b) 4 (c) 6 (d) 7

171. Scales found in chondrichthyes is/are
(a) placoid (b) cycloid (c) ctenoid (d) all

172. Which of the following is incorrect about Cartilaginous fish?
(a) Teeth are modified placoid scales which are backwardly directed
(b) 5 to 7 pair of gills for respiration but without operculum (i.e. gill cover)
(c) Air bladder absent so they have to swim constantly to avoid sinking
(d) In males pelvie fins claspers are absent

173. Select the total number of organism which posses two chambered heart and are poikilothermal.
Scoliodon, Pristis, Clarias, Betta, Pterophyllum, Echinus, Devil Fish, Cuttle fish, Sea lily, Hyla, Labeo, catla, Torpedo, Trygon
(a) 7 (b) 9 (c) 11 (d) 13

174. Select the difference which is wrongly written:

Cartilaginous fish		Bony fishes
(a) Operculum absent	–	Operculum present
(b) Fertilization internal	–	Fertilization external
(c) Posses 5–7 pair of gills	–	Posses 4 pair of gills
(d) Mostly oviparous	–	Mostly viviparous

175. Which fish possess poison sting?
(a) Scoliodon (dog fish) (b) Trygon
(c) Torpedo (d) Pristis (saw fish)

176. Which fish possess electric organs?
(a) Scoliodon (dog fish) (b) Trygon
(c) Torpedo (d) Pristis (saw fish)

177. Males possess claspers in pelvic fins in class _____
(a) cyclostomata (b) chondrichthyes (c) osteicthyes (d) amphibia

178. Select correct matching:
(a) Petromyzon – Hagfish
(b) Myxine – Lamprey
(c) Carcharodon – Great white shark
(d) Trygon – Torpedo

179. (1) Stream-lined body.
(2) Both marine and fresh water.
(3) Mouth terminal.
(4) Caudal fin Homocercal.
(5) 4 pair of gills with operculum.
Which class has the above characters?
(a) Cyclostomata (b) chondrichthyes (c) Osteichthyes (d) Amphibia

180. Osteicthyes possess which kind of scales?
(a) placoid (b) cycloid (c) ctenoid (d) both (b) and (c)

181. External fertilization is found in
(a) sting ray (b) flying fish (c) saw fish (d) dog fish

182. Select total number of bony fishes from the following:
Exocoetus, Hippocampus, Labeo, Catla, Clarias, Betta, Pterophyllum, Trygon, Torpedo, Pristis, Scolidon, Carcharodon.
(a) 6 (b) 7 (c) 8 (d) 12

183. Air bladder which regulate buoyancy is present in
(a) cyclostomata (b) cartilaginous fish (c) bony fishes (d) amphibians

184. Select correct matching:
(a) Betta – Fighting fish
(b) Hippocampus – Flying fish
(c) Pterophyllum – Fighting fish
(d) Clarias – Labeo

185. Select incorrect matching:
(a) Scoliodon – Dog fish
(b) pterophyllum – Angel fish
(c) Clarias – Magur
(d) Trygon – Torpedo

186. Select correct matching:
(a) Cyclostomata – gills (6–15 pairs)
(b) chondrichthyes – gills (5–7 pairs)
(c) Osteichthyes – gills (4 pairs)
(d) All are correct

187. Following are marine bony fishes:
(a) Exocoetus (flying fish) (b) Hippocampus (sea-horse)
(c) Both (a) and (b) (d) Saw fish (pristis)

188. Following are fresh water bony fishes:
(a) Labeo (rohu) (b) Catla (katla) (c) Clarias (magur) (d) All

189. Following are fresh water cartilaginous fishes
(a) Scoliodon (dog fish) (b) Trygon (sting ray)
(c) Torpedo (electric ray) (d) None

190. The name 'amphibian' indicate that they can live in
(a) aquatic habitat (b) terrestrial habitat
(c) both (a) and (b) (d) aerial habitat

191. Amphibian belong to super class
(a) pisces (b) agnatha (c) gnathostomata (d) tetrapoda

192. Following features belong to which class?
(1) Body in divisible into head and trunks, tail may be present in some.
(2) Skin is moist and act as respiratory organ.
(3) External skeleton is absent.
(4) Eye have eyelids.
(a) Cyclostomata (b) Amphibia (c) Reptilia (d) Osteichthyes

193. Respiration in adult frog is by
(a) Buccopharyngeal cavity (b) Skin
(c) Lungs (d) All

194. Respiration in tadpole larva is by
(a) gills (b) lungs (c) skin (d) all

195. Following tract open into a common chamber cloaca in amphibians
(a) Alimentary canal (b) Urinary tract
(c) Reproductive tract (d) All

196. Which type of dentition is found in amphibian?
(a) Homodont (b) Thecodont (c) Heterodont (d) Monophyodont

197. Three chambered heart, cold blooded, external fertilization and indirect development is seen in
(a) labeo (b) salpa (c) frog (d) myxine

198. Skin is moist and a tympanum represent ear is found in
(a) hyla (b) frog (c) Ichthyophis (d) all

199. Select correct matching:

Column I		**Column II**
A. Bufo	–	1. Salamander
B. Frog	–	2. Rana
C. Hyla	–	3. Limbless amphibian
D. Salamandra	–	4. Tree frog
E. Ichthyophis	–	5. Toad

(a) A–2, B–5, C–4, D–1, E–3
(b) A–5, B–2, C–4, D–1, E–3
(c) A–2, B–4, C–5, D–1, E–3
(d) A–5, B–4, C–2, D–1, E–3

200. Limbless amphibian is
(a) frog (b) tree frog (c) ichthyophis (d) bufo

201. First class of vertebrate, which are fully adopted for terrestrial life is
(a) amphibia (b) reptilia (c) aves (d) mammals

202. Reptilia means
(a) flying mode of locomotion (b) swim mode of locomotion
(c) saltation mode of locomotion (d) creeping or crawling mode of locomotion

203. Which of the following is incorrect about reptilia?
(a) Body is covered by dry and cornified skin, epidermal scales or scutes
(b) Body divisible into head, neck, trunk and tail
(c) Heart is usually three chambered
(d) Respiration occur through lungs and skin

204. Four chambered heart is present in all except
(a) crocodilus (b) alligator (c) corvus (d) calotes

205. Which of the following shed their scales as skin cast?
(a) Snakes (b) Lizards (c) Both (a) and (b) (d) Testudo

206. Sexes separate, internal fertilization, oviparous and direct development seen in case of
(a) Chelone (b) Testudo (c) Bangarus (d) All

207. Cloaca is seen in case of
(a) Amphibia (b) Reptiles (c) Aves (d) All

208. Select incorrect matching:
(a) Chelone – Turtle
(b) Testudo – Tortoise
(c) Chameleon – Tree lizard
(d) Calotes – Wall lizard

209. Select incorrect matching:
(a) Naja – Cobra
(b) Krait – Bangarus
(c) Vipera – Viper
(d) Hemidactylus – Garden lizard

210. Select the total number of lizards from the following:
Chelone, calotes, chameleon, crocodylus, hemidactylus, columba, neophron
(a) 2 (b) 3 (c) 4 (d) 5

211. Following are poisonous snakes
(a) cobra (b) krait (c) viper (d) all

212. Limbless reptile is
(a) chameleon (b) crocodile (c) chelone (d) snake

213. In birds
Forelimb are modified into _(1)_
Jaw modified into _(2)_
Bones are _(3)_
Heart is _(4)_
Fill in the blanks correctly:
(a) Wings, beak, solid, 3 chambered
(b) Wings, beak, pneumatic, 4 chambered
(c) Claws, beak, pneumatic, 3 chambered
(d) Wings, beak, solid, incompletely 4 chambered

214. First vertebrate which are warm-blooded
(a) reptilia (b) amphibian (c) birds (d) mammals

215. The aves have additional chamber in digestive tract and of which ____ is for food storage and ____ for food grinding.
(a) crop, gizzard (b) gizzard, crop
(c) crop, pharynx (d) pharynx, gizzard

216. All are flying birds from the following except
(a) corvus (b) columba (c) psittacula (d) aptenodytes

217. Pneumatic bones are present in
(a) corvus (b) neophron (vulture)
(c) pavo (peacock) (d) all

218. Which of the following is incorrect about birds?
(a) Air sacs connected to lungs help in respiration
(b) Hind limb posses scales and are modified for walking, swimming or clasping
(c) Separate sexes, internal fertilization, oviparous and direct development
(d) Endoskeleton is consist of feathers, scales, beak and claws

219. Mammalia means organism which possess
(a) exoskeleton (b) endoskeleton of bone
(c) mammary gland (d) two pair of limbs

220. Following features belong to
(1) Exoskeleton include hairs on body, horns and nail.
(2) Pinna present.
(3) Heart is four chambered.
(4) Warm-blooded (homoiotherm).
(5) Thecodont and Heterodont teeth.
(a) Reptilia (b) Aves
(c) Mammals (d) Amphibians

221. Mammals are adapted for
(a) walking and running (c) climbing and burrowing
(c) swimming and flying (d) any of the above

222. Mammals are mostly
(a) viviparous (b) oviparous (c) ovoviviparous (d) all

223. Oviparous mammal is
(a) canis (dog) (b) felis (cat)
(c) pteropus (flying fox (d) ornithorhynchus (platypus)

224. Select incorrect matching:
(a) Kangaroo – Macropus
(b) Blue whale – Balaenoptera
(c) Monkey – Macaca
(d) Elephas – Camel

225. Find out the incorrect matching:
(a) Reptiles – Chelone, Testudo, Chameleon
(b) Aves – Psittacula, Aptenodytes, Neophron
(c) Mammals – Elephas, Rattus, Delphinus
(d) Amphibian – Naja, bangarus, Calotes

226. Aquatic mammal is
(a) panthera tigris (b) balaenoptera (c) pteropus (d) macropus

227. Which of the following is a 'rat'?
(a) felis (b) canis (c) camelus (d) rattus

228. Which of the following mammal have aerial adaptation?
(a) felis (b) canis (c) bat (d) macropus

229. Basic fundamental features enabled us to broadlus classify the animal kingdom are
(a) Level of organisation, symmetry
(b) Cell organisation, coelom
(c) Segmentation of notochord
(d) All

230. Select total number of correct statement from the following:
(1) Coelenterates have tentacles and bear cnidoblasts
(2) Ctenophores are marine animals with comb plates
(3) Annelids are metamerically segmented animals with a true coelom
(4) The Echinoderm posses water vascular system
(5) Hemichordates are a small group of worm like marine animals characterized by cylindrical body with proboscis, collar and trunk
(a) 2 (b) 3 (c) 4 (d) 5

231. Most primitive chordates and are ectopariste on fishes belongs to class
(a) Chondrichthyes (b) Amphibia (c) Cyclostomata (d) Osteichthyes

232. Select incorrect matching: [A: Phylum, B: Segmentation, C: Circulatory system, D: Distinctive features] [A: Absent, P: Present]

	A	B	C	D
(a)	Ctenophore	A	A	Comb plates for locomotion
(b)	Aschelminthes	A	P	Often worm shaped, elongated
(c)	Annelid	P	P	Body segmentation like rings
(d)	Arthropoda	P	P	Jointed appendages

233. Below figure shows which type of symmetry

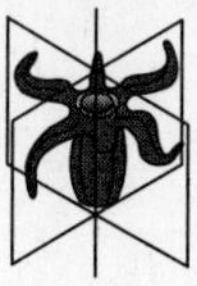

(a) Bilateral (b) Radial (c) Biradial (d) Asymmetry

234. Below diagram shows ____ symmetry, which is also found in following group of organism

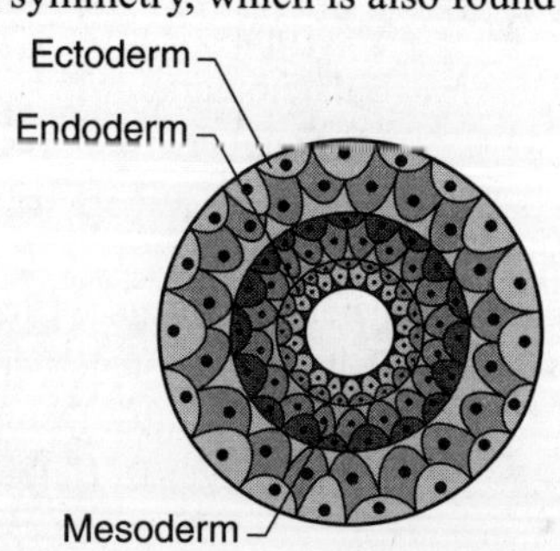

(a) Adamsia, Asterias, Aplysia (b) Salpa, Hyla, Calotes
(c) Taenia, Ctenoplana, Antedon (d) Doliolum, Gorgonia, Sycon

235. Excretory organ present in organism given in figure is

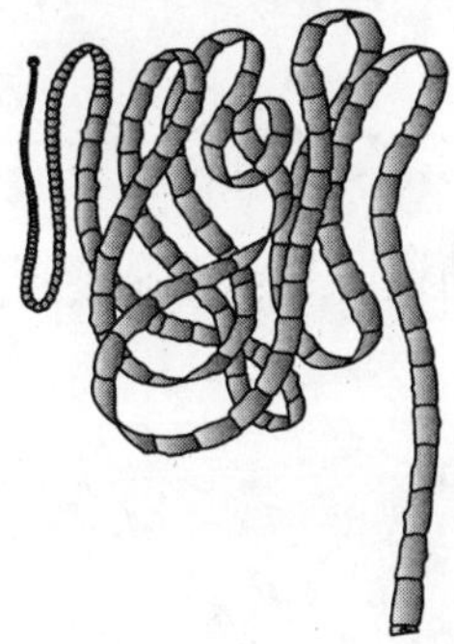

(a) Rennet cells (b) Protonephridia or flame cells
(c) Malpighian tubules (d) Kidney

236. All features given belongs to organism given in diagram except

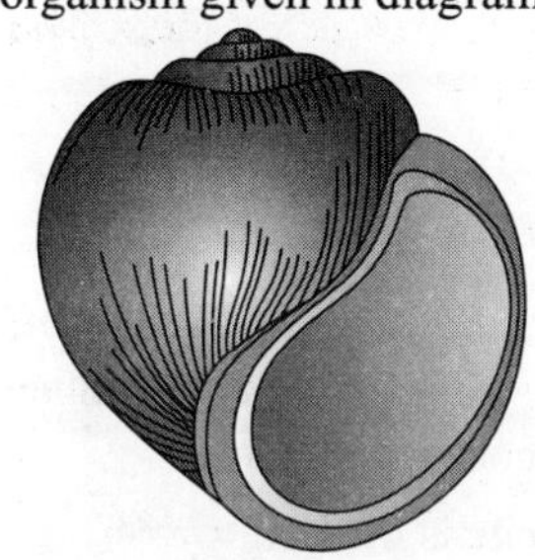

(a) It belongs to second largest animal phylum
(b) Body is segmented and covered by calcareous shell
(c) Triploblastic, Coelomate
(d) Mantle cavity is present

237. Find out total number of organism given in figure belongs to marine habitat:

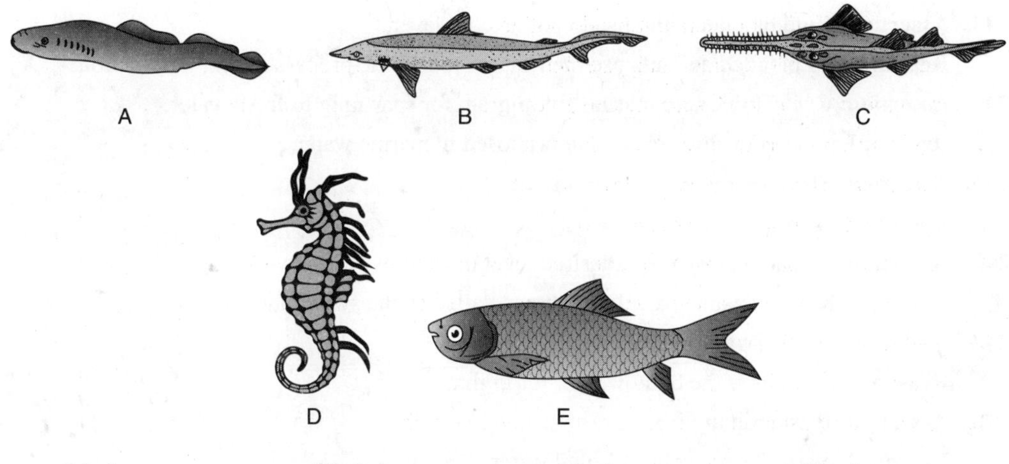

(a) 1 (b) 3 (c) 4 (d) 5

238. Organism given in figure is respire by

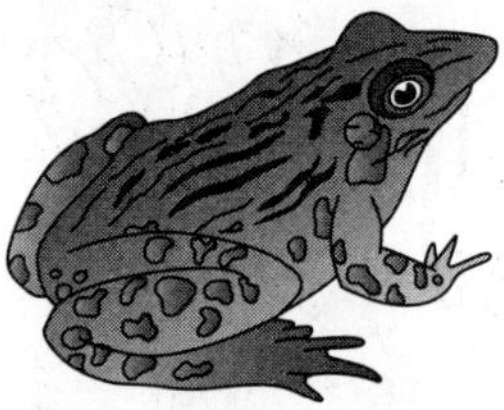

(a) Lungs (b) Skin (c) Buccopharyngeal cavity (d) All

Read the ***assertion*** *and* ***reason*** *carefully to mark the correct option out of the options given below:*

(a) If both the assertion and the reason are true and the reason is a correct explanation of the assertion

(b) If both the assertion and reason are true but the reason is not a correct explanation of the assertion

(c) If the assertion is true but the reason is false

(d) If both the assertion and reason are false

239. Assertion: A closed circulatory system is found in annelids.
Reason: Annelids posses true coelom.

240. Assertion: Fertilisation in sponge is internal.
Reason: Sponges are aquatic organisms.

241. Assertion: The skeleton of sponges is made up of spicules.
Reason: Composition of spicules help in classification of sponges.

242. Assertion: Acraniata is a group of organisms which do not have distinct cranium.
Reason: It includes small marine forms without head.

243. Assertion: Cold blooded animals do not have fat layer.
Reason: Cold blooded animals use their fat for metabolic process during hibernation.

244. Assertion: Cyclostomes are marine but migrate for spawning to fresh water.
Reason: Larvae of cyclostome metamorphosed in marine water.

245. Assertion: Sponges belong to Porifera.
Reason: Sponges have canal system.

246. Assertion: A shark can stay at a desired level in water without swimming.
Reason: It has a buoyancy-regulating organ called as the swim bladder.

247. Assertion: Birds have one ovary.
Reason: This reduces the body weight for flight.

248. Assertion: Plasmodium vivax is responsible for malaria.
Reason: Malaria is caused by polluted water.

249. **Assertion:** Birds are warm blooded.

Reason: Birds are able to maintain a constant body temperature.

250. **Assertion:** Systematics is the branch of biology that deals with classification of living organisms.

Reason: The aim of classification is to group the organisms.

251. **Assertion:** All birds, except the ones like koel (cuckoo) build nests for retiring and taking rest during night time (day time for nocturnal).

Reason: Koel lays its eggs in the nests of tailor bird.

252. **Assertion:** Bats and whales are classified as mammals.

Reason: Bats and whales have four-chambered heart.

253. **Assertion:** Tapeworm, roundworm and pinworm are endoparasites of human intestine.

Reason: Improperly cooked food is the source of all intestinal infections.

254. **Assertion:** The duck-billed Platypus and the spiny ant-eater, both are egg-laying animals yet they are grouped under mammals.

Reason: Both of them have seven cervical vertebrae and 12 pairs of cranial nerves.

AIPMT PREVIOUS YEAR QUESTIONS

1. Crocodile and penguin are similar to whale and dogfish in which one of the following features [AIPMT MAINS 2010]

   (a) Possess a solid single stranded central nervous system
   (b) Lay eggs and guard them till they hatch
   (c) Possess bony skeleton
   (d) Have gill slits at some stage

2. One example of animals having a single opening to the outside that serves both as mouth as well as anus is: [AIPMT PRE 2010]

   (a) Octopus (b) Asterias
   (c) Ascidia (d) Fasciola

3. Which one of the following statements about all the four of Spongilla, leech, dolphin and penguin is correct? [AIPMT PRE 2010]

   (a) Penguin is homoiothermic while the remaining three are poikilothermic
   (b) Leech is a fresh water form 'while all others are marine
   (c) Spongilla has special collared cells called choanocytes, not found in the remaining three
   (d) All are bilaterally symmetrical

4. Which one of the following kinds of animals are triploblastic? [AIPMT PRE 2010]

   (a) Flat worms (b) Sponges
   (c) Ctenophores (d) Corals

5. Which one of the following statements about certain given animals is correct? [AIPMT PRE 2010]

   (a) Round worms (Aschelminthes) are pseudocoelomates
   (b) Molluscs are acoelomates

(c) Insects are pseudocoelomates
(d) Flat worms (Platyhelminthes) are coelomates

6. Which one of the following statements is totally wrong about the occurrence of notochord, while the other three are correct?

[AIPMT MAINS 2011]

(a) It is present only in larval tail in ascidian
(b) It is replaced by a vertebral column in adult frog
(c) It is absent throughout life in humans from the very beginning
(d) it is present throughout life in Amphioxus

7. Frogs differ from humans in possessing

[AIPMT MAINS 2011]

(a) Paired cerebral hemispheres
(b) Hepatic portal system
(c) Nucleated red blood cells
(d) Thyroid as well as parathyroid

8. The figures (A-D) show four animals. Select the correct option with respect to a common characteristic of two of these animals.

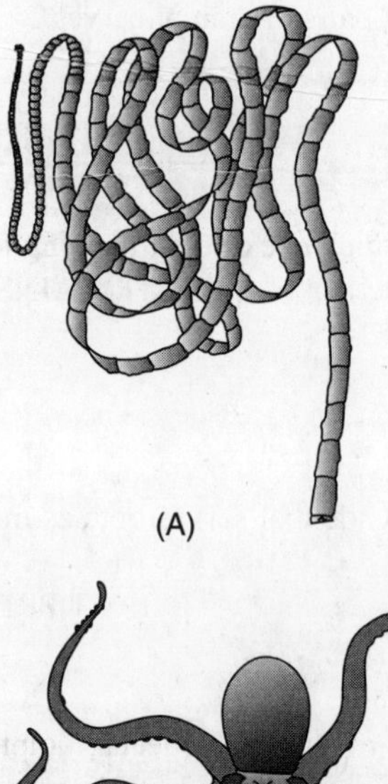

(A)

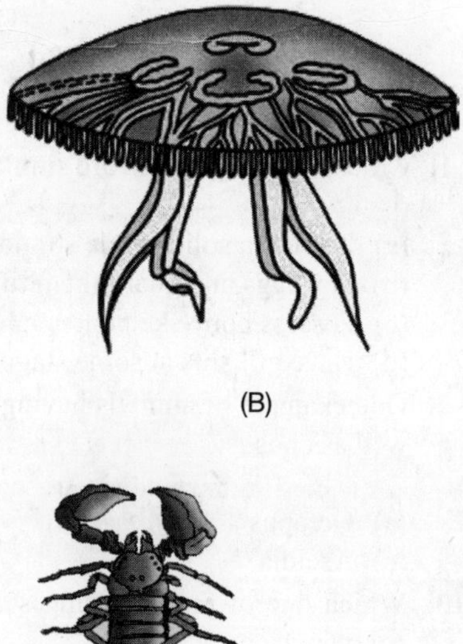

(B)

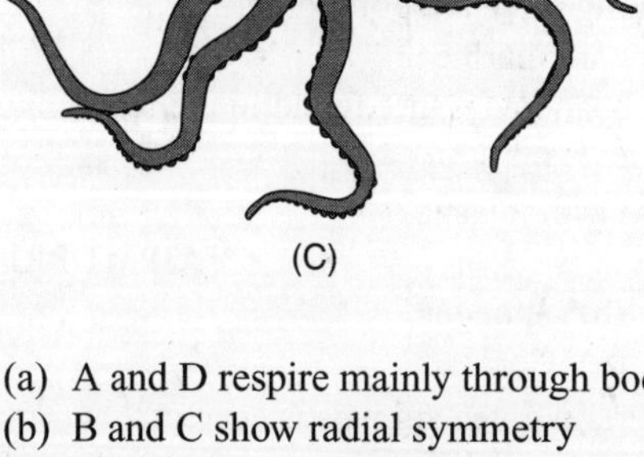

(C)

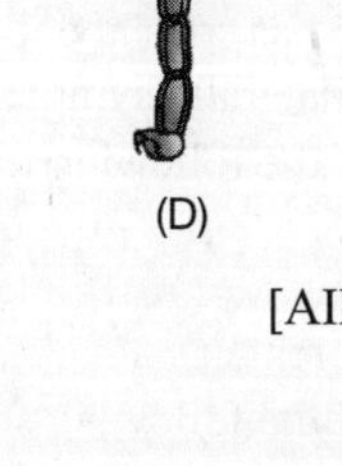

(D)

[AIPMT MAINS 2011]

(a) A and D respire mainly through body wall
(b) B and C show radial symmetry
(c) A and B have cnidoblasts for self-defence
(d) C and D have a true coelom.

9. Which one of the following have the highest number of species in nature? [AIPMT PRE 2011]

(a) Insects (b) Birds
(c) Angiosperms (d) Fungi

10. What will you look for to identify the sex of the following? [AIPMT PRE 2011]

(a) Male frog – A copulatory pad on the first digit of the hind limb
(b) Female cockroach – Anal cerci
(c) Male shark – Claspers borne on pelvic fin
(d) Female ascaris – Sharply curved posterior end

11. In which one of the following the genus name, its two characters and its class/phylum are correctly matched? [AIPMT PRE 2011]

	Genus	Two characters	Class/phylum
(a)	Salamander	(1) A tympanum represents ear (2) Fertilization is external	Amphibian
(b)	Pteropus	(1) Skin possesses hair (2) Oviparous	Mammalian
(c)	Aurelia	(1) Cnidoblast (2) Organ level of organization	Coelenterate
(d)	Ascaris	(1) Body segmented (2) Males and females distinct	Annelid

12. Which one of the following animals is correctly method with its particular named taxonomic category? [AIPMT PRE 2011]

(a) Cuttlefish – Mollusca, a class
(b) Humans – Primata, the family
(c) Housefly – Musca, an order
(d) Tiger – tigris, the species

13. Which one of the following groups of animals is correctly matched with its one characteristic feature without even a single exception? [AIPMT PRE 2011]

(a) Chordate – Possess a mouth provided with an upper and a lower jaw
(b) Chondrichthyes – Possess cartilaginous endoskeleton
(c) Mammalian – Give birth to young ones
(d) Reptilian – Possess 3 chambered heart with one incompletely divided ventricle

14. Which one of the following categories of animals, is correctly described with no single exception in it? [AIPMT MAINS 2012]

(a) All bony fishes have four pairs of gills and an operculum on each side
(b) All sponges are marine and have collared cells
(c) All mammals are viviparous and possess diaphragm for breathing
(d) All reptiles possess scales, have a three chambered heart and are cold blooded (poikilothermal)

15. Which one of the following pairs of animals are similar to each other pertaining to the feature stated against them?

[AIPMT MAINS 2012]

(a) Garden lizard and crocodile – Three chambered heart
(b) Ascaris and ancylostoma – Metameric segmentation
(c) Sea horse and flying fish – Cold blooded (poikilothermal)
(d) Pteropus and ornithorhyncus – Viviparity

16. In which one of the following, the genus name, its two characters and its phylum are not correctly matched, whereas the remaining three are correct?

[AIPMT PRE 2012]

Genus name	Two characters	Phylum
(a) Pila	(1) Body segmented (2) Mouth with radula	Mollusc
(b) Asterias	(1) Spiny skinned (2) Water vascular system	Echinodermata
(c) Sycon	(1) Pore bearing (2) Canal system	Porifera
(d) Periplaneta	(1) Jointed appendages (2) Chitinous exoskeleton	Arthropoda

17. Match the name of the animal (column I), with on characteristics (column II), and the phylum/class (column III) to which it belongs:

[AIPMT 2013]

Column-I	Column-II	Column-III
(a) Petromyzon	Ectoparasite	Cyclostomata
(b) Icthyophis	Terrestrial	Reptilian
(c) Limulus	Body covered by chitinous exoskeleton	Pisces
(d) Adamsia	Radially symmetrical	Porifera

18. Which of the following are correctly matched with respect to their taxonomic classification?

[AIPMT 2013]

(a) Flying fish, cattle fish, silverfish, Pisces
(b) Centipede, millipede, spider, scorpion Insecta
(c) House fly, butterfly, tsetse fly, silverfish Insecta
(d) Spiny anteato, sea urchin, sea cucumber echinodermata

19. Which group of animals belong to the same phylum?

[AIPMT 2013]

(a) Malarial parasite, Amoeba, Mosquito
(b) Earthworm, Pinworm, Tapeworm
(c) Prawn, Scorpion, Locusta
(d) Sponge, Sea anemone, Starfish

20. One of the sepresentatives of Phylum Arthropoda is: [AIPMT 2013]

(a) Cuttlefish (b) Silverfish
(c) Pufferfish (d) Flying fish

21. Select the Taxon mentioned that represent both marine and fresh water species: [AIPMT 2014]

(a) Echinoderms (b) Ctenophora
(c) Cephalochordata (d) Cnidaria

22. Which one of the following living organisms completely lack a cell wall? [AIPMT 2014]

(a) Cyanobacteria (b) Sea – fan (Gorgonia)
(c) Saccharomyces (d) Blue – green algae

23. Planaria posses high capacity of: [AIPMT 2014]

(a) Metamorphosis (b) Regeneration
(c) Alternation of generation (d) Bioluminescence

24. A marine cartilaginous fish that can produce electric current is: [AIPMT 2014]

(a) Pristis (b) Torpedo
(c) Trygon (d) Scoliodon

25. Which of the following represents the correct combination without any exception? [AIPMT 2015]

	Characteristics	Class
(a)	Mammary gland; hair on body pinnate two pairs of limbs.	Mammalian
(b)	Mouth ventral; gills without operculum skin with placoid scales; persistent notochord	Chondrichthyes
(c)	Sucking and circular mouth laws absent integument without scales; paired appendages	Cyclostomata
(d)	Body covered with feathers; skin most and glandular; fore limbs than wings; lungs with air sacs.	Aves

26. Which of the following animals is not viviparous? [AIPMT 2015]

(a) Flying fox (Bat) (b) Elephant
(c) Platypus (d) Whale

27. Metagenesis refers to: [RE-AIPMT 2015]

(a) Alternation of generation between asexual and sexual phases of an organism
(b) Occurrence of a drastic change in form during post-embryonic development
(c) Present of a segmented body and parthenogenetic mode of reproduction
(d) Presence of different morphic forms

28. A jawless fish, which lays eggs in fresh water and whose ammocoets larvae after metamorphosis return to the ocean is: [RE-AIPMT 2015]

(a) Myxine (b) Neomyxine
(c) Petromyzon (d) Eptatrelus

29. Body having meshwork of cells, internal cavities lined with food filtering flagellated cells and indirect developments are the characteristics of phylum: [RE-AIPMT 2015]

(a) Porifera (b) Mollusca
(c) Protozoa (d) Coelenterata

Answer Keys

1. (d)	2. (d)	3. (c)	4. (d)	5. (d)	6. (c)	7. (d)	8. (d)	9. (d)	10. (a)
11. (d)	12. (d)	13. (a)	14. (b)	15. (d)	16. (b)	17. (c)	18. (a)	19. (b)	20. (d)
21. (d)	22. (d)	23. (b)	24. (b)	25. (b)	26. (c)	27. (d)	28. (c)	29. (a)	30. (a)
31. (d)	32. (b)	33. (c)	34. (a)	35. (a)	36. (b)	37. (b)	38. (b)	39. (c)	40. (d)
41. (d)	42. (a)	43. (d)	44. (a)	45. (d)	46. (b)	47. (b)	48. (d)	49. (c)	50. (d)
51. (c)	52. (c)	53. (d)	54. (d)	55. (b)	56. (a)	57. (c)	58. (c)	59. (c)	60. (b)
61. (b)	62. (a)	63. (c)	64. (b)	65. (c)	66. (c)	67. (c)	68. (d)	69. (c)	70. (a)
71. (d)	72. (d)	73. (a)	74. (d)	75. (b)	76. (b)	77. (a)	78. (d)	79. (d)	80. (d)
81. (c)	82. (d)	83. (b)	84. (c)	85. (b)	86. (b)	87. (d)	88. (d)	89. (c)	90. (d)
91. (c)	92. (b)	93. (a)	94. (d)	95. (c)	96. (c)	97. (b)	98. (c)	99. (c)	100. (d)
101. (c)	102. (c)	103. (d)	104. (d)	105. (c)	106. (c)	107. (d)	108. (d)	109. (a)	110. (b)
111. (d)	112. (d)	113. (c)	114. (b)	115. (c)	116. (d)	117. (c)	118. (a)	119. (d)	120. (c)
121. (d)	122. (d)	123. (b)	124. (d)	125. (a)	126. (c)	127. (c)	128. (c)	129. (c)	130. (d)
131. (c)	132. (c)	133. (d)	134. (d)	135. (d)	136. (c)	137. (d)	138. (d)	139. (b)	140. (c)
141. (d)	142. (a)	143. (d)	144. (d)	145. (c)	146. (a)	147. (b)	148. (c)	149. (d)	150. (d)
151. (d)	152. (c)	153. (c)	154. (d)	155. (c)	156. (b)	157. (c)	158. (a)	159. (c)	160. (d)
161. (d)	162. (d)	163. (d)	164. (d)	165. (c)	166. (d)	167. (a)	168. (b)	169. (a)	170. (b)
171. (a)	172. (d)	173. (b)	174. (d)	175. (b)	176. (c)	177. (b)	178. (c)	179. (c)	180. (d)
181. (b)	182. (b)	183. (c)	184. (a)	185. (d)	186. (d)	187. (c)	188. (d)	189. (d)	190. (c)
191. (d)	192. (b)	193. (d)	194. (a)	195. (d)	196. (a)	197. (c)	198. (d)	199. (b)	200. (c)
201. (b)	202. (d)	203. (d)	204. (d)	205. (c)	206. (d)	207. (d)	208. (d)	209. (d)	210. (b)
211. (d)	212. (d)	213. (b)	214. (c)	215. (a)	216. (d)	217. (d)	218. (d)	219. (c)	220. (c)
221. (d)	222. (a)	223. (d)	224. (d)	225. (d)	226. (b)	227. (d)	228. (c)	229. (d)	230. (d)
231. (c)	232. (b)	233. (b)	234. (b)	235. (b)	236. (b)	237. (c)	238. (d)	239. (b)	240. (b)
241. (b)	242. (b)	243. (b)	244. (c)	245. (b)	246. (d)	247. (a)	248. (c)	249. (a)	250. (b)
251. (b)	252. (b)	253. (b)	254. (a)						

AIPMT Previous Year Questions

1. (d)	2. (d)	3. (c)	4. (a)	5. (a)	6. (c)	7. (c)	8. (d)	9. (a)	10. (c)
11. (a)	12. (d)	13. (b)	14. (a)	15. (c)	16. (a)	17. (a)	18. (c)	19. (c)	20. (b)
21. (d)	22. (b)	23. (b)	24. (b)	25. (a)	26. (c)	27. (a)	28. (c)	29. (a)	

Unit II

Structural Organization in Plants and Animals

Unit II includes morphology and anatomy of living organism, mainly higher plants and animals. In this unit, the chapter on plant morphology is the most important chapter and demands special attention. It should be studied in more detail then the rest of the chapters in this book because of the variety of questions **(for example, how many of the following have marginal type of placentation and then with the given examples, you have to find out numbers of plants having that type of placentation)** that can be prepared. Hence pay careful attention to all the questions of this unit. You should also focus a lot on diagram of family, placentaion, and aestivation. For structural organization and anatomy of plant, this book is more than sufficient and by solving the questions present in this book, you should have excellent command on these chapters.

CHAPTER 5

Plant Morphology

1. Angiosperms are characterized by the presence of
   (a) roots and stem (b) leaf and flowers (c) fruit (d) all
2. In majority of dicot, the direct elongation of the radicle leads to the formation of
   (a) primary root (b) secondary root (c) tertiary root (d) none
3. The primary root and its branches constitute
   (a) fibrous root system (b) tap root system
   (c) both (d) none
4. In wheat (monocot)
   (a) primary root is short lived
   (b) primary root replaced by fibrous roots
   (c) fibrous roots arises from the base of stem
   (d) all are correct
5. Adventitious roots are found in
   (a) grass (b) monestra (c) banyan tree (d) all
6. Adventitious roots arise from part other than
   (a) hypocotyl (b) epicotyl (c) plumule (d) radicle
7. Functions of root are
   (a) absorption of water and mineral from soil
   (b) anchoring of plant in soil
   (c) storage of food material and synthesis of plant growth regulator
   (d) all
8. What is the number of regions in which a root is divided?
   (a) 1 (b) 2 (c) 3 (d) 4
9. Root is covered at the apex by a thimble-like structure called
   (a) root cap (b) radicle (c) coleorhiza (d) coleoptile
10. Root region are arranged proximal to distal part in following manner
    (a) zone of cell elongation–zone of cell maturation–zone of cell division
    (b) zone of cell division–zone of cell elongation–zone of cell maturation
    (c) zone of cell maturation–zone of cell elongation–zone of cell division
    (d) zone of cell maturation–zone of cell division–zone of cell elongation
11. Root hairs arise from
    (a) zone of cell division (b) zone of cell elongation
    (c) one of cell maturation (d) all

12. Find out the incorrect statement:
    (a) Root hair absorb water and mineral from the soil
    (b) Root increase in length due to region of elongation
    (c) Meristematic region have thin walled cell with dense cytoplasm
    (d) Root cannot synthesize plant growth regulators
13. Which of the following is an exception for the modification of the tap root?
    (a) carrot (b) turnip (c) sweet potato (d) all
14. Prop or pillar roots are found in
    (a) carrot (b) sweet potato (c) banyan tree (d) maize
15. Maize and sugarcane contain
    (a) storage root (b) stilt root (c) pneumatophores (d) prop roots
16. Find out incorrect statement:
    (a) Sweet potato has root modification for storage of food
    (b) Still root arises from lower nodes of the stem
    (c) Rizophora posses pneumatophores
    (d) Pneumatophores are meant for anaerobic respiration
17. Which of the following is incorrect of stem?
    (a) It is developed from plumule of embryo of a germinating seed
    (b) It bears nodes and internodes
    (c) It bears only terminal bud not axillary bud
    (d) Its main function is spreading of branches and bear leaves, flowers and fruits
18. Functions of stem are
    (a) conduct water, mineral and photosynthates
    (b) some perform storage food, support and protection
    (c) some perform function of vegetative propagation
    (d) all
19. Young stems are generally
    (a) woody (b) dark brown in color
    (c) green and photosynthetic (d) all
20. Underground stem store food in following except
    (a) zaminkand (b) colocasia (c) ginger (d) sugarcane
21. Which stem act as organ of perennation?
    (a) potato (b) ginger (c) colocasia (d) all
22. Which of the following is a gourd?
    (a) cucumber (b) pumpkins (c) watermelon (d) all
23. Which of the following is correct about gourds?
    (a) stem tendril develop from apical bud
    (b) stem tendril are slender and spirally coiled
    (c) stem tendril doesn't help in climbing
    (d) stem tendril develop from radicle
24. Select incorrect matching:
    (a) thorn–citrus, bougainvillea (b) flattened stem–opuntia
    (c) underground stem–turmeric (d) stem tendril–colocasia
25. The lateral branches original from basal and underground portion of the main stem, grow horizontally beneath the soil and then come out obliquely upward giving rise to leafy shoots seen in case of
    (a) banana (b) pineapple (c) chrysanthemum (d) all

26. A slender lateral branch arises from the base of the main axis and after growing aerially for sometime arch downward to touch the ground seen in case of
(a) mint (b) jasmine (c) pistia (d) both (a) and (b)

27. A lateral branch with short internodes and each node bearing a rosette of leaves and a tuft of roots are found in aquatic plants like
(a) pistia (b) eichhornia (c) wolffia (d) both (a) and (b)

28. Select the correct statement from the following:
A. Fleshy cylindrical stem in Euphorbia carry out photosynthesis.
B. Pistia and Eichhornia are example of offset.
C. Underground stem of grass and strawberry spread to new niche and when older part die new plants are formed.
D. Thorns are woody, straight and pointed.
(a) A and B only (b) B and D only (c) B and C only (d) All

29. Most important vegetative organ for photosynthesis is
(a) stem (b) leaf (c) root (d) all

30. Which of the following is correct about leaf?
(a) It has originated from root apical meristem
(b) It is arranged in basipetal order
(c) It arises from axillary bud
(d) It bears a bud in its axil

31. Which of the following is incorrect about leaf?
(a) It is arranged in acropetal order (b) It develops from node
(c) It is generally flattened in shape (d) It is arranged in basipetal order

32. Typical leaf consist of
(a) petiole (b) leaf base (c) lamina (d) all

33. The leaf is attached to the stem by the leaf base and may bear two lateral small leaf like structure called
(a) leaflet (b) lamina (c) stipule (d) leaf blade

34. Select the correct statement from the following:
A. In monocot leaf base expand into a sheath covering the stem partially or wholly
B. In all leguminous plants the leaf base may become swollen, which is called the pulvinus
C. The lamina or leaf blade is the green expanded part of the leaf with veins and veinlets
D. Veins provide rigidity to leaf blade
(a) A and B only (b) C and D only (c) All except B (d) All except D

35. Leaf can be differentiated by
(a) shape (b) margin and apex (c) surface (d) all

36. Long thin ________ petiole allow leaf blade to flutter in wind, thereby cooling of the leaf and bringing ________ air to leaf surfaces.
(a) hard, fresh (b) flexible, fresh (c) hard, fresh (d) rigid, fresh

37. The arrangement of arteries and arterioles in the lamina of leaf is termed as
(a) venation (b) phyllotaxy (c) inflorescence (d) none

38. Which of the following is correct about venation?
A. Parallel venation generally found in monocot
B. Parallel venation generally found in dicot
C. Reticulate venation generally found in monocot
D. Reticulate venation generally found in dicot
(a) A and D only (b) B and C only (c) B and D only (d) A and C only

39. Bud is present in axil
(a) simple leaf (b) compound leaf (c) leaflet (d) both (a) and (b)
40. Pinnately compound leaf found in
(a) lemon (b) bombax (c) desmodium (d) neem
41. Palmately compound leaf found in
(a) neem (b) rose (c) silk cotton (d) mimosa pudica
42. Find out correct matching:
A. Palmately compound leaves – Leaf let attached to common axis rachis
B. Phyllotaxy – Pattern of arrangement of leaves on stemor branch
C. Pinnately compound leaves – Leaflet attached to a common point i.e. at the tip of petiole
D. Venation – Arrangement of veins and veinlets in the lamina of leaf
(a) A and B only (b) B and C only (c) C and D only (d) B and D only
43. Phyllotaxy usually of three types, namely,
(a) alternate (b) whorled (c) opposite (d) all
44. Select correct matching:

Column I	Column II	Column II
A. Alternate	X. Single leaf arises at each node	1. China rose, mustard, sunflower
B. Whorled	Y. More than 2 leaf arises at node	2. Alstonia
C. Opposite	Z. Pair of leaf arises at node	3. Calotropis and guava

(a) A–X–1, B–Y–2, C–Z–3 (b) A–Y–3, B–Z–2, C–X–1
(c) A–Y–3, B–Z–1, C–Y–2 (d) A–Z–3, B–Y–2, C–X–1
45. Following posses alternate phyllotaxy except
(a) mustard (b) china rose (c) sunflower (d) calotropis
46. In which plant the leaves are small and short-lived. The petiole in these plant expand, become green and synthesize food, such petiole is known as phyllode?
(a) sweat peat (b) clematis (c) Australian acacia (d) eichhornia
47. Select incorrect matching:
(a) leaf into tendril–pea (b) leaf into spine–cacti
(c) fleshy leaf–onion and garlic (d) whorled phyllotaxy–Calotropis
48. Following pair represent insectivorous plant
(a) pitcher plant, australian acacia
(b) venus fly trap, calotropis
(c) pitcher plant, venus fly trap
(d) silk cotton, neem
49. In pitcher plant, pitcher is modified
(a) root (b) stem (c) leaf (d) flower
50. In floral meristem
(a) internode do not elongate
(b) axis get condensed
(c) the apex produced different kinds of floral appendages laterally at successive nodes instead of leaves
(d) all
51. The arrangement of flowers on the floral axis is termed as
(a) phyllotaxy (b) aestivation (c) inflorescence (d) placentation

52. In cymose type of inflorescence
A. Main axis terminates into flower.
B. Flower born in basipetal order.
C. Main axis not terminates into flower.
D. Flower born in acropetal order.
(a) A and B only (b) C and D only (c) A and C only (d) B and C only

53. In racemose-type of inflorescence,
A. Main axis terminates into flower.
B. Flower born in basipetal order.
C. Main axis not terminates into flower.
D. Flower born in acropetal order.
(a) A and B only (b) C and D only (c) A and C only (d) B and C only

54. Which of the following is correct about flower?
A. Reproductive unit in angiosperm
B. Calyx and corolla are reproductive organ
C. Typical flower has four kinds of whorls
D. Whorls arranged successively on thalamus or receptacle
(a) All except C (b) All except D (c) All except B (d) All except A

55. Select incorrect matching:

A. Actinomorphic	–	When flower can be divided into two equal radial halves in any radial plane passing through the centre
B. Zygomorphic	–	When flower can be divided into two similar halves only in one particular vertical plane
C. Asymmetric	–	When flower cannot be divided into two similar halves by any vertical plane passing through centre.

D. All are correct

56. Asymmetric flower is found in
(a) pea (b) datura (c) bean (d) canna

57. How many of following contain zygomorphic flower?
Pea, Gulmohur, bean, Cassia, Mustard, Datura, Chilli, Sesbania, lupin, Muliathi
(a) 6 (b) 7 (c) 4 (d) 8

58. Reduced leaf found at base of the pedicel is known as
(a) leaflet (b) stipule (c) bract (d) calyx

59. Based on the position of calyx, corolla and androecium in respect of the ovary on thalamus, the flower is of how many types
(a) 1 (b) 2 (c) 3 (d) 4

60. Select the correct matching:

Column I	Column II	Column III
1. Hypogynous	A. Gynoecium occupy highest position	X. Mustard, Brinjal, China rose
2. Epigynous	B. Gynoecium situated in the centre	Y. Plum, peach, rose
3. Perigynous	C. Margin of thalamus grows upward enclosing ovary completely	Z. Guava, cucumber, ray florets of sunflower

(a) 1–A–X, 2–B–Y, 3–C–Z (b) 1–A–X, 2–C–Z, 3–B–Y
(c) 1–B–Y, 2–A–X, 3–C–Z (d) 1–A–X, 2–B–Z, 3–C–Y

61. Which flower posses superior ovary?
(a) Mustard (b) China rose (c) Brinjal (d) All
62. Select correct matching:
(a) gamosepalous–sepal united (b) polysepalous–sepals free
(c) gamopetalous–petals united (d) all
63. Shape of corolla may be
(a) tubular (b) funnel-shaped (c) bell-shaped (d) all
64. The mode of arrangement of sepals or petals in floral bud with respect is the other members of the same whorl are known as
(a) phyllotaxy (b) inflorescence (c) aestivation (d) hibernation
65. Sepals or petals in a whorl just touch one another at the margin, without overlapping is found in
(a) china rose (b) pea (c) cassia (d) calotropis
66. Twisted aestivation found in all except
(a) cotton (b) china rose (c) lady's finger (d) gulmohur
67. If the margins or sepals or petals overlap one another but not in any particular direction is known as _________ aestivation
(a) vexillary (b) twisted (c) imbricate (d) gulmohur
68. Which is false for vexillary or papilionaceous aestivation?
(a) Two smallest anterior petals are known as keel
(b) Two lateral petals are known as wing
(c) The largest standard petal is posterior
(d) The largest standard petal is anterior and overlaps wing
69. Select the correct matching:

Aestivation		Example
(a) Valvate	–	Cassia
(b) Twisted	–	China rose, ladyfinger, calotropis
(c) Imbricate	–	Cassia and Gulmohar
(d) Vexillary	–	Pea, bean, Aloe, Tulip

70. Stamen consist of
(a) stalk or filament (b) stigma (c) anther (d) both (a) and (c)
71. Anther usually posses
(a) one sac (b) two sacs (c) three sacs (d) four sacs
72. A sterile stamen is called
(a) monoadelphous (b) epipetalous (c) epiphyllous (d) staminode
73. Epiphyllous stamens are found in
(a) sunhemp (b) ashwagandha (c) mustard (d) lily
74. Epipetalous stamens are found in
(a) Trifolium (b) Brinjal (c) Asparagus (d) Indigofera
75. The stamens are united into one bunch (Monoadelphous) condition is found in
(a) pea (b) citrus (c) arhar (d) china rose
76. Diadelphous condition is found
(a) citrus (b) pea (c) china rose (d) tomato
77. A carpet consists of
(a) stigma (b) ovary (c) style (d) all
78. Which of the following is incorrect about carpet?
(a) ovary is enlarged basal portion (b) stigma is usually at tip of style
(c) style is elongated tube over ovary (d) style is the receptive surface for pollen grains

79. Apocarpous condition is found in
(a) Mustard (b) Tomato (c) Lotus (d) All

80. Syncarpous condition is found in
(a) Mustard (b) Lotus (c) Rose (d) All

81. After fertilization
(a) ovule develop into seed (b) ovary matures to fruit
(c) ovary wall changes to fruit wall (d) all

82. Arrangement of ovules within the ovary is known as
(a) placentation (b) aestivation (c) fragmentation (d) hibernation

83. Match the column:

Column I	–	Column II
A. Marginal	–	1. Pea
B. Parietal	–	2. Mustard and Argemone
C. Axile	–	3. Dianthus and Primrose
D. Central and free central	–	4. China rose, tomato, lemon
E. Basal	–	5. Sunflower and marigold

(a) A–1, B–2, C–4, D–3, E–5 (b) A–2, B–1, C–3, D–4, E–5
(c) A–4, B–1, C–3, D–5, E–4 (d) A–5, B–2, C–4, D–2, E–3

84. Ovary is one-chambered but it becomes two chambered due to formation of false septum is found in
(a) argemone and mustard (b) dianthus and primrose
(c) rose and tomato (d) pea

85. A placentation in which ovule are born on central axis and septa are absent, is found in
(a) argemone and mustard (b) dianthus and primrose
(c) rose and tomato (d) pea

86. A placentation, in which placenta develops at the base of ovary and a single ovule is attached, is found in
(a) argemone and mustard (b) dianthus and primrose
(c) rose and tomato (d) sunflower and marigold

87. Fruit is
(a) the resultant ripened ovary (b) formed generally after fertilization
(c) a characteristic feature of flowing plant (d) all

88. What is the name of the pericarp when it is thick and fleshy?
(a) Epicarp (b) Mesocarp (c) Endocarp (d) All

89. In which fruit mesocarp is fibrous?
(a) Mango (b) Coconut (c) Both (d) None

90. Which is the edible part in mango?
(a) Thin epicarp (b) Fleshy mesocarp
(c) Stony hard endocarp (d) All

91. In coconut and mango, the fruit is known as
(a) legume (b) pod (c) drupe (d) samara

92. If fruit is develop without fertilization of the ovary, it is called
(a) parthenocarpic fruit (b) apomictic fruit
(c) fleshly fruit (d) polyembryomic fruit

93. Mango is develop from
(a) monocarpellary inferior ovary
(b) monocarpellary superior ovary
(c) multicarpellary inferior ovary
(d) multi carpellary superior ovary

94. Seed is made up of
(a) seed coat (b) embryo (c) both (d) none

95. Embryo is made up of
(a) a radicle
(b) embryonal axis
(c) one or two cotyledons
(d) all

96. Following are monocots except
(a) wheat (b) maize (c) sugar cane (d) gram

97. Following are dicot except
(a) bean (b) gram (c) pea (d) maize

98. Which of the following is correct about dicot seed?
A Micropyle is present above the hilum.
B. At the ends of embryonal axis radicle and plumule is present.
C. Seed coat has 3 layers.
D. Cotyledons are generally without food reserve.
(a) A and B only (b) B and C only (c) C and D only (d) A and D only

99. Following are the non-endospermic seed except
(a) bean (b) gram (c) pea (d) castor

100. Which layer is called aleurone layer?
(a) Protein (b) Carbohydrate (c) Lipid (d) All

101. The plumule and radical in monocot seed are enclosed in sheaths which are called _________ and _________ respectively.
(a) coleoptile and scutellum
(b) scutellum and coleorhiza
(c) coleoptile and coleorhiza
(d) coleorhiza and Coleoptile

102. Select the incorrect statement among the following:
A. Monocot seeds are generally endospermic.
B. In maize seed coat is membranous and generally fused with fruit wall.
C. In monocot seed single large shield shape cotyledon is known as scutellum.
D. In orchids seeds are non-endospermic.
(a) A and B only (b) C only (c) D only (d) None

103. Which family is known as the 'potato' family?
(a) Fabaceae
(b) Solanaceae
(c) Liliaceae
(d) Cruciferae (Brassicaceae)

104. Find out the correct matching:

A. Br	–	1.	Bracteate
B. K	–	2.	Calyx
C. C	–	3.	Corolla
D. A	–	4.	Gynoecium
E. G	–	5.	Androecium
F. G	–	6.	Superior ovary
G. ♂	–	7.	Male
H. ⚥	–	8.	Bisexual
I. ⊕	–	9.	Actinomorphic
J. %	–	10.	Zygomorphic
K. ♀	–	11.	Female

(a) 1–B, 2–C, 3–E, 4–K, 5–A, 6–J, 7–I, 8–F, 9–H, 10–D, 11–G
(b) 1–C, 2–A, 3–B, 4–E, 5–D, 6–G, 7–I, 8–H, 9–F, 10–J, 11–K
(c) 1–K, 2–J, 3–I, 4–H, 5–G, 6–F, 7–D, 8–E, 9–C, 10–B, 11–A
(d) 1–A, 2–B, 3–C, 4–E, 5–D, 6–F, 7–G, 8–H, 9–I, 10–J, 11–K

105. Stem of fabaceae are
(a) Erect or climber
(b) Herbaceous rarely woody, aerial; erect, cylindrical, branched solid
(c) Herbaceous with underground bulb/corms/rhizomes
(d) All

106. Find out from the following total number of plants with stipulate leaves.
Gram, Arhar, Moong, Sesbania, Lupin, Muliathi, Soyabean, Tomato, Brinjal, Belladona, Petunia, Tobacco, Tulip, Aloe, Colchicine, Asparagus, Chilli, Ground nuts, Indigofera, Sunhemp
(a) 7 (b) 10 (c) 15 (d) 20

107. Select the incorrect pair:
(a) Indigofera – Sepals five (Gamosepalous), corolla (Vexillary aestivation)
(b) Brinjal – Sepals five united (persistent, valvate aestivation) Petals five united (valvate aestivation)
(c) Asparagus – Sepals three often united into tube (valvate aestivation)
(d) Colchicine – Perianth present tepals six (valvate aestivation)

108. Select from the following total no of plant showing tricarpellary gynoceium.
Gram, Arhar, Moong, Sesbania, Lupin, Muliathi, Soyabean, Tomato, Brinjal, Belladona, Petunia, Tobacco, Tulip, Aloe, Colchicine, Asparagus, Chilli, Ground nuts, Indigofera, Sunhemp
(a) 7 (b) 10 (c) 4 (d) 6

109. Select from the flowing, total number of plant having epipetalous stamens.
Gram, Arhar, Moong, Sesbania, Lupin, Muliathi, Soyabean, Tomato, Brinjal, Belladona, Petunia, Tobacco, Tulip, Aloe, Colchicine, Asparagus, Chilli, Ground nuts, Indigofera, Sunhemp
(a) 7 (b) 6 (c) 8 (d) 10

110. Fruit of Liliaceae is mainly
(a) Drupe (b) Ovary (c) Legume (d) Capsule

111. Which is correct for the gynoecium of Liliaceae?
(a) Tricarpellary, syncarpous, superior ovary, trilocular with many ovule, axile placenation
(b) Bicarpellary, syncarpous, superior ovary, bilocular, swollen placenta with many ovule
(c) Superior ovary, monocarpellary, unilocular with many ovules
(d) Tricarpellary, inferior ovary, syncarpous, trilocular with many ovules, axile placentation

112. Select from the following the total number of plant showing axile placentation.
Dianthus, primrose, china rose, tomato, lemon, tulip, aloe, asparagus, cholchicine, trifolium, lupin, arhar
(a) 6 (b) 7 (c) 8 (d) 9

113. Select the incorrect matching:
(a) Ornamental – Tulip, gloriosa, lupin, sweet pea, petunia
(b) Medicine – Muliathi, belladonna, aloe
(c) Fodder – Sesbania, trifolium
(d) Edible oil – Soyabean, groundnut, colchicine

114. Select from the following total number of plant having non-endospermic seed.
Gram, Arhar, Moong, Sesbania, Lupin, Muliathi, Soyabean, Tomato, Brinjal, Belladona, Petunia, Tobacco, Tulip, Aloe, Colchicine, Asparagus, Chilli, Ground nuts, Indigofera, Sunhemp
(a) 10 (b) 15 (c) 20 (d) 6

115. Diadelphous condition seen in all except
(a) Soyabean (b) Lupin (c) Brassica rapa (d) China rose

116. Inflorescence in makoi is
(a) Racemose (b) Cymose (c) Catkin (d) None

117. Zygomorphic flower is found in
(a) Aloe (b) Potato (c) Sesbania (d) Ashwagandha

118. Botanical name of onion is
(a) Allium sativum (b) Solanum melogena
(c) Allium cepa (d) Brassica rapa

119. Which of the following is correct about chilli?
(a) Gamosepalous (C), gamopetalous (K), epipetalous, stamen, superior ovary
(b) Gamosepalous (C), Stamen five, ovary superior
(c) Gamosepalous (C), Polypetalous (K), diadelphous (A), Superior ovary
(d) Poly seplous (C), gamopetalous (K), epipetalous stamen, superior ovary

120. 'Lily' family stands for
(a) Solanaceae (b) Liliaceae (c) Fabaceae (d) Brassicaeae

121. Select correct matching:
(a) Vegetable–Colchicine (b) Medicine–Tulip
(c) Ornamental–Asparagus (d) Medicine–Belladonna, ashwagandha

122. Floral formula of Brassicaceae is
(a) $\oplus ⚥ K_{2-2} C_4 A_{2+4} \underline{G}_{(2)}$ (b) $\oplus ⚥ K_{2+2} C_4 A_{2+4} \underline{G}_{(2)}$
(c) $\oplus ⚥ K_{2+(2)} C_4 A_{2-4} \underline{G}_{(2)}$ (d) $\oplus ⚥ K_{2+2} C_{(4)} A_{2+4} \underline{G}_2$

123. Select dye from the following:
(a) Sesbania (b) Sunhemp (c) Lupin (d) Indigofera

124. Monocarpellary condition is found in
(a) Groundnut (b) Petunia (c) Lily (d) Allium cepa

125. Floral formula of Liliaceae is
(a) $\oplus ⚥ P_{3+3} A_{3+3} \underline{G}_{(3)}$ (b) $\oplus ⚥ P_{3-3} A_{3+3} \underline{G}_{(3)}$
(c) $P_{3+3} A_{3+3} \underline{G}_{(3)} \oplus$ (d) $\oplus ⚥ P_{3+3} A_{3+3} G_{(3)}$

126. Which of the following is a source of medicine?
(a) Petunia (b) Asparagus (c) Gloriosa (d) Aloe

127. Floral formula of solanaceae is
(a) $\oplus ⚥ \overparen{C_{(5)} A_{(5)}} \underline{G}_{(2)} K_{(5)}$ (b) $\oplus ⚥ K_{(5)} \overparen{C_{(5)} A_{(5)}} \underline{G}_{(2)}$
(c) $\oplus ⚥ K_{(5)} \overparen{C_{(5)} A_{(5)}} G_{(2)}$ (d) $\oplus ⚥ K_{(5)} \overparen{C_{(5)} A_{(5)}} G_{(2)}$

128. Floral formula of fabaceae is
(a) $\oplus ⚥ K_{(5)} C_{1+2+(2)} A_{(9)+1} \underline{G}_1$ (b) $\oplus ⚥ K_{(5)} C_{1+2-(2)} A_{(9)+1} G_1$
(c) $\oplus ⚥ K_{(5)} C_{1+2} A_{9+1} G_1$ (d) $\oplus ⚥ K_{(5)} C_{1+2+2} A_{(9)-1} G_1$

129. Select incorrect statement for liliaceae from following:
(a) Bisexual, zygomorphic flower
(b) Bisexual, actinomorphic flower

(c) Leaves are mostly basal, exstipulate with parallel venation
(d) Tepal shows valvate aestivation

130. Tomato, Brinjal and potato belongs to the family called
(a) Brassicaceae (b) Solanaceae (c) Liliaceae (d) Fabaceae

131. Botanical name of makoi is
(a) Solanum tuberosum (b) Solanum melongena
(c) Solanum lycopersicum (d) Solanum nigrum

132. What indicates A to E in below figure.

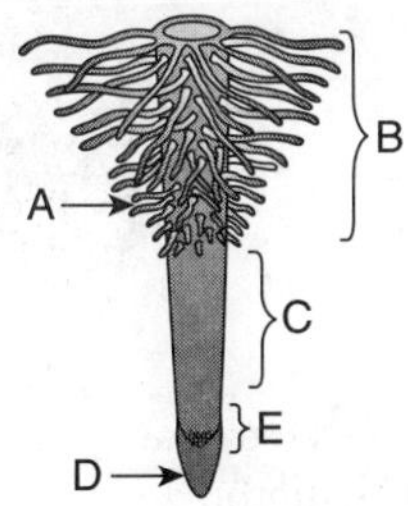

(a) A–Region of maturation, B–Root cap, C–Region of meristematic activity, D–Root hair, E–Region of elongation
(b) A–Root hair, B–Region of maturation, C–Region of elongation, D–Root cap, E–Region of meristematic activity
(c) A–Root cap, B–Region of maturation, C–Region of elongation, D–Root hair, E–Region of meristemetic activity
(d) A–Region of meristematic activity, B–Region of elongation, C–Region of maturation, D–Root hair, E–Root cap

133. Identify the A to E in below figure?

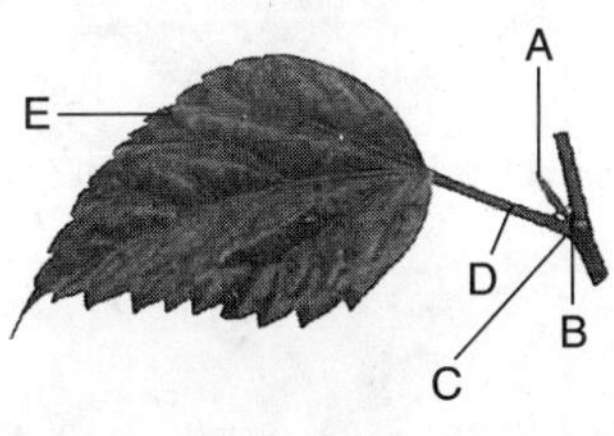

(a) A–Leaf base, B–Petiole, C–Stipule, D–Lamina, E–Axillary bud
(b) A–Stipule, B–Axillary bud, C–Leaf base, D–Petiole, E–Lamina
(c) A–Lamina, B–Stipule, C–Petiole, D–Leaf base, E–Axillary bud
(d) A–Stipule, B–Leaf base, C–Axillary bud, D–Lamina, E–Petiole

134. What indicates A to E in below figure.

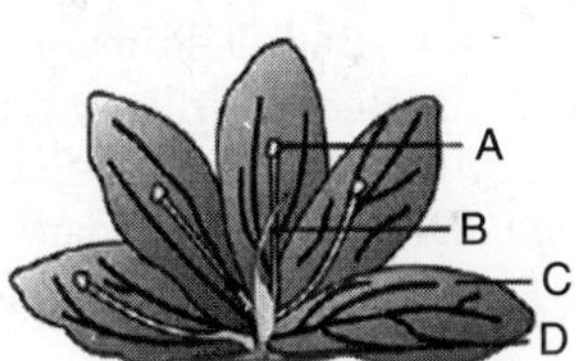

(a) A–Gynoecium, B–Calyx, C–Corolla, D–Pedicel, E–Androecium
(b) A–Corolla, B–Calyx, C–Gynoecium, D–Androecium, E–Pedicel
(c) A–Androecium, B–Gynoecium, C–Corolla, D–Calyx, E–Pedicel
(d) A–Calyx, B–Gynoecium, C–Pedicel, D–Androecium, E–Corolla

135. Identify the A to C in dicotyledonous seed

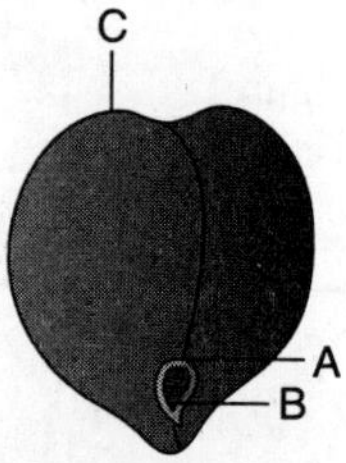

(a) A–Hilum, B–Micropyle, C–Seed coat
(b) A–Seed coat, B–Hilum, C–Micropyle
(c) A–Micropyle, B–Seed coat, C–Hilum
(d) A–Micropyle, B–Hilum, C–Seed coat

136. Identify the A to F in this figure.

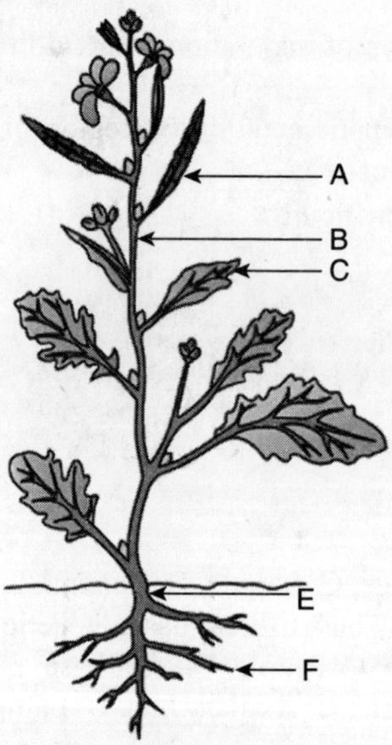

(a) A–Stem, B–Secondary root, C–Bud, D–Primary root, E–Leaf, F–Fruit
(b) A–Fruit, B–Stem, C–Leaf, D–Bud, E–Primary root, F–Secondary root
(c) A–Bud, B–leaf, C–Primary root, D–Fruits, E–Secondary root, F–Stem
(d) A–Fruit, B–Leaf, C–Stem, D–Bud, E–Secondary root, F–Primary root

137. Identify the A, B and C in this figure.

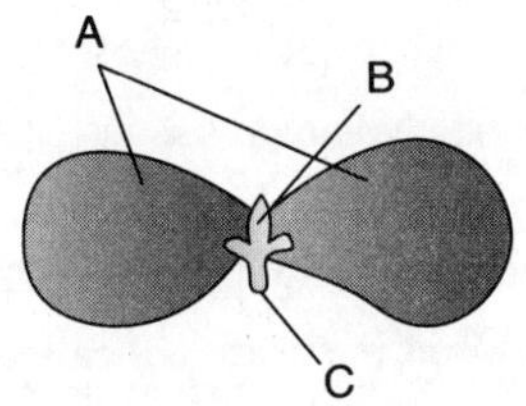

(a) A–Plumule, B–Cotyledon, C–Radicle
(b) A–Radicle, B–Cotyledon, C–Plumule
(c) A–Cotyledon, B–Plumule, C–Radicle
(d) A–Radicle, B–Plumule, C–Cotyledon

138. Identify the A to D in this figure.

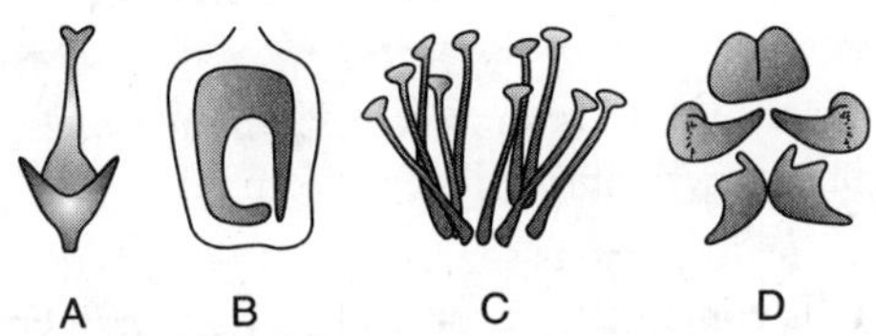

(a) A–Petals, B–Carpel, C–Basal, D–Androecium
(b) A–Androecium, B–Basal, C–Carpel, D–Petals
(c) A–Basal, B–Androecium, C–Petals, D–Carpel
(d) A–Carpel, B–Basal, C–Androecium, D–Petals

*Read the **assertion** and **reason** carefully to mark the correct option out of the options given below:*

(a) If both the assertion and the reason are true and the reason is a correct explanation of the assertion
(b) If both the assertion and reason are true but the reason is not a correct explanation of the assertion
(c) If the assertion is true but the reason is false
(d) If both the assertion and reason are false

139. Assertion: Old root hairs are replaced by new ones.
Reason: Outer cells of root gives rise to root hairs.

140. Assertion: Adventitious roots develop from any part of plant.
Reason: In such plants, tap root is not developed.

141. Assertion: Generally,dicotyledonous plants have tap roots while monocotyledonous plants have fibrous roots.
Reason: The roots in some plants get modified for storage of food, mechanical support and respiration.

142. Assertion: Assimilatory roots can photosynthesize.
Reason: Asimilatory roots possess chlorophyll.

143. Assertion: Epiphytes are called space parasites.
Reason: Epiphytic roots possess velamen tissue.

144. Assertion: The flower is modified shoot meant for sexual reproduction.
Reason: Flowers are arranged in different types of inflorescence.

145. Assertion: The plumule enclosed in sheath are called coleoptile.
Reason: The radicle enclosed in sheath are called coleorhiza.

146. Assertion: In plants such as bean,gram and pea seeds are called non-endospermous.
Reason: The endosperm inis not present in mature seeds of above plants.

147. Assertion: Sucker is an underground stem.
Reason: Sucker stem never comes above the ground.

148. Assertion: In mango and coconut , the fruit is known as drupe.
Reason: The fruit develope in above plant are monocarpellary superior ovary and are one seeded.

149. Assertion: Actinomorphic flowers show radial symmetry.
Reason: Zygomorphic flowers have bilateral symmetry.

150. Assertion: Maize is an albuminous seed.
Reason: Endosperm is completely absorbed by its growing embryo.

AIPMT PREVIOUS YEAR QUESTIONS

1. Which one of the following is a xerophytic plant in which the stem is modified into the flat green and succulent structure?

[AIPMT MAINS 2010]

(a) Opuntia
(b) Casuarina
(c) Hydrilla
(d) Acacia

2. Aestivation of petals in the flower of cotton is correctly shown in

[AIPMT MAINS 2010]

(a) 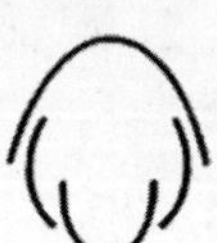

(b) 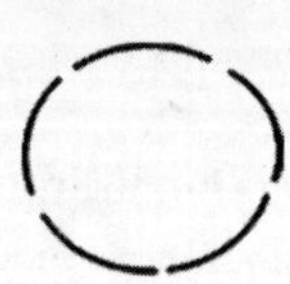

(c) 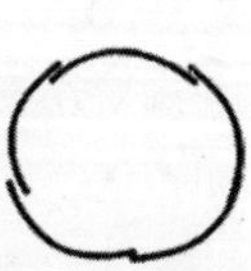

(d) 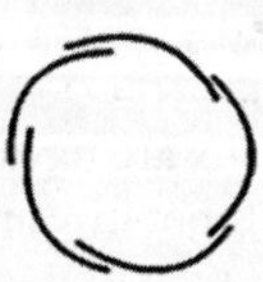

3. The correct floral formula of soyabean is

[AIPMT MAINS 2010]

(a) $\oplus ⚥ K_{(5)} C_{1+(2)+2} A_{(9)+1} \underline{G}_1$
(b) $\oplus ⚥ K_5 C_{1+(2)+2} A_{(9)+1} \underline{G}_1$
(c) $\oplus ⚥ K_{(5)} C_{1+2+(2)} A_{(9)+1} \underline{G}_1$
(d) $\oplus ⚥ K_{(5)} C_{1+2+(2)} A_{1+(9)} \underline{G}_1$

4. Consider the following four statements (a), (b), (c) and (d) and select the right option for two correct statements.

Statements:

(a) In vexillary aestivation, the large posterior petal is called- standard, two lateral ones are wings and two small anterior petals are termed keel

(b) The floral formula for liliaceae is $\oplus ⚥\ P_{3+3}A_{3+3}\underline{G}_3$

(c) In pea flower the stamens are monadelphous

(d) The floral formula for Solanaceae is $\oplus ⚥\ K_{(3)}C_{(3)}A_{(4)}\underline{G}_{(2)}$

The correct statements are

[AIPMT MAINS 2010]

(a) (a) & (c)   (b) (a) & (b)
(c) (b) & (c)   (d) (c) & (d)

5. In unilocular ovary with a single ovule, the placentation is

[AIPMT PRE 2010]

(a) Marginal   (b) Basal
(c) Free central   (d) Axile

6. Keel is characteristic of the flowers of

[AIPMT PRE 2010]

(a) Gulmohur   (b) Cassia
(c) Calotropis   (d) Bean

7. Ovary is half-inferior in the flowers of

[AIPMT PRE 2010]

(a) Guava   (b) Plum
(c) Brinjal   (d) Cucumber

8. The technical term used for the androecium in a flower of China rose (Hibiscus rosa sinensis) is

[AIPMT PRE 2010]

(a) Monadelphous   (b) Diadelphous
(c) Polyandrous   (d) Polyadelphous

9. Coiling of garden pea tendrils around any support is an example of

[AIPMT PRE 2010]

(a) Thigmotaxis   (b) Thigmonasty
(c) Thigmotropism   (d) Thermotaxis

10. Which one of the following figures represents the placentation in Dianthus?

[AIPMT MAINS 2011]

(a) 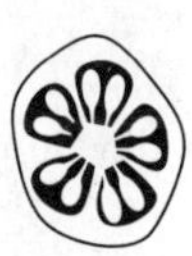   (b) 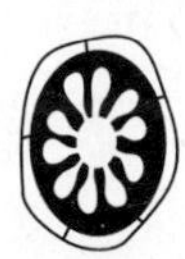

(c) 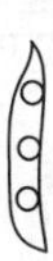   (d) 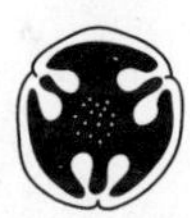

11. Whorled, simple leaves with reticulate venation are present in

[AIPMT MAINS 2011]

(a) Calotropis (b) Neem
(c) China rose (d) Alstonia

12. Which one of the following statements is correct?

[AIPMT PRE 2011]

(a) Seeds of orchids have oil-rich endosperm
(b) Placentation in primrose is basal
(c) Flower of tulip is a modified shoot
(d) In tomato, fruit is a capsule

13. The 'Eyes' of the potato tuber are:

[AIPMT PRE 2011]

(a) Flower buds (b) Shoot buds
(c) Axillary buds (d) Root buds

14. Flowers are zygomorphic in:

[AIPMT PRE 2011]

(a) Gulmohur (b) Tomato
(c) Datura (d) Mustard

15. A drupe developed in

[AIPMT PRE 2011]

(a) Wheat (b) Pea
(c) Tomato (d) Mango

16. Which one of the following is wrongly matched?

[AIPMT PRE 2011]

(a) Puccinia - Smut
(b) Root - Exarch protoxylem
(c) Cassia - Imbricate aestivation
(d) Root pressure - Guttation

17. The ovary is half inferior in flowers of:

[AIPMT PRE 2011]

(a) Cucumber (b) Cotton
(c) Guava (d) Peach

18. The correct floral formula of chilli is:

(a) $\oplus$⚥ $K_{(5)}\overset{\frown}{C_{(5)}\,A_5}G_{(2)}$ (b) $\oplus$⚥ $K_{(5)}C_{(5)}A_{(5)}G_2$

(c) $\oplus$⚥ $K_5\overset{\frown}{C_5\,A_{(5)}}G_2$ (d) $\oplus$⚥ $K_{(5)}C_5A_5G_{(2)}$

[AIPMT PRE 2011]

19. How many plants in the list given below have composite fruits that develop from an inflorescence?
Walnut, poppy, radish, fig, pineapple, apple, tomato, mulberry.

[AIPMT PRE 2012]

(a) Four (b) Five
(c) Two (d) Three

20. How many plants in the list given below have marginal placentation?
Mustard, Gram, Tulip, Asparagus, Arhar, Sun hemp, Chilli, Colchicine, Onion, Moong, Pea, Tobacco, Lupin

[AIPMT MAINS 2012]

(a) Five
(b) Six
(c) Three
(d) Four

21. Which one of the following organisms is correctly matched with its three characteristics?

[AIPMT MAINS 2012]

(a) Tomato: Twisted aestivation, Axile placentation, Berry
(b) Onion: Bulb, Imbricate aestivation, Axile placentation
(c) Maize: C_3 pathway, closed vascular bundles, Scutellum
(d) Pea: C_3 pathway, Endospermic seed, Vaxillary aestivation

22. Cymose inflorescence is present in:

[AIPMT PRE 2012]

(a) Solanum
(b) Sesbania
(c) Trifolium
(d) Brassica

23. Phyllode is present in

[AIPMT PRE 2012]

(a) Asparagus
(b) Euphorbia
(c) Australian Acacia
(d) Opuntia

24. Placentation in tomato and lemon is:

[AIPMT PRE 2012]

(a) Parietal
(b) Free central
(c) Marginal
(d) Axile

25. Vexillary aestivation is characteristic of the family:

[AIPMT PRE 2012]

(a) Fabaceae
(b) Asteraceae
(c) Solanaceae
(d) Brassicaceae

26. Among bitter gourd, mustard, brinjal, pumpkin, china rose, lupin, cucumber, sunhemp, gram, guava, bean, chilli, plum, petunia, tomato, rose, withania, potato, onion, aloe and tulip how many plants have hypogynous flower?

[AIPMT 2013]

(a) Six
(b) Ten
(c) Fifteen
(d) Eighteen

27. In China rose the flowers are:

[AIPMT 2013]

(a) Actinomorphic, hypogynous with twisted aestivation
(b) Actinomorphic, epigynous with valvate aestivation
(c) Zygomorphic, hypogynous with imbricate aestivation
(d) Zygomorphic, egigynous with twisted aestivation

28. Seed coat is not thin, membranous in:

[AIPMT 2013]

(a) Maize
(b) Coconut
(c) Groundnut
(d) Gram

29. Placenta and pericarp are both edible portions in: [AIPMT 2014]

(a) Apple (b) Banana
(c) Tomato (d) Potato

30. When the margins of sepals or petals overlap one another without any particular direction, the condition is termed as: [AIPMT 2014]

(a) Vexillary (b) Imbricate
(c) Twisted (d) Valvate

31. Which one of the following statements is correct? [AIPMT 2014]

(a) The seed in grasses is not endospermic
(b) Mango is a parthenocarpic fruit
(c) A Proteinaceous aleurone layer is present in maize grain
(d) A sterile pistil is called a staminode

32. An example of edible underground stem is: [AIPMT 2014]

(a) Carrot (b) Groundnut
(c) Sweet potato (d) Potato

33. An aggregate fruit is one which develops from [AIPMT 2014]

(a) Multicarpellary syncarpous gynoecium
(b) Multicarpellary apocarpous gynoecium
(c) Complete inflorescence
(d) Multicarpellary superior ovary

34. $\oplus ⚥ K_{(5)} \widehat{C_{(5)} A_{(5)}} \underline{G}_{(2)}$ is the floral formula of [AIPMT 2015]

(a) Alium (b) Serbia
(c) Petunia (d) Brassica

35. Keel is the characteristic feature flower of [AIPMT 2015]

(a) Tulip (b) Indigofera
(c) Aloe (d) Tomato

36. Perigynous flowers are found in: [AIPMT 2015]

(a) Guava (b) Cucumber
(c) China rose (d) Rose

37. The Hilum a scar on the [AIPMT 2015]

(a) Seed, where uncle was attached
(b) Fruit, where it was attaché to pedicel
(c) Fruit, where style was present
(d) Seed, where micropyle was present

38. Among china rose, mustard, brinjal, potato, guava, cucumber, onion and tulip, how many plants have superior ovary? [RE-AIPMT 2015]

(a) Six (b) Three
(c) Four (d) Four

39. The wheat grain has an embryo with one large, shield-shaped cotyledon known as: [RE-AIPMT 2015]

(a) Coleorrhiza (b) Scutellum
(c) Coleoptile (d) Epiblast

40. Axile placentation is present in: [RE-AIPMT 2015]

(a) Lemon (b) Pea
(c) Argemone (d) Dianthus

41. Flowers are unisexual in [RE-AIPMT 2015]

(a) Cucumber (b) China rose
(c) Onion (d) Pea

Answer Keys

1. (d)	2. (a)	3. (b)	4. (d)	5. (d)	6. (d)	7. (d)	8. (c)	9. (a)	10. (c)
11. (c)	12. (d)	13. (c)	14. (c)	15. (b)	16. (d)	17. (c)	18. (d)	19. (c)	20. (d)
21. (d)	22. (d)	23. (b)	24. (d)	25. (d)	26. (d)	27. (d)	28. (d)	29. (b)	30. (d)
31. (d)	32. (d)	33. (c)	34. (c)	35. (d)	36. (b)	37. (d)	38. (a)	39. (d)	40. (d)
41. (c)	42. (d)	43. (d)	44. (a)	45. (d)	46. (c)	47. (d)	48. (c)	49. (c)	50. (d)
51. (c)	52. (a)	53. (b)	54. (c)	55. (d)	56. (d)	57. (b)	58. (c)	59. (c)	60. (b)
61. (d)	62. (d)	63. (d)	64. (c)	65. (d)	66. (d)	67. (c)	68. (d)	69. (c)	70. (d)
71. (d)	72. (d)	73. (d)	74. (b)	75. (d)	76. (b)	77. (d)	78. (d)	79. (c)	80. (a)
81. (d)	82. (a)	83. (a)	84. (a)	85. (b)	86. (d)	87. (d)	88. (d)	89. (b)	90. (b)
91. (c)	92. (a)	93. (b)	94. (c)	95. (d)	96. (d)	97. (d)	98. (a)	99. (d)	100. (a)
101. (c)	102. (d)	103. (b)	104. (d)	105. (a)	106. (a)	107. (c)	108. (c)	109. (b)	110. (d)
111. (a)	112. (b)	113. (d)	114. (a)	115. (d)	116. (b)	117. (c)	118. (c)	119. (a)	120. (b)
121. (d)	122. (b)	123. (d)	124. (a)	125. (a)	126. (d)	127. (b)	128. (a)	129. (a)	130. (b)
131. (d)	132. (b)	133. (b)	134. (c)	135. (a)	136. (b)	137. (c)	138. (d)	139. (b)	140. (c)
141. (c)	142. (a)	143. (b)	144. (b)	145. (b)	146. (a)	147. (c)	148. (b)	149. (b)	150. (c)

AIPMT Previous Year Questions

1. (a)	2. (d)	3. (b)	4. (b)	5. (b)	6. (d)	7. (b)	8. (a)	9. (c)	10. (b)
11. (d)	12. (c)	13. (c)	14. (a)	15. (d)	16. (a)	17. (d)	18. (a)	19. (d)	20. (b)
21. (b)	22. (a)	23. (c)	24. (d)	25. (a)	26. (c)	27. (a)	28. (a)	29. (c)	30. (b)
31. (c)	32. (d)	33. (b)	34. (c)	35. (b)	36. (d)	37. (a)	38. (a)	39. (b)	40. (a)
41. (a)									

CHAPTER 6

Anatomy of Flowering Plants

1. Study of internal structure of plants is called
   (a) morphology (b) physiology (c) anatomy (d) autotomy
2. Find out incorrect statement:
   (a) Monocot and dicot are anatomically different
   (b) Internal structures also show adaptations to diverse environment
   (c) Basic unit of plant is made up of cells
   (d) Different organs of plants are similar in their internal structure
3. A tissue is a group of cells having a
   (a) common origin and always a common function
   (b) common origin and always a different function
   (c) common origin and usually a common function
   (d) different origin and a different function
4. Depending on whether the cells being formed are capable of dividing or not, plant tissues are classified into how many types?
   (a) 1 (b) 2 (c) 3 (d) 4
5. Find the example of primary meristem.
   (a) Apical meristem (b) Intercalary meristem
   (c) Lateral meristem (d) Both (a) and (b)
6. Apical meristem is present at
   (a) root and shoot apex (b) place between mature tissue
   (c) vascular cambium (d) cork cambium
7. Axillary bud is
   (a) present in axil of leaf (b) capable of forming branch
   (c) capable of forming flower (d) all
8. Which tissue occurs in grasses and regenerate parts removed by the grazing herbivores?
   (a) Apical meristem (b) Lateral meristem
   (c) Intercalary meristem (d) All
9. The meristem that occurs in the mature regions of roots and shoots of many plants, particularly those that produce woody axis and appear later than primary meristem, is called
   (a) Intercalary meristem
   (b) Apical meristem
   (c) Secondary or lateral meristem
   (d) All
10. Find the example of lateral meristem.
   (a) Fascicular cambium (b) Interfascicular cambium
   (c) Cork-cambium (d) All

11. Newly-formed cells from primary and secondary meristem, which becomes structurally and functionally specialized and lose the ability to divide, are known as
(a) permanent cells (b) mature cells (c) both (d) none
12. During the formation of the primary plant body, specific regions of the apical meristem produces
(a) dermal tissues (b) ground tissues (c) vascular tissues (d) all
13. Permanent tissues, which have all cell similar in structure and function, are called
(a) complex tissues (b) simple tissues
(c) meristematic tissues (d) all
14. Permanent tissues, which have many different types of cells are called
(a) complex tissues (b) simple tissues
(c) meristematic tissues (d) all
15. Which tissue is the most abundant in plant organ?
(a) Parenchyma (b) Collenchyma
(c) Sclerenchyma (d) Sclereids
16. Following features belong to
I. Cells are generally isodiametric. They may be spherical, oval, round, polygonal, or elongated in shape.
II. Cells have thin wall and are made up of cellulose.
III. Cells may be closely packed or may have intercellular spaces.
IV. Tissue perform various kind of functions like photosynthesis, storage and secretion.
(a) collenchyma (b) parenchyma (c) xylem (d) sclerenchyma
17. Following features belong to
I. Cells are thick at corner due to deposition of cellulose, hemicelluloses and pectin.
II. Cells may contain chloroplast and gets assimilated.
III. Intercellular spaces are absent.
IV. Provide mechanical support to growing parts of the plant such as young stem and petiole of leaf.
(a) collenchyma (b) parenchyma (c) xylem (d) sclerenchyma
18. Which simple tissue is characterized by pits?
(a) Collenchyma (b) Parenchyma
(c) Sclerenchyma (d) All
19. ________ are spherical, oval, cylindrical, highly thickened dead cell with very narrow cavities.
(a) Sieve tube (b) Companion cell (c) Fibres (d) Sclereids
20. Secondary thickening in collenchyma is of
(a) cellulose (b) hemicellulose (c) pectin (d) all
21. On what basis we classify sclerenchyma into fibres or sclereids?
(a) Structure (b) Origin (c) Development (d) All
22. Sclereids are present in the pulp of
(a) guava (b) pear (c) sapota (d) all
23. Sclereids are present in
(a) fruit wall of nuts (b) seed coat of legumes
(c) leaves of tea (d) all
24. Which tissue is usually dead and without protoplast?
(a) Parenchyma (b) Collenchyma (c) Sclerenchyma (d) All

25. Collenchyma tissue is characterized by
(a) elongated cells with thickness at the corners
(b) isodiametric cells with deposits of cellulose and pectin at the corners
(c) elongated cells with deposits of cellulose and pectin all over the wall
(d) isodiametric cells with thickness all over the cell wall

26. In which way collenchyma differs from sclerenchyma?
(a) Retaining protoplasm at maturity (b) Having thick walls
(c) Having wide lumen (d) Being meristematic

27. Walls of sclerenchyma are
(a) rigid (b) lignified (c) pectinised (d) suberised

28. Collenchyma differs from parenchyma in having
(a) living protoplasm (b) cellulose walls
(c) vacuoles (d) pectin deposits at corners

29. Which of the following are simple tissues?
(a) Parenchyma, xylem and phloem
(b) Parenchyma, collenchyma and sclerenchyma
(c) Parenchyma, xylem and collenchymas
(d) Parenchyma, xylem and sclerenchyma

30. What is the most common type of permanent tissue found in almost all plants?
(a) Sclerenchyma (b) Collenchyma
(c) Parenchyma (d) Xylem

31. Which of the following tissues gives tensile strength against bending and swaying?
(a) Parenchyma (b) Collenchyma (c) Sclereids (d) All

32. A simple mechanical tissue devoid of lignin is
(a) parenchyma (b) collenchymas (c) sclerenchyma (d) chlorenchyma

33. Primary plant body is made up of
(a) meristematic tissues (b) simple tissues
(c) complex tissues (d) all the above

34. Hard lignified thick-walled long and pointed cells of a plant are
(a) parenchyma (b) sclerenchyma fibers
(c) collenchymas (d) sclereids

35. A thick-walled lignified simple mechanical tissue is
(a) parenchyma (b) collenchymas (c) sclerenchyma (d) chlorenchyma

36. How many types of cells consist in complex tissue?
(a) More than one (b) More than three
(c) One type (d) None of the above

37. Function of xylem are
(a) conduct water from root to stem and leaves
(b) conduct mineral from root to stem and leaves
(c) provide mechanical strength to plant
(d) all

38. Xylem is composed of how many different elements?
(a) 1 (b) 2 (c) 3 (d) 4

39. Gymnosperm lacks _________ in their xylem.
(a) tracheids (b) vessels
(c) xylem fibres (d) xylem parenchyma

40. Select the correct matching

Column I		Column II
A. Tracheids	–	1. Elongated and tube like cells with thick and lignified wall and tapering ends.
B. Vessels	–	2. Tube like structure made up of many cells, each cell with lignified wall and large central cavity.
C. Xylem fibre	–	3. Highly thickened walls and obliterated central humans.
D. Xylem parenchyma	–	4. Living cell with thin cell wall made up of cellulose.

(a) A–2, B–1, C–3, D–4 (b) A–3, B–1, C–2, D–4
(c) A–1, B–2, C–3, D–4 (d) A–3, B–2, C–1, D–4

41. Xylem parenchyma stores
(a) starch (b) fat (c) tannins (d) all

42. Phloem parenchyma stores
(a) resins (b) latex (c) mucilage (d) all

43. Select the incorrect statement from the following:
(a) Vessel members are interconnected through perforations in their common walls
(b) Presence of vessel is a characteristic feature of angiosperms
(c) Radial conduction of water takes place by the ray parenchymatous cells
(d) Tracheids, vessel, xylem sclerenchyma and parenchyma are without protoplast

44. Protoplast is absent in all except
(a) tracheids (b) vessels
(c) xylem sclerenchyma (d) xylem parenchyma

45. The primary xylem elements formed are called _________ and the secondary xylem formed is called _________.
(a) protoxylem, protoxylem (b) metaxylem, metaxylem
(c) protoxylem, metaxylem (d) metaxylem, protoxylem

46. In stem
(a) protoxylem lies towards pith (centre)
(b) metaxylem lies towards periphery of the organs
(c) endarch arrangement present
(d) all

47. In root
(a) endarch arrangement is present (b) exarch arrangement is present
(c) protoxylem lies towards the centre (d) metaxylem lies towards the periphery

48. Phloem transports
(a) water (b) mineral (c) food materials (d) all

49. How many elements are composed in phloem in angiosperm?
(a) 1 (b) 2 (c) 3 (d) 4

50. Phloem is composed of all except
(a) sieve tube elements (b) companion cells
(c) phloem parenchyma and sclerenchyma (d) vessels

51. Gymnosperm posses
(a) sieve tubes (b) companion cells
(c) albuminous cell and sieve cells (d) all

52. Select the incorrect statement from the following:
(a) End walls of sieve tube have sieve plates
(b) Sieve tube and companion cell are connected by pit present between common longitudinal wall
(c) Companion cells are specialized parenchymatous cells having nucleus which control function of sieve tubes
(d) Phloem parenchyma is present in most of monocots

53. Following are live components of phloem except
(a) sieve tube (b) companion cell
(c) phloem parenchyma (d) phloem fibre (bast fibre)

54. Following are dead components of xylem except
(a) tracheids (b) vessels
(c) xylem sclerenchyma (wood fibres) (d) xylem parenchyma

55. Select the correct statement from the following:
(a) Companion cells help in maintaining pressure gradients in the sieve tubes
(b) Phloem parenchyma stores food material
(c) Bast fibres are generally absent in the primary phloem but are found in secondary phloem
(d) All

56. Following are the features of phloem fibres except
(a) pointed apices (b) more elongated (c) branched (d) unbranched

57. Phloem fibre, which is commercially used, is actually
(a) jute (b) flax (c) hemp (d) all

58. Select the incorrect matching:
(a) Protophloem – Narrow sieve tubes
(b) Metaphloem – Bigger sieve tubes
(c) Gymnosperm – Albuminous cells and sieve cells
(d) Gymnosperm – Vessels in xylem

59. A mature sieve tube differs from vessel in
(a) being nearly dead (b) lacking cytoplasm
(c) lacking a functional nucleus (d) absence of lignified walls

60. In pteridophyta and gymnosperms, which cells are present in place of companion cell?
(a) Sclereids (b) Albuminous cells
(c) Idioblasts (d) None of the above

61. Both vessels and companion cells are absent in
(a) angiosperms (b) pteridophyta (c) gymnosperms (d) both (b) and (c)

62. The only plant cells without nuclei among the following are
(a) cambium cells (b) cells of pericycle
(c) xylem parenchyma (d) sieve tubes

63. Vessels differ from tracheids
(a) in being derived from single cell
(b) in having vertical rows of cells with cross walls dissolved
(c) in being alive
(d) in helping in the conduction of water

64. Companion cells are usually seen associated with
(a) fibres (b) vessels (c) tracheids (d) sieve tubes

65. Sieve tubes are better-suited for translocation because they
(a) possess broader lumen and perforated cross walls
(b) are broader than long
(c) possess bordered pits
(d) possess no end walls

66. Lignified cell wall is the characteristic feature of
(a) phloem cells (b) epidermal cells
(c) cambial cells (d) xylem cells

67. The chief function of sieve tube is
(a) to translocate the organic materials manufactured in the leaves
(b) to conduct minerals
(c) to transport water from root to leaves
(d) to help the plant in forming wood

68. Function of storage is performed by
(a) parenchyma (b) sclerenchyma (c) phloem (d) all

69. Which is present in the vascular bundles of gymnosperms?
(a) Tracheids (b) Vessels (c) Companion cells (d) All

70. How many types of tissue systems are present in plant depending on their structure and function?
(a) 1 (b) 2 (c) 3 (d) 4

71. Tissue system include
(a) epidermal tissue system
(b) ground tissue system or fundamental tissue system
(c) vascular tissue system
(d) all

72. Epidermal tissue system is made up of
(a) epidermal cells (b) stomata
(c) epidermal appendages (d) all

73. Which of the following is epidermal appendage?
(a) Trichome (b) Guard cell
(c) Sclereid (d) Subsidiary cell

74. Select T/F (True/False).
(a) Epidermis is usually single-layered.
(b) Epidermal cells are parenchymatous cell with abundant cytoplasm.
(c) Vessel members of xylem are interconnected through perforation in their common walls.
(d) Sclerenchyma provides mechanical support to organs.
(a) TTTT (b) TFFT (c) TFTT (d) FFTT

75. The epidermis is generally covered with a waxy thick layer called the ________ which prevents the loss of water.
(a) suberin (b) tunicin (c) cuticle (d) chitin

76. Which of the following is true about stomata?
(a) Formed by guard cells
(b) Regulate process of transpiration and gaseous exchange
(c) Mainly present on epidermis of leaves
(d) All

77. Which of the following is true about guard cells?
(a) Outer wall is thin
(b) Inner wall (towards stomatal pore) is thick
(c) Bean-shaped in dicots and dumb-bell-shaped in grasses
(d) All

78. Which of the following cell posses chloroplast?
(a) Mesophyll cells of leaf (b) Guard cells
(c) Sometimes in cells of collenhcyma (d) All

79. Stomatal apparatus consists of
(a) subsidiary cells (b) guard cells (c) stomatal aperture (d) all

80. Stem hairs are
(a) unicellular (b) acellular (c) multicellular (d) any of them

81. Trichomes are
(a) epidermal hair of stem (b) either soft or stiff
(c) branched or unbranched (d) all

82. Select the incorrect statement from the following:
(a) Trichomes help in preventing water loss due to transpiration
(b) Cuticle prevents loss of water
(c) Cuticle is absent in roots
(d) Epidermis is made up of elongated, loosely arranged cell, which forms continuous layer

83. Ground tissue is made up of
(a) parenchyma (b) collenchyma (c) sclerenchyma (d) all

84. Parenchymatous cells are usually present in
(a) cortex, pericycle (b) pith and medullary rays
(c) primary stem and roots (d) all

85. Thin-walled chloroplast containing mesophyll cells are present in
(a) root (b) stem (c) leaf (d) all

86. Vascular system consist of
(a) simple tissue (b) complex tissue (c) xylem (d) phloem

87. Closed vascular bundle is present in
(a) monocot (b) dicot (c) both (d) none

88. Conjoint vascular bundle is present in
(a) monocot stem (b) dicot stem (c) leaf (d) all

89. A root hair is formed by
(a) epidermal cell (b) endodermal cell (c) cortical cell (d) pericycle cell

90. Epidermal outgrowths are known as
(a) stomata (b) leaves (c) trichomes (d) flower buds

91. Vascular bundles having xylem and phloem which lie at the same radius is termed as
(a) concentric (b) radial (c) collateral (d) amphicribral

92. Which of the following would not secrete a cuticle?
(a) Root epidermis (b) Leaf epidermis (c) Xerophytes (d) Stem epidermis

93. Which one of the following is a type of tissue system?
(a) Parenchyma (b) Sclerenchyma (c) Vascular (d) All

94. Root hairs are
(a) acellular (b) unicellular
(c) multicellular (d) multicellular and unicellular

95. Vascular bundles of roots are
(a) conjoint (b) concentric (c) bicollateral (d) radial

96. Radial vascular bundle can be seen in
(a) leaf (b) dicot root (c) stem (d) flower

97. When xylem and phloem are separated by a strip of cambium it is called
(a) collateral and open (b) collateral and closed
(c) bicollatoral and open (d) concentric and closed

98. Vascular bundle is closed when
(a) cambium is present (b) cambium is absent
(c) pericycle is absent (d) none

99. Following features belong to which option?
I. Cortex is made up of several layers of thin-walled parenchyma cells with intercellular spaces.
II. Endoderm is made up of single layer of barrel-shaped cells without any intercellular spaces.
III. Few layers of thick-walled parenchymatous cell forms pericycle.
IV. Pith is small or inconspicuous.
V. Conjuctive tissue present 2 to 4 xylem and phloem patches.
(a) dicot root (b) dicot stem (c) monocot root (d) monocot stem

100. Stele is made up of (in dicot root)
(a) pericycle (b) vascular bundle (c) pith (d) all

101. Outside to inside the layer of monocot root are
(a) Endodermis–Epidermis–Cortex–Pith–Vascular bundle–Pericycle
(b) Pith–Epidermis–Endodermis–Cortex–Pericycle–Vascular bundle
(c) Epidermis–Cortex–Endodermis–Pericycle–Vascular bundle–Pith
(d) Pericycle–Vascular bundle–Cortex–Pith–Epidermis–Endodermis

102. Following features belong to which option?
I. Epidermis may bear trachoma and few stomata.
II. Cortex is divided into three sub-zones.
III. Hypodermis made up of collenchymas starch sheath.
IV. Pericycle above phloem in form of semilunar patches of sclerenchyma.
(a) dicot root (b) dicot stem
(c) monocot root (d) monocot stem

103. Select the incorrect statement among the following:
(a) Ring arrangement of vascular bundle is a characteristic of dicot stem
(b) Phloem parenchyma is absent in monocot stem
(c) Monocots have sclerenchymatous hypodermis
(d) In monocot peripheral, vascular bundle, which are generally large and centrally located, are small and water-containing cavities are present within the vascular bundle

104. Which of the following is correct about dorsiventral leaf?
(a) The veins vary in thickness in the reticulate venation
(b) Palisade parenchyma is abaxially placed
(c) Abaxial surface bears no stomata
(d) The size of vascular bundles are independent on the size of veins

105. Which of the following is incorrect about isobilateral leaf?
(a) Stomata present on both surfaces
(b) Undifferentiated mesophyll
(c) Nearly same size vascular bundle present all over leaf
(d) It is monocot leaf

106. The growth of the roots and stems in length with the help of apical meristem is called
(a) secondary growth (b) primary growth (c) both (d) none

107. Dicot plant exhibits an increase in girth. It is an example of
(a) secondary growth (b) primary growth (c) both (d) none

108. Cells of cambium present between primary xylem and primary phloem forms
(a) interfascicular cambium
(b) intrafascicular cambium (fascicular cambium)
(c) cork cambium
(d) none

109. Vascular cambium is formed by
I. interfascicular cambium.
II. intrafascicular cambium.
III. cork cambium.
(a) I and III only (b) II and III only (c) I, II and III only (d) I and II only

110. Cambium wing forms cells towards
(a) inner side of ring (b) outer side of ring
(c) both side of ring (d) they do not form cells

111. Vascular Cambium activity is
(a) more on inner side than outer (b) more on outer side than inner
(c) equal on outer and inner side (d) none of the above

112. Following will not happen during secondary growth by cambium ring:
(a) Secondary xylem produced is more than secondary phloem
(b) Primary and secondary phloem crushed due to continued formation and accumulation of secondary xylem
(c) Primary xylem remain more or less intact in or around centre
(d) The cells cut off towards pith mature into secondary phloem and cells cut off towards periphery mature into secondary xylem

113. During secondary growth all occur except
(a) secondary medullar rays forms (b) phloem crushed
(c) primary phloem forms (d) secondary xylem forms

114. Activity of cambium is under control of
(a) physiological factor (b) environmental factor
(c) both (d) none

115. Select total number of correct statements from the following:
(1) In spring season cambium is active and produces a large number of xylary elements having vessels with wider lumen.
(2) Spring wood is also known as early wood.
(3) In winter cambium is less active and forms few xylary elements having narrow vessels this is called autumn wood or late wood.
(4) Spring wood is lighter in color and has lower density.
(5) Autumn wood is darker and has higher density.
(6) Annual ring (autumn wood and spring wood) used to estimate the age of plant.
(a) 3 (b) 4 (c) 5 (d) 6

116. In older trees greater part of secondary xylem is dark brown due to deposition of
(a) tannins and resins (b) oil and gums
(c) aromatic substance and essential oil (d) all

117. Dark brown deposition of organic compound in heartwood will make it
(a) hard (b) durable
(c) resistant to microbes and pest (d) all

118. Heartwood contain
(a) live lignified element (b) dead highly lignified element
(c) live non-lignified element (d) dead non-lignified elements

119. Function of heartwood is
(a) conduction of water (b) conduction of mineral
(c) conduction of food (d) mechanical support

120. Peripheral region of secondary xylem, which is light in color, is known as
(a) heartwood (duramen) (b) sapwood (alburnum)
(c) spring wood (d) autumn wood

121. The cells of secondary cortex are
(a) parenchymatous (b) sclerenchymatous
(c) collenchymatous (d) meristems

122. Bark refers to
(a) periderm (b) secondary phloem
(c) both (d) none

123. At certain region, the phellogen cuts off closely arranged parenchymatous cells on the outer side instead of cork cells. These parenchymatous cells soon rupture epidermis, forming a lens-shaped opening called
(a) hydathodes (b) stomata (c) lenticels (d) none

124. Which of the following is correct about lenticels?
(a) It is present in most woody trees (b) It helps in gaseous exchange
(c) It is formed by activity of phellogen (d) All

125. In dicot root vascular cambium is
(a) completely primary in origin (b) partly primary and partly secondary
(c) completely secondary in origin (d) none

126. Initially formed cambium in dicot root is
(a) circular (b) rectangular (c) oval (d) wavy

127. Secondary growth occur in
(a) dicot root (b) dicot stem
(c) stem and root of gymnosperm (d) all

128. Which of the following is incorrect?
(a) Wood is actually a secondary xylem
(b) Different type of woods are found on basis of their composition and time of production
(c) Monocot and dicot show marked variation in their internal structure
(d) Increase in girth of dicot stem by vascular cambium only

129. Main functions of plant tissues are
(a) assimilation of food and its storage
(b) transportation of water, mineral and photosynthates
(c) mechanical support
(d) all

130. Cambium causes growth in
(a) circumference (b) width (diameter)
(c) leaves (d) length

131. The function of cork cambium (phellogen) is to produce
(a) cork and secondary cortex (b) secondary xylem and secondary phloem
(c) cork (d) secondary cortex and phloem

132. Other names of secondary cortex, cork cambium and cork are
(a) phellem, phelloderm and phellogen (b) phellogen, phellem and phelloderm
(c) phelloderm, phellogen and phellem (d) phellogen, phelloderm and phellem

133. In dicot roots, vascular cambium is derived from
(a) epidermis (b) hypodermis (c) cortex (d) pericycle

134. Periderm is made up of
(a) phellem (b) phellogen (c) phelloderm (d) all

135. Cork cells are
(a) dead (b) photosynthetic
(c) elongated and participate in movement (d) meristematic

136. Annual rings are distinct in plants growing in
(a) tropical regions (b) arctic region
(c) grasslands (d) temperate region

137. Xylem, which is functional in a dicot tree, is
(a) spring wood (b) sap wood (c) autumn wood (d) heart wood

138. External protective tissues of plants (of dicot stem are)
(a) cork and pericycle (b) cortex and epidermis
(c) pericycle and cortex (d) epidermis and cork

139. Cork cambium is a
(a) secondary meristem (b) apical meristem
(c) intercalary meristem (d) primary meristem

140. Cambium, which produces cork, is known as
(a) phelloderm (b) phellogen (c) periblem (d) periderm

141. Dendrochronology is the study of
(a) height of a tree
(b) diameter of a tree
(c) age of a tree by counting the number of annual rings in the main stem
(d) none

142. The tissue made up of thin-walled rectangular cells responsible for the secondary growth is
(a) cortex (b) xylem (c) cambium (d) pith

143. In old dicot stems, a major part of the wood is filled up with tannins, resins, gums etc. This part of wood is called
(a) hard wood (b) heart wood (c) sap wood (d) soft wood

144. Lenticel develops through the activity of
(a) vascular cambium (b) dermatogens
(c) phellogen (d) intercalary meristem

145. The waxy substance associated with cell walls of cork cells are impervious to water because of the presence of ________, which gets deposited on cork cells
(a) cutin (b) suberin (c) lignin (d) hemicellulose

146. Growth rings determine
(a) age (b) length
(c) breadth (d) number of branches of a plant

147. Lenticels are formed in bark, which are
(a) aerating pores
(b) made up of phloem
(c) made up of xylem
(d) found in monocot plants

148. Heart wood or duramen is
(a) outer region of secondary xylem
(b) inner region of secondary xylem
(c) outer region of secondary phloem
(d) inner region of secondary phloem

149. The bark of tree comprises
(a) all the tissues outside the vascular cambium
(b) all the tissues outside the cork cambium
(c) only the cork
(d) the cork and secondary cortex

150. Layer of cells between endodermis and vascular bundles is called
(a) epidermis
(b) pericycle
(c) hypodermis
(d) pith

151. Bulliform or motor cells are present in
(a) dicot stem
(b) upper epidermis of dicot leaves
(c) lower epidermis of monocot leaves
(d) upper epidermis of monocot leaves

152. Exarch and polyarch vascular bundles occur in
(a) monocot stem
(b) monocot root
(c) dicot stem
(d) dicot root

153. In root, xylem is
(a) mesarch
(b) exarch
(c) placed at different places in different plants
(d) endarch

154. In monocot leaf
(a) bulliform cells are absent from the epidermis
(b) veins form a network
(c) mesophyll is well differentiated into these parts
(d) mesophyll is not differentiated into palisade and spongy parenchyma

155. In dicot root
(a) vascular bundles are scattered and with cambium
(b) vascular bundles are arranged in a ring and have cambium
(c) xylem and phloem are radially arranged
(d) xylem is always endarch

156. Well-developed pith is found in
(a) monocot stem and dicot root
(b) monocot and dicot stems
(c) dicot stem and dicot root
(d) dicot stem and monocot root

157. The correct situation of mesophyll in isobilateral grass leaf is shown by
(a) palisade towards adaxial surface
(b) palisade towards abaxial surface
(c) undifferentiated mesophyll
(d) palisade along both the surface

158. Monocot root differs from dicot root in having
(a) open vascular bundles
(b) scattered vascular bundles
(c) well-developed pith
(d) radially arranged vascular bundles

159. Vascular bundles are scattered in
(a) bryophytes
(b) dicot root
(c) dicot stem
(d) monocot stem

160. Generally hypodermis in monocots is composed of
(a) parenchyma (b) sclerenchyma
(c) collenchymas (d) chlorenchyma

161. Polyarch condition is seen in
(a) monocot stem (b) monocot root
(c) dicot root (d) dicot stem

162. Which of the following is not a characteristic feature of the anatomy of dicotyledonous root?
(a) Radial vascular bundles (b) Secondary growth
(c) Pith little or absent (d) conjoint collateral

163. Endodermis of dicot stem is also called
(a) bundle sheath (b) starch sheath (c) mesophyll (d) pith

164. The cell layer located at the periphery in the cross-section of the root is called
(a) endodermis (b) epiblema (c) pericycle (d) xylem

165. Exarch xylem is found in
(a) root (b) stem (c) leaf (d) rachis

166. Two to four xylem bundle are found in
(a) monocot root (b) monocot stem (c) dicot stem (d) dicot root

167. Collenchymatous hypodermis is characteristics of
(a) dicot stem (b) monocot stem
(c) monocot as well as dicot stem (d) hydrophytes

168. Vascular bundles in dicot stem are
(a) conjoint and collateral (b) conjoint and closed
(c) conjoint, collateral and open (d) collateral and open

169. Cortex and pith are not distinguished in
(a) dicot stem (b) monocot stem (c) dicot root (d) monocot root

170. In a dorsiventral leaf, location of palisade tissue and phloem are known as
(a) abaxial and abaxial (b) adaxial and abaxial
(c) adaxial and adaxial (d) abaxial and adaxial

171. Which of the following is seen in a monocot root?
(a) Large pith (b) Vascular cambium
(c) Endarch xylem (d) Medullary ray

172. In what respect, the pericycle of a root differs from that of the stem?
(a) Sclerenchymatous in root and collenchymatous in stem
(b) Collenchymatous in root and parenchymatous in stem
(c) Parenchymatous in root and sclerenchymatous in stem
(d) Parenchymatous in root and collenchymatous in stem

173. Collenchyma generally occurs
(a) in scattered dicot roots
(b) in a ring in monocot roots
(c) in patches under epidermis in dicot stem
(d) in all of the above

174. Phloem parenchyma is absent in
(a) dicot root (b) dicot leaf
(c) monocot stem (d) dicot stem

175. Collenchyma tissue is present in
(a) dicot stem (b) monocot stem
(c) dicot root (d) flowers

176. The vascular bundles in the stem of monocots are typically
(a) collateral (b) bicollateral
(c) concentric (d) radial

177. Sclerenchymatous sheath is present in vascular bundles of
(a) monocot root (b) dicot root
(c) dicot stem (d) monocot stem

178. In monocot roots which types of vascular bundles are found?
(a) Collateral, conjoint and closed
(b) Radial V.B. with exarch xylem
(c) Bicollateral, conjoint and closed
(d) Radial V.B. with endarch xylem

179. Lateral roots arise from
(a) pericycle (b) pith (c) stem (d) root

180. In dicot roots, cells of which region show casparian strips?
(a) Cambium (b) Endodermis (c) Pericycle (d) Hypodermis

181. In the diagram of T.S. of Stele of Dicot Root, the different parts have been indicated by alphabets. Choose the answer in which these alphabets correctly match with the parts they indicate.

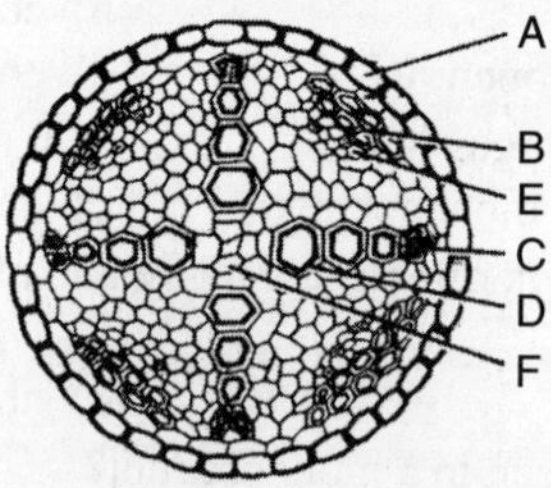

(a) A – Endodermis, B – Conjunctive tissue, C – Metaxylem, D – Protoxylem, E – Phloem, F – Pith
(b) A – Endodermis, B – Pith, C – Protoxylem, D – Metaxylem, E – Protoxylem, F – Conjuctive tissue
(c) A – Pericycle, B – Conjuctive tissue, C – Metaxylem, D – Protoxylem, F : Endodermis
(d) A – Endodermis, B – Conjuctive tissue, C – Protoxylem, D – Metaxylem, E – Phloem F – Pith

182. In grasses,
(a) certain adaxial epidermal cells along the veins modify themselves into large, empty, colourless cells. These are called bulliform cells
(b) when the bulliform cells in the leaves absorb water and are turgid, the leaf surface is exposed
(c) when bulliform cells are flaccid due to water stress, they make the leaves curl inwards to minimise water loss
(d) all are correct

*Read the **assertion** and **reason** carefully to mark the correct option out of the options given below:*

(a) If both the assertion and the reason are true and the reason is a correct explanation of the assertion

(b) If both the assertion and reason are true but the reason is not a correct explanation of the assertion

(c) If the assertion is true but the reason is false

(d) If both the assertion and reason are false

183. Assertion: All tissues lying inside vascular cambium are called as bark.
Reason: Bark is made up of phellogen, phellem and phelloderm lying inside secondary phloem.

184. Assertion: Stomata are absent in submerged hydrophytes.
Reason: Respiration occurs by means of air chambers in submerged plants.

185. Assertion: Cambium is a lateral meristem and cause growth in width.
Reason: Cambium is made up of fusiform and ray initials in stem.

186. Assertion: Higher plants have meristematic regions for indefinite growth.
Reason: Higher plants have root and shoot apices.

187. Assertion: In collateral vascular bundles phloem is situated towards inner side.
Reason: In monocot stem, cambium is present.

188. Assertion: Thick cuticle is mostly present in disease resistant plants.
Reason: Disease causing agents cannot grow on cuticle and cannot invade the cuticle.

189. Assertion: Quiescent centre is found in the centre of the root apex.
Reason: It consists of actively dividing cells.

190. Assertion: Permanent tissue is composed of mature cells.
Reason: Meristematic tissue is a group of actively dividing cells.

191. Assertion: Intercalary meristem increase length of plant like apical meristems.
Reason: Intercalary meristem originates from the apical meristems.

192. Assertion: The lenticel is meant for gaseous exchange.
Reason: Lenticel checks excessive evaporation of water.

193. Assertion: Xerophytic leaves may contain stomatal crypts or sunken stomata.
Reason: Spongy parenchyma is more in xerophytic leaves.

194. Assertion: Isobilateral leaves are amphistomatic.
Reason: Mesophyll is not differentiated into palisade and spongy.

195. Assertion: Trichomes helps in preventing water loss due to transpiration.
Reason: On the stem epidermal hairs are called trichomes.

196. Assertion: Growth rings are also called as annual rings.
Reason: Generally growth ring is formed in each year.

197. Assertion: Heartwood is more durable than the sapwood.
Reason: Heartwood contain organic compound like tannins,resins,oil,gumsaromatic substances and essential oils make it hard and more durable.

198. Assertion: Sugarcane shows Kranz anatomy.
Reason: In diocot leaves, bundle sheath cells lack chloroplasts.

AIPMT PREVIOUS YEAR QUESTIONS

1. Kranz anatomy is one of the characteristics of the leaves of [AIPMT MAINS 2010]
   (a) Potato (b) Wheat
   (c) Sugarcane (d) Mustard
2. Give below is the diagram of a stomatal apparatus. In which of the following, all the four parts labelled as A, B, C, D are correctly identified?

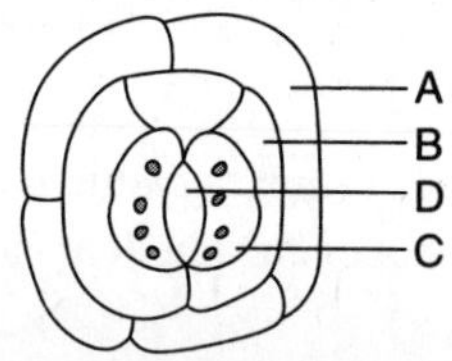

[AIPMT MAINS 2010]
   (a) A: Subsidiary cell, B: Epidermal cell, C: Guard cell, D: Stomatal aperture
   (b) A: Guard cell, B: Stomatal aperature, C: Subsidiary cell, D: Epidermal cell
   (c) A: Epidermal cell, B: Guard cell, C: Stomatal aperture, D: Subsidiary cell
   (d) A: Epidermal cell, B: Subsidiary cell, C: Guard cell, D: Stomatal aperture
3. The chief water conducting elements of xylem in gymnosperms are [AIPMT PRE 2010]
   (a) Vessels (b) Fibres
   (c) Transfusion tissue (d) Tracheids
4. Which one of the following is not a lateral meristem? [AIPMT PRE 2010]
   (a) Intrafascicular cambium (b) Interfascicular cambium
   (c) Phellogen (d) Intercalary meristem
5. Heartwood differs from sapwood in: [AIPMT PRE 2010]
   (a) Presence of rays and fibres
   (b) Absence of vessels and parenchyma
   (c) Having dead and non-conducting elements
   (d) Being susceptible to pests and pathogens
6. Some vascular bundles are described as open because these: [AIPMT MAINS 2011]
   (a) Are surrounded by pericycle but no endodermis
   (b) Are capable of producing secondary xylem and phloem
   (c) Possess conjunctive tissue between xylem and phloem
   (d) Are not surrounded by pericycle
7. In Kranz anatomy, the bundle sheath cells have [AIPMT MAINS 2011]
   (a) Thin walls, many intercellular spaces and no chloroplasts
   (b) Thick walls, no intercellular spaces and large number of chloroplasts
   (c) Thin walls, no intercellular spaces and several chloroplasts
   (d) Thick walls, many intercellular spaces and few chloroplasts

8. Ground tissue includes: [AIPMT PRE 2011]
   (a) All tissues except epidermis and vascular bundles
   (b) Epidermis and cortex
   (c) All tissues internal to endodermis
   (d) All tissues external to endodermis
9. In land plants, the guard cells differ from other epidermal cells in having: [AIPMT PRE 2011]
   (a) Mitochondria (b) Endoplasmic reticulum
   (c) Chloroplasts (d) Cytoskeleton
10. The cork cambium, cork and secondary cortex are collectively called: [AIPMT PRE 2011]
   (a) Phellogen (b) Periderm
   (c) Phellem (d) Phelloderm
11. As compared to a dicot root, a monocot root has: [AIPMT MAINS 2012]
   (a) Many xylem bundles
   (b) Inconspicuous annual rings
   (c) Relatively thicker periderm
   (d) More abundant secondary xylem
12. The common bottle cork is a product of: [AIPMT PRE 2012]
   (a) Dermatogen (b) Phellogen
   (c) Xylem (d) Vascular Cambium
13. Closed vascular bundles lack: [AIPMT PRE 2012]
   (a) Ground tissue (b) Conjunctive tissue
   (c) Cambium (d) Pith
14. Water containing cavities in vascular bundles are found in: [AIPMT PRE 2012]
   (a) Sunflower (b) Maize
   (c) Cycas (d) Pinus
15. Gymnosperms are also called soft wood spermatophytes because they lack: [AIPMT PRE 2012]
   (a) Cambium (b) Phloem fibres
   (c) Thick – walled tracheids (d) Xylem fibres
16. Interfascicular cambium develops from the cells of: [AIPMT 2013]
   (a) Medullary rays (b) Xylem parenchyma
   (c) Endodermis (d) Pericycle
17. Lenticels are involved in: [AIPMT 2013]
   (a) Transpiration (b) Gaseous exchange
   (c) Food transport (d) Photosynthesis

18. Age of a tree can be estimated by:

[AIPMT 2013]

(a) Its height and girth
(b) Biomass
(c) Number of annual rings
(d) Diameter of its heartwood

19. You are given a fairly old piece of dicot stem and a dicot root. Which of the following anatomical structures will you use to distinguish between the two?

[AIPMT 2014]

(a) Secondary xylem
(b) Secondary phloem
(c) Protoxylem
(d) Cortical cells

20. Tracheids differ from other tracheary element in:

[AIPMT 2014]

(a) Having casparian strips
(b) Being imperforate
(c) Lacking nucleus
(d) Being lignified

21. Vascular bundles in monocotyledons are considered closed because:

[AIPMT 2015]

(a) A bundle sheath surrounds each bundles
(b) Cambium is absent
(c) There are no vessels with perforations
(d) Xylem is surrounded all around by phloem

22. A major characteristic of the monocot root is the presence of:

[AIPMT 2015]

(a) Open vascular bundles
(b) Scattered vascular bundles
(c) Vasculature without cambium
(d) Xylem along the radius

23. Read the different components from (a) to (d) in the list given below and tell the correct order of the components with reference to their arrangement from outer side to inner side in a woody dicot stem:

(a) Secondary cortex
(b) Wood
(c) Secondary cortex
(d) Phellem

The correct order is:

[RE-AIPMT 2015]

(a) (A), (b), (d), (c)
(b) (d), (a), (c), (b)
(c) (d), (c), (a), (b)
(d) (c), (d), (b), (a)

Answer Keys

1. (c)	2. (d)	3. (c)	4. (b)	5. (d)	6. (a)	7. (d)	8. (c)	9. (c)	10. (d)
11. (c)	12. (d)	13. (b)	14. (a)	15. (a)	16. (b)	17. (a)	18. (c)	19. (d)	20. (d)
21. (d)	22. (d)	23. (d)	24. (c)	25. (b)	26. (a)	27. (b)	28. (d)	29. (b)	30. (c)
31. (b)	32. (b)	33. (d)	34. (b)	35. (c)	36. (a)	37. (d)	38. (d)	39. (b)	40. (c)
41. (d)	42. (d)	43. (d)	44. (d)	45. (c)	46. (d)	47. (b)	48. (c)	49. (d)	50. (d)
51. (c)	52. (d)	53. (d)	54. (d)	55. (d)	56. (c)	57. (d)	58. (d)	59. (d)	60. (b)
61. (d)	62. (d)	63. (b)	64. (d)	65. (a)	66. (d)	67. (a)	68. (a)	69. (a)	70. (c)
71. (d)	72. (d)	73. (a)	74. (c)	75. (c)	76. (d)	77. (d)	78. (d)	79. (d)	80. (c)

81. (d) 82. (d) 83. (d) 84. (d) 85. (c) 86. (b) 87. (a) 88. (d) 89. (a) 90. (c)
91. (c) 92. (a) 93. (c) 94. (b) 95. (d) 96. (b) 97. (a) 98. (b) 99. (a) 100. (d)
101. (c) 102. (b) 103. (d) 104. (a) 105. (c) 106. (b) 107. (a) 108. (b) 109. (d) 110. (c)
111. (a) 112. (d) 113. (c) 114. (c) 115. (d) 116. (d) 117. (d) 118. (b) 119. (d) 120. (b)
121. (a) 122. (c) 123. (c) 124. (d) 125. (c) 126. (d) 127. (d) 128. (d) 129. (d) 130. (b)
131. (a) 132. (c) 133. (d) 134. (d) 135. (a) 136. (d) 137. (b) 138. (d) 139. (a) 140. (b)
141. (c) 142. (c) 143. (b) 144. (c) 145. (b) 146. (a) 147. (a) 148. (b) 149. (a) 150. (b)
151. (d) 152. (b) 153. (b) 154. (d) 155. (c) 156. (d) 157. (c) 158. (c) 159. (d) 160. (b)
161. (b) 162. (d) 163. (b) 164. (b) 165. (a) 166. (d) 167. (a) 168. (c) 169. (b) 170. (b)
171. (a) 172. (c) 173. (c) 174. (c) 175. (a) 176. (a) 177. (d) 178. (b) 179. (a) 180. (b)
181. (d) 182. (d) 183. (d) 184. (b) 185. (b) 186. (a) 187. (d) 188. (a) 189. (c) 190. (a)
191. (a) 192. (b) 193. (c) 194. (b) 195. (b) 196. (a) 197. (a) 198. (c)

AIPMT Previous Year Questions

1. (c) 2. (d) 3. (d) 4. (d) 5. (c) 6. (b) 7. (b) 8. (a) 9. (c) 10. (b)
11. (a) 12. (b) 13. (c) 14. (b) 15. (c) 16. (a) 17. (b) 18. (c) 19. (c) 20. (b)
21. (b) 22. (c) 23. (b)

CHAPTER 7

Structural Organization in Animals

1. What do you call an organization of group of similar cells along with intercellular substances?
(a) Organ (b) System (c) Tissue (d) Cell membrane
2. To establish a system of organ system what kind of interaction occurs to form a common function?
(a) Physical (b) Chemical (c) Both (d) Symbiotic
3. Which of the following is correct for epithelial tissue?
(a) It is present only inner lining (b) It is present only as outer lining
(c) Contains very less intracellular matrix (d) All
4. Which of the following contain simple epithelium as their lining?
(a) Ducts (b) Tubes (c) Both (a) and (b) (d) Skin of mouth
5. Which of the following tissue has a free surface?
(a) Connective tissue (b) Muscular tissue (c) Epithelial tissue (d) Neural tissue
6. Which of the following is not a simple epithelium?
(a) Squamous (b) Cuboidal (c) Columnar (d) None
7. Which of the following sites contain squamous epithelium as its living?
(a) Blood vessel (b) Air sac in lungs (c) Nasal cavity (d) Both (a) and (b)
8. Secretion and absorption is done by what kind of epithelium?
(a) Squamous epithelium (b) Cuboidal epithelium
(c) Columnar epithelium (d) Ciliated columnar epithelium
9. Which of the following epithelium is irregularly shaped?
(a) Squamous epithelium (b) Cuboidal epithelium
(c) Columnar epithelium (d) Ciliated columnar epithelium
10. Cuboidal epithelium can be found in
(a) Distal convoluted tubule (b) Proximal convoluted tubule
(c) Henle's loop (d) Both (a) and (b)
11. In columnar epithelium, where is nucleus located?
(a) At the base (b) In the middle
(c) At the top (d) No nucleus present
12. If the cuboidal epithelium turns out to have microvilli on it, what will it be called?
(a) Ciliated columnar epithelium (b) Pseudo ciliated epithelium
(c) Both (d) Ciliated epithelium

13. Where is columnar epithelium found?
(a) Lining of intestine (b) Outer wall of stomach
(c) Proximal convoluted tubule (d) All
14. Where is ciliated epithelium found?
(a) Bronchioles (b) Fallopian tubes (c) Both (d) Lungs
15. Cuboidal or columnar epithelium specialized for secretion are called _________.
(a) ciliated epithelium (b) glandular epithelium
(c) both (d) none
16. Which of the following is unicellular glandular epithelium?
(a) Salivary gland (b) Islets of langer han's
(c) Goblet cells (d) All
17. Which of the following is not secreted by exocrine glands?
(a) Earwax (b) Oil (c) Milk (d) None
18. Whose products are called hormone and where are they secreted?
(a) Exocrine, Blood (b) Endocrine, Blood
(c) Exocrine, lymph (d) Endocrine, Fluid bathing the gland
19. Which of the following functions of compound epithelium is minimal?
(a) Protection (b) Secretion (c) Absorption (d) Both (b) and (c)
20. Where we will not find the compound epithelium?
(a) Dry skin surface (b) Moist surface of mouth
(c) Pharynx (d) Pancreas
21. What is the function of tight junction?
(a) Protect from bacterial infection (b) Stop substance leaking across the tissue
(c) Both (d) Elasticity to the tissue
22. What is the function of Adhering junction?
(a) Cementing to keep neighbouring cells together
(b) Give rigidity to tissue
(c) Stop leaking substance across the tissue
(d) All
23. Which of the following junctions facilitate the cells to communicate with each other by connecting the cytoplasm of adjoining cells?
(a) Tight junction (b) Adhering junction
(c) Gap junction (d) Both (b) and (c)
24. Big molecules can be transported to the neighbouring cell by which of the following junction?
(a) Adhering junction (b) Gap junction
(c) Both (a) and (b) (d) Not possible for big molecules
25. Which tissue links and supports other tissues/organs of the body?
(a) Epithelial tissue (b) Connective tissue (c) Neural tissue (d) All
26. In which of the following connective tissues elastin fibres are absent?
(a) Bone (b) Cartilage (c) Blood (d) Both (a) and (b)
27. Matrix or ground substance in connective tissues are made up of _________ .
(a) thick proteins (b) elastin fibres
(c) modified polysaccharides (d) modified triglycerides
28. Which of the following possess semi-fluid ground substance?
(a) Aerolar tissue (b) Adipose tissue (c) Blood (d) Both (a) and (b)

29. Which of the following is not a part of aerolar tissue?
(a) Fibroblasts (b) Mast cells (c) Fibro clasts (d) All

30. Where is the excess unused nutrition stored in our body?
(a) Aerolar tissue (b) Adipose tissue (c) Both (d) Blood

31. In which tissue Fibres and fibroblasts are completely packed?
(a) Dense regular connective tissue (b) Dense irregular connective tissue
(c) Both (d) Cartilage

32. Which structures are joined by tendons?
(a) Skeletal muscles to bones (b) Skeletal muscles to ligaments
(c) Both (a) and (b) (d) Bones to ligaments

33. Which of the following tissue is not present in skin?
(a) Epithelial tissue (b) Dense connective (c) Aerolar tissue (d) All

34. Which of the following is/are example of dense connective tissue?
(a) Tendon (b) Cartilage (c) Ligament (d) All

35. What kind of tissue is goblet cells?
(a) Epithelial tissue (b) Connective tissue (c) Neural tissue (d) All

36. Which portion of cartilage provides it with solidity, pliability and resistance to compression?
(a) Collagen fibres (b) Calcium content
(c) Intracellular material (d) Chondrocytes

37. What provides bone with hard and non-pliable properties?
(a) Collagen fibres (b) Calcium salts (c) Both (d) None

38. Where are osteocytes located?
(a) Entire bone (b) In lacunae (c) Both (d) None

39. Which of the following is not true?
(a) Limb bones are long bones
(b) The function of long bones is weight bearing and bringing out movement
(c) Bone marrows in all such long bones are site of blood cells production
(d) All

40. What is the main function of blood?
(a) Protection of body (b) Transport of various substances
(c) pH buffering (d) Maintaining osmocarity balance

41. The long cylindrical fibres that form a muscle is made up of________ .
(a) tinofibriles (b) collagen fibres (c) fibroblasts (d) myofibrils

42. When muscle cells receive stimulus, they get _________ .
(a) shortend (b) lengthend (c) elongated (d) all

43. Muscular movement are intended to _________ .
(a) move the body to adjust to changes in environment
(b) maintain position of various body parts
(c) both
(d) none

44. Which of the following is a typical skeletal muscle?
(a) Biceps (b) Triceps (c) Both (d) None

45. The sheath enclosing the several bundles of muscle fibres is _________ tissue.
(a) epithelial (b) connective (c) both (d) neural

46. Which of the following is a fusiform muscle?
(a) Cardiac muscle (b) Smooth muscle (c) Both (a) and (b) (d) Skeletal muscle

47. Smooth muscles are held together by _________ .
(a) connective tissue (b) cell junctions (c) epithelial tissue (d) none

48. Where can we find smooth muscles?
(a) Artery (b) Vein (c) Stomach (d) All

49. Fusion of what sticks the cardiac muscles together?
(a) Cell junctions (b) Plasma membranes
(c) Intercalated disc (d) All

50. Intercalated discs in cardiac muscles provide _________ .
(a) tight junctions (b) communication junction
(c) flexible junction (d) all

51. Which of the following is not true for intercalated discs?
(a) Found only in heart
(b) All the fusion points form intercalated disc
(c) One stimulus is enough for multiple muscle
(d) None

52. Which of the following are excitable cells?
(a) Muscle cells (b) Neural cells (c) Both (d) None

53. Which of the following cells are found in neural tissue?
(a) Neuron (b) Neuroglia (c) Both (d) None

54. What is the function of Neuroglia?
(a) Protect and support neurons (b) Act as intracellular matrix
(c) Both (d) None

55. The electrical disturbance generated in neurons travels through _________ .
(a) neuroglial cell (b) cytoplasm (c) plasma membrane (d) all

56. What kind of action can be caused by neurons?
(a) Stimulatory (b) Inhibitory (c) Both (a) and (b) (d) Excitatory

57. What is the importance of organized organ system?
(a) Optimum efficiency of cells (b) Co-ordinated activity of cells
(c) Both (a) and (b) (d) None

58. Heart contains which of the following kind of tissue?
(a) Epithelial tissue (b) Cardiac muscular tissue
(c) Connective tissue (d) All

59. What is discernable trend?
(a) Complexity of organ system (b) Evolutionary trend
(c) Inheritance trend (d) All

60. What do you call the study of form or externally visible features?
(a) Physiology (b) Morphology (c) Anthropology (d) None

61. What do you call the study of morphology of internal organs in the animals?
(a) Physiology (b) Anatomy (c) Internal morphology
(d) None

62. Earthworm can be traced by faecal deposits. What are they called?
(a) Worm deposits (b) Worm castings (c) Both (d) None

63. Which of the following type are of Indian earthworms?
(a) Pheretima (b) Lumbricus (c) Lumbricoidus (d) Both (a) and (b)

64. Size of cockroach ranges from
(a) ¼" to 3" (b) 1 to 3" (c) 2 to 3" (d) ¼" to ¾"

65. Cockroach is
(a) Omnivores (b) Nocturnal (c) Cursorial (d) All
66. Which one is correct about cockroach?
(a) Generally brown and black color (b) Pest and vectors of several disease
(c) Found in damp places (d) All
67. Zoological name of cockroach is
(a) Periplaneta americana (b) Pheretima posthuma
(c) Rana tigrina (d) Maja maja
68 In each segment exoskeleton has hardened plates in cockroach known as
(a) Sclerites (b) Sternum (c) Carapace (d) All
69 Body of cockroach is segmented and divisible into three distinct region known as
(a) Head (b) Thorax (c) Abdomen (4) All
70. Head of cockroach is formed by fusion of how many segments
(a) 4 (b) 5 (c) 6 (d) 8
71. Cockroach has which type of mouth parts
(a) Biting and chewing type (b) Siphoning type
(c) Sponging type (d) All
72. How many filamentous Malpighian tubules are found in cockroach?
(a) 100–150 (b) 50–100 (c) 150–200 (d) 200–250
73. A ring of 6–8 blind tubules are present at the junction of foregut and midgut in cockroach is known as
(a) Hepatic caecae (b) Gastric caecae
(c) Both (a) and (b) (d) Malpighian tubules
74. It midget of cockroach contain
(a) ileum (b) colon (c) rectum (d) all
75. Heamolymph of cockroach consist of
(a) Plasma (b) Haemocyte
(c) Both (a) and (b) (d) None
76. Alary muscles one found in
(a) Frog (b) Earthworm
(c) Cockroach (d) Hookworm
77. How many pairs of spiracles present on surface of cockroach
(a) 5 Pairs (b) 15 Pairs (c) 10 Pairs (d) 20 Pairs
78. In cockroach following organ help in excretion
(a) Fat body (b) Nephrocyte
(c) Urecose gland (d) All
79. How many ganglia lie in thorax and abdomen of cockroach
(a) 3 and 6 (b) 6 and 3 (c) 2 and 1 (d) 1 and 2
80. If the head of cockroach is cut off, it will live for as long as
(a) 2 week (b) 1 week (c) 3 week (d) 4 week
81. Mosaic vision means
(a) More sensitivity and less resolution
(b) More sensitivity and more resolution
(c) Less sensitivity and less resolution
(d) Less sensitivity and more resolution

82. A pair of testes in cockroach lie in
(a) 2–4 abdominal segment (b) 4–6 abdominal segment
(c) 4–7 abdominal segment (d) 6–8 abdominal segment

83. External genitalia in cockroach in represented by
(a) Male gonophysis (b) Phallomere
(c) Ejaculatory duct (d) Both (a) and (b)

84. Each ovary in cockroach is made up of how many ovarian tubules or ovarioles
(a) 6 (b) 4 (c) 8 (d) 10

85. Match the column:

Column I		Column II
1. Pair of spermatheca	–	A. 2–6th segment (Abdominal)
2. Ovary	–	B. 6th segment (Abdominal)
3. Mushroom shaped accessory reproductive gland	–	C. 6–7th segment (Abdominal)
4. Anal cerci	–	D. 10th segment

(a) 1–B, 2–A, 3–C, 4–D (b) 1–C, 2–B, 3–D, 4–A
(c) 1–D, 2–C, 3–A, 4–B (d) 1–A, 2–D, 3–B, 4–C

86. How many oothecae produced by female cockroach?
(a) 9–10 (b) 14–16 (c) 13 (d) 1–2

87. Nymph of cockroach grow by moulting about _______ times to reach the adult form
(a) 12 (b) 11 (c) 13 (d) 10

88. Which one of the following is incorrect statement about cockroach?
(a) They are pest because they destroy food and contaminate it with their smelly excreta
(b) All species have economic importance
(c) Development in P. americana is paurometabolus type
(d) Next to last nymphal stage has wing pads

89. Which one of the following is correct correct statement about cockroach?
(a) Anal style is present only in male cockroach
(b) Anal cerci are present only in female cockroach
(c) Each eye consist of about 1000 hexagonal ommatidia
(d) Each oothecae contain 12–14 eggs

90. What indicate A to C in given below figure.

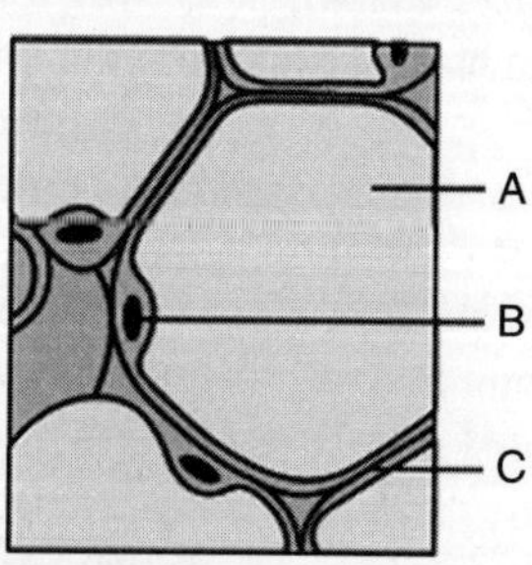

(a) A–Nucleus, B–Fat storage area, C–Plasma membrane
(b) A–Fat storage area, B–Nucleus, C–Plasma membrane
(c) A–Plasma membrane, B–Fat storage area, C–Nucleus
(d) A–Plasma membrane, B–Nucleus, C–Fat storage area

91. Identify A to D given in the figure.

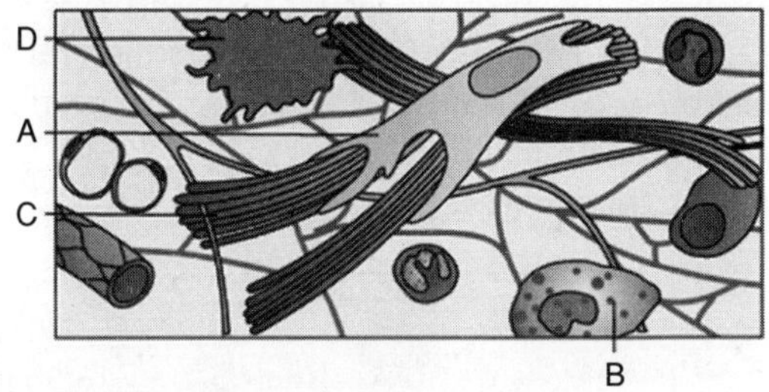

(a) A–Collagen fibres, B–Macrophage, C–Mast cell, D–Fibroblast
(b) A–Macrophage, B–Fibroblast, C–Mast cell, D–Collagen fibres
(c) A–Mast cell, B–Collagen fobres, C–Macrophage, D–Fibroblast
(d) A–Fibroblast, B–Mast cell, C–Collagen fibres, D–Macrophage

92. Identify A, B, C, D, E and F given in the figure.

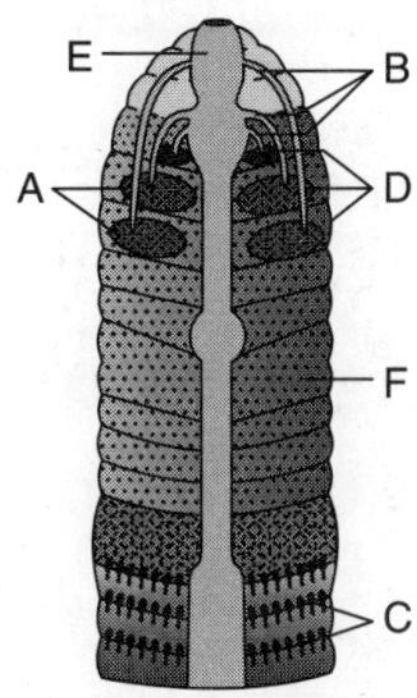

(a) A–Blood glands, B–Ducts of pharyngeal nephridia, C–Septal nephridia, D–Tufts of pharyngeal nephridia, E–Buccal cavity, F–Ingergumentary nephridia
(b) A–Ingergumentary nephridia, B–Blood glands, C–Tufts of pharyngeal nephridia, D–Buccal cavity, E–Septal nephridia, F–Ducts of pharyngeal nephridia
(c) A–Ducts of pharyngeal nephridia, B–Ingergumentary nephridia, C–Blood gland, D–Septal nephridia, E–Buccal cavity, F–Tufts of pharyngeal nephridia
(d) A–Blood glands, B–Septal nephridia, C–Buccal cavity, D–Ducts of pharngeal nephridia, E–Ingergumentary nephridia, F–Tufts of pharyngeal nephridia

93. Identify A, B and C given in the figure.

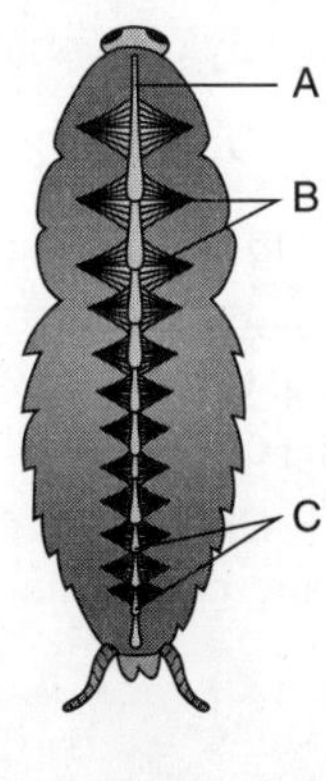

(a) A–Chambers of heart, B–Anterior aorta, C–Alary muscles
(b) A–Alary muscles, B–Chembers of heart, C–Anerior aorta
(c) A–Anterior aorta, B–Chambers of heart, C–Alary muscles
(d) A–Anterior aorta, B–Alary muscles, C–Chembers of heart

94. Identify the A, B, C, D and E in this figure.

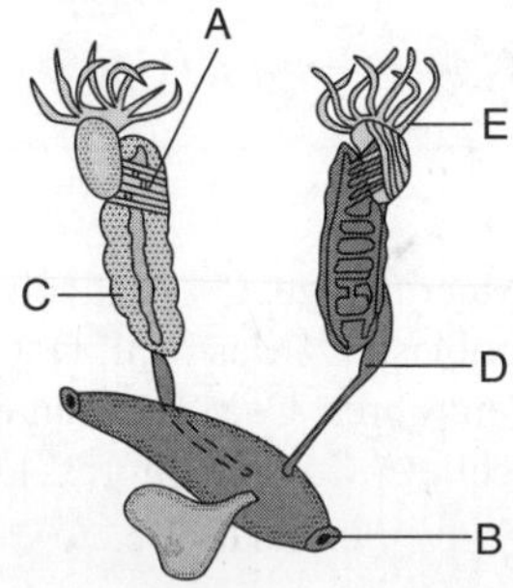

(a) A–Vasa efferentia, B–Cloacal aperture, C–Adrenal gland, D–Urino genital duct, E–Fat bodies
(b) A–Urini genital duct, B–Vasa efferentia, C–Fat bodies, D–Clocal aperture, E–Adrenal gland
(c) A–Adrenal gland, B–Urino genital duct, C–Cloacal aperture, D–Vasa efferentia, E–Fat bodies
(d) A–Fat bodies, B–Adrenal gland, C–Cloacal aperture, D–Vasa efferentia, E–Urino genital duct

*Read the **assertion** and **reason** carefully to mark the correct option out of the options given below:*

(a) If both the assertion and the reason are true and the reason is a correct explanation of the assertion
(b) If both the assertion and reason are true but the reason is not a correct explanation of the assertion
(c) If the assertion is true but the reason is false
(d) If both the assertion and reason are false

95. **Assertion:** Ciliated epithelium mainly present in the inner surface of hollow organs like bronchioles and fallopian tube.
Reason: cilia are microvilli.

96. **Assertion:** Muscle fibres are said to be contractile in nature.
Reason: Cells of muscle tissues can shorten forcefully and again return to the relaxed state.

97. **Assertion:** Gap junctions facilitate the cells to communicate with each other.
Reason: Gap junction connect the cytoplasm of adjoining cells .

98. **Assertion:** Skeletal muscle fibres appear to be striated.
Reason: This is due to regular alternate arrangement of thick and thin filaments is smooth muscle fibre.

99. **Assertion:** Non-striated muscles are said to be voluntary in nature.
Reason: Non-striated muscles can be moved according to will.
100. **Assertion:** Intercalated discs are important regions of cardiac muscle cells.
Reason: Intercalated discs function as communication junction for muscle contraction waves.
101. **Assertion:** Neurons are said to possess the property of excitability.
Reason: Neurons can get excited by a given stimulus.
102. **Assertion:** Extracellular materials help in separation of cells.
Reason: Cell junctions are formed by extra cellular materials.
103. **Assertion:** Epithelial tissues protect the under lying and over lying tissues.
Reason: Materials are exchanged at the surfaces across the epithelial tissues.
104. **Assertion:** The cells of columnar epithelium in absorptive surfaces often bears microvilli on their free ends.
Reason: Microvilli on their free ends.
105. **Assertion:** Ciliated epithelium helps in movement of particles.
Reason: Cilia help in movement.
106. **Assertion:** Extracellular materials are important for cells.
Reason: Intercellular materials surround the cells & bind them together.
107. **Assertion:** Urinary bladder can considerably expand to accommodate urine.
Reason: It is lined by stretchable transitional epithelium.

AIPMT PREVIOUS YEAR QUESTIONS

1. The kind of epithelium which forms the inner walls of blood vessels is [AIPMT PRE 2010]
(a) Cuboidal epithelium
(b) Columnar epithelium
(c) Ciliated columnar epithelium
(d) Squamous epithelium
2. If for some reason our goblet cells are non-functional, this will adversely affect [AIPMT PRE 2010]
(a) Production of somatostatin
(b) Secretion of sebum from the sebaceous glands
(c) Maturation of sperms
(d) Smooth movement of food down the intestine
3. The cells lining the blood vessels belong to the category of [AIPMT MAINS 2011]
(a) Smooth muscle tissue (b) Squamous epithelium
(c) Columnar epithelium (d) Connective tissue
4. Consider the following four statements (A–D) related to the common frog *Rana tigrina*, the select the correct option stating which ones are true (T) and which ones are false (F) statement?
(A) On dry land it would die due to lack of O_2 if its mouth is forcibly kept closed for a few days.
(B) It has four-chambered heart.
(C) On dry land it turns uricotelic from ureotelic.
(D) Its life-history is carried out in pond water.

[AIPMT MAINS 2011]

	A	B	C	D
(a)	T	F	F	T
(b)	T	T	F	F
(c)	F	F	T	T
(d)	F	T	T	F

5. Which one of the following structures in Pheretima is correctly matched with its function?

[AIPMT MAINS 2011]

(a) Clitellum – secretes cocoon
(b) Gizzard – absorbs digested food
(c) Setae – defence against predators
(d) Typhlosole – storage of extra nutrients

6. Ureters act as urinogenital ducts in

[AIPMT MAINS 2011]

(a) Human males
(b) Human females
(c) Both male and female frogs
(d) Male frogs

7. The type of muscle present in our

[AIPMT MAINS 2011]

(a) Heart is involuntary and unstriated smooth muscle
(b) Intestine is striated and involuntary
(c) Thigh is striated and involuntary
(d) Upper arm is smooth muscle and fusiform in shape

8. One very special feature in the earthworm Pheretima is that:

[AIPMT PRE 2011]

(a) The typhlosole greatly increases the effective absorption area of the digested food in the intestine
(b) The S-shaped setae embedded in the integument are the defensive weapons used against the enemies
(c) It has a long dorsal tubular heart
(d) Fertilization of eggs occurs inside the body

9. The ciliated columnar epithelial cells in humans are known to occur in

[AIPMT PRE 2011]

(a) Bronchioles and fallopian tubes
(b) Bile duct and oesophagus
(c) Fallopian tubes and urethra
(d) Eustachian tube and stomach lining

10. Which of the following is correctly states as it happen in the common cockroach?

[AIPMT PRE 2011]

(a) Oxygen is transported by haemoglobin in blood
(b) Nitrogenous excretory product is urea
(c) The food is ground by mandibles and gizzard
(d) Malpighian tubules are excretory organs projecting out from the colon

11. The supportive skeletal structures in the human external ears and in the nose tip are examples of:

[AIPMT MAINS 2012]

(a) Areolar tissue
(b) Bone
(c) Cartilage
(d) Ligament

12. Given below is the diagrammatic sketch of a certain type of connective tissue identify the parts labelled A, B, C and D and select the right option about them

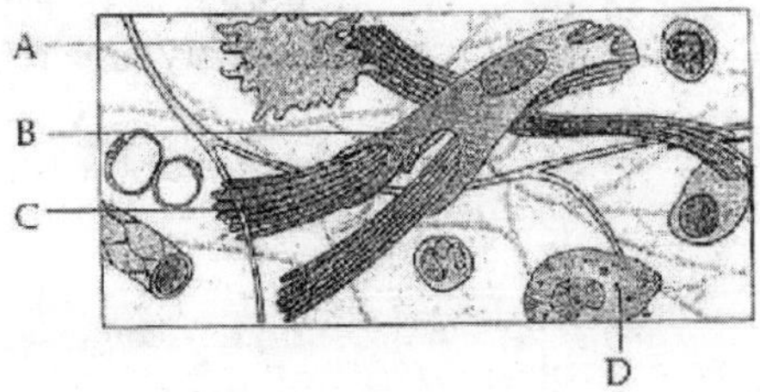

[AIPMT MAINS 2012]

Options:

(a) A: Mast cell, B: Marcophage, C: Fibroblast, D: Collagen fibres
(b) A: Macrophage, B: Collagen fibres, C: Fibroblast, D: Mast cell
(c) A: Mast cell, B: Collagen fibres, C: Fibroblast, D: Macrophage
(d) A: Macrophage, B: Fibroblast, C: Collagen fibres, D: Mast cell

13. Which one of the following characteristics is common both in humans and adult frogs? [AIPMT MAINS 2012]

(a) Internal fertilization
(b) Nucleated RBCs
(c) Ureotelic mode of excretion
(d) Four – chambered heart

14. The four sketches (A, B, C and D) given below, represent four different types of animal tissues. Which one of these is correctly identified in the options given, along with its correct location and function?

[AIPMT MAINS 2012]

(a) 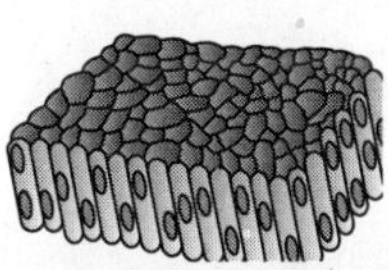

(b) 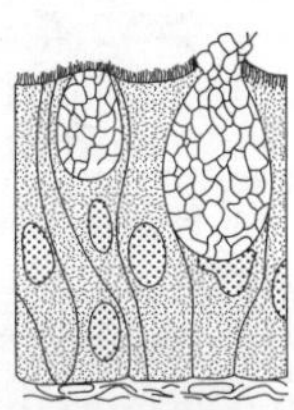

(c) 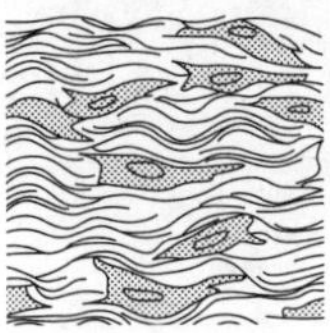

(d) 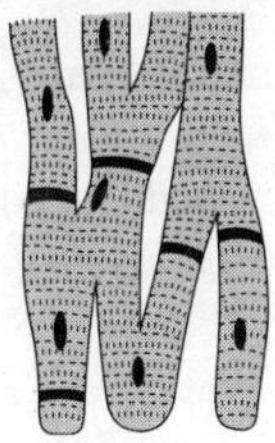

	Tissue	Location	Function
(a)	(C) Collagen fibres	Cartilage	Attach skeletal muscles to bones
(b)	(D) Smooth muscle tissue	Heart	Heart contraction
(c)	(A) Columnar epithelium	Nephron	Secretion and absorption
(d)	(B) Glandular epithelium	Intestine	Secretion

15. Pheretima and its close relatives derive nourishment from:

[AIPMT PRE 2012]

(a) Sugarcane roots
(b) Decaying fallen leaves and soil organic matter
(c) Soil insects
(d) Small pieces of fresh of fresh fallen leaves of maize, etc.

16. Compared to those of humans, the erythrocytes in frog are:

[AIPMT PRE 2012]

(a) Without nucleus but with haemoglobin
(b) Nucleated and with haemoglobin
(c) Very much smaller and fewer
(d) Nucleated and without haemoglobin

17. Select the correct statement from the ones given below with respect to Periplaneta americana.

[AIPMT PRE 2012]

(a) Nervous system located dorsally, consists of segmentally arranged ganglia joined by a pair of longitudinal connectives.
(b) Males bear a pair of short thread like anal styles
(c) There are 16 very long Malpighian tubules present at the junctions of midgut and hindgut.
(d) Grinding of food is carried out only by the mouth parts.

18. What external changes are visible after the last moult of a cockroach nymph?

[AIPMT 2013]

(a) Mandibles become harder
(b) Anal cerci develop
(c) Both fore wings and hind wings develop
(d) Labium develops

19. Choose the correctly matched pair:

[AIPMT 2014]

(a) Tendon – Specialized connective tissue
(b) Adipose tissue – Dense connective tissue
(c) Areolar tissue – Loose connective tissue
(d) Cartilage – Loose connective tissue

20. Choose the correctly matched pair:

[AIPMT 2014]

(a) Inner lining of salivary ducts – Ciliated epithelium
(b) Moist surface of buccal cavity – Glandular epithelium
(c) Tubular parts of nephrons – Cuboidal epithelium
(d) Inner surface of bronchioles – Squamous epithelium

21. The terga, sterna and pleura of cockroach body are joined by:

[AIPMT 2015]

(a) Cementing glue
(b) Muscular tissue
(c) Arthrodial membrane
(d) Cartilage

22. The function of the gap junction is to:

[RE-AIPMT 2015]

(a) Facilitate communication between adjoining cells by connecting the cytoplasm for rapid transfer of ions, small molecules and some large molecules.
(b) Separate two cells from each other
(c) Stop substance from leaking across a tissue
(d) Performing cementing to keep neighboring cells together.

23. The body cells in cockroach discharge tier nitrogenous waste in the haemolymph mainly in the form of:

[RE-AIPMT 2015]

(a) Potassium urate
(b) Urea
(c) Calcium carbonate
(d) Ammonia

Answer Keys

1. (c)	2. (c)	3. (c)	4. (c)	5. (c)	6. (d)	7. (d)	8. (b)	9. (a)	10. (b)
11. (a)	12. (d)	13. (a)	14. (c)	15. (b)	16. (c)	17. (d)	18. (d)	19. (d)	20. (d)
21. (b)	22. (a)	23. (c)	24. (b)	25. (b)	26. (c)	27. (c)	28. (d)	29. (c)	30. (b)
31. (c)	32. (a)	33. (c)	34. (a)	35. (a)	36. (c)	37. (c)	38. (b)	39. (c)	40. (b)
41. (d)	42. (a)	43. (c)	44. (c)	45. (b)	46. (b)	47. (b)	48. (d)	49. (b)	50. (b)
51. (b)	52. (b)	53. (c)	54. (c)	55. (c)	56. (c)	57. (c)	58. (d)	59. (b)	60. (b)
61. (b)	62. (b)	63. (d)	64. (a)	65. (d)	66. (d)	67. (a)	68. (a)	69. (d)	70. (c)
71. (a)	72. (a)	73. (c)	74. (d)	75. (c)	76. (c)	77. (c)	78. (d)	79. (a)	80. (b)
81. (a)	82. (b)	83. (d)	84. (c)	85. (a)	86. (a)	87. (c)	88. (b)	89. (a)	90. (b)
91. (d)	92. (a)	93. (d)	94. (a)	95. (c)	96. (a)	97. (a)	98. (a)	99. (d)	100. (a)
101. (a)	102. (b)	103. (c)	104. (a)	105. (a)	106. (a)	107. (a)			

AIPMT Previous Year Questions

1. (d)	2. (d)	3. (b)	4. (a)	5. (a)	6. (d)	7. (c)	8. (a)	9. (a)	10. (c)
11. (c)	12. (d)	13. (c)	14. (d)	15. (b)	16. (d)	17. (b)	18. (c)	19. (c)	20. (c)
21. (c)	22. (a)	23. (a)							

Unit III

Cell: Structures and Functions

Unit III includes cytology and biomolecules. This unit is important in AIPMT because its contribution in the exam is more than plant physiology. Diagrams like biomolecules chemical structures are important. If you can solve all problems given in book, you can crack various question of this unit.

CHAPTER 8

Cell: The Unit of Life

1. Which of the following organisms are not composed of cells?
   (a) Amoeba (b) Paramecium
   (c) Euglena (d) None
2. Unicellular organisms are not capable of
   (a) independent existence
   (b) performing essential functions of life
   (c) both
   (d) none
3. Who was the first one to see a live cell?
   (a) Robert Hook (b) Leeuwenhoek
   (c) Robert Brown (d) None
4. Who was the Germen botanist to study different cells forming plant tissues?
   (a) Schleiden (b) Schwann
   (c) Rudolf Virchow (d) None
5. In which year Matthias Schleiden examined a large number of plants and observed that all plants are composed of different kinds of cells which form the tissues of the plant?
   (a) 1638 (b) 1738 (c) 1838 (d) 1938
6. In which year Schwann studied different types of animal cells?
   (a) 1839 (b) 1739 (c) 1639 (d) 1938
7. Cell had a thin outer layer which is known as 'Plasma membrane'. Who reported this?
   (a) Schleiden (b) Schwann
   (c) Virchow (d) Robert Hooke
8. 'Cell wall is a unique structure of plant cells'. Who concluded this?
   (a) Schleiden (b) Schwann
   (c) Both (d) None
9. Who proposed the hypothesis that the bodies of animals and plants are composed of cells and product of cells?
   (a) Schleiden (b) Schwann (c) Both (d) None
10. Who formulated the cell theory?
    (a) Schleiden (b) Schwann (c) Both (d) None
11. 'Omnis Cellula-e cellula' was given in the year _________
    (a) 1756 (b) 1855 (c) 1945 (d) 1839
12. Who was the one to describe that cells divided and new cells are formed from pre-existing cells?
    (a) Schleiden (b) Schwann (c) Virchow (d) All

13. Which of the following statement is not a part of final cell theory?
    (a) Cell has a thin outer layer called plasma membrane
    (b) All living organisms are made up of cells and products of cells
    (c) All cells arise from pre-existing cells
    (d) All
14. What is the outer covering of typical plant cell?
    (a) Cell wall externally
    (b) Plasma membrane externally
    (c) Cell wall internally
    (d) Cell wall externally, plasma membrane internally
15. Identify the A, B, C and D in the given figure.

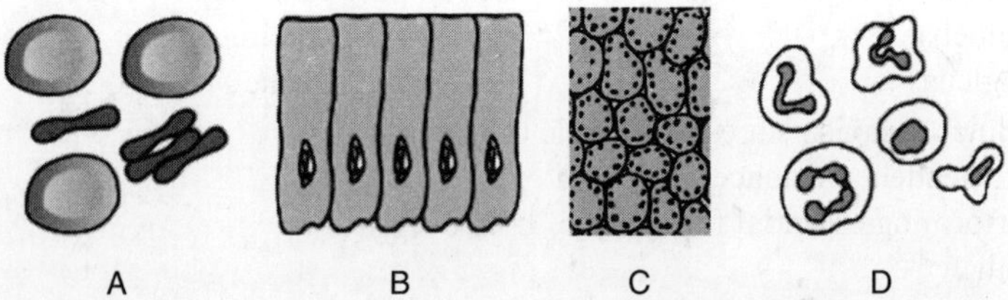

    (a) A–WBC, B–Mesophyll cell, C–RBC, D–Columnar Epithelial cells
    (b) A–Columnar epithelial cells, B–Mesophyll cell, C–WBC, D–RBC
    (c) A–Mesophyll cell, B–WBC, C–Columnar epithelial cells, D–WBC
    (d) A–RBC, B–Columnar epithelial cells, C–Mesophyll Cell, D–WBC
16. In each cheek cell, there is a dense membrane bound structure which contains chromosome. This structure is
    (a) Endoplasmic reticulum (b) Golgi bodies
    (c) Nucleus (d) Mitochondria
17. What does a nucleus of a typical animal cell contain?
    (a) Chromosomes (b) Genes (c) DNA (d) All
18. Cell containing membrane bound nucleus can be called
    (a) eukaryotic (b) prokaryotic (c) both (d) none
19. Identify the figure given below.

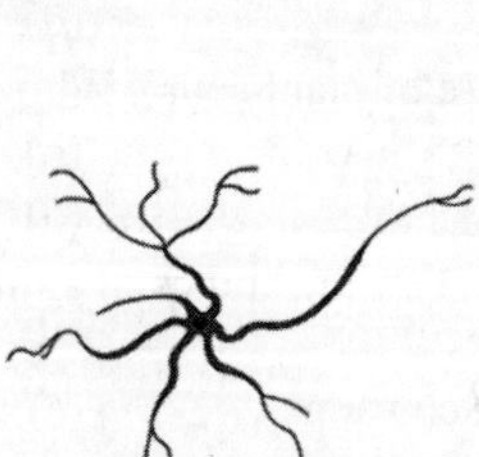

    (a) Tracheid (b) Nerve Cell (c) Lipid bilayer (d) None
20. If volume of the cell is filled with semi-fluid matrix called cytoplasm, what kind of cell is it?
    (a) Eukaryotic (b) Prokaryotic (c) Both (d) None

21. Identify the given below figure.

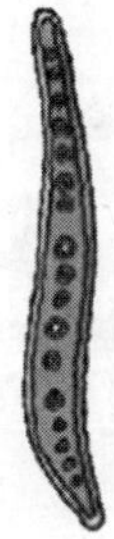

(a) A tracheid (b) A vessel
(c) A parenchyma cell (d) A sieve cell

22. What is the main arena of cellular activities in eukaryotic cells?
(a) Nucleus (b) Cytoplasm
(c) Plasma membrane (d) All

23. In a eukaryotic cell, where does the various chemical reactions occur to keep cell in living state?
(a) Nucleus (b) Cytoplasm (c) Mitochondria (d) All

24. How many of the following organelles are found in prokaryotic cells?
ER, Golgi complex, Lysosome, Mitochondria, Microbodies, Vacuoles
(a) 1 (b) 3 (c) 4 (d) 0

25. Where are ribosomes found in prokaryotic cells?
(a) Cytoplasm (b) Mitochondria
(c) Chloroplast (d) All

26. Where are ribosomes found in eukaryotic cells?
(a) Cytoplasm (b) Mitochondria
(c) Chloroplast (d) All

27. How many of the following are membrane bound organelles?
Lysosomes, Ribosomes, Mitochondria, Vacuoles
(a) 2 (b) 3 (c) 4 (d) 0

28. Which of the following organelle is exclusively found in animal cells?
(a) Mitochondria (b) Chloroplast (c) Vacuole (d) Centriole

29. Which of the following is incorrect?
(a) Smallest cell → Mycoplasma (b) Smallest cell → Bacteria
(c) Largest single cell → Ostrich's egg (d) None

30. What is the length of mycoplasm cell?
(a) 300 mm (b) 0.3 μm (c) 3000 cm (d) All

31. What could be the length of bacterial cell?
(a) 3 to 5 mm (b) 3 to 5 μm (c) 3.5 cm (d) None

32. Diameter of an RBC is
(a) 7 μm (b) 700 mm
(c) 6 μm (d) 6000 mm

33. Longest cells in human body are
(a) muscle cells (b) cardiac muscle cells
(c) neurons (d) none

34. Which of the following is incorrect matching?
(a) Round and biconcave – RBC
(b) Amoeboid – WBC
(c) EElongated – Tracheid
(d) Long and narrow - Nerve cells

35. Identify the A, B, C, D and E in this figure.

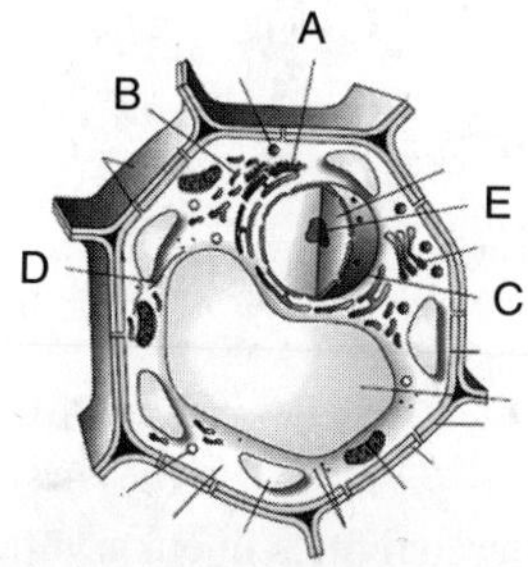

(a) A–Rough endoplasmic reticulum, B–Smooth endoplasmic reticulum, C–Nuclear envelope, D–Microtubule, E–Nucleolus
(b) A–Smooth endoplasmic reticulum, B–Rough endoplasmic reticulum, C–Microtubule, D–Nuclear envelope, E–Nucleolus
(c) A–Nucleolus, B–Microtubule, C–Smooth endoplasmic reticulum, D–Nuclear envelope, E–Rough endoplasmic reticulum
(d) A–Rough endoplasmic reticulum, B–Nucleolus, C–Microtubule, D–Smooth endoplasmic reticulum, E–Microtubule

36. Which of the following cells are round and oval?
(a) RBCs
(b) WBCs
(c) Columnar cells
(d) Mesophyll cells

37. Which of the following are long and narrow cells?
(a) Nerve cells
(b) WBC
(c) Columnar epithelial cells
(d) Tracheid

38. Which of the following represent prokaryotic cell?
(a) Blue-green algae
(b) PPLO
(c) Bacteria
(d) All

39. Identify the A, B, C, D and E in this figure.

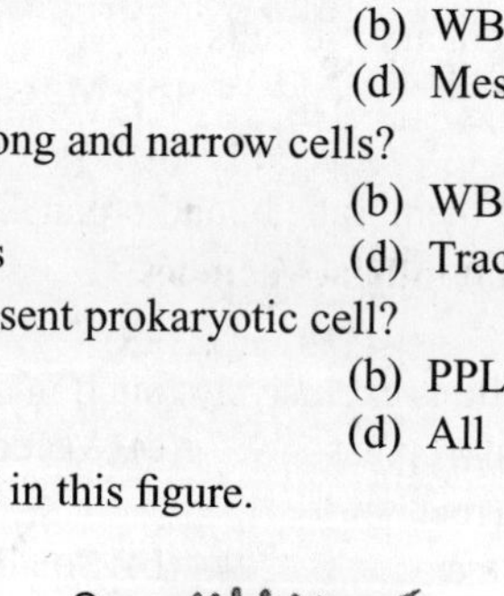

(a) A–Smooth endoplasmic reticulum, B–Centriole, C–Golgi apparatus, D–Rough endoplasmic reticulum, E–Ribosomes

(b) A–Centriole, B–Smooth endoplasmic reticulum, C–Golgi apparatus, D–Ribosomes, E–Rough endoplasmic reticulum
(c) A–Rough endoplasmic reticulum, B–Smooth endoplasmic reticulum, C–Ribosomes, D–Centriole, E–Golgi apparatus,
(d) A–Centriole, B–Rough endoplasmic reticulum, C–Golgi apparatus, D–Smooth endoplasmic reticulum, E–Ribosomes

40. What is true for a prokaryotic cell?
(a) They are smaller in size (b) Multiply much rapidly than eukaryotes
(c) Greatly very in shape and size (d) All

41. What is the size of a typical eukaryotic cell?
(a) 1–2 μm (b) 10–20 μm (c) 10–20 mm (d) 1–2 mm

42. How much is the size of typical bacteria?
(a) 1–2 μm (b) 10–20 μm (c) 10–20 mm (d) 1–2 mm

43. How much is the size of viruses?
(a) 0.02–0.2 μm (b) 0.2–0.4 μm (c) 0.02–0.04 μm (d) None

44. What is a genomic DNA of bacteria?
(a) Circular DNA (b) Single stranded DNA
(c) Both (d) ds DNA, linear

45. Where is genetic material located in prokaryotes?
(a) Nucleus (b) Enveloped by nuclear membrane
(c) Naked in cytoplasm (d) None

46. What are plasmids?
(a) Naked genomic DNA (b) Smaller DNA than genomic DNA
(c) Enveloped DNA (d) None

47. Resistance to antibiotics is conferred by
(a) Plasmid DNA (b) Chromosome
(c) Both (d) None

48. Which is the common organelles that are found in both eukaryotes and prokaryote?
(a) Lysosome (b) Ribosome
(c) Vacuole (d) Mitochondria

49. What is a specialized differentiated form of cell membrane?
(a) Plasmid (b) Nucleosome
(c) Mesosome (d) All

50. Infoldings of cell membrane in prokaryotic is called
(a) mesosomes (b) lysosomes
(c) both (d) none

51. What is external to cell wall in a prokaryotic cell?
(a) Glycocalyx layer (b) Plasma membrane
(c) Both (d) None

52. Select the incorrect statement:
(a) Glycocalyx differs in composition and thickness among different bacteria
(b) All organism are made of cells or aggregates of cells
(c) ER helps in synthesis of proteins, lipoproteins and glycogen
(d) Cells of all living organisms have nuclues

53. What is external to plasma membrane in prokaryotic cell like bacteria?
(a) Glycocalyx layer (b) Cell wall (c) Both (d) None

54. What is external to glycocalyx layer in prokaryotic cell like bacteria?
(a) Cell wall
(b) Plasma membrane
(c) Both
(d) None

55. What is external to plasma membrane and internal to glycocalyx layer?
(a) Capsule
(b) Cell wall
(c) Cellular matrix
(d) None

56. What is the basis of classification of bacteria's into gram the or gram –ve?
(a) Cell wall
(b) Glycocalyx layer
(c) Plasma membrane
(d) All

57. A bacterial cell was taken and gram staining was done and observed that it did not take up gram stain such a bacteria is known as
(a) gram positive
(b) gram negative
(c) non-effective to gram stain
(d) none

58. Which of the following statement is not true?
(a) Response to gram stain is due to the cell envelop
(b) The cell envelope act as single protective unit
(c) Glycocalyx layer is similar in all the bacteria
(d) None

59. A loose sheath of glycocalyx layer is called
(a) plasma membrane
(b) capsule
(c) slime layer
(d) cell wall

60. What is a thick, tough, layer of glycocalyx known as?
(a) Slime layer
(b) Capsule
(c) Cell wall
(d) Cell envelope

61. Which of the following is not the function of cell wall?
(a) Interaction with outside world
(b) Provide structural support and shape
(c) Prevent from bursting and collapsing
(d) Exchange of nutrition takes place through it

62. Which of the following is a form of mesosome?
(a) Vesicles
(b) Tubules
(c) Lamellae
(d) All

63. Which of the following is a function of mesosome?
(a) Cell wall formation
(b) DNA replication and its distribution to daughter cells
(c) Both
(d) None

64. Which of the following help in respiration, secretion process, and increase surface area for enzymatic content?
(a) Plasma membrane
(b) Cell wall
(c) Mesosomes
(d) Glycocalyx layer

65. In which organisms pigment containing chromatophores are found?
(a) Algae
(b) Cyanobacteria
(c) Green algae
(d) Amoeba

66. A thin, filamentous extension of cell wall required for a bacteria motility is called ________.
(a) hook (b) flagella (c) tail (d) mesosome

67. Which of the following is not a part of bacteria flagellum?
(a) Filament (b) Hook
(c) Basal body (d) None
68. Of all the parts of flagellum, which one is the longest?
(a) Filament (b) Hook (c) Basal body (b) Fimbriae
69. Which of the following surface structure of bacteria which do not take part in motility?
(a) Flagella (b) Pilli (c) Fimbriae (d) Both (b) and (c)
70. Which is the elongated tubular structure made of special protein on surface of bacterial cell?
(a) Flagella (b) Fimbriae (c) Pilli (d) All
71. What is small bristle like structures or fibres sprouting out of the cell?
(a) Flagella (b) Fimbriae (c) Pilli (d) All
72. In prokaryotes, ribosomes are associated with which structure of cell?
(a) Cell wall (b) Mesosome
(c) Lysosomes (d) Plasma membrane
73. What is the size of ribosomes?
(a) 10–20 μm (b) 15–20 nm (c) 10–20 nm (d) 15–20 cm
74. In a 70S prokaryotic ribosomes, what are the sub units present in them?
(a) 50S and 20S (b) 50S and 30S (c) 40S and 30S (d) 60S and 30S
75. A polysome is a chained structure of which organelle?
(a) Lysosome (b) Mesosome (c) Ribosome (d) All
76. In polyribosome riboromes attach to which RNA?
(a) m-RNA (b) t-RNA (c) r-RNA (d) All
77. In what form, reserve material in prokaryotic cells are stored in cytoplasm?
(a) Lysosome (b) Mesosome
(c) Ribosome (d) Inclusion bodies
78. Which of the following are not inclusion bodies?
(a) Phosphate granules (b) Cyanophycean granules
(c) Glycogen granules (d) Glucose granules
79. Gas vacuoles are found in
(a) blue green bacteria (b) purple bacteria
(c) green photosynthetic, bacteria (d) all
80. Which of the following do not belong to eukaryote?
(a) Protists (b) Bacteria (c) Fungi (d) All
81. In eukaryotic cells, why there is a extensive compartmentalization of cytoplasm?
(a) Due to the presence of fibres
(b) Due to the presence of so many organelles
(c) Due to the presence of membranous organelles
(d) All
82. Chemical studies on cell membrane to deduce its possible structure was mostly done on which cells?
(a) WBC (b) Human erythrocytes
(c) Platelets (d) Cheek cells
83. In plasma membrane, lipids have their polar heads facing
(a) outer side (b) inner side
(c) in the middle (d) stable facing no where
84. Lipid component of plasma membrane will be mainly constituted of
(a) glycolipids (b) glycogen (c) phosphoglycerides (d) all

85. Identify the A, B, C and D in this figure.

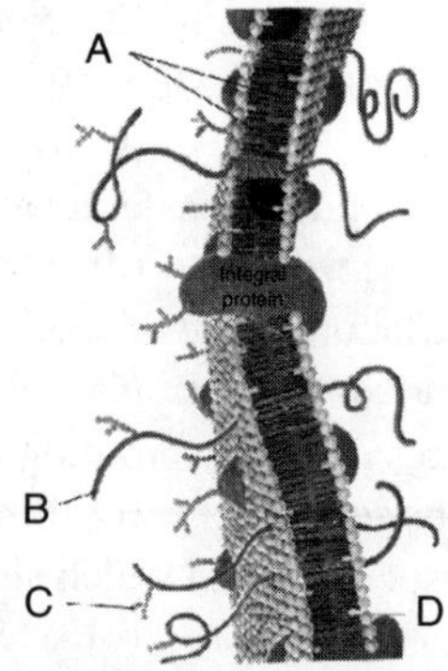

(a) A–Lipid bilayer, B–Protein, C–Sugar, D–Cholesterol
(b) A–Protein, B–Lipid bilayer, C–Cholesterol, D–Sugar
(c) A–Protein, B–Sugar, C–Lipid bilayer, D–Cholesterol
(d) A–Cholesterol, B–Protein, C–Sugar, D–Lipid bilayer

86. Which of the following are not the component of plasma membrane?
(a) Sugar (b) Protein (c) Cholesterol (d) None

87. What is the percentage of protein and lipids in an RBC membrane respectively?
(a) 52%, 40% (b) 50%, 40% (c) 50%, 42% (d) 52%, 42%

88. Which of the following membrane proteins lie on the surface of the cell?
(a) Integral proteins (b) Peripheral proteins
(c) Both (a) and (b) (d) Glycoproteins

89. Which of the following membrane proteins are partially or totally buried in cell membrane?
(a) Integral proteins (b) Peripheral proteins (c) Both (d) Glycoproteins

90. Fluid mosaic model was given by Singer and Nicolson in the year ______
(a) 1972 (b) 1976 (c) 1982 (d) 1986

91. The ability of proteins to move laterally within the membrane is measured as
(a) mobility (b) flexibility (c) fluidity (d) none

92. For what reason, fluid nature of membrane is important?
(a) Cell growth (b) Secretions (c) Endocytosis (d) All

93. The most important function of plasma membrane is that it
(a) divides the cell (b) gives shape to the cell
(c) transport molecules across (d) both (a) and (b)

94. In which kind of transport, molecules move across without the utilization of energy?
(a) Passive transport (b) Osmosis
(c) Both (a) and (b) (d) Active transport

95. Movement of water across the plasma membrane occurs by
(a) passive transport (b) osmosis (c) active transport (d) all

96. In which kind of transport, molecules will go against the concentration gradient?
(a) Passive transport (b) Active transport
(c) Facilitated transport (d) All

97. In which of the following does active transport take place?
(a) Pumps (b) Carrier protein transport
(c) Ion channels (d) Diffusion

98. Functions of cell wall in eukaryotic cells
(a) give shape to cell (b) prevent from mechanical damage
(c) protect from infection (d) all

99. Which of the following organisms have cell wall made up of cellulose, galactans, mannans, and minerals like calcium carbonates?
(a) Fungi (b) Plants (c) Algae (d) All

100. Which of the following organisms have cell wall made up of cellulose, hemicelluloses, pectins and proteins?
(a) Fungi (b) Plants (c) Algae (d) All

101. Which of the following wall is capable of growth in a plant cell?
(a) Primary wall (b) Secondary wall
(c) Both (d) Middle lamella

102. What is the component of middle lamella that puts the different binds neighbouring cells together?
(a) Calcium phosphate (b) Sodium pectate
(c) Calcium pectate (d) Sodium phosphate

103. A structure that is traversing the middle lamella and connecting the cytoplasm of neighbouring cells is called
(a) primary wall junction (b) plasmodesmata
(c) desmosomes (d) secondary wall

104. Identify the A, B, C and D in this figure.

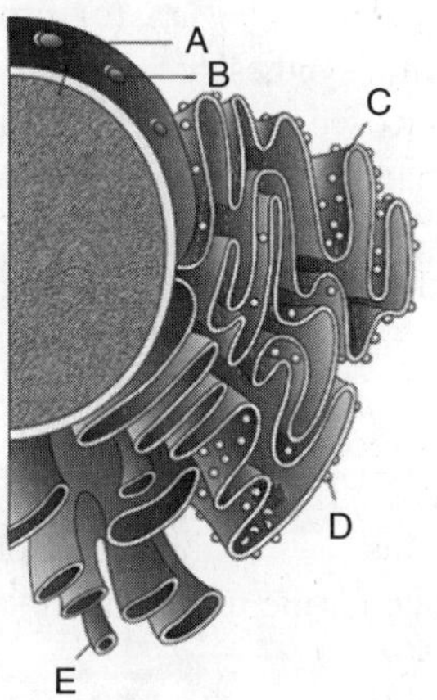

(a) A–Nuclear pore, B–Nucleus, C–Ribosome, D–Smooth endoplasmic reticulum, E–Rough endoplasmic reticulum
(b) A–Rough endoplasmic reticulum, B–Nuclear pore, C–Ribosome, D–Smooth endoplasmic reticulum, E–Nucleus
(c) A–Ribosome, B–Nuclear pore, C–Nucleus, D–Smooth endoplasmireticulum, E–Rough endoplasmic reticulum
(d) A–Nucleus, B–Nuclear pore, C–Rough endoplasmic reticulum, D–Ribosome, E–Smooth endoplasmic reticulum

105. How many of the following are not included in endomembrane system?
Endoplasmic Reticulum, Golgi complex, Lysosome, Mitochondria, Chloroplast, Vacuoles, Peroxisomes
(a) 2 (b) 3 (c) 4 (d) 5

106. What is the network of tiny tubular structures scattered in cytoplasm as seen from electron microscope?
(a) Golgi complex (b) Microtubules
(c) Endoplasmic reticulum (d) Mitochondria

107. What indicates A in the figure?

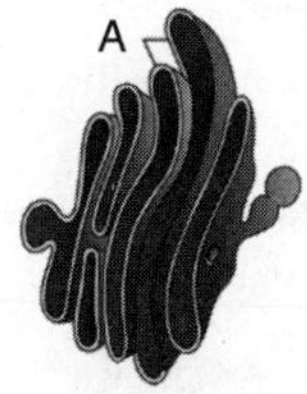

(a) Cisternae (b) Nuclear pore (c) Crista (d) Thylakoid

108. Which side in a cell does luminal and extra luminal compartments are situated respectively?
(a) Cytoplasm, inside ER (b) Inside ER, cytoplasm
(c) cytoplasm, plasma membrane (d) Nucleus, cytoplasm

109. Rough endoplasmic reticulum is called so due to the presence of
(a) lysosome (b) golgi granules
(c) ribosomes (d) protein granules

110. RER is frequently seen in cells associated with frequent synthesis and secretion of
(a) lipid (b)glucose (c) protein (d) all

111. SER is frequently associated with synthesis of
(a) lipid (b) glucose (c) protein (d) all

112. What is the diameter of cisternae
(a) 0.5–1 μm (b) 0.5–1 mm (c) 0.5–2 μm (d) 5–11 μm

113. Cis and trans face of golgi body are ____ and ____ respectively
(a) Convex, Concave (b) Concave, Convex
(c) Convex, Convex (d) Concave, Concave

114. Which face of golgi apparatus receives the materials packaged in the form of vesicles from the ER?
(a) Cis (b) Trans (c) Both (d) None

115. Golgi apparatus is important site for the formation of
(a) protein and lipids
(b) glycoproteins and glycolipids
(c) carbohydrates and proteins
(d) glucose and lipids

116. Which structure is formed by the process of packaging in golgi apparatus?
(a) Ribosomes (b) Protein granules (c) Lysosomes (d) Centrosomes

117. Which of the following are not hydrolytic enzyme?
(a) Lipase (b) Proteases (c) Carbohydrases (d) Ligases

118. Hydrolytic enzymes are activated at _______ pH.
(a) acidic (b) neutral (c) 0 basic (d) all

119. Which of the following cannot be digested by hydrolytic enzymes?
(a) DNA (b) Immunoglobulins
(c) Glucose (d) Insulin

120. Which of the following are not the contents of vacuole?
(a) Water (b) Enzymes
(c) Sap (d) Excretory products

121. Which of the following is correct about vacoule?
(a) Vacuole contain water Sap, excretory product and other material not useful for the cell
(b) In plant cell the vacuole can occupy up to 90% of the volume of the cell
(c) Vacuole is bounded by tonoplast
(d) All

122. Tonoplast membrane is important for
(a) transporting ions along concentration gradient
(b) transporting ions against concentration gradient
(c) providing rigidity to structure
(d) all

123. Contractile vacuole present in amoeba is useful for
(a) ingestion (b) locomotion (c) both (a) and (b) (d) excretion

124. Amount or number of mitochondria in a cell depends on
(a) anatomical structure of cell (b) size of the cell
(c) colour and contour of the cell (d) physiological activity of cell

125. What is the main function of cristae?
(a) To hold the vesicles formed (b) Increase the surface area
(c) Increase the density of organelle (d) All

126. What kind of ribosome is seen in mitochondria?
(a) 80 S (b) 70 S (c) Both (d) None

127. How is new mitochondria formed by the pre-existing ones?
(a) Mitosis (b) Fission (c) Conjugation (d) Budding

128. What does a chloroplast contain?
(a) Chlorophyll (b) Carotenoid (c) Both (a) and (b) (d) Anthocyanin

129. Select the incorrect pair:
(a) Leucoplast–Carotene (b) Amyloplast–Starch
(c) Elaioplast–Oils (d) Aleuroplasts–Proteins

130. In 30 S and 40 S ribosomes, 'S' stands for
(a) sub-unit (b) Svedberg's unit (c) single unit (d) size

131. Identify A, B, C, D and E in the given figure.

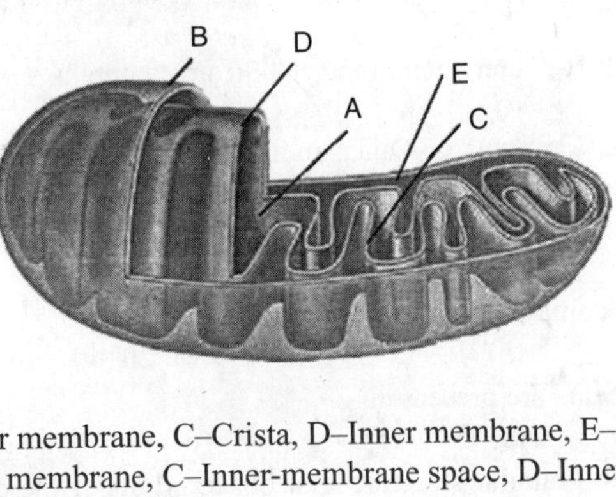

(a) A–Matrix, B–Outer membrane, C–Crista, D–Inner membrane, E–Inner-membrane space
(b) A–Crista, B–Outer membrane, C–Inner-membrane space, D–Inner membrane, E–Matrix

(c) A–Matrix, B–Inner membrane, C–Inner-membrane space, D–Crista, E–Outer membrane
(d) A–Inner-membrane space, B–Outer membrane, C–Matrix, D–Crista, E–Inner membrane

132. What kind of ribosome is present in mitochondria?
(a) 70 S (b) 80 S (c) 40 S (d) 60 S

133. Plastids are found in:
(a) All plant cells (b) All animal cells (c) Euglenoids (d) Both (a) and (c)

134. Based on the type of pigments plastid can be classified into how many types
(a) 1 (b) 2 (c) 3 (d) 4

135. Which of the following is type of plastid?
(a) Chloroplast (b) Chromoplast (d) Leucoplast (d) All

136. Select correct matching:

Column I (Type of leucoplast)	**Column II (Stored food)**
A. Amyloplast	1. Oil and fat
B. Elaioplast	2. Protein
C. Aleuroplasts	3. Carbohydrate

(a) A–3, B–1, C–2 (b) A–1, B–2, C–3 (c) A–3, B–2, C–1 (d) A–2, B–3, C–1

137. Select the incorrect statement:
(a) The chloroplast contain chlorophyll and carotenoid pigments
(b) Chromoplast contain water soluble carotenoid pigments like carotene, xanthophylls
(c) Plastid is easily observed under microscope
(d) Chloroplast is double membrane bound organelle

138. Number of chloroplast in alga chlamydomonas is:
(a) 2 (b) 1 (c) 20–40 (d) 5–10

139. Indentify A–F in the given figure.

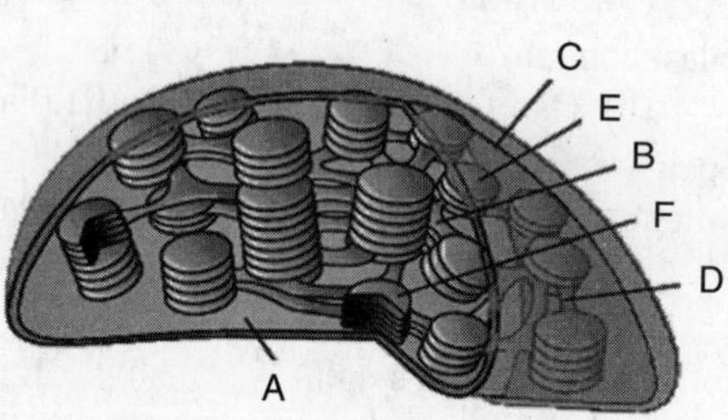

(a) A–Outer membrane, B–Thylakoid, C–Stroma lamella, D–Inner membrane, E–Granum, F–Stroma
(b) A–Thylakoid, B–Outer membrane, C–Stroma lamella, D–Inner membrane, E–Stroma, F–Granum
(c) A–Stroma, B–Granum, C–Outer membrane, D–Stroma lamella, E–Inner membrane, F–Thylakoid
(d) A–Inner membrane, B–Thylakoid, C–Stroma lamella, D–Outer membrane, E–Stroma, F–Granum

140. A mesophyll cell contain how many chloroplast
(a) 5–10 (b) 10–15 (c) 20–40 (d) > 100

141. Chlorophyll pigments are present in
(a) Thylakoid (b) Stroma (c) Outer membrane (d) Inner membrane

142. Ribosomes are the granular structure first observed under the electron microscope as dense particle by which scientist

(a) Robert Brown (1831) (b) George Palade (1953)
(c) Camillo Golgi (1898) (d) Singer and Nicolson (1972)

143. Type of ribosome present in eukaryote cell
(a) 70 s (b) 80 s (c) Both (d) None

144. A elaborate network of filamentous proteinaceous structures present in the cytoplasm is collectively known as
(a) Cilia (b) Flagella (c) Cytoskeleton (d) ER

145. Cytoskeleton helps in
(a) Mechanical support to cell (b) Providing mobility to cell
(c) Maintenance of shape of cell (d) All

146. The central part of the proximal region of the centriole is also proteinaceous and is called
(a) Spokes (b) Doublet (c) Hub (d) Linkers

147. Find out the incorrect statement:
(a) Centrioles forms basal bodies of cilia or flagella
(b) Centriole gives rise to spindle fibres at the time of cell division in animal cell
(c) Centrosome is an organelle usually containing two cylindrical structures called centrioles
(d) Peripheral fibril of centriole is doublet

148. Identify A, B, C, D, E and F given in the figure.

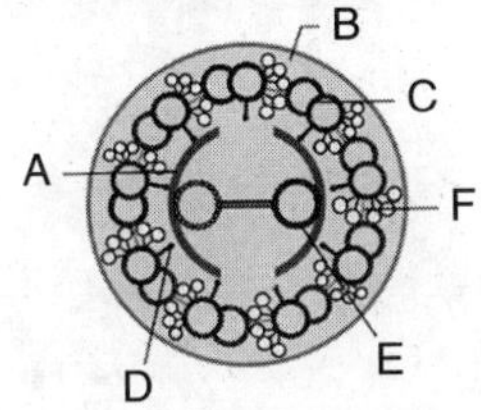

(a) A–Interdoublet bridge, B–Peripheral microtubules (doublets), C–Central microtubule, D–Plasma membrane, E–Central bridge, F–Radial spoke
(b) A–Central sheath, B–Radial spoke, C–Interdoublet bridge, D–Central microtubule, E–Plasma membrane, F–Peripheral microtubules (doublets)
(c) A–Central sheath, B–Plasma membrane, C–Peripheral microtubules (doublets), D–Radial spoke, E–Central microtubule, F–Interdoublet bridge
(d) A–Plasma membrane, B–Radial spoke, C–Peripheral microtubules (doublets), D–Central sheath, E–Central microtubule, F–Interdoublet bridge

149. Select the incorrect statement:
(a) Cilia and flagella are hair-like outgrowths of the cell membrane
(b) Cilia causes the movement of either the cell or the surrounding medium
(c) Bacterial flagella are structurally similar to eukaryotic flagella
(d) Flagella responsible for cell movement

150. About internal structure of axoneme
(a) Central sheath connected to one of the tubule of each peripheral doublets by a radial spoke
(b) Axoneme is not covered by plasma membrane at all
(c) Then are only and radial spokes are found
(d) Peripheral doublets are not connected with each other

151. Both cilium and flagellum emerges from centriole like structure is called
(a) Basal granules (b) Basal bodies (c) Basal lamina (d) Basal ganglion

152. Chromatin name was given by
(a) Robert Brown (b) Fleming (c) Schwann (d) Ramchandran

153. Outer membrane of nucleus remains continuous with which cell organelle
(a) ER (b) Golgi body (c) Lysosome (d) All

154. Perinuclear space is about
(a) 1–5 nm (b) 5–10 nm (c) 10–50 nm (d) > 100 nm

155. Following cells are without nucleus
(a) Erythrocytes of many mammals (b) Sieve tube cells of vascular plant
(c) Bacterial cell (d) All

156. Site of active ribosomal RNA synthesis
(a) Nucleolus (b) Mitochondria (c) Cytoplasm (d) All of above

157. Chromatin contains
(a) DNA (b) Basic protein histone
(c) Some non histone protein and RNA (d) All

158. How long a DNA is distributed in our forty six chromosomes?
(a) 1 meter (b) 3 meter (c) 2 meter (d) 4 meter

159. Based on the position of centromere chromosomes are classified into how many types?
(a) 1 (b) 3 (c) 2 (d) 4

160. Identify A, B, C, D, E and F given in the figure.

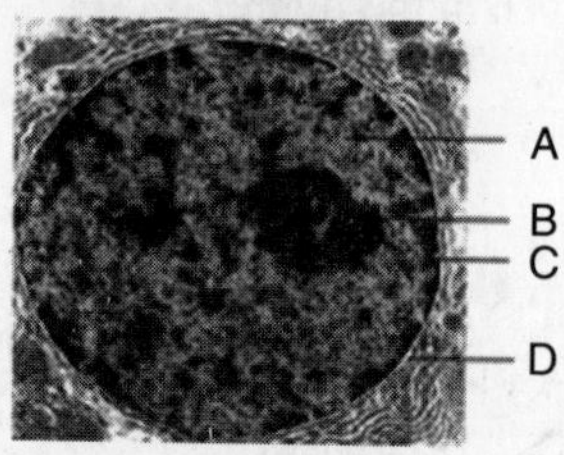

(a) A–Nucleoplasm, B–Nucleolus, C–Nuclear pore, D–Nuclear membrane
(b) A–Nucleolus, B–Nucleoplasm, C–Nuclear membrane, D–Nuclear pore
(c) A–Nuclear pore, B–Nuclear membrane, C–Nucleoplasm, D–Nucleolus
(d) A–Nuclear membrane, B–Nucleoplasm, C–Nuclear pore, D–Nuclear membrane

161. Match the column:

Column I	**Column II**
A) Metacentric chromosomal	1) Middle centromere
B) Sub-metacentric	2) Centromere slightly way from middle
C) Acrocentric	3) Centromere close to its end
D) Telocentric	4) Terminal centromere

(a) A–1, B–2, C–3, D–4 (b) A–2, B–1, C–3, D–4
(c) A–1, B–2, C–4, D–3 (d) A–4, B–3, C–2, D–1

162. Diagram shows a chromosome. A is

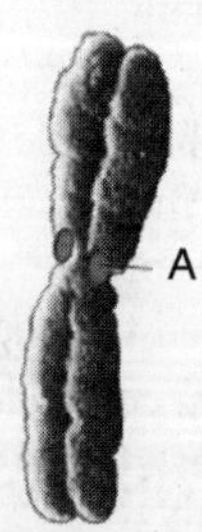

(a) Chromosomes (b) Kinetichore (c) Centromere (d) Acrocentric

163. Select the incorrect statement:
(a) Micro bodies contain various enzyme and are present in both plant and animal cells
(b) Few chromosome have non-staining secondary constriction of constant location. This give the appearance of a small fragment called the satellite
(c) Nuclei are spherical structures present in nucleoplasm and it is a site for ribosomal RNA synthesis
(d) Every chromosome essentially has a secondary constriction or the centromere on the sides of which disc shaped structures called kinetochores are present

164. Identify A, B, C, D, E, F and G given in the figure.

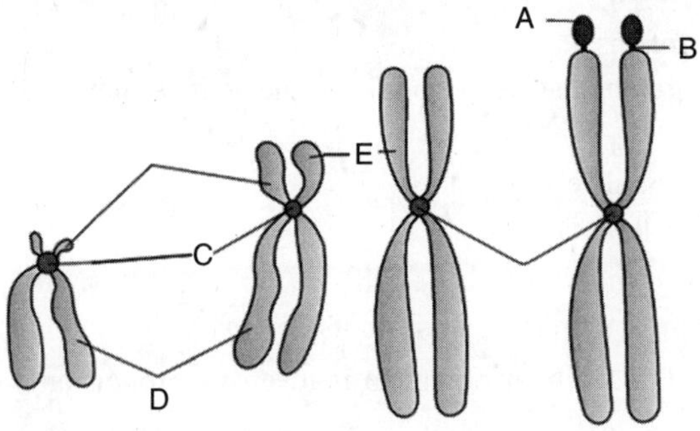

(a) A–Satellite, B–Secondary constriction, C–Centromere, D–Long arm, E–Short arm
(b) A–Secondary constriction, B–Satellite, C–Long arm, D–Centromere, E–Short arm
(c) A–Centromere, B–Satellite, C–Long arm, D–Short arm, E–Secondary constriction
(d) A–Satellite, B–Short arm, C–Long arm, D–Centromere, E–Secondary constriction

*Read the **assertion** and **reason** carefully to mark the correct option out of the options given below:*
(a) If both the assertion and the reason are true and the reason is a correct explanation of the assertion
(b) If both the assertion and reason are true but the reason is not a correct explanation of the assertion
(c) If the assertion is true but the reason is false
(d) If both the assertion and reason are false

165. **Assertion:** Bacterial cells may be motile or non motile.
Reason: Bacterial cells may or may not posses cilia.

166. **Assertion:** Bacterial cell walls are not like the plant cell.
Reason: Bacterial cell wall is not made up of cellulose.

167. **Assertion:** Membrane transport occurs through the carrier proteins.
Reason: The transport carried by carrier proteins is always passive.

168. **Assertion:** Cristae are the infoldings of outer membrane of mitochondria.
Reason: Electron transport occurs in mitochondrial stroma.

169. **Assertion:** Eukaryotic cells have more DNA than prokaryotic cells.
Reason: Eukaryotes are genetically more complex than prokaryotes.

170. Assertion: Schleiden and Schwann were the first to observe the cells and to put forward cell theory.
Reason: The cells are always living unit.

171. Assertion: In animal cells lipid – like steroidal hormones are synthesized in SER.
Reason: The smooth ER is major site for synthesis of lipid.

172. Assertion: Lysosomes help in photorespiration.
Reason: Lysosome have basic enzyme.

173. Assertion: Mitochondria is known as power house of cell.
Reason: ATP production takes place here.

174. Assertion: DNA is associated with proteins.
Reason: DNA binds around histone protein that form a pool and the entire structure is called a nucleosome.

175. Assertion: Cell wall is not found in animal cell.
Reason: Animal cells are covered by cell membrane.

176. Assertion: It is important that the organisms should have cell.
Reason: A cell keeps its chemical composition steady within its boundary.

177. Assertion: The number of cells in a multicellular organism is inversely proportional to the size of body.
Reason: All the cells in the biological world are of same size.

178. Assertion: A cell membrane shows fluid behaviour.
Reason: A membrane is a mosaic or composite of diverse lipids and proteins.

179. Assertion: Mitochondria and chloroplasts are semiautonomous organelles.
Reason: mitocondria and chloroplast are devoid of ribosomes

AIPMT PREVIOUS YEAR QUESTIONS

1. Identify the components labelled A, B, C and D in the diagram below from the list (i) to (vii) given along with:

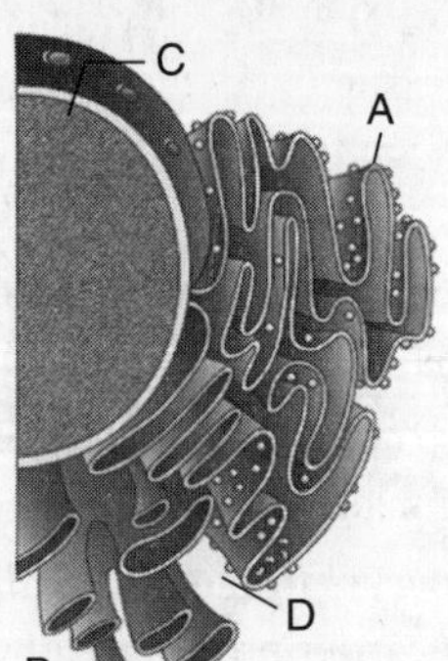

Components:

(i) Cristae of mitochondria
(ii) Inner membrane of mitochondria
(iii) Cytoplasm
(iv) Smooth endoplasmic reticulum

(v) Rough endoplasmic reticulum (vi) Mitochondrial matrix
(vii) Cell vacuole (viii) Nucleus

[AIPMT MAINS 2010]

The correct components are:

	A	B	C	D
(a)	(v)	(iv)	(viii)	(iii)
(b)	(i)	(iv)	(viii)	(vi)
(c)	(vi)	(v)	(iv)	(vii)
(d)	(v)	(i)	(iii)	(ii)

2. Membrane-bound organelles are absent in:

[AIPMT PRE 2010]

(a) Saccharomyces (b) Streptococcus
(c) Chlamydomonas (d) Plasmodium

3. Which one of the following has its own DNA?

[AIPMT PRE 2010]

(a) Mitochondria (b) Dictyosome
(c) Lysosome (d) Peroxisome

4. The main arena of various types of activities of a cell is

[AIPMT PRE 2010]

(a) Plasma membrane (b) Mitochondrion
(c) Cytoplasm (d) Nucleus

5. The plasma membrane consists mainly of

[AIPMT PRE 2010]

(a) Phospholipids embedded in a protein bilayer
(b) Proteins embedded in a phospholipid bilayer
(c) Proteins embedded in a polymer of glucose molecules
(d) Proteins embedded in a carbohydrate bilayer

6. The figure below shows the structure of a mitochondrion with its four parts labelled A, B, C and D. select the part

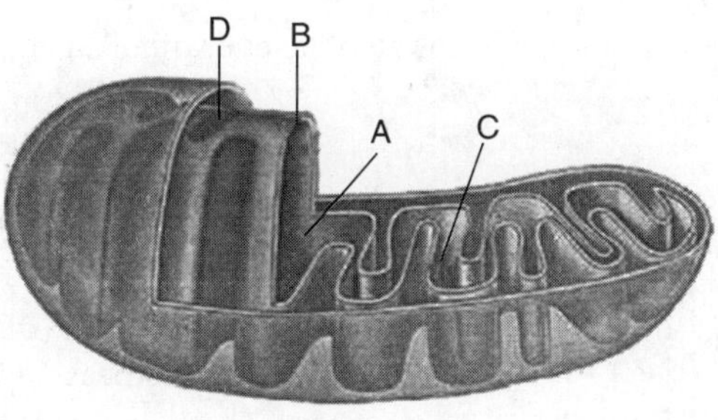

[AIPMT MAINS 2011]

(a) D (outer membrane) – gives rise to inner membrane by splitting
(b) B (inner membrane) – forms infolding called cristae
(c) C (crista) – possesses single circular DNA molecule and ribosomes
(d) A (matrix) – major site for respiratory chain enzymes

7. In mitochondria, protons accumulate in the

[AIPMT MAINS 2011]

(a) Outer membrane (b) Inner membrane
(c) Intermembrane space (d) Matrix

8. Which one of the following is not considered as a part of the endomembrane system? [AIPMT MAINS 2011]
   (a) Golgi complex (b) Peroxisome
   (c) Vacuole (d) Lysosome

9. Which one of the following organisms is not an example of eukaryotic cells? [AIPMT PRE 2011]
   (a) Escherichia coli (b) Euglena viridis
   (c) Amoeba proteus (d) Paramecium caudatum

10. Important site for formation of glycoproteins and glycolipids is: [AIPMT PRE 2011]
    (a) Golgi apparatus (b) Plastid
    (c) Lysosome (d) Vacuole

11. In eubacteria, a cellular component that resembles eukaryotic cells is: [AIPMT PRE 2011]
    (a) Nucleus (b) Ribosomes
    (c) Cell wall (d) Plasma membrane

12. Peptide synthesis inside a cell takes place in: [AIPMT PRE 2011]
    (a) Mitochondria (b) Chromoplast
    (c) Ribosomes (d) Chloroplast

13. Which one of the following cellular parts is correctly described? [AIPMT MAINS 2012]

(a)	Centrioles	–	Sites for active RNA synthesis
(b)	Ribosomes	–	Those on chloroplasts are larger (80S) while those in the cytoplasm are smaller (70S)
(c)	Lysosomes	–	Optimally active at a pH of about 8.5
(d)	Thylakoids	–	Flattened membranous sacs forming the grana of chloroplasts

14. Which one of the following structures is an organelle within an organelle? [AIPMT MAINS 2012]
    (a) Peroxisome (b) ER
    (c) Mesosome (d) Ribosome

15. Ribosomal RNA is actively synthesized in: [AIPMT PRE 2012]
    (a) Lysosomes (b) Nucleolus
    (c) Nucleoplasm (d) Ribosomes

16. What is true about ribosomes? [AIPMT PRE 2012]
    (a) The prokaryotic ribosomes are 80S, where “S” stands for sedimentation coefficient
    (b) These are composed of ribonucleic acid and proteins
    (c) These are found only in eurkaryotic cells
    (d) These are self-splicing introns of some RNAs

17. Nuclear membrane absent in: [AIPMT PRE 2012]
    (a) Penicillium (b) Agaricus
    (c) Volvox (d) Nostoc

18. Select the correct statement from the following regarding cell membrane. [AIPMT PRE 2012]

(a) NA^+ and K^+ ions move across cell membrane by passive transport.
(b) Proteins make up 60 to 70% of the cell membrane.
(c) Lipids are arranged in a bilayer with polar heads towards the inner part.
(d) Fluid mosaic model of cell membrane was proposed by Singer and Nicolson.

19. A major site for synthesis of lipids is: [AIPMT 2013]

(a) RER (b) SER
(c) Symplast (d) Nucleoplasm

20. The Golgi complex plays a major role: [AIPMT 2013]

(a) In trapping the light and transforming it into chemical energy
(b) In digesting proteins and carbohydrates
(c) As energy transferring organelles
(d) In post translational modification of proteins and glycosidation of lipids

21. Which one of the following organelle in the figure correctly matches with its function?

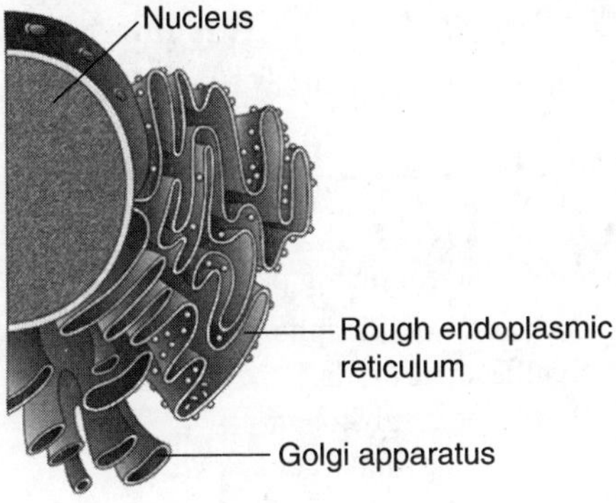

[AIPMT 2013]

(a) Rough endoplasmic reticulum, formation of glycoproteins
(b) Golgi apparatus, protein synthesis
(c) Golgi apparatus, formation of glycolipids
(d) Rough endoplasmic reticulum, protein synthesis

22. Which structures perform the function of mitochondria in bacteria? [AIPMT 2014]

(a) Nucleoid (b) Ribosomes
(c) Cell wall (d) Mesosomes

23. The solid linear cytosketetal elements having a diameter of 6 nm and made up of a single type of monomer are known as: [AIPMT 2014]

(a) Microtubules (b) Microfilaments
(c) Intermediate filaments (d) Lamins

24. Match the following and select the correct answer: [AIPMT 2014]

(A) Centriole	(1) Infoldings in mitochondria
(B) Chlorophyll	(2) Thylakoids
(C) Cristae	(3) Nucleic acids
(D) Ribozymes	(4) Basal body cilia or flagella

(a) A:4, B:2, C:1, D:3
(b) A:1, B:2, C:4, D:3
(c) A:1, B:3, C:2, D:4
(d) A:4, B:3, C:1, D:2

25. The motile bacteria are able to move by: [AIPMT 2014]
(a) Fimbriae
(b) Flagella
(c) Cilia
(d) Pili

26. The chromosomes in which Centromere is situated close to one end are: [AIPMT 2015]
(a) Metacentric
(b) Acrocentric
(c) Telocentric
(d) Sub-metacentric

27. Nuclear envelope is a derivative of :
(a) Smooth endoplasmic reticulum
(b) Membrane of Golgi complex
(c) Microtubules
(d) Rough endoplasmic reticulum

28. The structures that are formed by stacking of organized flattened membranous sacs in the chloroplast are [AIPMT 2015]
(a) Cristae
(b) Grana
(c) Stroma lamellae
(d) Stroma

29. Select the correct matching in the following pairs [AIPMT 2015]
(a) Smooth ER Oxidation of phospholipids
(b) Smooth ER Synthesis of lipids
(c) Rough ER Synthesis of glycogen
(d) Rough ER Oxidation of fatty acid

30. True nucleus is absent in [AIPMT 2015]
(a) Anabaena
(b) Mucor
(c) Vaucheria
(d) Volvox

31. Which one of the following is not an inclusion body found in prokaryotes? [AIPMT 2015]
(a) Phosphate granule
(b) Cyanophycean granule
(c) Glycogen granule
(d) Polysome

32. DNA is not present in
(a) Chloroplast
(b) Ribosomes
(c) Nucleus
(d) Mitochondria

33. Which of the following are not membrane-bound? [RE-AIPMT 2015]
(a) Ribosomes
(b) Lysosomes
(c) Mesosomes
(d) Vacuoles

34. Which of the following structures is not found in a prokaryotic cell? [RE-AIPMT 2015]

(a) Ribosome (b) Mesosome
(c) Plasma membrane (d) Nuclear envelope

35. The structures that help some bacteria to attach to rocks and/or host tissues are: [RE-AIPMT 2015]

(a) Fimbriae (b) Mesosomes
(c) Holdfast (d) Rhizoids

36. Match the columns and identify the correct option. [RE-AIPMT 2015]

	Column I		Column II
(a)	Thylakoids	(i)	Disc-shaped sacs in Golgi apparatus
(b)	Cristae	(ii)	Condensed structure of DNA
(c)	Cisternae	(iii)	Flat membranous sacs in stroma
(d)	Chromatic	(iv)	Infoldings in mitochondria

	(a)	(b)	(c)	(d)
(a)	(iii)	(iv)	(i)	(ii)
(b)	(iii)	(i)	(iv)	(ii)
(c)	(iii)	(iv)	(ii)	(i)
(d)	(iv)	(iii)	(i)	(ii)

37. Cellular organelles with membranes are: [RE-AIPMT 2015]

(a) Chromosomes, ribosomes and endoplasmic reticulum
(b) Endoplasmic reticulum, ribosomes and nuclei
(c) Lysosomes, Golgi apparatus and mitochondria
(d) Nuclei, ribosomes and mitochondria

Answer Keys

1. (d)	2. (d)	3. (b)	4. (a)	5. (c)	6. (a)	7. (b)	8. (b)	9. (b)	10. (c)
11. (b)	12. (c)	13. (a)	14. (d)	15. (d)	16. (c)	17. (d)	18. (a)	19. (b)	20. (c)
21. (a)	22. (b)	23. (b)	24. (d)	25. (a)	26. (d)	27. (b)	28. (d)	29. (b)	30. (b)
31. (b)	32. (a)	33. (c)	34. (d)	35. (a)	36. (d)	37. (c)	38. (d)	39. (b)	40. (d)
41. (b)	42. (a)	43. (a)	44. (a)	45. (c)	46. (b)	47. (a)	48. (b)	49. (c)	50. (a)
51. (a)	52. (d)	53. (c)	54. (d)	55. (b)	56. (d)	57. (b)	58. (c)	59. (c)	60. (b)
61. (d)	62. (d)	63. (c)	64. (c)	65. (b)	66. (b)	67. (d)	68. (a)	69. (d)	70. (c)
71. (b)	72. (d)	73. (b)	74. (b)	75. (c)	76. (a)	77. (d)	78. (d)	79. (d)	80. (b)
81. (c)	82. (b)	83. (a)	84. (c)	85. (a)	86. (d)	87. (a)	88. (b)	89. (a)	90. (a)
91. (c)	92. (d)	93. (c)	94. (c)	95. (b)	96. (b)	97. (a)	98. (d)	99. (c)	100. (b)
101. (a)	102. (c)	103. (b)	104. (d)	105. (b)	106. (c)	107.(a)	108. (b)	109. (c)	110. (c)
111. (a)	112. (a)	113. (a)	114. (a)	115. (b)	116. (c)	117. (d)	118. (a)	119. (c)	120. (b)

121. (d) 122. (b) 123. (d) 124. (d) 125. (b) 126. (b) 127. (b) 128. (c) 129. (a) 130. (b)
131. (a) 132. (a) 133. (d) 134. (c) 135. (d) 136. (a) 137. (b) 138. (b) 139. (c) 140. (c)
141. (a) 142. (b) 143. (c) 144. (c) 145. (d) 146. (c) 147. (d) 148. (c) 149. (c) 150. (a)
151. (b) 152. (b) 153. (a) 154. (c) 155. (d) 156. (a) 157. (d) 158. (c) 159. (d) 160. (a)
161. (a) 162. (b) 163. (d) 164. (a) 165. (c) 166. (a) 167. (c) 168. (d) 169. (a) 170. (d)
171. (b) 172. (d) 173. (a) 174. (a) 175. (a) 176. (a) 177. (d) 178. (a) 179. (c)

AIPMT Previous Year Questions

1. (a) 2. (b) 3. (a) 4. (c) 5. (b) 6. (b) 7. (c) 8. (b) 9. (a) 10. (a)
11. (d) 12. (c) 13. (d) 14. (d) 15. (b) 16. (b) 17. (d) 18. (d) 19. (b) 20. (d)
21. (d) 22. (d) 23. (b) 24. (a) 25. (b) 26. (b) 27. (d) 28. (b) 29. (b) 30. (a)
31. (d) 32. (b) 33. (a) 34. (d) 35. (a) 36. (d) 37. (c)

CHAPTER

9 Biomolecules

1. Which elements are abundantly found in living organism in comparison to earth crust?
(a) Carbon (b) Hydrogen (c) Oxygen (d) All
2. To analyze chemical composition of living tissue we solubilise them in
(a) HNO_3 (b) HCl (c) CF_3COOH (d) CCl_3COOH
3. Percentage of oxygen in human body is
(a) 65% (b) 46.6% (c) 18.5% (d) 3.3%
4. Chemical analysis of living tissue
(Vegetable or piece of liver + CCl_3COOH)

Acid soluble pool (Filterate)
1. mol. wt (a) ______

Acid insoluble pool (retentate)
1. It contain 4 type of organic compound
a. Protein
b. Polysaccharides
c. (b) ______
d. Lipids

Fill in the blanks in (1) and (2) in above flowchart.
(a) a → greater than 1000 Dalton b → Nucleotide
(b) a → 18–800 Da b → Nucleic acid
(c) a → greater than 10,000 Da b → Oligosaccharides
(d) a → greater than 1000 Dalton b → Nucleoside
5. All the carbon compounds that we get from living tissues can be called
(a) bio-resource (b) bio-informatics (c) bio-war (d) bio-molecules
6. Select the incorrect compounds that we get from living tissues can be called:
(a) Elemental analysis of living tissues gives elemental composition of living tissue
(b) Analysis of chemical compound of living tissue gives idea of organic and inorganic constituent of living tissue
(c) Weight of small amount of living fresh tissue is known as wet weight
(d) Acid soluble pool contain lipids, nucleic acid, polysaccharide only
7. The biomolecule whose weight is less than_____ dalton (Da) is referred to as biomicromolecule.
(a) 800 (b) 18 (c) 1000 (d) 10,000
8. Which of the following is not a macromolecule?
(a) Nucleic acid (b) Polysaccharides (c) Lipids (d) Proteins

9. Lipids are extracted with acid insoluble fraction because
   (a) its molecular weight is less than 800 Da
   (b) it form vesicle or micelle which are not water soluble
   (c) it is polymer
   (d) it is not a polymer
10. Select the incorrect matching for component % in living cell:
   (a) Water – 70–90%
   (b) Proteins – 10–15%
   (c) Carbohydrate – 2%
   (d) Nucleic Acid – 5–7%
11. ________ of the total cell mass is formed by ions.
   (a) 1% (b) 2% (c) 3% (d) 4%
12. Monomeric unit of cellulose is
   (a) glucose (b) fructose (c) mannose (d) ribose
13. Monomeric unit of inulin is
   (a) glucose (b) fructose (c) mannose (d) ribose
14. Which of the following is homopolysaccharide?
   (a) Cellulose (b) Inulin (c) Starch (d) All
15. Starch forms helical ________ structure that can hold ________ molecule and gives blue colour.
   (a) primary, I_2 (b) secondary, I_2 (c) tertiary, I_2 (d) quaternary, I_2
16. Select the incorrect statement from the following:
   (a) Cellulose does not contain complex helices
   (b) Cellulose does not give colour with I_2
   (c) Cotton fibre, plant cell wall are made up of cellulose
   (d) Cellulose is heteropolysaccharide
17. Which of the following is amino-sugar?
   (a) Glucosamine (b) Galactosamine (c) Both (d) None
18. Chitin is
   (a) homopolysaccharide (b) heteropolysaccharide
   (c) oligosaccharide (d) monosaccharide
19. Chitin is present in
   (a) exoskeleton of arthropods (b) cell wall of fungus
   (c) seate of earthworm (d) all
20. In glycogen, which kind of linkage is found between adjacent glucose molecule?
   (a) 1, 4 (b) 1, 6 (c) both (d) 1, 2
21. Which of the following is incorrect about glycogen?
   (a) It is a stored form of glucose in animals
   (b) In glycogen, right end is reducing and left end is non-reducing
   (c) It is a branched polymer of glucose
   (d) It is a stored form of glucose in plants
22. Bond formed between two adjacent monosaccharide is
   (a) peptide bond (b) ester bond (c) glycosidic bond (d) ionic bond
23. Blood concentration of glucose in normal healthy individual is
   (a) 2–3 mM (b) 4.5–5 mM (c) 6–7 mM (d) 1 mM

24. Which is the correct Haworth structure of glucose?

(a) 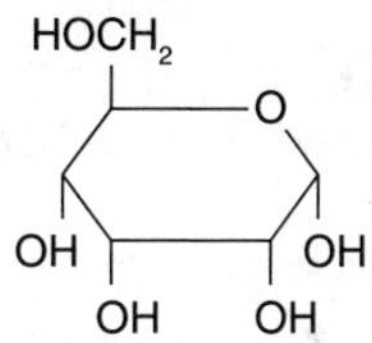 (b) 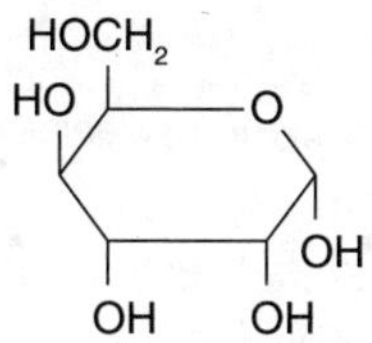 (c) 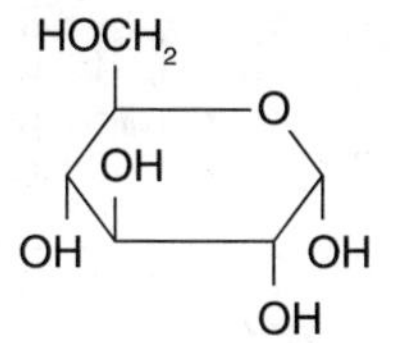 (d) All

25. Which is the correct representation of ribose?

(a) 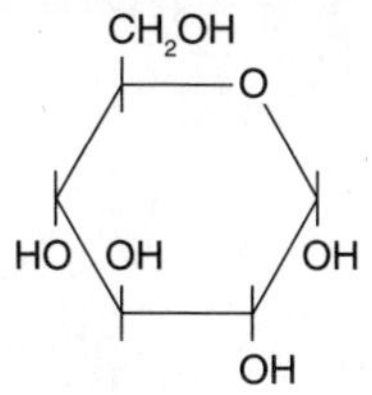

(b) 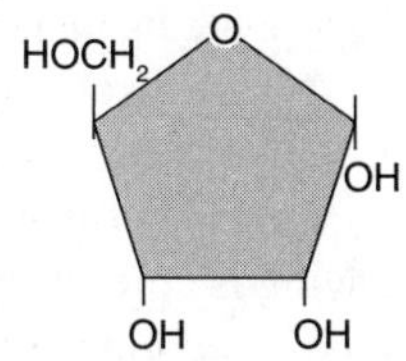

(c) 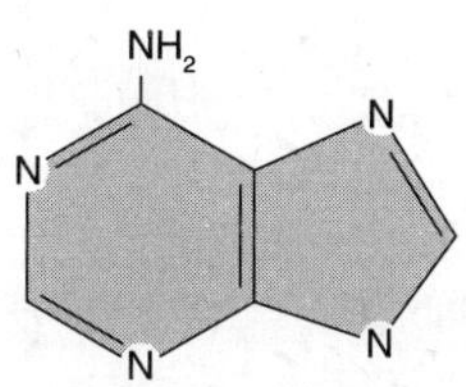

(d) 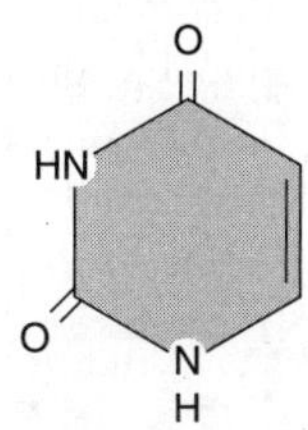

26. Which of the following is a stored form of energy in plant?
(a) starch (b) cellulose (c) glycogen (d) chitin

27. Lipids are
(a) compounds of carbon, hydrogen and oxygen
(b) compounds of glycerol and fatty acid
(c) insoluble in water
(d) all

28. Lipids may be
(a) fatty acid (b) glycerol
(c) compound respectively of both (d) all

29. What is the number of carbon atoms which palmitic and arachidonic acid contain (including carboxyl carbon)?
(a) 16, 19 (b) 15, 19 (c) 16, 20 (d) 18, 20

30. Fats or oils are
(a) monoglycerides (b) diglycerides (c) triglycerides (d) any of the above

31. Which of following is an example of phospholipid?
(a) Palmitic acid (b) Arachidonic acid
(c) Lecithin (d) Glycerol

32. Which of the following is correct about lipids?
(a) On basis on melting points they are divided into fats and oils
(b) Neural tissues are made up of simple lipids only
(c) Phospholipids are never form part of cell membrane
(d) Lipids are strictly macromolecule

33. Select the incorrect matching regarding following diagram:

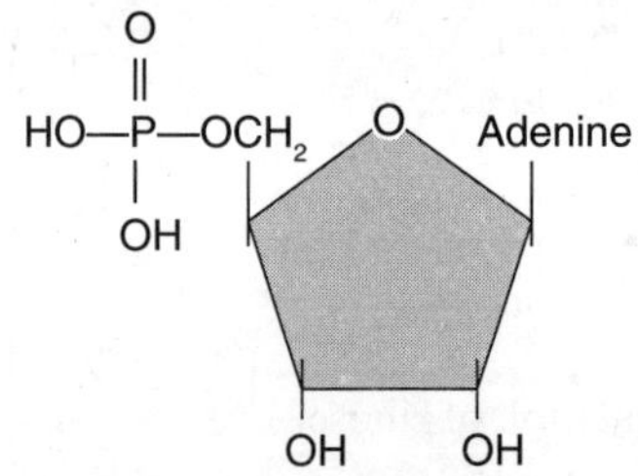

(a) Purine – Its metabolism forms uric acid
(b) Uracil – Exclusively found in RNA only
(c) Adenylic acid – Monomer of both RNA and DNA
(d) Cholesterol – Forms part of cell membrane

34. Which of the following is correct about amino acid?
(a) It is a compound containing amino and acidic group (–COOH)
(b) It is a substitute and is methane
(c) It is based on nature of 'R' group they are of many types
(d) All

35. How many amino-acids are used to form protein?
(a) 18 (b) 20 (c) 21 (d) 22

36. COOH | $H—C—NH_2$ | ® is a structure of α–amino acid. Based on different ® groups the following amino acids are formed. Select the correct amino acid according to different ® group.
(a) R→H (glycine),
(b) R→CH_3 (alanine),
(c) R→CH_2OH (serine)
(d) All

37. Chemical and Physical property of amino acid is based on
(a) $–NH_2$ group (b) –COOH group (c) –R group (d) All

38. Match the column:

Column I		Column II
A. Acidic	–	1. Valine
B. Basic	–	2. Lysine
C. Neural	–	3. Glutamic acid
D. Aromatic	–	4. Tyrosine, phenylalanine, tryptophan

(a) A–3, B–2, C–1, D–4 (b) A–2, B–3, C–4, D–1
(c) A–4, B–1, C–2, D–3 (d) A–1, B–2, C–2, D–4

39. Which of the following is a Zwitter-ionic form of amino acid?
(a) R | $H_3\overset{+}{N}—CH—COOH$ (b) R | $H_3\overset{+}{N}—CH—COO^-$ (c) R | $H_2N—CH—COO^-$ (d) All

40. Protein is
(a) homopolymer (b) heteropolymer (c) polypeptide (d) both (b) and (c)

41. Essential amino acids are those which are
(a) not synthesized by our body
(b) not required by our body
(c) synthesized by our body
(d) only used to form proteins

42. The most abundant protein in animal world is
(a) RuBisCO (b) collagen (c) elastin (d) albumin

43. The most abundant protein in whole biosphere is
(a) RuBisCO (b) collagen (c) elastin (d) albumin

44. Protein acts as a
(a) enzyme (b) receptor (c) antibody (d) all

45. Match the column:

Column I		Column II
A. Collagen	–	1. Hormone
B. Trypsin	–	2. Enzyme
C. Insulin	–	3. Fight Infectious agent
D. Receptor	–	4. Enable glucose transport into cells
E. GLUT–4	–	5. Sensory reception (smell, taste hormone)
F. Antibody	–	6. Intercellular ground substance

(a) A–3, B–2, C–4, D–1, E–6, F–5 (b) A–6, B–2, C–1, D–5, E–4, F–3
(c) A–1, B–4, C–2, D–5, E–3, F–6 (d) A–2, B–4, C–5, D–3, E–1, F–6

46. Which one is correct about macromolecular fraction is comprised of
(a) poly nucleotides (b) poly peptides (c) polysaccharides (d) all

47. Protein is described by biologists at _________ levels.
(a) 1 (b) 2 (c) 3 (d) 4

48. Sequence or positional information of amino acid is given by the
(a) 2° structure (b) 1° structure
(c) tertiary structure (d) quaternary structure

49. In primary structure of protein
(a) Left end represent → 1st amino acid (C-terminal amino acid)
(b) Right end represent → Last amino acid (N terminal amino acid)
(c) Left end represent → 1st amino acid (N-terminal amino acid)
(d) Right end represent → 1st amino acid (C-terminal amino acid)

50.

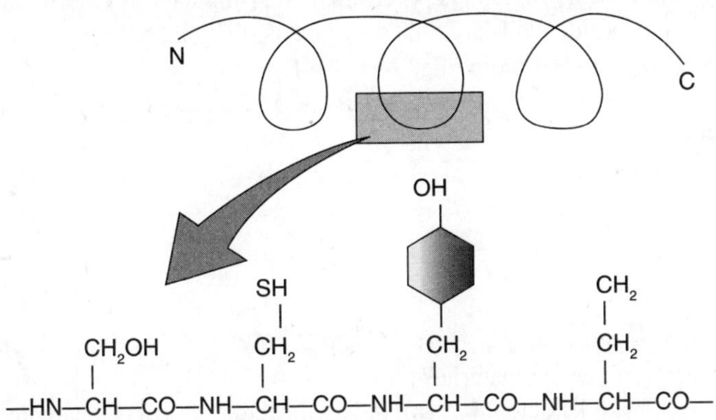

Name the used amino acid in above diagram.
(a) Serine–Cysteine–Tyrosine–Glutamic acid
(b) Serine–Methionin–Tryptophan–Glutamic acid
(c) Serine–Methionin–Tyrosine–Aspartic acid
(d) Serine–Cysteine–Tyrosine–Aspartic acid

51. Which of the following is correct about secondary structure?

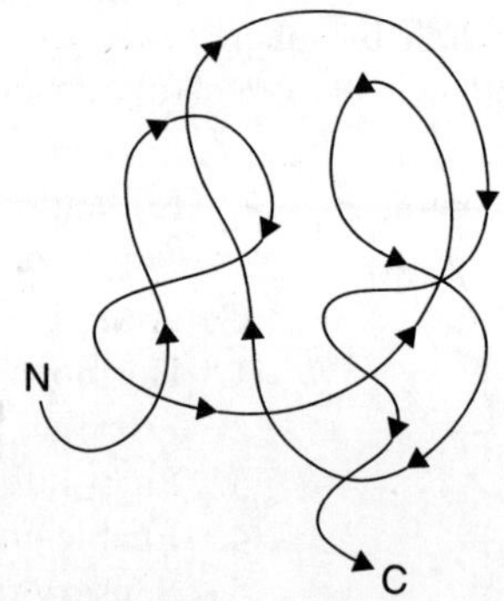

(a) Helix is primary structure
(b) In proteins only left handed helices are observed
(c) In proteins only right handed helices are observed
(d) None

52. Which structure is absolutely necessary for the many biological activities of proteins?
(a) 1° (b) 3° (c) 2° (d) 4°

53. When assembly of more than one poly peptide occur it is known as _____ structure of protein.
(a) 1° (b) 2° (c) 3° (d) 4°

54. Which of the following is correct about human Haemoglobin (Hb)?
(a) Made up to 2-α and 2-β subunits (b) Present in RBC
(c) Use to carry O_2 and CO_2 (d) All

55. Select incorrect statement from the following:
(a) Most of the enzymes are protein
(b) 'Hb' is example of quaternary structure of protein
(c) In primary structure of protein, left hand is N-terminal and right hand is C-terminal
(d) In protein or polypeptide, amino acids are linked by glycosidic bond

56. Which of the following possess heterocyclic ring?
(a) Adenine (b) Guanine and Cytosine
(c) Thymine and Uracil (d) All

57. Identify the nucleoside from the following:
A. Adenosine
B. Uridylic acid
C. Uridine
D. Cytidylic acid
(a) A and B only (b) A and C only (c) C and D only (d) B and C only

58. Which of the following act as a genetic material?
(a) DNA and RNA (b) Uridylic acid (c) Adenylic acid (d) Gunanylic acid

59. Sugar + Nitrogen bases form
(a) Nucleoside (b) Nucleotide
(c) Peptide (d) Glycoside

60. Sugar + Nitrogen bases + Phosphate forms
(a) Nucleoside (b) Nucleotide
(c) Peptide (d) Glycoside

61. How many Nitrogen atoms are present in adenine?
(a) 3 (b) 4 (c) 5 (d) 6

62.

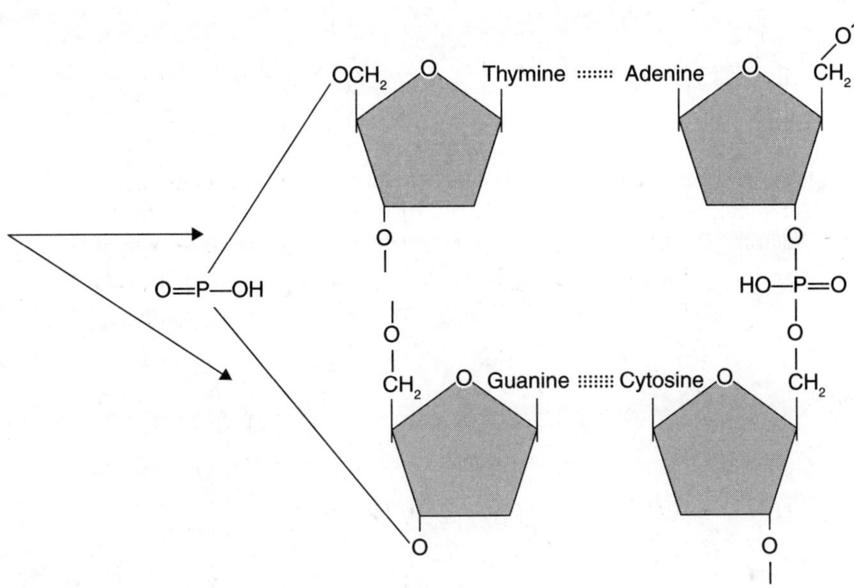

Linkage represented by arrow is
(a) Peptide linkage (b) Phosphodiester linkage
(c) Glycosidic linkage (d) N-glycosidic linkage

63. DNA and RNA are
(a) polypeptide (b) polynucleotide (c) polysaccharide (d) all

64. How much percentage of total cellular mass is formed by nucleic acid?
(a) 3 (b) 2 (c) 5–7 (d) 10–15

65. Following are purines
(a) Adenine (b) Guanine (c) Cytosine (d) Both (a) and (b)

66. Following are pyramidine (substituted):
(a) Cytosine (b) Thymine
(c) Uracil (d) All

67. DNA contains
(a) ribose (b) 3' deoxyribose (c) 5' deoxyribose (d) 2' deoxyribose

68. The bond present between two nucleotides is known as
(a) phosphoester linkage (b) phosphodiester linkage
(c) gycosidic linkage (d) peptide linkage

69. Watson–Crick Structure of DNA is
(a) 1° structure (b) 2° structure (c) 3° structure (d) 4° Structure

70. Which of the following is correct about DNA?
(a) Double helical structure in which two strands of polynucleotide runs antiparallel
(b) Bank-bone is formed by Sugar–Phosphate–Sugar chain
(c) N_2-bases projected more or less perpendicular to back bone and faces inside
(d) All

71.

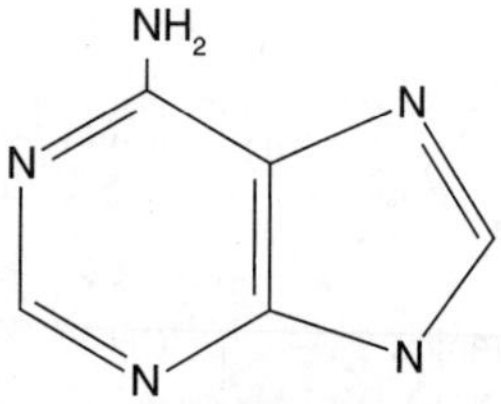

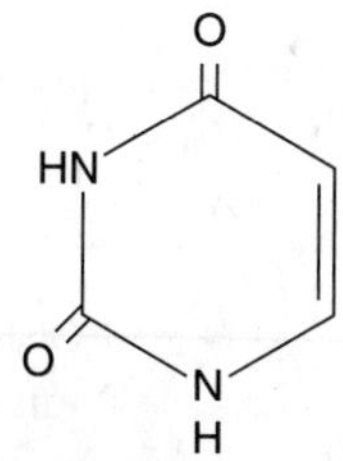

The diagrams represent the nitrogenous bases. Identify the correct combination.
(a) A→Adenine; B→Thymine
(b) A→Guanine; B→Uracil
(c) A→Adenine; B→Uracil
(d) A→Guanine; B→Thymine

72. Which one of the following is the diagrammatic representation of a nucleotide?

(a)

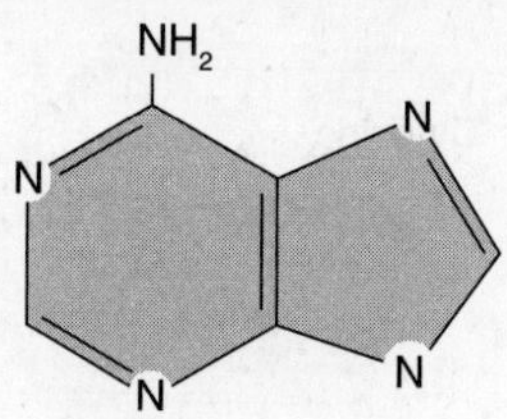

(b)

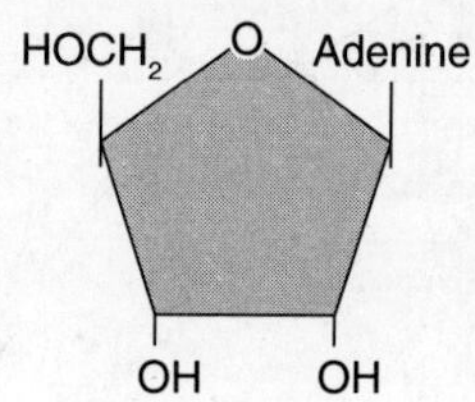

(c)

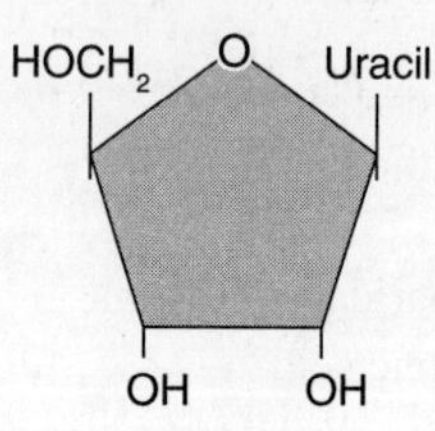

(d)

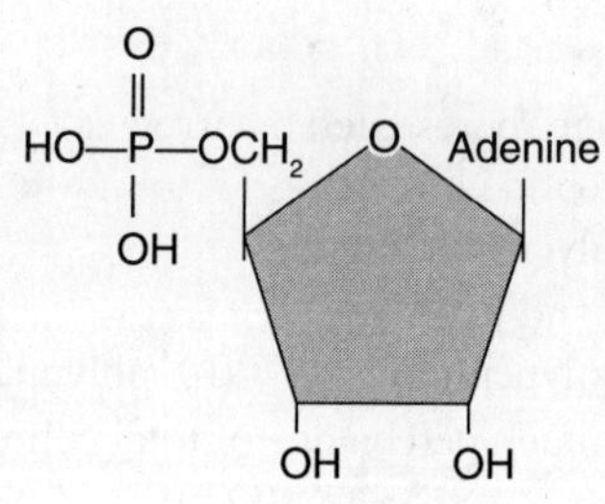

73. Which one is correct about following diagram?

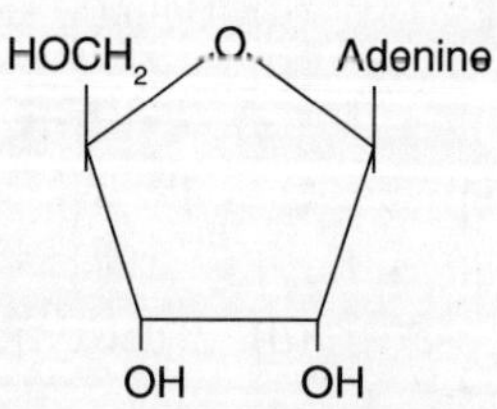

(a) It is a nucleotide
(b) It contain pyrimidine nitrogen base
(c) It is used to form DNA
(d) It is used to form RNA

74. Which one is correct about DNA?
(a) DNA exist as double helix
(b) Two strands of polynucleotide in DNA are antiparallel
(c) The nitrogen bases are projected more or less perpendicular to this backbone but face inside
(d) All

75. At each step of ascent in a B-DNA double helical structure, the strand turn ________.
(a) 36° (b) 72°
(c) 90° (d) 18°

76. One full turn of B-DNA helix strand would involve how many base pairs?
(a) 12 (b) 8
(c) 10 (d) 20

77. Select the incorrect statement from the following:
(a) N_2-bases (A, G, C, T, U) have heterocyclic rings
(b) In most of organism DNA is genetic material
(c) Adenylic acid is nucleoside
(d) The rise per base pair in B-DNA is 3.4A°

78. There are _____ hydrogen bond between A and T, and _____ hydrogen bond between G and C.
(a) 2,2 (b) 3,3 (c) 2,3 (d) 3,2

79. Plants produce an enormous diversity of substances that have no apparent roles in growth and development processes and are classified under the heading of
(a) primary metabolites (b) secondary metabolites
(c) necessary metabolites (d) tertiary metabolites

80. Which one of the following is secondary metabolite?
(a) Amino acid (b) Sugar
(c) Flavonoides and autibiotics (d) Protein

81. Which one of the following statement is incorrect?
(a) Primary metabolites have indenfiable functions
(b) Some secondary metabolites have ecological importance
(c) Secondary metabolites like rubber, drugs, spices, scents and pigments are useful to human welfare
(d) Secondary metabolites are not found in fungi, microbes and plants

82. Following are pigments
(a) Morphine (b) Vinblastin
(c) Carotenoids and anthocyanin (d) Ricin

83. Which one of the following is not a polymeric substance?
(a) Rubber (b) Morphine (c) Protein (d) Cellulose

84. Which of the following secondary metabolites are used as drugs?
(a) Abrin + Ricin (b) Vinblastin + Curcumin
(c) Anthocyanins (d) Monoterpenes

85. Which one of the following is a secondary metabolite?
(a) Lemon oil grass (b) Sucrose (c) Lactose (d) Glycine

86. Match the Column

Column I (Category)		Column II (Secondary Metabolites)
A. Pigments	–	1. Concanavalin A
B. Terpenoides	–	2. Monoterpenes, Diterpenes
C. Alkaloids	–	3. Morphine, Codeine

D. Lectins – 4. Carotenoids, Anthocyanine
E. Toxins – 5. Abrin and Ricin
F. Drugs – 6. Vinblastin, Curcumin
(a) A–1, B–2, C–6, D–4, E–5, F–6 (b) A–4, B–2, C–3, D–1, E–5, F–6
(c) A–3, B–4, C–6, D–5, E–1, F–2 (d) A–2, B–1, C–4, D–6, E–5, F–6

87. Which one(s) is (are) secondary metabolites?
(a) Flavonoids and Rubber
(b) Antibiotics, coloured pigments and essential oils
(c) Scents, gums, spices
(d) All

88. Select the incorrect statement from the following:
(a) All biomolecules have turnover in cell
(b) Metabolic reaction does not occur in isolation
(c) Metabolic pathways are either linear or circular
(d) Metabolites flow is a steady state of body constituent

89. Select the incorrect statement from the following:
(a) Acetic acid becoming cholesterol is an example of biosynthetic or anabolic pathway
(b) Glucose becoming lactic acid in our skeletal muscles is an example of degradation or catabolic pathway
(c) Flow of metabolite through metabolic pathway does not have a definite rate and direction
(d) Anabolic pathway requires energy whereas catabolic pathway releases energy

90. Bond energy, which is stored in our body in the form of ATP, is utilized in
(a) biosynthetic phase (b) osmotic work (c) mechanical work (d) all

91. Living state is
(a) non-equilibrium, non-steady state (b) equilibrium, steady state
(c) non-equilibrium, steady state (d) equilibrium, non-steady state

92. Select the correct statement from the following:
(A) Biomolecules are in metabolic flux in living state.
(B) Living process is a constant effort to prevent falling into equilibrium.
(C) Metabolism provides a mechanism for the production of energy.
(D) Living state and metabolism is synonymous.
(a) All except A (b) All except B (c) All except D (d) All

93. In how many metabolic steps degradation of glucose to lactic acid occurs?
(a) 8 (b) 9 (c) 10 (d) 2

94. How do living organisms derive their energy? What strategies have they evolved? How do they store this energy and in what form? How do they convert this energy into work? These aspects are studied under a sub-discipline called
(a) Biowar (b) Bioinformatics (c) Bioenergetics (d) Biosynthesis

95. Almost all enzymes are
(a) proteins (b) nucleic acid (c) carbohydrates (d) vitamins

96. There are some nucleic acids that behaves like enzymes and are called
(a) DNAase (b) RNAase (c) endonuclease (d) ribozymes

97. ________ of an enzyme is a crevices or pocket into which substrate fit.
(a) Inactive site (b) Active site (c) Allosteric site (d) Any of the above

98. Select the incorrect statement from the following:
(a) Active enzyme has tertiary structure having many active sites (substrate binding sites)
(b) Enzymes are biocatalyst

(c) Enzymes occur in viruses
(d) Enzyme are mainly protein in nature

99. Select the correct statement from the following:
(a) Inorganic catalysts work efficiently at high temperature and high pressure while enzymes get damaged at high temperature (above 40°C)
(b) Ribozymes are nucleic acids behaving like enzyme
(c) Thermophilic organisms living in hot vents and sulphur springs have enzymes that are stable and retain their catalytic power even at high temperature (80–90°C)
(d) All

100. Select the incorrect statement from the following:
(a) A physical change simply refers to a change in shape without breaking of bonds
(b) Change is state of matter is also physical change
(c) Hydrolysis of starch into glucose is an inorganic chemical reaction
(d) Catalyzed reactions proceed at rates vastly higher than that of uncatalyzed ones

101. $CO_2 + H_2O \Leftarrow H_2CO_3$
Carbonic acid

Which one of the following statement is incorrect about the above reaction?
(a) In the absence of enzyme, the rate of H_2CO_3 formation is about 200 molecules per hour
(b) When carbonic anhydrase catalyses the same reaction, there is no change in the rate of H_2CO_3 formation
(c) The reaction catalyzed by the enzyme shows dramatically higher decrease speed about 600,000 molecules being formed every second. (rate becomes 10 million times more)
(d) The enzymes carbonic anhydrase occurs in abundance in RBC

102. Fill in the blanks in below statements:
A. A multistep chemical reaction, when each of the steps is catalyzed by the same enzyme complex or different enzymes, is called a _________ 1 _________ pathway
B. In our skeletal muscle, under anaerobic conditions, _________ 2 _________ is formed.
C. In yeast, during fermentation, the gylcolytic pathway leads to the production of _________ 3 _________.

(a) 1-metabolic pathway 2-acetic acid 3-ethanol
(b) 1-glycolytic pathway 2-lactic acid 3-ethanol
(c) 1-glycolytic pathway 2-ethanol 3-ethanol
(d) 1-metabolic pathway 2-lactic acid 3-ethanol

103. There could be many more 'altered structural states' (like transition state) between the stable substrate and the product in enzymatic reaction. These structural states are
(a) stable
(b) unstable
(c) metastable
(d) of lower energy then both substrate and product

104. Which one of the following statement about enzymes is true?
1. Enzymes are proteins whose three dimensional shape is key to their functions.
2. Enzymes speed up reactions by lowering activation energy.
3. Enzymes are highly specific for reactions.
4. Enzyme activity affected by change in temperature and pH.

(a) All except 2 (b) All except 1 (c) All except 3 (d) All

105. Which of the following is a unique feature about the enzyme?
(a) They are not consumed by the enzyme-mediated reaction
(b) They are not altered by the enzyme-mediated reaction

(c) They lower the activation energy
(d) All

106. The catalytic cycle of an enzyme action can be described in the following steps. Arrange them in sequence accordingly.

1. The binding of the substrate induces the enzyme to alter its shape, fitting more tightly around the substrate.
2. The substrate binds to the active site of the enzyme, fitting into the active site.
3. The enzyme releases the products of the reaction and the free enzyme is ready to bind to another molecule of the substrate and run through the catalytic cycle once again.
4. The active site of the enzyme, now in close proximity of the substrate breaks the chemical bonds of the substrate and the new enzyme product complex is formed.

(a) $1 \rightarrow 2 \rightarrow 3 \rightarrow 4$ (b) $2 \rightarrow 1 \rightarrow 4 \rightarrow 3$
(c) $1 \rightarrow 2 \rightarrow 4 \rightarrow 3$ (d) $2 \rightarrow 1 \rightarrow 3 \rightarrow 4$

107. Activation energy for given reaction is (i.e. reactant $\rightarrow$ product):
(a) Energy of transition state – Energy of substrate
(b) Energy of transition state – Energy of product
(c) Threshold energy – Energy of transition state
(d) All are correct

108. Which one is correct?
(a) $E + S \rightarrow ES \rightarrow EP \rightarrow EP$ (b) $E + S \rightarrow ES \rightarrow EP \rightarrow E + P$
(c) $E + S \rightarrow ES \rightarrow EP \rightarrow E - P$ (d) $E + S \rightarrow ES \rightarrow EP \rightarrow E - P$

109. Which one of the graphs shows the effect of pH on the enzymatic activity (EA)?

(a) 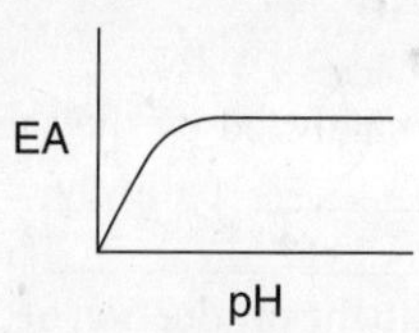

(b) 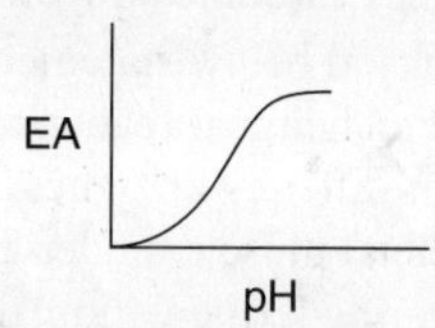

(c) 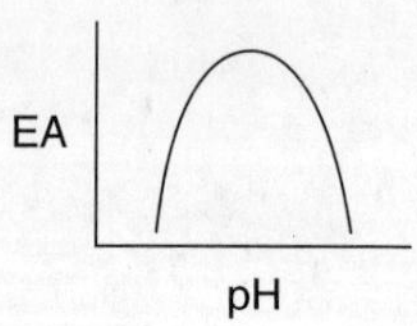

(d) 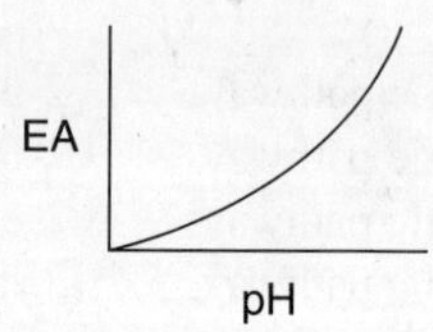

110. Which one of the graphs shows the effect of temperature on the enzymatic activity?

(a) 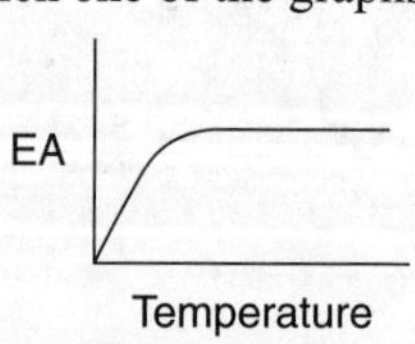

(b) 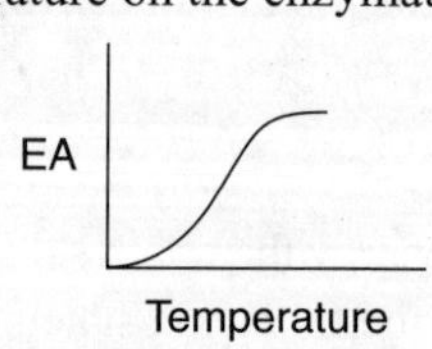

(c) 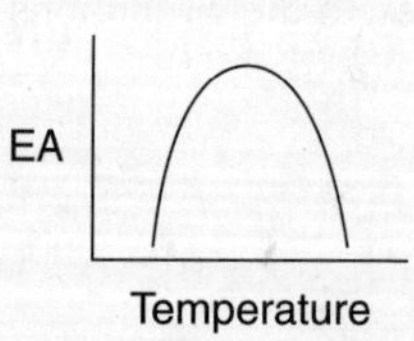

(d) 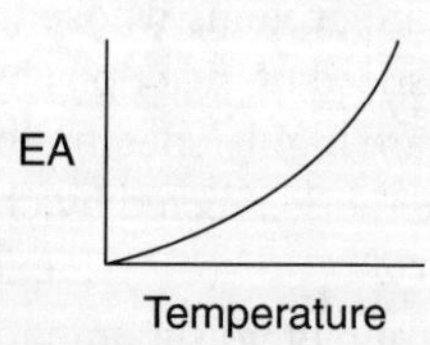

111. Which one of the following graphs show the relationship between the of an enzymatic activity and substrate conc.(S)?

(a) 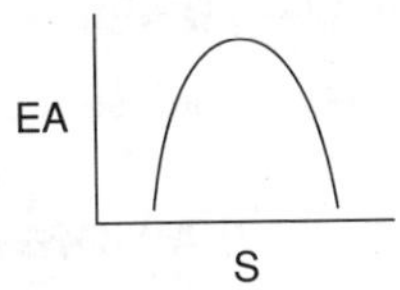

(b) 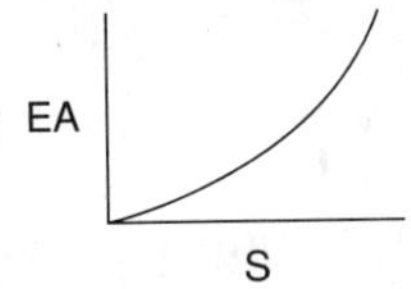

(c) 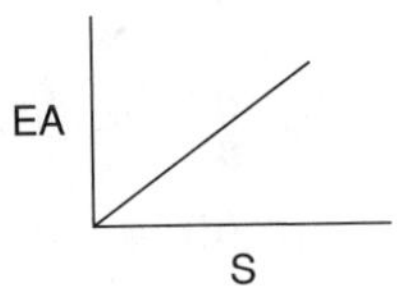

(d) 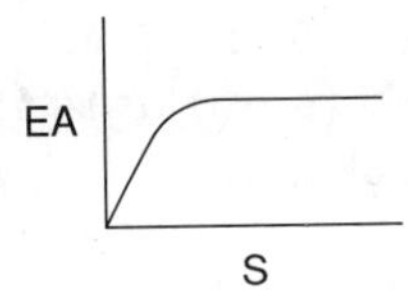

112. Each enzyme shows its highest activity at particular temperature and pH called the __(1)__ temperature and __(2)__ pH. These (1) and (2) are respectively.
(a) optimum, optimum
(b) minimum, minimum
(c) maximum, maximum
(d) minimum, maximum

113. Select the correct statement:
(a) Low temperature preserves the enzyme in a temporarily inactive state
(b) Higher temperature destroys enzymatic activity because proteins are denatured by heat
(c) Activity of enzymes declines both below and above the optimum value
(d) All

114. Select the correct statement:
(a) Increase in substrate concentration, increases velocity of enzymatic reaction at first than it reaches maximum and further increment not occur
(b) In competitive inhibition inhibitor closely resembles the substrate in its molecular structure
(c) Competitive inhibition are often used in the control of bacterial pathogens
(d) All

115. The activity of an enzyme is also sensitive to the presence of specific chemicals that bind to the enzyme. When the binding of the chemical shuts off enzyme activity, the process is called ________ and the chemical is called an ________ .
(a) activation, activator
(b) inhibition, inhibitor
(c) Inhibition, promoter
(d) activation, inhibitor

116. Inhibition of succinate dehydrogenase by malonate is an example of
(a) non-competitive inhibition
(b) negative feed back
(c) allosteric inhibition
(d) competitive inhibition

117. Enzymes are divided into
(a) 6 classes, each with 4–13 subclasses and named accordingly by a four-digit number
(b) 7 classes, each with 3–13 subclasses and named accordingly by a four-digit number
(c) 7 classes, each with 4–13 subclasses and named accordingly by a three-digit number
(d) 6 classes, each with 4–20 subclasses and named accordingly by a four-digit number

118. Enzymes which catalyze oxidoreduction between two substrate belongs to class
(a) oxidoreductase (b) transferase (c) hydrolase (d) ligase

119. Enzymes which catalyze transfer of group other than hydrogen belongs to the class
(a) oxidoreductase (b) transferase (c) hydrolase (d) ligase

120. Enzymes which catalyze hydrolysis of ester, ether, peptide, glycosidic bond belongs to class
(a) oxidoreductase (b) transferase (c) hydrolase (d) ligase

121. Enzymes that catalyze removal of groups from substrates by mechanisms other than hydrolysis leaving double bonds is known as
(a) oxidoreductase (b) transferase (c) hydrolase (d) lyase

122. Enzymes which catalyze inter-conversion of optical, geometric or positional isomers belongs to the class of class
(a) isomerase (b) transferase (c) hydrolase (d) ligase

123. Enzymes catalyzing the linking together of two compounds, for e.g. enzymes which catalyse joining of C-O, C-S, C-N, P-O etc. bonds, belongs to the class of
(a) isomerases (b) transferases (c) hydrolases (d) ligases

124. How many types of cofacter can be identified?
(a) 1 (b) 2 (c) 3 (d) 4

125. The suffix '–' added to substrate for naming the enzyme is
(a) –ase (b) –in (c) –zyme (d) –ose

126. Ptylin is an example of
(a) oxidoreductase (b) transferase (c) hydrolase (d) ligase

127. When Apoenzyme is separated from its metal component, its activity is
(a) decreased (b) increased
(c) lost (d) remains unaffected

128. Cofactors are
(a) prosthetic groups (b) co-enzymes
(c) metallic ions (d) all

129. Which of the following combinations is correct?
(a) Metal ions loosely attached with Apoenzyme–Activators
(b) Nonprotein organic part attached tightly to Apoenzyme–Prosthetic group
(c) Nonprotein organic part attached loosely to Apoenzyme–Coenzyme
(d) All

130. Which one of the following is not cofactor?
(a) Co-enzyme (b) Metal ions (c) Prosthetic group (d) Apoenzyme

131. Haem is prosthetic group of ________ enzyme
(a) peroxidase (b) catalase (c) both (d) none

132. Zn is activator of ________ enzyme
(a) carbonic anhydrase (b) carboxypeptidase
(c) carboxylases (d) all

133. Which of the following statement is correct?
(1) Catalytic activity is lost when the co-factor is removed from the enzyme
(2) Coenzyme nicotinamide adenine dinucleotide (NAD) and NADP contain the vitamin niacin.
(3) Biomacromolecules have a hierarchy of structures–primary, secondary, tertiary and quaternary
(4) Enzymes lower activation energy of reactions and enhance greatly the rate of the reactions.
(5) Nucleic acids carry hereditary information and are passed on from parental generation to progeny.
(a) 1,5 only (b) 2,3 only (c) 2,5 only (d) All

134. The figure given below shows the conversion of a substrate into product by an enzyme. In which one of the options (a–d) the components of reaction labelled as A, B, C and D are identified correctly?

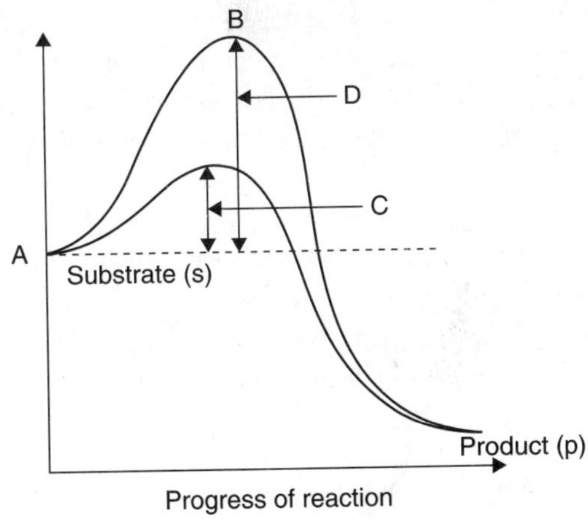

	A	B	C	D
(a)	Potential energy	Transition state	Activation energy with enzyme	Activation energy without enzyme
(b)	Transition state	Potential energy	Activation energy without enzyme	Activation energy with enzyme
(c)	Potential energy	Transition state	Activation energy without enzyme	Activation energy with enzyme
(d)	Activation energy with enzyme	Transition state	Activation energy without enzyme	Potential energy

*Read the **assertion** and **reason** carefully to mark the correct option out of the options given below:*

(a) If both the assertion and the reason are true and the reason is a correct explanation of the assertion
(b) If both the assertion and reason are true but the reason is not a correct explanation of the assertion
(c) If the assertion is true but the reason is false
(d) If both the assertion and reason are false

135. **Assertion:** Arachidonic acid is an unsaturated fatty acid.
Reason: There are present one or more double bonds between carbon atoms in unsaturated fatty acids.

136. **Assertion:** Amino acids are amphoteric in their function.
Reason: All amino acids are necessary for our body.

137. **Assertion:** Coenzyme is a nonprotein group without which enzymes are inactive or incomplete.
Reason: Coenzymes not only provide a point of attachment for the chemical group being transformed but also influence the properties of the group.

138. **Assertion:** Activity of an enzyme is pH dependent.
Reason: Change in pH affects the solubility of the enzyme in water.

139. **Assertion:** A coenzymes or metal ions that is very tightly bound to enzyme protein is called prosthetic group.
Reason: A complete, catalytically active enzyme together with its bound prosthetic group is called apoenzyme.

140. **Assertion:** Enzymes are proteins which catalyse biochemical reactions.
Reason: The enzymes itself unchanged in the reaction, its presence allows the reaction to take place.

141. **Assertion:** Simple carbohydrates having free aldose or ketose group are called reducing sugars.
Reason: They can reduce cupric icon to cuprous state.

142. **Assertion:** Protein amino acids possess an amino group attached to a corbon (α amino acid).
Reason: Proline and hydrolyproline have NH (imino group) so they are imino acids.

143. **Assertion:** Linolenic acid is precursor of arachidonic acid.
Reason: Ascorbic acid is sugar acid having NH_2 group.

144. **Assertion:** Protein is a heteropolymer.
Reason: Protein is made up of amino acid.

145. **Assertion:** Watson–Crick model of DNA is secondary structure of DNA.
Reason: It contain covalent as well as hydrogen bond.

146. **Assertion:** Total number of amino acids involved in protein synthesis in plants is 20.
Reason: Only 20 amino acids have been discovered so far.

147. **Assertion:** In human body collagen is the most abundent protein.
Reason: Scleroproteins occure in hard parts of animals body for providing support and protection.

148. **Assertion:** Living state is a non–equilibrium dteady state to be able to perform work.
Reason: System at equilibrium can not perform work.

AIPMT PREVIOUS YEAR QUESTIONS

1. The figure given below shows the conversion of a substate into product by an enzyme. In which one of the four options (a-d) the components of reaction labelled as A, B, C and D are identified correctly?

[AIPMT MAINS 2010]

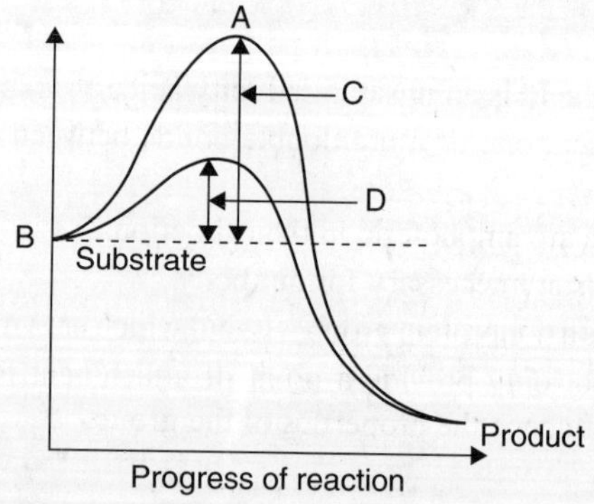

(a) A: Potential energy, B: Transition state, C: Activation energy with enzyme, D: Activation energy without enzyme
(b) A: Transition state, B: Potential energy, C: Activation energy without enzyme, D: Activation energy with enzyme
(c) A: Potential energy, B: Transition state, C: Activation energy with enzyme, D: Activation energy without enzyme
(d) A: Activation energy with enzyme, B: Transition state, C: Activation energy without enzyme, D: Potential energy

2. Three of the following statements about enzymes are correct and one is wrong. Which one is wrong?

[AIPMT MAINS 2010]

(a) Enzymes require optimum pH for maximal activity
(b) Enzymes are denatured at high temperature but in certain exceptional organisms they are effective even at temperatures 80°–90°C
(c) Enzymes are highly specific
(d) Most enzymes are proteins but some lipids

3. Which one of the following structural formulae of two organic compounds is correctly identified along with its related function?

[AIPMT PRE 2011]

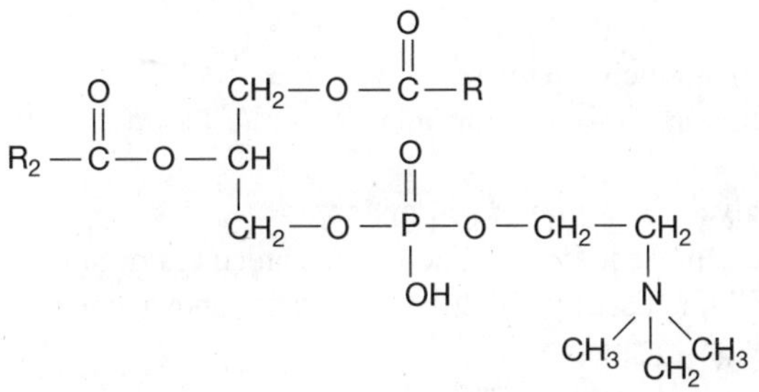

(A)

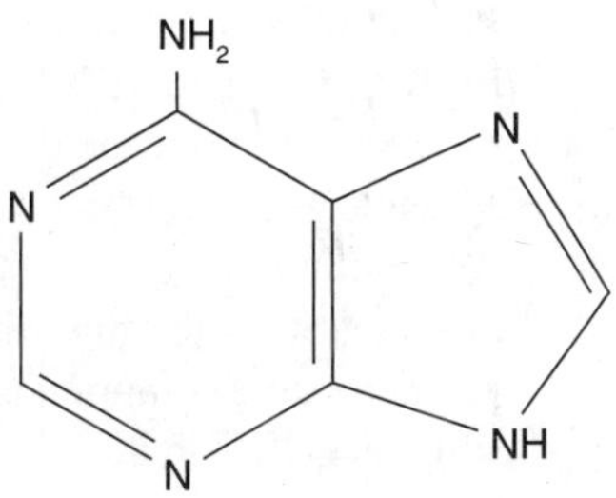

(B)

(a) A: Triglyceride — Major source of energy
(b) B: Uracil — A component of DNA
(c) A: Lecithin — A component of cell membrane
(d) B: Adenine — A nucleotide that makes up nucleic acids

4. Select the correct option with respect to mitosis.

[AIPMT PRE 2011]

(a) Chromatids start moving towards opposite poles in telophase
(b) Golgi complex and endoplasmic reticulum are still visible at the end of prophase
(c) Chromosomes move to the spindle equator and get aligned along equatorial plate in metaphase
(d) Chromatids separate but remains in the centre of the cell in anaphase

5. The curve given below shows enzymatic activity with relation to three conditions (pH, temperature and substrate concentration)

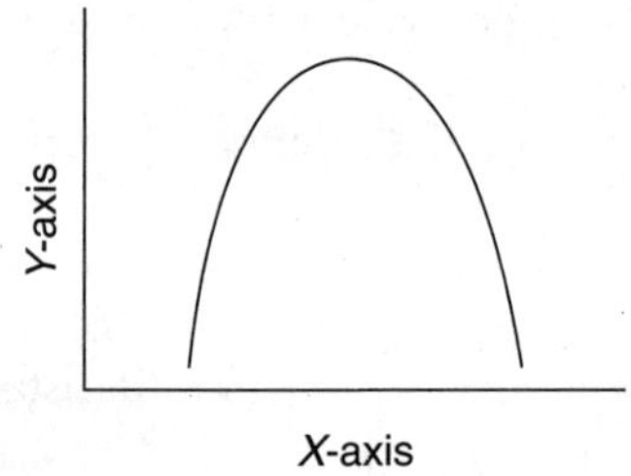

What do the two axises (X and Y) represent?

[AIPMT PRE 2011]

	X-axis	**Y-axis**
(a)	Temperature	Enzyme activity
(b)	Substrate concentration	Enzymatic activity
(c)	Enzymatic activity	Temperature
(d)	Enzymatic activity	pH

6. Which one of the following biomolecules is correctly characterised?

[AIPMT MAINS 2012]

(a) Palmitic acid - an unsaturated fatty acid with 18 carbon atoms
(b) Adenylic acid - adenosine with a glucose phosphate molecule
(c) Alanine amino acid - Contains an amino group and an acidic group anywhere in the molecule
(d) Lecithin - a phosphorylated glyceride found in cell membrane

7. Given below is the diagrammatic representation of one of the categories of small molecular weight organic compounds in the living tissues. Identify the category shown and the one blank component "X" in it.

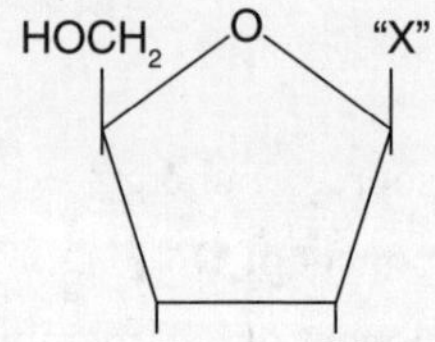

[AIPMT PRE 2012]

	Category	**Component**
(a)	Cholesterol	Guanin
(b)	Amino acid	NH_2
(c)	Nucleotide	Adenine
(d)	Nucleoside	Uracil

8. Which one is the most abundant protein in the animal world?

[AIPMT PRE 2012]

(a) Trypsin (b) Haemoglobin
(c) Collagen (d) Insulin

9. Which one out of A. D given below correctly represents the structural formula of the basic amino acid?

(A) (B) (C) (D)

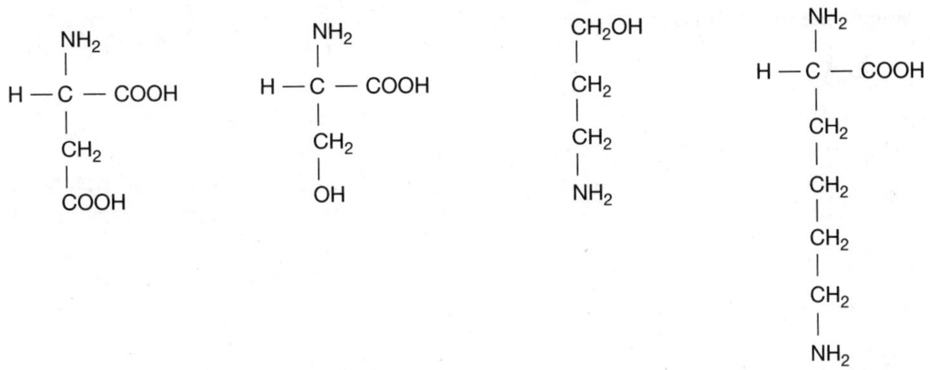

[AIPMT PRE 2012]

Options:

(a) C (b) D (c) A (d) B

10. Transition state structure of the substrate formed during an enzymatic reaction is: [AIPMT AIPMT 2013]

(a) Transient but stable
(b) Permanent but unstable
(c) Transient and unstable
(d) Permanent and stable

11. A phosphoglyceride always made up of: [AIPMT AIPMT 2013]

(a) Only a saturated fatty acid esterified to a glycerol molecule to which a phosphate group is also attached
(b) Only an unsaturated fatty acid esterified to a glycerol molecule to which a phosphate group is also attached
(c) A saturated or unsaturated fatty acid esterified to a glycerol molecule to which a phosphate group is also attached
(d) A saturated or unsaturated fatty acid esterified to a phosphate group which is also attached to a glycerol molecule

12. Macro molecule chitin is [AIPMT 2013]

(a) Nitrogen containing polysaccharide
(b) Phosphorus containing polysaccharide
(c) Sulphur containing polysaccharide
(d) Simple polysaccharide

13. The essential chemical components of many coenzymes are: [AIPMT 2013]

(a) Proteins
(b) Nucleic acids
(c) Carbohydrates
(d) Vitamins

14. Select the option which is not correct with respect to enzyme action [AIPMT 2014]

(a) Substrate binds with enzyme at its active site
(b) Addition of lot of succinate does not reverse the inhibition of Succinic dehydrogenase by malonate

(c) A non – competitive inhibitor binds the enzyme at a site distinct from that which binds the substrate
(d) Malonate is a competitive inhibitor of Succinic dehydrogenase

15. Which one of the following is non reducing carbohydrate?

[AIPMT 2014]

(a) Maltose (b) Sucrose
(c) Lactose (d) Ribulose 5 – phosphate

16. Which one of the following statement is incorrect?

[AIPMT 2015]

(a) A competitive inhibitor reacts reversibly with the enzyme to form an enzyme inhibitor complex
(b) In competitive inhibition, the inhibitor molecule is not chemically change by the enzyme
(c) The competitive inhibitor does not affect the rate of breakdown of the enzyme subtract complex
(d) The present of the competitive inhibitor decreases the K_m of the enzyme for the substrate.

17. The chitinous exoskeleton of arthropods is formed by the polymerization of:

[RE-AIPMT 2015]

(a) D – glucosamine (b) N – acetyl glucosamine
(c) Lipoglycans (d) Keratin sulphate and chondroitin sulphate

18. Which of the following biomolecules does have a phosphodiester bond?

[RE-AIPMT 2015]

(a) Monosaccharides in a polysaccharide (b) Amino acids in a polypeptide
(c) Nucleis acids in a nucleotide (d) Fatty acids in a diglycerides

Answer Keys

1. (d)	2. (d)	3. (a)	4. (b)	5. (d)	6. (d)	7. (c)	8. (c)	9. (b)	10. (c)
11. (a)	12. (a)	13. (b)	14. (d)	15. (b)	16. (d)	17. (c)	18. (b)	19. (d)	20. (c)
21. (d)	22. (c)	23. (b)	24. (c)	25. (b)	26. (a)	27. (d)	28. (d)	29. (c)	30. (d)
31. (c)	32. (a)	33. (c)	34. (d)	35. (b)	36. (d)	37. (d)	38. (a)	39. (b)	40. (d)
41. (a)	42. (b)	43. (a)	44. (d)	45. (b)	46. (d)	47. (d)	48. (b)	49. (c)	50. (a)
51. (c)	52. (b)	53. (d)	54. (d)	55. (d)	56. (d)	57. (b)	58. (a)	59. (a)	60. (b)
61. (c)	62. (b)	63. (b)	64. (c)	65. (d)	66. (d)	67. (d)	68. (b)	69. (b)	70. (d)
71. (c)	72. (d)	73. (d)	74. (d)	75. (a)	76. (c)	77. (c)	78. (c)	79. (b)	80. (c)
81. (d)	82. (c)	83. (b)	84. (b)	85. (a)	86. (b)	87. (d)	88. (d)	89. (c)	90. (d)
91. (c)	92. (d)	93. (c)	94. (c)	95. (a)	96. (d)	97. (b)	98. (c)	99. (d)	100. (c)
101. (b)	102. (d)	103. (b)	104. (d)	105. (d)	106. (b)	107. (a)	108. (b)	109. (c)	110. (c)
111. (d)	112. (a)	113. (d)	114. (d)	115. (b)	116. (d)	117. (a)	118. (a)	119. (b)	120. (c)
121. (d)	122. (a)	123. (d)	124. (c)	125. (a)	126. (c)	127. (c)	128. (d)	129. (d)	130. (d)
131. (c)	132. (d)	133. (d)	134. (a)	135. (a)	136. (b)	137. (a)	138. (a)	139. (c)	140. (b)
141. (a)	142. (b)	143. (c)	144. (b)	145. (a)	146. (c)	147. (b)	148. (a)		

AIPMT Previous Year Questions

1. (b)	2. (d)	3. (c)	4. (c)	5. (a)	6. (d)	7. (d)	8. (c)	9. (b)	10. (c)
11. (c)	12. (a)	13. (d)	14. (b)	15. (b)	16. (d)	17. (b)	18. (c)		

CHAPTER

10 Cell Cycle and Cell Division

1. All organism starts its life with
   (a) single cell (b) many cells (c) few cells (d) few organs
2. The sequence of events by which a cell duplicates its genome, synthesize the other constituent of cells and eventually divides itself into two daughter cells is termed as
   (a) cytology (b) cell division (c) cell cycle (d) cell biology
3. Which of the following is correct about cell cycle?
   (a) All events occur in coordinated manner
   (b) All events are under genetic control
   (c) DNA synthesis occurs only during one specific stage in the cell cycle
   (d) All
4. Cell growth (increase in cytoplasm) is a
   (a) continuous process (b) discontinuous process
   (c) irregular process (d) retrogressive process
5. Our cell can divide itself once approximately in
   (a) 24 hours (b) 24 minutes (c) 24 seconds (d) 24 days
6. Duration of cell cycle in yeast is approximately
   (a) 90 seconds (b) 90 minutes (c) 20 minutes (d) 45 minutes
7. Identify A, B, C, D in below diagram

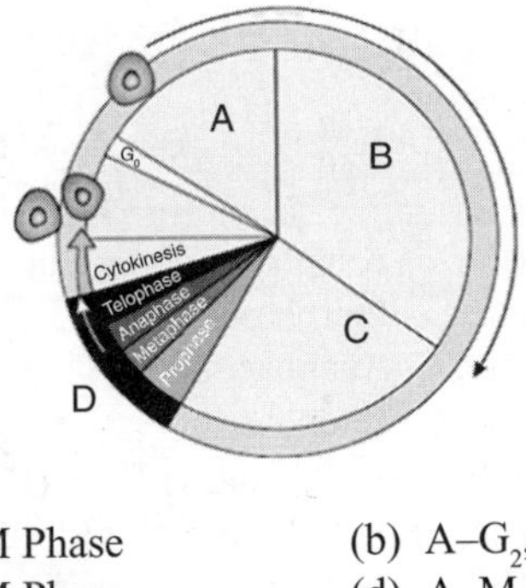

   (a) A–G_1, B–S, C–G_2, D–M Phase (b) A–G_2, B–M Phase, C–G_1, D–S
   (c) A–S, B–G_2, C–G_1, D–M Phase (d) A–M Phase, B–G_1, C–G_1, D–S
8. M-phase in human cell lasts for
   (a) 1 hour (b) 2 hours (c) 23 hours (d) 4 hours
9. Which of the following is correct about Interphase?
   (a) It is the phase present between two successive M-phase
   (b) It lasts for more than 95% in duration of cell cycle in human cell

(c) It is also known as resting phase
(d) All

10. Select correct matching:

Column I		**Column II**
A. G_1 Phase	–	1. Gap 1 Phase
B. Cytokinesis	–	2. Nuclear division
C. Karyokinesis	–	3. Cytoplasmic division
D. S phase	–	4. Synthesis phase

(a) B–1, C–2, A–3, D–4 (b) A–1, C–2, B–3, D–4
(c) D–1, C–2, B–3, A–4 (d) A–1, D–2, B–3, C–4

11. G_1-phase is not characterized by
(a) continuous growth (b) active metabolism
(c) DNA replication (d) non-replication of DNA

12. S-phase is not characterized by
(a) DNA duplication
(b) no increase in chromosome number
(c) DNA replication
(d) duplication of centriole in nucleus of eukaryotic animal cell

13. Which is continuously occurring in dividing G_1, S, and G_2 phase?
(a) DNA Replication (b) DNA Duplication
(c) Centriole duplication (d) Growth of cell

14. If a cell has 2n number of chromosome in G_1-phase, what is the number of chromosome in cell after S-phase?
(a) n (b) 4n (c) 2n (d) 8n

15. Identify A, B, C in below diagram.

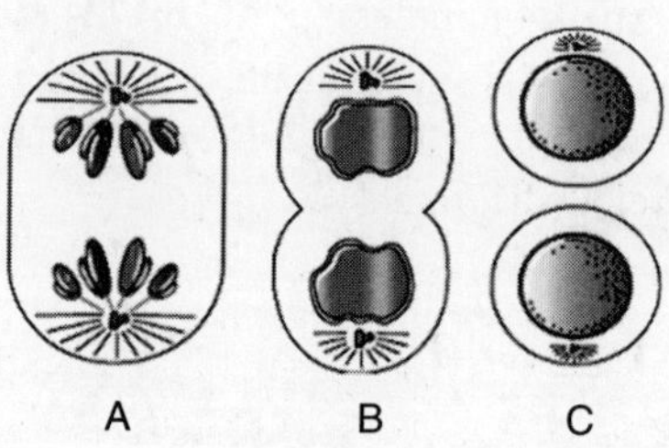

(a) A–Interphase, B–Telophase, C–Anaphase
(b) A–Anaphase, B–Telophase, C–Interphase
(c) A–Telophase, B–Interphase, C–Anaphase
(d) A–Interphase, B–Anaphase, C–Telophase

16. Those cells which do not divide enter ____ phase from G_1-phase.
(a) S-phase (b) Directly G_2-phase (c) G_0-phase (d) Any one of these

17. G_0-phase is characterized by
(a) DNA duplication (b) Active metabolism
(c) S-phase (d) M-phase

18. Select the incorrect statement from the following:
(a) In animals, mitotic cell division is only seen in the diploid somatic cells
(b) Plant can show mitotic division in both haploid and diploid cells

(c) In an adult's heart, cells do not divide
(d) All organisms starts their life cycle from multiple cell

19. Mitosis is further divided in ____ stages of cytoplasmic division?
(a) 1 (b) 2 (c) 3 (d) None

20. Prophase is characterized by
(a) initiation of condensation of chromosomal material
(b) centrioles moving towards opposite pole
(c) initiation of the assembly of mitotic spindle
(d) all

21. Cells at the end of prophase, when viewed under the microscope, do not show
(a) golgi body and ER (b) nucleolus
(c) nuclear envelop (d) all

22. Which of the following initiates the start of metaphase?
(a) Completion of bivalent chromosome formation
(b) Assemblage of microtubules of nucleoplasm
(c) Complete disintegration of nuclear envelope
(d) Duplication of chromosome

23. Metaphase is not characterized by
(a) complete condensation of chromosome
(b) alignment of chromosome on metaphase plants
(c) attachment of spindle fibre to kinetochore
(d) splitting of chromosome

24. Indentify A, B, C, D in the below mitosis diagram.

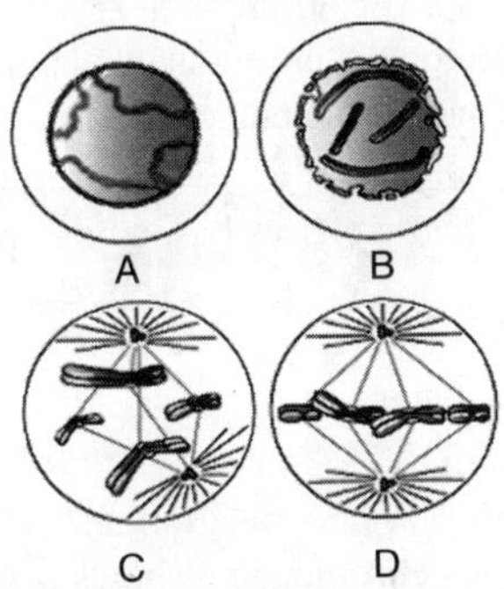

(a) A–Transition to Metaphase, B–Metaphase, C–Early Prophase, D–Later Prophase
(b) A–Late Prophase, B–Transition to Metaphase, C–Metaphase, D–Early Prophase
(c) A–Early Prophase, B–Late Prophase, C–Transition to Metaphase, D–Metaphase
(d) A–Metaphase, B–Early Prophase, C–Late Prophase, D–Transition to Metaphase

25. Anaphase is characterized by
(a) splitting of centromere (b) separation of chromatids
(c) movement of chromatid to opposite pole (d) all

26. Events of telophase are
(a) chromosomes cluster at opposite spindle poles and their identity is lost as discrete elements
(b) nuclear envelope assembles around the chromosome cluster

(c) nucleolus, Golgi complex and ER reforms
(d) all

27. Furrow formation does not occur in plant cell during cytokinesis because of
(a) extensible cell wall (b) inextensible cell wall
(c) extensible plasma membrane (d) inextensible plasma membrane

28. Select the total number of correct statement:
I. Cell-plate formation occur in plant cell during cytokinesis
II. During cytokinesis mitochondria & plastid get distributed between two daughter cells in mitosis
III. Liquid endosperm in coconut is syncytium
IV. Furrow formation occur in Animal cell during cytokinesis
(a) 1 (b) 2 (c) 3 (d) 4

29. Cell which divide by mitosis is
(a) upper layer of epidermis (b) cells lining gut
(c) stem cells (d) all

30. Plant shows continuous growth throughout their life because of
(a) mitosis (b) amitosis (c) meiosis (d) all

31. Mitosis helps
(a) growth (b) repair (c) both (d) none

32. Which of the following holds true about meiosis?
I. It ensure production of haploid phase is the life cycle of sexually reproducing organism where fertilization restores the diploid phase.
II. It involved two sequential cycle of nuclear and cell division called meiosis I and II but only a single cycle of DNA replication.
III. It involves pairing of homologous chromosomes and recombination between them.
IV. Four haploid cells are formed at the end of meiosis.
(a) I, II, IV only (b) IV only (c) I and III only (d) All

33. Prophase I is divided into how many phases based on chromosomal behaviour?
(a) 1 (b) 2 (c) 4 (d) 5

34. Synaptonemal complex formes in
(a) zygotene (b) pachytene (c) diplotene (d) dikinesis

35. Select the correct statement from the following:
(a) In leptotene stage chromosomes become gradually visible under light microscope
(b) During zygotene heterologus chromosome shows pairing
(c) Chiaswater is a J-shape structure formed in diplotene
(d) Pachytene is characterized by the formation of synaptonemal complex

36. Recombination is seen in
(a) diplotene (b) zygotene or synaptotene
(c) pachytene (d) dikinesis

37. Synaptonemal complex is visible in
(a) compound microscope (b) simple microscope
(c) hand lens (d) electron microscope

38. Crossing over is an exchange of genetic material between
(a) homologous chromosome (b) heterologus chromosome
(c) non-homologous chromosome (d) all

39. Beginning of diplotene is characterized by
(a) recombination (b) synapsis
(c) dissolution of synaptonemal complex (d) formation of tetrad

40. Diakinesis is characterized by
(a) condensation of chromosome
(b) assemblage of spindle
(c) disappearance of nucleous and nuclear membrane
(d) all

41. Homologous chromosomes separate during
(a) Metaphase-I (b) Anaphase-I (c) Anaphase-II (d) Telophase-I

42. The stage between two meiosis is
(a) M-phase (b) interphase (c) S-phase (d) interkinesis

43. Which of the following statement is incorrect?
(a) Prophase II is simpler than prophase I
(b) Prophase I is longer and complex than prophase of mitosis
(c) Nuclear membrane reappear in telophase I
(d) Anaphase II is not characterized by splitting of centromere

44. Meiosis is significant because it
(a) increases genetic variability
(b) helps in the conservation of specific chromosome number
(c) is important for evolution
(d) all

45. Most of the cell organelle duplicate during
(a) G_1-phase (b) S-phase (c) G_2-phase (d) M-phase

46. Reduction of the division is
(a) meiosis (b) mitosis (c) both (d) none

47. The main difference between dividing an animal and plant cell lies in
(a) cell plate formation (b) chromosome movement
(c) coiling of chromosome (d) chromosome division

48. Which of the following cells do not divide once it is differentiated?
(a) Interstitial cells (b) Nerve cells (c) Myeloid cells (d) Glial cells

49. Mitosis occurs in
(a) haploid cells only (b) diploid cells only
(c) triploid cells only (d) both (a) and (b)

50. Interphase is also called resting stage because
(a) cell has stopped differentiation
(b) cell is metabolically inactive
(c) no visible changes occur in the nucleus
(d) cell does not grow

51. Diploid somatic cells is divided by
(a) meiosis (b) mitosis only
(c) both meiosis and mitosis. (d) none

52. Cell division takes place when the cell
(a) is haploid (b) becomes diploid
(c) attains optimum growth (d) any time

53. Before cell division, the entire DNA content of the cell gets doubled during interphase.This doubling takes place
(a) throughout the interphase
(b) at the beginning of the interphase
(c) at the end of the interphase
(d) somewhere during the middle of the interphase

54. Cell cycle is divisible into
(a) karyokinesis and cytokinesis. (b) interphase and prophase
(c) interphase and mitotic phase. (d) M-phase and S-phase

55. Correct sequence of stages in cell cycle is
(a) G_1, S, G_2, M (b) G_1, G_2, S, M (c) M, S, G_1, G_2 (d) G_2, G_1, M, S

56. Condensation of chromosome with visible centromere occurs during
(a) G_1-phase (b) G_2-phase (c) S-phase (d) M-phase

57. Synthesis of RNA and proteins takes place in
(a) M-phase (b) S-phase
(c) G_1-phase (d) G_1 and G_2-phases

58. Mitosis is
(a) karyokinesis
(b) cytokinesis
(c) reduction in chromosome number
(d) both (a) and (b)

59. As compared to meiosis, in mitosis
(a) homologous chromosomes form pairs
(b) daughters have half chromosome number
(c) telophase stage is absent
(d) prophase is shorter

60. Cellular structure which always disappears during mitosis or meiosis is
(a) plastids (b) plasma membrane
(c) nucleolus and nuclear envelope. (d) none of the above

61. Chromosomes arrange at equatorial plate of division spindle in
(a) prophase (b) metaphase (c) anaphase (d) telophase

62. Chromosomes can be counted best at the stage of
(a) prophase (b) anaphase (c) metaphase (d) telophase

63. Best stage to observe shape, size and number of chromosomes is
(a) interphase (b) metaphase (c) prophase (d) telophase

64. Spindle fibres are made up of
(a) proteins (b) lipids (c) cellulose (d) pectin

65. Mitotic spindle is mainly composed of the protein
(a) actin (b) actomyosin (c) tubulin (d) myoglobin

66. Separation of daughter chromosomes occurs in
(a) the beginning of anaphase (b) metaphase
(c) late prophase (d) early prophase

67. At which stage of mitosis, chromatids separate and start moving towards poles?
(a) Prophase (b) Metaphase (c) Anaphase (d) Telophase

68. Mitotic anaphase differs from metaphase in possessing
(a) same number of chromosomes and half number of chromatids
(b) half number of chromosomes and same number of chromatids

(c) half number of chromosomes and half number of chromatids
(d) same number of chromosomes and same number of chromatid

69. Animal cells undergo cytokinesis by
(a) furrowing
(b) cell plate
(c) both (a) and (b)
(d) furrowing and followed by deposition of special materials

70. Significance of mitosis lies in
(a) producing cells genetically similar to parent cell
(b) occurrence in energy tissue of body
(c) increasing cellular mass
(d) swift division

71. Mitosis differs from meiosis in
(a) forming four haploid cells
(b) pairing of homologous chromosomes and their subsequent separation
(c) doubling of each chromosome and each pair showing four chromatids
(d) duplication of chromosomes and subsequent separation of the duplicates

72. Number of chromosomes present in pollen grains is six. What shall be their number in leaf cells?
(a) 12 (b) 24 (c) 6 (d) 3

73. Meiosis occurs in
(a) liver (b) kidney (c) gonad (d) brain

74. Meiosis is
(a) disjunctional division (b) equational division
(c) multiplicational division. (d) reductional division

75. Following diagram shows modification of the meiosis I. Indentify A, B, C, D.

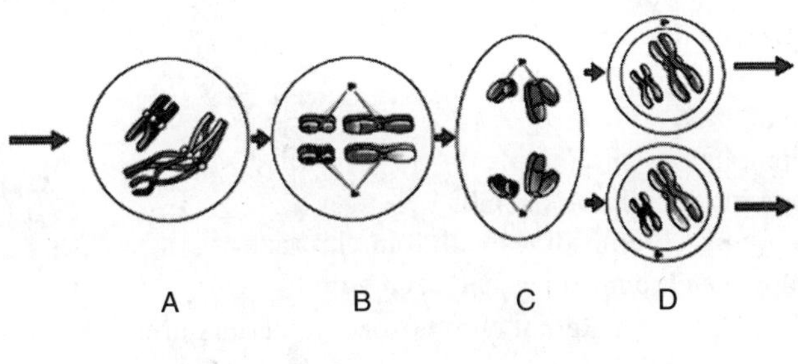

(a) A–Telophase I, B–Anaphase I, C–Metaphase I, D–Prophase I
(b) A–Prophase I, B–Metaphase I, C–Anaphase I, D–Telophase I
(c) A–Metaphase I, B–Telophase I, C–Prophase I, D–Anaphase I
(d) A–Anaphase I, B–Prophase I, C–Telophase I, D–Metaphase I

76. Meiosis involves
(a) two nuclear divisions and two chromosome divisions
(b) two nuclear divisions and one chromosome division
(c) one nuclear division and one chromosome division
(d) one nuclear division and two chromosome divisions

77. Meiosis occurs in
(a) haploid cells (b) diploid cells
(c) both haploid and diploid cells (d) triploid cells

78. Which of the following statements is correct for meiosis?
(a) First division is equational and second reductional
(b) First division is reductional and second equational
(c) Both divisions are equational
(d) Both divisions are reductional

79. Meiosis can be studied in angiosperm in
(a) root apical meristem (b) shoot apical meristem
(c) dividing cells of vascular cambium (d) dividing pollen mother cells in anther

80. How many meiotic divisions are necessary to produce 600 pollen grains?
(a) 50 (b) 100 (c) 150 (d) 300

81. Before undergoing meiosis, the amount of DNA of a cell
(a) become halves (b) become doubles
(c) remains same (d) become quadruples

82. Which of the following represents the correct order in Prophase I?
(a) Zygotene, diplotene, pachytene, leptotene, diakinesis
(b) Diakinesis, diplotene, leptotene, pachytene, zygotene
(c) Leptotene, zygotene, pachytene, diplotene, diakinesis
(d) Pachytene, leptotene, zygotene, diplotene, diakinesis

83. In which stage of meiosis, chromosome is thin, long, and thread-like?
(a) Leptotene (b) Zygotene (c) Pachytene (d) Diakinesis

84. Synaptonemal complex has a role in
(a) chromosome pairing (b) chromosome movement
(c) chromosome segregation. (d) chromosome organization

85. Synaptonemal complex is formed during
(a) cytokinesis (b) amitosis (c) mitosis (d) meiosis

86. Bivalents are formed during
(a) diplotene (b) pachytene (c) zygotene (d) leptotene

87. Tetrad is made of
(a) four nonhomologous chromatids
(b) four nonhomologous chromosomes
(c) four homologous chromosomes with four chromatids
(d) two homologous chromosomes and each with two chromatids

88. Exchange of paternal and maternal chromosome material during cell division is
(a) dyad formation (b) crossing over
(c) synapsis (d) bivalent formation

89. Transfer of genes from one chromosome to another and vice versa during synapsis is called
(a) crossing over (b) exchange (c) Chiasmata (d) translocation

90. Repulsion of homologous chromosomes takes place in
(a) diplotene (b) zygotene (c) diakinesis (d) leptotene

91. When are chromatids clearly visible in meiosis?
(a) Zygotene (b) Pachytene (c) Diplotene (d) Diakinesis

92. Chiasma formation occurs in
(a) leptotene (b) zygotene (c) pachytene (d) diplotene

93. Cross-like configuration when nonsister chromatids of a bivalent come in contact during first meiotic division are
(a) chiasmata (b) bivalents (c) chromomeres (d) centromeres

94. Terminalisation occurs during
(a) mitosis (b) diakinesis (c) cytokinesis (d) meiosis II

95. Number of chromosome groups at equatorial plate of metaphase I of a plant body having 2n = 50 chromosomes shall be
(a) 100 (b) 75 (c) 50 (d) 25

96. In meiosis I, the centromere undergoes
(a) no division
(b) division between anaphase and interphase
(c) division between prophase and metaphase
(d) division but the daughter chromosomes do not separate

97. Meiosis II performs
(a) synthesis of DNA and centromere
(b) separation of sex chromosomes
(c) separation of chromatids
(d) separation of homologous chromosomes

98. Significance of meiosis lies in the
(a) reduction of chromosome number to one half
(b) maintaining constancy of chromosome number during sexual reproduction
(c) production of genetic variability
(d) all of these

99. 200 egg cells are produced by (in meiosis)
(a) 50 divisions (b) 100 divisions (c) 200 divisions (d) 400 divisions

100. A cell has 23 pairs of chromosomes just after the completion of mitotic telophase. The number of chromatids at the preceding metaphase was
(a) 23 (b) 46 (c) 69 (d) 92

101. In plant cells, cytokinesis occurs by
(a) furrowing (b) invagination
(c) anticlinal division (d) cell plate formation

102. The phase of cell cycle during which 'DNA polymerase' is functionally active is
(a) S (b) G_2 (c) G_1 (d) M

103. The number of mitotic divisions required to produce 128 cells from a single cell is
(a) 7 (b) 14 (c) 8 (d) 36

104. Which statement is correct for meiosis?
(a) Meiosis I is reduction division
(b) Meiosis II is reduction division
(c) Meiosis I and II are both reduction divisions
(d) None of the above

105. Which of the following is the longest phase of meiosis?
(a) Prophase I (b) Anaphase I (c) Prophase II (d) Metaphase II

106. Following diagram shows modification of the meiosis II for storage. Indentify A, B, C, D

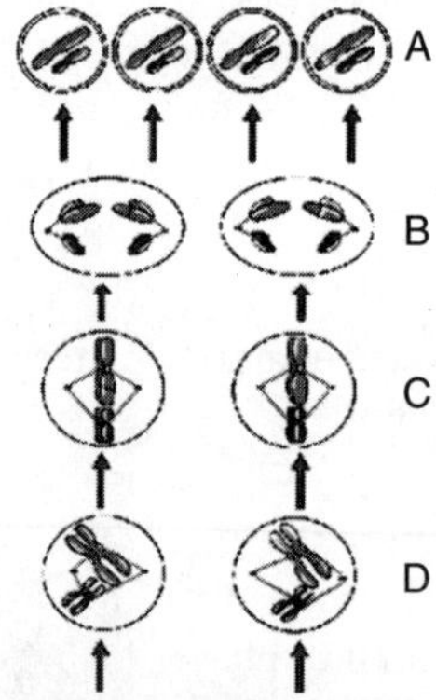

(a) A–Prophase II, B–Metaphase II, C–Anaphase II, D–Telophase II
(b) A–Anaphase II, B–Prophase II, C–Telophase II, D–Metaphase II
(c) A–Metaphase II, B–Telophase II, C–Prophase II, D–Anaphase II
(d) A–Telophase II, B–Anaphase II, C–Metaphase II, D–Prophase II

107. G_1-phase is
(a) end of mitosis and start of S-phase
(b) end of S-phase and start of mitosis
(c) start of S-phase and start of mitosis
(d) end of S-phase and end of mitosis

108. At which stage of mitosis chromatids separate and pass to different poles?
(a) Prophase (b) Metaphase (c) Anaphase (d) Telophase

109. During meiosis, crossing over occurs between
(a) sister chromatids of homologous chromosomes
(b) non-sister chromatids of homologous chromosomes
(c) sister chromatids of non-homologous chromosomes
(d) non-homologous chromatids of homologous chromosomes

110. Which of the following is not true for anaphase?
(a) Golgi body and ER are reformed
(b) Spindle poles move farther apart
(c) Chromosomes move to opposite poles
(d) Centromeres split and chromatids separate

111. The longest phase of meiosis I is
(a) Metaphase-I (b) Prophase-I (c) Anaphase-I (d) Telophase-I

112. Cyclin protein is required for cell cycle. Which other molecule is essential for the completion of cell cycle?
(a) CCK (b) CKc (c) CdK (d) CKd

113. Pick out the correct statements from the following:
I. Synapsis of homologous chromosomes takes place during prophase I of meiosis.
II. Division of centromeres takes place during anaphase I of meiosis.
III. Spindle fibres disappear completely in telophase of mitosis.
IV. Nucleoli reappear at telophase I of meiosis.
(a) I only (b) III only (c) I and II only (d) I, III and IV only

*Read the **assertion** and **reason** carefully to mark the correct option out of the options given below:*

(a) If both the assertion and the reason are true and the reason is a correct explanation of the assertion

(b) If both the assertion and reason are true but the reason is not a correct explanation of the assertion

(c) If the assertion is true but the reason is false

(d) If both the assertion and reason are false

114. **Assertion:** The comple formed by a pair of synapsed homologous chromosome is called a bivalent or a tetrad.
Reason: The first two stages of prophase I are relatively short lived in compared to the next stage that is pachytene.

115. **Assertion:** In oocytes of of some vertebrates, diplotene can last for months or years.
Reason: The final stage of meiotic prophase I is dikinesis.

116. **Assertion:** Variartions are are very important for the process of evolution.
Reason: Most of the organelle duplication occur in G_1 phase of cell cycle.

117. **Assertion:** Liquid endosperm in coconut is multinucleated.
Reason: Karyokinesis is not followed by cytokinesis.

118. **Assertion:** Karyokinesis occurs in S-phase
Reason: Cell division stops in M-phase

119. **Assertion:** Interphase is resting stage.
Reason: The interphase cell is metabolically inactive.

120. **Assertion:** DNA synthesis occurs in G_1 and G_2 periods of cell cycle.
Reason: During G_1 and G_2 phase the DNA contents become double.

121. **Assertion:** Mitosis maintains the genetic similarity of somatic cells.
Reason: Chromosomes do not undergo crossing over.

122. **Assertion:** Chiasmata is formed during diplotene.
Reason: Chiasmata are formed due to deposition of nucleoproteins.

123. **Assertion:** During zygotene, chromosomes show bivalent stage.
Reason: Bivalent is half the number of chromosomes.

124. **Assertion:** Meiosis takes place in pollen mother cells.
Reason: Each pollen mother cell produce 4 haploid pollen grains.

125. **Assertion:** Meiotic division results in the production of haploid cells.
Reason: Synapsis occurs during zygotene of meiosis.

AIPMT PREVIOUS YEAR QUESTIONS

1. An elaborate network of filamentous proteinaceous structures present in the cytoplasm which helps in the maintenance of cell shape is called.

[AIPMT MAINS 2010]

(a) Thylakoid
(b) Endoplasmic reticulum
(c) Plasmalemma
(d) Cytoskeleton

2. During mitosis ER and nucleolus begin to disappear at

[AIPMT PRE 2010]

(a) Late prophase
(b) Early metaphase
(c) Late metaphase
(d) Early prophase

3. Which stages of cell division do the following figures A and B represent respectively?

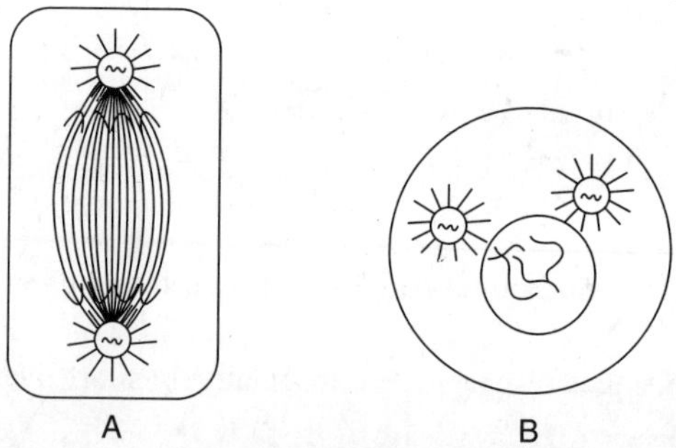

[AIPMT PRE 2010]

	A		B
(a)	Metaphase	-	Telophase
(b)	Telophase	-	Metaphase
(c)	Late anaphase	-	Prophase
(d)	Prophase	-	Anaphase

4. At metaphase, chromosomes are attached to the spindle fibres by their

[AIPMT MAINS 2011]

(a) Satellites
(b) Secondary constrictions
(c) Kinetochores
(d) Centromeres

5. Identify the meiotic stage in which the homologous chromosomes separate while the sister chromatids remain associated at their centromeres:

[AIPMT MAINS 2012]

(a) Metaphase-II
(b) Anaphase-I
(c) Anaphase-II
(d) Metaphase-I

6. During gamete formation the enzyme recombinase participates during:

[AIPMT PRE 2012]

(a) Metaphase – I
(b) Anaphase – II
(c) Prophase – I
(d) Prophase – II

7. Given below is the representation of a certain event at a particular stage of a type of cell division. Which is this stage?

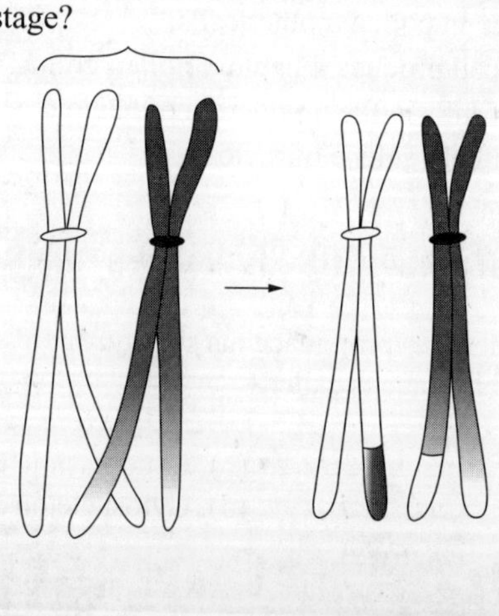

[AIPMT PRE 2012]

(a) Prophase I during meiosis (b) Prophase II during meiosis
(c) Prophase of Mitosis (d) Both prophase and metaphase of mitosis

8. The complex formed by a pair of synapsed homologous chromosomes is called: [AIPMT 2013]

(a) Equatorial plate (b) Kinetochore
(c) Bivalent (d) Axoneme

9. A stage in cell division is shown in the figure. Select the answer which gives correct identification of the stage with its characteristics.

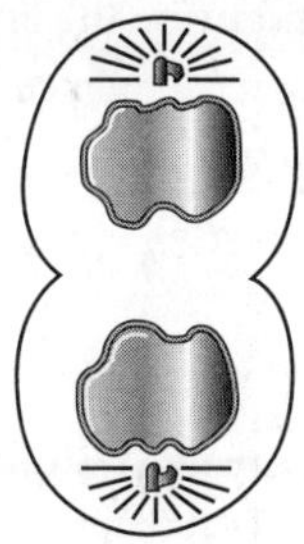

[AIPMT 2013]

(a) Telophase — Nuclear envelope reforms, Golgi complex reforms
(b) Late anaphase — Chromosomes move away from equatorial plate, Golgi complex not present
(c) Cytokinesis — Cell plate formed mitochondria distributed between two daughter cells.
(d) Telophase — Endoplasmic reticulum and nucleolus not reformed yet.

10. During which phase(s) of cell cycle, amount of DNA in a cell remains at 4C level if the initial amount is denoted as 2C? [AIPMT 2014]

(a) G_0 and G_1 (b) G_1 and S
(c) Only G_2 (d) G_2 and M

11. In 'S' phase of the cell cycle: [AIPMT 2014]

(a) Amount of DNA doubles in each cell
(b) Amount of DNA remains same in each cell
(c) Chromosome number is increased
(d) Amount of DNA is reduced to half in each cell

12. The enzyme recombinase is required at which state of meiosis [AIPMT 2014]

(a) Pachytene (b) Zygotene
(c) Diplotene (d) Diakinesis

13. Select the correct option.

Column I		**Column II**
A. Synapsis aligns homologous chromosomes	–	1. Anaphase - II
B. Synthesis of RNA and protein	–	2. Zygotene
C. Action of enzyme recombinase	–	3. G_2-phase
D. Centromeres do not separate but chromatids move towards opposite poles	–	4. Anaphase - I

[AIPMT 2015]

(a) A:2, B:1, C:3, D:4
(b) A:2, B:3, C:5, D:4
(c) A:1, B:2, C:5, D:4
(d) A:2, B:3, C:4, D:5

14. A somatic cell that has just completed the S phase of its cell cycle as compared to gamete of the same species has:

[AIPMT 2015]

(a) Twice the number of chromosomes and twice the amount of DNA
(b) Same number of chromosomes but twice the amount of DNA
(c) Twice the number of chromosomes and four times the amount of DNA
(d) Four times the number of chromosomes and twice the amount of DNA

15. Arrange the following events of meiosis in correct sequence:

[RE-AIPMT 2015]

(A) Crossing over
(B) Synapsis
(C) Terminalisation of chiasmata
(D) Disappearance of nucleolus

(a) (b), (a), (c), (d)
(b) (a), (b), (c), (d)
(c) (b), (c), (d), (a)
(d) (b), (a), (d), (c)

Answer Keys

1. (a)	2. (c)	3. (d)	4. (a)	5. (a)	6. (b)	7. (a)	8. (a)	9. (d)	10. (b)
11. (c)	12. (d)	13. (d)	14. (c)	15. (b)	16. (c)	17. (b)	18. (d)	19. (d)	20. (d)
21. (d)	22. (c)	23. (d)	24. (c)	25. (d)	26. (d)	27. (b)	28. (d)	29. (d)	30. (a)
31. (c)	32. (d)	33. (d)	34. (a)	35. (a)	36. (c)	37. (d)	38. (a)	39. (c)	40. (d)
41. (b)	42. (d)	43. (d)	44. (d)	45. (a)	46. (a)	47. (a)	48. (b)	49. (d)	50. (c)
51. (b)	52. (c)	53. (d)	54. (c)	55. (a)	56. (d)	57. (d)	58. (d)	59. (d)	60. (c)
61. (b)	62. (c)	63. (b)	64. (a)	65. (c)	66. (a)	67. (c)	68. (a)	69. (a)	70. (a)
71. (d)	72. (a)	73. (c)	74. (d)	75. (b)	76. (b)	77. (b)	78. (b)	79. (d)	80. (c)
81. (b)	82. (c)	83. (a)	84. (a)	85. (d)	86. (c)	87. (d)	88. (b)	89. (a)	90. (a)
91. (b)	92. (d)	93. (a)	94. (b)	95. (d)	96. (a)	97. (c)	98. (d)	99. (c)	100. (d)
101. (d)	102. (a)	103. (a)	104. (a)	105. (a)	106. (d)	107. (a)	108. (c)	109. (b)	110. (a)
111. (b)	112. (c)	113. (d)	114. (b)	115. (b)	116. (b)	117. (a)	118. (d)	119. (c)	120. (d)
121. (a)	122. (c)	123. (b)	124. (a)	125. (a)					

AIPMT Previous Year Questions

1. (d)	2. (a)	3. (c)	4. (c)	5. (b)	6. (c)	7. (a)	8. (c)	9. (a)	10. (d)
11. (a)	12. (a)	13. (b)	14. (c)	15. (a)					

Unit IV

Plant Physiology

Unit IV includes plant physiology. In this unit, more questions are asked from the chapter on plant water relationship and mineral nutrition. In AIPMT, three to five questions are asked from this unit. For these chapters, textbook is more than sufficient.

CHAPTER 11

Transport in Plants

1. In flowering plant, we need to transport
   (a) water and mineral nutrients
   (b) organic nutrients
   (c) plant growth regulators
   (d) all
2. For covering a small distance, substances move by
   (a) diffusion
   (b) cytoplasmic streaming
   (c) active transport
   (d) all
3. Transport over longer distance is known as
   (a) translocation
   (b) transformation
   (c) transduction
   (d) diffusion
4. Which of the following undergo multidirectional transport?
   (a) Water
   (b) Mineral nutrients
   (c) Organic nutrients
   (d) Both (b) and (c)
5. Transport of which substance is essentially unidirectional in xylem?
   (a) Water
   (b) Mineral nutrients
   (c) Organic nutrients
   (d) Both (a) and (b)
6. Select the correct statement from the following:
   (a) Mineral nutrients taken up by the roots and transported upward into stem, leaves and growing region
   (b) When a plant part undergoes senescence, nutrient always remain in the senescence part and gets lost from the plant
   (c) In flowering plant complex traffic of compound in unorderly manner moving in different direction
   (d) All hormones shows polarised movement
7. Diffusion can occur between
   (a) one part of cell to other part
   (b) cell to cell
   (c) intercellular space to outside of leaf
   (d) all
8. Only mode of gaseous movement in plant body is
   (a) diffusion
   (b) osmosis
   (c) facilitated transport
   (d) all
9. Which of the following is incorrect about diffusion?
   (1) Molecules move in random fashion.
   (2) It occurs from higher to lower concentration.
   (3) It is a slow process.
   (4) It does not depend on living system.

(5) Protein carriers are required.
(6) It is a passive process.
(a) Only 1 and 5 (b) Only 5 (c) 1, 3, 5 only (d) Only 4

10. Diffusion rate is affected by
(a) Concentration gradient
(b) Membrane permeability through which it occur
(c) Pressure and temperature
(d) All

11. Find out total number of false statements from the following.
(1) The diffusion rate depends on size of substrate.
(2) Diffusion across membrane depends upon solubility a lipids.
(3) Membrane protein provide sites for hydrophilic substance to cross membrane.
(4) Facilitated diffusion do not require concentration gradient.
(a) 1 (b) 2 (c) 3 (d) 4

12. Facilitated diffusion require __________ to transport substance across membrane.
(a) Special membrane protein (b) ATP
(c) Protein inhibitor (d) All

13. Which process undergo saturation?
(a) Facilitated diffusion (b) Active transport
(c) Simple diffusion (d) Both (a) and (b)

14. Which of the following transport is not highly selective?
(a) Facilitated diffusion (b) Active transport
(c) Simple diffusion (d) All

15. Identify A, B and C in the given figure.

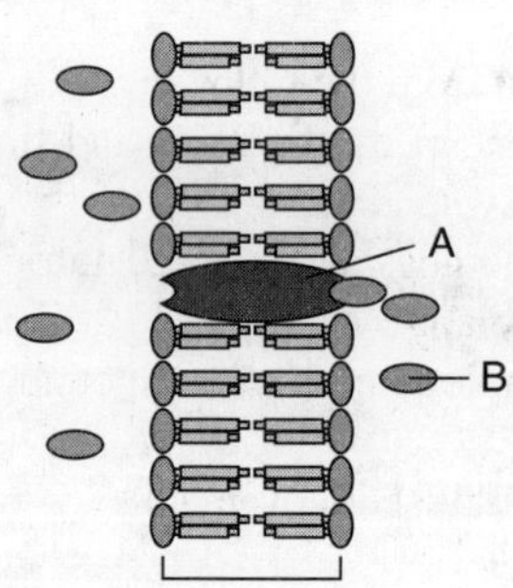

(a) A–Transported molecule, B–Inner side of cell, C–Transport protein
(b) A–Transport protein, B–Transported molecule, C–Membrane
(c) A–Inner side of cell, B–Membrane, C–Transported molecule
(d) A–Membrane, B–Transport protein, C–Transported molecule

16. Where poring proteins are present?
(a) Outer membrane of plastid (b) Inner membrane of mitochondria
(c) Inner membrane of some bacteria (d) Outer membrane of ribosomes

17. Choose total number of correct statements from the following:
(1) Some channels in membrane are always open.
(2) Porins allow passes of molecule of size up to small protein.

(3) Water channel made up of eight different type of aquaporins.
(4) Facilitated diffusion is very specific.
(a) 1 (b) 2 (c) 3 (d) 4

18. Some transport proteins allow diffusion only. If two type of molecules move together in same direction. Such type of transport is known as
(a) symport (b) antiport (c) uniport (d) all

19. If two move together in opposite direction. If two type of molecules move together in opposite direction. Such type of transport is known as
(a) symport (b) antiport (c) uniport (d) all

20. When molecule move across in a membrane independent of other molecules through carrier protein the process is known as
(a) symport (b) antiport (c) uniport (d) all

21. A transport which uses energy to pump molecules against a concentration gradient is known as
(a) diffusion (b) facilitated diffusion
(c) active transport (d) all

22. Proteins in the membrane, responsible for facilitated diffusion and active transport, show some common characteristic like.
(1) being highly selective. (2) being liable to saturate.
(3) responding to inhibitor. (4) being regulated by hormones.
(a) 1, 2 only (b) 2, 3 only (c) 3, 4 only (d) all

23. Identify A–E given in the figure.

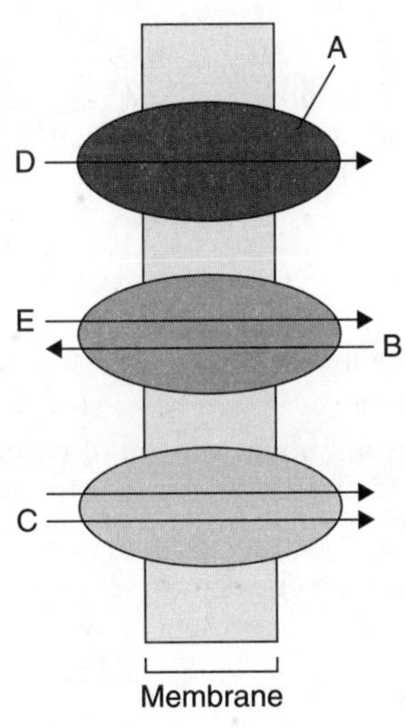

(a) A–Antiport B, B–Uniport A, C–Antiport A, D–Symport B, E–Carrier point
(b) A–Carrier point, B–Antiport A, C–Uniport A, D–Symport B, E–Antiport B
(c) A–Carrier point, B–Antiport B, C–Symport B, D–Uniport A, E–Antiport A
(d) A–Symport B, B–Antiport A, C–Antiport B, D–Carrier point, E–Uniport A

24. Identify A, B and C shown in this table:

Property	Simple Diffusion	Facilitated Transport	Active Transport
Requires special membrane proteins	A	Yes	Yes
Highly selective	No	Yes	Yes
Transport Saturates	No	B	Yes
Uphill transport	No	No	C
Requires ATP energy	No	No	Yes

(a) A–Yes, B–Yes, C–Yes (b) A–Yes, B–No, C–Yes
(c) A–No, B–Yes, C–Yes (d) A–No, B–No, C–Yes

25. Select the incorrect statement from the following:
(1) A watermelon has over 92% water.
(2) Most herbaceous plants have only about 10–15% of its fresh water as dry matter.
(3) Woody parts of the plant have very little water.
(4) Seed is without water.
(5) Mature corn plant absorb almost three litres of water in a day.
(6) Mustered plant absorb water epical to its own weight in about 5 hours.
(a) All except 6 (b) All except 5 (c) Only 4 (d) Only 3

26. Water is often a limitary factor for plant growth and _________ in both _________ and _________ environments.
(a) productivity, agricultural, natural
(b) movement, agricultural, artificial
(c) photosynthesis, aquatic, terrestrial
(d) senescence, agricultural, natural

27. Major similarity between active transport and facilitated diffusion is that
(a) both consume ATP
(b) both are passive
(c) both are non-selective
(d) both require membrane proteins

28. A watermelon has approximately _________ of water.
(a) 20% (b) 80% (c) 100% (d) 92%

29. Which of the following has minimum amount of water?
(a) Leaf (b) Flower
(c) Epidermal cell of root (d) Cork

30. Select from the following which one is move by active transport
(1) Na^+ amino acid, in proximal convoluted tubules.
(2) Absorption of most minerals by epidermal cells of root.
(3) Na^+ K^+ pump.
(4) Loading of sucrose from companion cell to sieve tube cells.
(a) All except 4 (b) All except 3 (c) All except 1 (d) All

31. Two main components which determine water potential are
(a) solute potential (b) pressure potential
(c) matric potential (d) both (a) and (b)

32. Which of the following has the maximum water potential?
(a) 1 M of NaCl (b) 0.5 M of glucose (c) Pure water (d) 0.001 M of HCl

33. Three solutions in container are given under one similar condition. Which solution posses greater kinetic energy in water molecules?

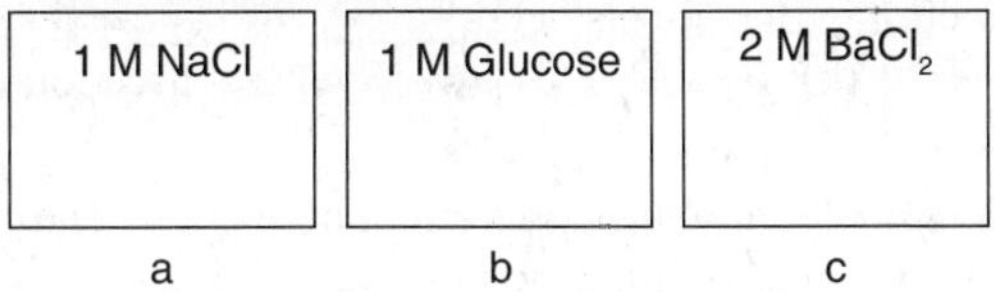

(a) A (b) B
(c) C (d) All solution possess same energy

34. What is the condition for pure water having zero water potential?
(a) Standard temperature (b) No pressure
(c) At 1 atm pressure (d) Only (a) and (b)

35. Which is always negative (under natural condition)?
(1) ψ_s (2) ψ_w of solution (3) ψ_p (4) ψ_p of solution
(a) 1, 2 only (b) 1 only (c) 4 only (d) 3 only

36. The relationship between ψ_w, ψ_s and ψ_p is
(a) $\psi_s = \psi_w + \psi_p$ (b) $\psi_p = \psi_w + \psi_s$ (c) $\psi_w = \psi_p + \psi_s$ (d) All

37. Which is important to determine that which is going in or out of plant cell?
(a) Cell membrane only (b) Tonoplast only
(c) Both together (d) Cell wall only

38. Cell wall is
(a) permeable (b) impermeable
(c) semi-permeable (d) selectively permeable

39. Osmosis means diffusion of water across
(a) semi-permeable membrane (b) differentially permeable membrane
(c) permeable membrane (d) both (a) and (b)

40. Water will move from
(a) higher pressure potential to lower (b) higher solute potential to lower
(c) higher water potential to lower (d) lower water potential to higher

41.

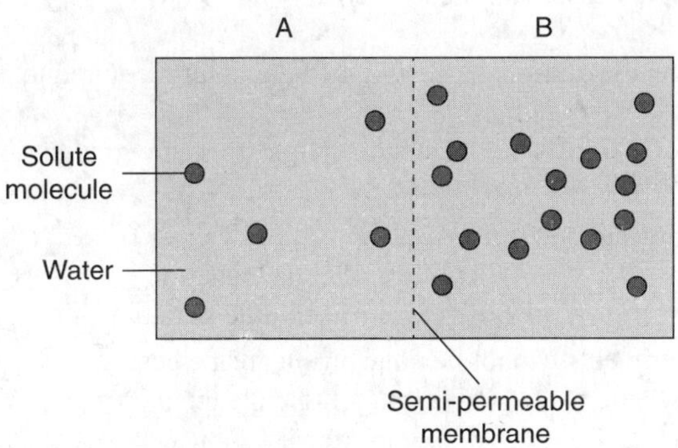

Answer the Question with respect to above diagram:
(1) Solution of which chamber has a lower water potential?
(a) A (b) B (c) Both have same (d) Cannot predict

(2) Solution of which chamber has a lower solute potential?
(a) A (b) B (c) Both have same (d) Cannot predict
(3) In which direction will osmosis occur?
(a) None (b) B to A (c) Both the direction (d) A to B

42. How we can get egg membrane?
(a) Remove yolk and albumin through a small hole at one end of the egg
(b) Place the shell in dilute HCl for few hours
(c) Both
(d) None

43. Identify A–D in the given figure.

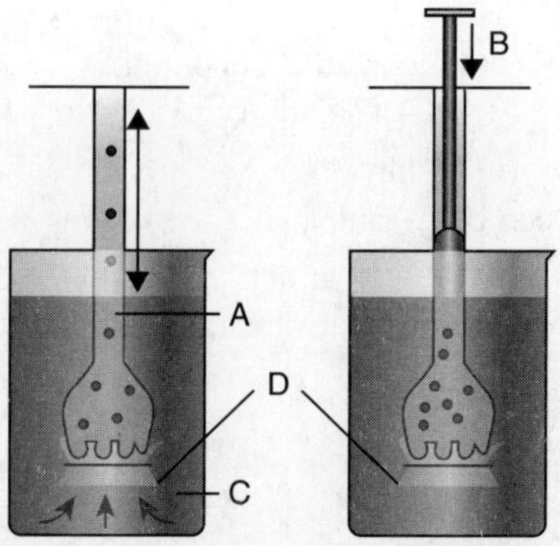

(a) A–Pressure, B–Membrane, C–Water, D–Sucrose solution
(b) A–Sucrose solution, B–Pressure, C–Water, D–Membrane
(c) A–Membrane, B–Sucrose solution, C–Pressure, D–Water
(d) A–Sucrose solution, B–Membrane, C–Water, D–Pressure

44. Select the correct statement from the following:
(a) Osmotic pressure is the negative pressure applied
(b) Osmotic potential is positive
(c) More is the solute concentration of solution, more will be the pressure required to prevent water from diffusing in
(d) The net direction and rate of osmosis not depend on the pressure gradient nor on concentration gradient

45. Which portion of root absorbs both water and minerals?
(a) Terminal portion of roots (b) Zone of cell elongation
(c) Zone of cell formation (d) Zone of cell differentiation

46. Meaningful girdling (ringing) experiments cannot be done on sugarcane because
(a) phloem is present inside the xylem (b) it cannot tolerate the injury
(c) vascular bundles are scattered (d) plants are very delicate

47. Some leaves are removed from the stem cuttings planted for vegetative propagation. This is done
(a) to increase water uptake (b) because it helps in rooting of cuttings
(c) to reduce water loss (d) because the cuttings need less food

48. In terms of permeability, the cell wall and plasmalemma are
(a) permeable and differentially permeable respectively

(b) both semi permeable
(c) semi permeable and differentially permeable
(d) both differentially permeable

49. The process of osmosis involves
(a) movement of solute through semi permeable membrane
(b) movement of solvent through a semi permeable membrane
(c) movement of solution through a semi permeable membrane
(d) none

50. Dry seeds when placed in water swells due to
(a) imbibitions (b) absorption (c) diffusion (d) adsorption

51. A cell placed in strong solution will shrink because
(a) cytoplasm will decompose (b) mineral salt will break the cell wall
(c) salt water enter the cell (d) water comes out by exosmosis

52. A cell increases in volume if the external medium is
(a) hypotonic (b) hypertonic (c) isotonic (d) none

53. All the following involves osmosis except
(a) water from soil entering a root hair
(b) water passing from root hair to adjacent cells
(c) water passing up a xylem vessel element to xylem vessel element above it
(d) water entering a mesophyll cell from xylem vessel element

54. A cell is plasmolysed after being kept in a hypertonic solution. What will be present between cell wall and plasmalemma?
(a) Isotonic solution (b) Hypertonic solution
(c) Air (d) Hypotonic solution

55. Wilting of a plant results from excessive
(a) respiration (b) photosynthesis
(c) absorption (d) transpiration

56. Water moves across a selectively permeable membrane:

	From	To
(a)	Region of higher water-potential	Region of lower water potential
(b)	Lower water concentration	Higher water concentration
(c)	Higher solute concentration	Lower solute concentration
(d)	Region of higher osmotic potential	Region of lower osmotic potential

57. In seed germination, the first phenomenon which takes place is called
(a) diffusion (b) osmosis (c) imbibitions (d) all

58. Deplasmolysis occurs in a cell when it is placed in
(a) hypotonic solution (b) hypertonic solution
(c) isotonic solution (d) buffer solution

59. Grapes immersed in water would shrink if
(a) water contains salts (b) water contains starch
(c) water is cold (d) water is hot

60. Plant cells submerged in distilled water will become
(a) turgid (b) flaccid (c) plasmolysed (d) impermeable

61. The plants face water stress due to the use of excessive fertilizers because of
(a) exosmosis (b) endosmosis (c) imbibitions (d) nonc

62. You are given three cells—a root hair, a cell of the inner cortical layer and a cell of the mesophyll. Arrange them in the ascending order of DPD.
    (a) Root hair < Cortical cell < Mesophyll (b) Cortical cell < Mesophyll < Root hair
    (c) Mesophyll < Root hair < Cortical cell (d) Root hair < Mesophyll < Cortical cell
63. What will be the direction of movement of water, when solution A having water potential of –9 bars and another solution B of –4 bars is separated by a semipermeable membrane
    (a) B to A (b) A to B
    (c) Both directions (d) None
64. If the external solution is more dilute than cytoplasm, the external solution is said to be
    (a) hypotonic (b) hypertonic (c) isotonic (d) isothermal
65. During plasmolysis
    (a) cell membrane of a plant cell shrinks away from its cell wall
    (b) water first lost from the cytoplasm and then from the vacuoles
    (c) area between cell wall and shrunken protoplast is occupied by outer solution
    (d) all
66. When plant cell is put in hypotonic solution:
    (a) cell swells up (b) cell undergo plasmolysis
    (c) cell wall shrinks (d) cell will burst
67. The pressure exerted by the protoplast due to the entry of water against the rigid cell wall is called
    (a) osmotic potential (b) pressure potential
    (c) water potential (d) matrix potential
68. Imbibition is
    (a) special type of diffusion (b) osmosis
    (c) facilitated diffusion (d) active transport
69. Imbibition is characterized by
    (a) increase in volume (b) release of energy
    (c) increase in pressure (d) all
70. Best example of imbibitions is
    (a) absorption of water by seed (b) absorption of water by dry wood
    (c) both (d) none
71. Which of the following is correct about imbibitions?
    (a) It require ψω gradient between the absorbent and the liquid imbibed
    (b) It require affinity between the absorbent and the liquid
    (c) Imbibition pressure is produced by the swelling of wood and in turn used by prehistonic man to split rocks and boulders
    (d) All
72. The path of the movement of water is demonstrated by using
    (a) solution containing pure water (b) solution of water and mineral
    (c) dye (colour) dissolve in water (d) all
73. Simple long distance transport cannot be achieved by
    (a) diffusion (b) facilitated diffusion
    (c) active transport (d) all
74. Water, mineral, and food are generally moved by over large distance by
    (a) simple diffusion (b) facilitated diffusion
    (c) active transport (d) bulk flow or mass flow

75. Identify A–D in the given figure.

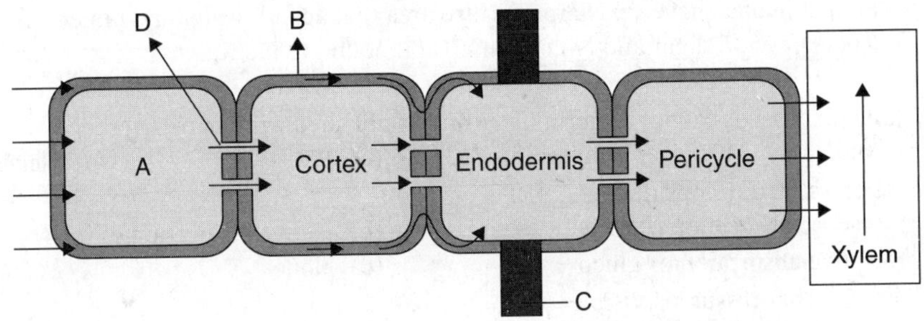

(a) A–Plasma membrane, B–Plasmodesmata, C–Epidermis, D–Casparian strip
(b) A–Casparian strip, B–Epidermis, C–Plasmodesmata, D–Plasma membrane
(c) A–Plasmodesmata, B–Epidermis, C–Casparian strip, D–Plasma membrane
(d) A–Epidermis, B–Plasma membrane, C–Casparian strip, D–Plasmodesmata

76. Bulk flow can be achieved by
(a) positive hydrostatic pressure gradient
(b) negative hydrostatic pressure gradient (suction)
(c) both
(d) none

77. Xylem is associated with the translocation of
(a) water (b) mineral
(c) some organic nitrogen and hormone (d) all

78. Which of the following is incorrect about apoplastic pathway?
(a) Movement of water takes place through intercellular spaces and the walls of cells
(b) Movement depend on gradient
(c) Mass flow occur due to adhesive and cohesive property of water
(d) This pathway provide barrier to water movement

79. During symplastic pathway water moved through
(a) cytoplasm (b) plasmodesmata (c) cell membrane (d) all

80. Which of the following is incorrect about symplastic pathway?
(a) Movement of water is relatively slower
(b) Movement is down the concentration gradient
(c) It may be aided by cytoplasmic streaming
(d) Most of water flow in root occur by this pathway

81. Cytoplasmic streaming is easily seen in
(a) leaf of hydrilla (b) leaf of mango
(c) stem cells of sunflower (d) pollen grains

82. Movement of water is correctly represented by
(a) Cortex → Root hair (Epidermis) → Xylem → Endodermis → Pericycle
(b) Root hair (Epidermis) → Endodermis → Xylem → Pericycle → Cortex
(c) Root hair (Epidermis) → Cortex → Endodermis → Pericycle → Xylem
(d) Xylem → Cortex → Endodermis → Pericycle → Root hair (Epidermis)

83. Where is apoplastic movement shifted to symplastic pathway?
(a) Cortex (b) Endodermis (c) Pericycle (d) Xylem

84. Which of the following is true about mycorrhizae?
(a) Association between roots and fungus
(b) Fungal hyphae have very large surface area that absorb water and mineral from the soil
(c) Roots provide sugar and N-containing compound to the fungus
(d) All

85. Which plant seeds cannot be germinated and established without the presence of mycorrhizae?
(a) Mango (b) Pulses (c) Pinus (d) Selaginella

86. Root pressure develops due to
(a) Passive absorption of ions (b) Active absorption of ions
(c) Active absorption of glucose (d) None

87. Effect of root pressure is visible
(a) at night (b) at early morning
(c) when evaporation is low (d) all

88. Guttation seen in
(a) vein opening near tip of grass blade (b) leaves of many herbaceous plant
(c) both (a) and (b) (d) leaves of trees

89. Root pressure contributes to the
(a) ascent of sap in small herbaceous plants
(b) re-establishment of continuous chains of water molecules in the xylem which often breaks down under the enormous tension created by transpiration
(c) guttation
(d) all

90. What is the approximate rate of the ascent of sap?
(a) 5 m/hr (b) 15 m/hr (c) 40 m/hr (d) 2 m/hr

91. How much % of water is used for photosynthesis?
(a) 1% (b) 2% (c) 3% (d) 4%

92. Stomata helps in
(a) transpiration (b) exchanges of gases
(c) both (d) none

93. Transpiration is affected by
(a) humidity (b) wind speed
(c) light and temperature (d) all

94. Plant factor which affects transpiration are
(a) number and distribution of stomata (b) number of stomata open
(c) water status of plant (d) all

95. Transpiration driven ascent of sap depends mainly on the _________ physical properties of water.
(a) Cohesion (b) Adhesion (c) Surface tension (d) All

96. Properties of water which provide high tensile strength (i.e. ability to resist a pulling force) are:
(a) cohesion (b) adhesion (c) surface tension (d) all

97. Force generated by transpiration creates pressure sufficient to lift a xylem-sized column of water over _________ meters.
(a) 130 (b) 200 (c) 400 (d) 500

98. Sap ascends in woody stems because of root pressure and
(a) transpiration pull (b) capillarity
(c) molecular adhesion (d) photosynthesis

99. Identify A–E parts in the given figure.

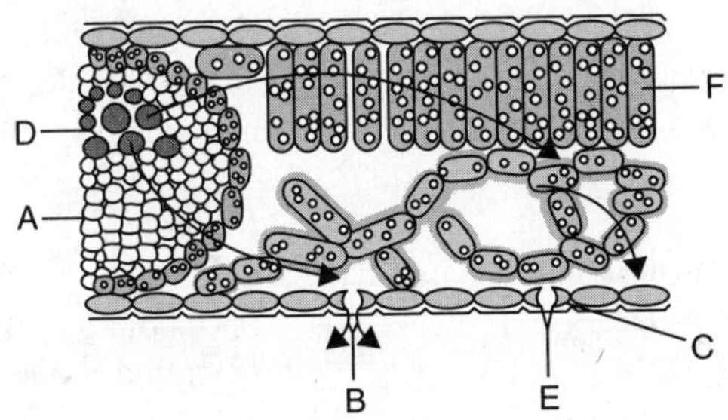

(a) A–Phloem, B–Diffusion into surrounding air, C–Guard cell, D–Xylem, E–Stomatal pore, F–Palisade
(b) A–Palisade, B–Guard cell, C–Phloem, D–Xylem, E–Diffusion into surrounding air, F–Stomatal pore
(c) A–Stomatal pore, B–Xylem, C–Palisade, D–Diffusion into surrounding air, E–Guard cell, F–Phloem
(d) A–Guard cell, B–Phloem, C–Xylem, D–Stomatal pore, E–Diffusion into surrounding air, F–Palisade

100. Most widely accepted explanation for the ascent of sap in tree is
(a) capillarity
(b) roll of atmospheric pressure
(c) pulsating action of living cells
(d) transpiration cohesion theory of Dixon

101. The path of water from soil up to secondary xylem is
(a) Soil → Root hair cell wall → Cortex → Endodermis → Pericycle → Protoxylem → Metaxylem
(b) Metaxylem → Protoxylem → Cortex → Soil → Root hair
(c) Cortex → Root hair → Endodermis → Pericycle → Protoxylem → Metaxylem
(d) Pericycle → Soil → Root hair → Cortex → Endodermis → Protoxylem → Metaxylem

102. A plant with well-washed roots is placed in a beaker of water diluted with red ink. The red colour travelled up the stem and into the leaf veins. Which of the following should be the correct explanation of the uptake of red ink into the roots?
(a) The red ink entered the root hairs by osmosis
(b) The molecules of red ink diffused into the root hairs
(c) The membranes of the root hairs are destroyed and red ink could enter
(d) The molecules of red ink passed from a region of low concentration to one of high concentration

103. Exudation of xylem is due to
(a) passive absorption
(b) root pressure
(c) guttation
(d) present of transpiration

104. By what mechanism does water moves through vessels and tracheids of root stem and leaves?
(a) Osmotic flow
(b) Bulk flow
(c) Gravity flow
(d) Imbibition

105. When cut end of a shoot is placed in a solution of safranin, the presence of dye could be located in
(a) cortex
(b) tracheid elements

(c) phloem (d) pith

106. Bulk flow of water occurs through
(a) living cells (b) cell vacuoles
(c) apparent free spaces (d) plasmodesmata

107. The continuity of water column in xylem is maintained due to the
(a) presence of air bubbles (b) cohesive property of water
(c) evaporation power of water (d) none

108. The chief role of transpiration in plants is to cause
(a) loss of surplus water (b) cooling of the plant
(c) rapid ascent of sap (d) rapid rise of minerals

109. The loss of water in the form of vapour from aerial plant parts is known as
(a) osmosis (b) respiration (c) photosynthesis (d) transpiration

110. Guard cells are found in
(a) stomata (b) root tips (c) ovary (d) lenticels

111. Position and frequency of stomata can be determined by
(a) calculating the loss of water (b) cobalt chloride paper method
(c) photometer (d) porometer

112. In both transpiration and evaporation, water is lost in the form of vapour yet they differ, because
(a) both transpiration and evaporation are similar but the rate of water loss differs
(b) frequency of water loss is different in both of them
(c) transpiration is a physical process and evaporation is a physiological process
(d) transpiration is a physiological process and evaporation is a physical process

113. Out of the following, which one is the most common type of transpiration?
(a) Foliar (b) Stomatal (c) Lenticular (d) Cuticular

114. In a hot summer day, a plant cools itself due to
(a) loss of water vapours from leaf (b) transport of water in plant
(c) loss of liquid water (d) loss of water from entire plant

115. Guard cells are surrounded by
(a) epidermal hairs (b) mesophyll cells (c) palisade cells (d) subsidiary cells

116. Which of the following is an adaptation to reduce water loss?
(a) Presence of thick cuticle (b) Change of leaf into spine
(c) Change of leaf into phylloclade (d) All

117. Which of the following is called necessary evil?
(a) Osmosis (b) Absorption (c) Transpiration (d) Photosynthesis

118. Which of the following plants economizes the transpirational loss of water?
(a) C_3 (b) C_4 (c) Both equally (d) C_2

119. The condition under which transpiration would be most rapid is
(a) high humidity
(b) excess of water in soil
(c) low humidity, high temperature, guard cells are turgid (open) and moist soil
(d) low velocity of wind

120. The transpiration in plants will be the lowest
(a) when there is high humidity in the atmosphere
(b) high wind velocity
(c) there is excess of water in the cell

(d) environmental conditions are very dry

121. Under what conditions the rate of transpiration increases?
(a) Increase of humidity (b) Increase of atmospheric pressure
(c) Decrease of temperature (d) Decrease of humidity

122. Transpiration increase with an increase in
(a) humidity (b) temperature (c) minerals (d) soil moisture

123. Stomata in angiosperms open and close due to
(a) their genetic constitution
(b) effect of hormones
(c) changes of turgor pressure in guard cells
(d) pressure of gases inside the leaves

124. Stomata open because of
(a) oxygen in the air
(b) increased turgidity of the guard cells brought about by the exposure to light
(c) vacuoles in guard cells
(d) all

125. The transpiration is regulated by the movements of
(a) subsidiary cells of the leaves (b) guard cells of the stomata
(c) mesophyll tissue cells (d) epidermal cells of the leaves

126. Guttation is caused due to
(a) imbibitions (b) osmosis
(c) positive root pressure (d) transpiration

127. Guttation usually occurs when the plant is put in a
(a) more saturated atmosphere (b) more humid soil
(c) dry condition (d) desert

128. Guttation is the process of elimination of water from plants. It occurs from the pores in leaves through which water comes out in the form of droplets or a specialized multicellular structure in leaves which excretes water droplets. The pores are called
(a) stomata (b) hydathodes (c) lenticels (d) wounds

129. Guttation is found mostly in
(a) herbaceous plants (b) shrubs
(c) wood plants (d) none

130. Water lost by guttation is
(a) pure (b) mixed with salts
(c) sometimes pure and sometimes impure (d) none

131. Guttation occurs in
(a) morning (b) night
(c) evening (d) morning 10 o'clock

132. Select from the following (in numbers) the correct function which are performed by transpiration.
(1) Creates transpiration pull for absorption and transport of water in plant.
(2) Transport minerals from the soil to all parts of the plant.
(3) Cools the leaf surface (sometime 10–15°C).
(4) Supplies water for photosynthesis.
(5) Maintain shape and structure of plants by keeping cells turgid.
(a) 1 (b) 3 (c) 4 (d) 5

133. C_4 plants are more evolved than C_3 plants because
(a) C_4 plants are twice efficient in terms of carbon fixing

(b) C_4 plants loose only half of its water as C_3 plants for same amount of CO_2 fixed
(c) both
(d) none

134. Plant obtain most of its carbon from
(a) atmosphere (b) water (c) soil (d) all

135. Minerals are mostly absorbed by
(a) active transport (b) facilitated diffusion
(c) simple diffusion (d) all

136. Ions are absorbed from soil by
(a) active transport (b) passive transport (c) both (d) none

137. Where is the control point for minerals, where a plant adjust the quantity and types of solutes that reach the xylem?
(a) Epidermal cell (b) Cortical cell
(c) Endodermal cell (d) Pericycle cell

138. Endodermis Actively transport ion in one direction because
(a) it is inner to epidermis
(b) cell wall is suberised
(c) cell wall is lignified
(d) its cell membrane has special transport proteins

139. Chief sink of minerals are
(a) apical and lateral meristem
(b) young leafs and storage organs
(c) developing flower, fruits and seeds
(d) all

140. Unloading of mineral occurs at the fine vein endings through
(a) diffusion (b) active uptake (c) both (d) none

141. All elements are remobilized except
(a) P (b) N (c) K (d) Ca

142. Which of the following helps in transportation of minerals?
(a) Xylem (b) Phloem (c) Both (d) None

143. Sink and source in sucrose transport may be reversed depending on
(a) plant's need (b) season (c) both (d) none

144. Phloem sap is mainly composed of
(a) Water + Glucose (b) Water + Fructose
(c) Water + Cellulose (d) Water + Sucrose

145. Which of the following is translocated through phloem?
(a) Sugar (b) Amino acid (c) Hormone (d) All

146. The accepted mechanism for the translocation of sugar from source to sink is called
(a) pressure flow hypothesis (b) mass flow hypothesis
(c) transpiration pull hypothesis (d) both (a) and (b)

147. What is the means of transport through which sucrose move into sieve tube of source and out of sieve tube at sink?
(a) Simple diffusion (b) Facilitated diffusion
(c) Active transport (d) Passive transport

148. When sugar is added at source water potential of sucrose _________ and when sugar is removed from sink, the water potential of sink _________.

(a) ↑es, ↑es (b) ↑es, ↓es (c) ↓es, ↓es (d) ↓es, ↑es

149. Which of the following experiment showed that food in plant is transported through phloem?
(a) Avena curvature experiment (b) Girdling experiment
(c) Bell-jar experiment (d) None

150. Select the incorrect statement from the following:
(a) The portion of bark above the ring in girdling experiment gets swollen after few weeks
(b) Translocation in phloem is bidirectional
(c) Phloem tissue is composed of sieve tube cells, which form long coloumns with holes in the walls called sieve plates

*Read the **assertion** and **reason** carefully to mark the correct option out of the options given below:*

(a) If both the assertion and the reason are true and the reason is a correct explanation of the assertion
(b) If both the assertion and reason are true but the reason is not a correct explanation of the assertion
(c) If the assertion is true but the reason is false
(d) If both the assertion and reason are false

(d) The process of loading at the source which produces a hypotonic condition in the phloem

151. Assertion: Phloem is principal food conducting tissue.
Reason: It has been recognised by girdling or ringing experiment.

152. Assertion: Water and mineral uptake by root hairs from the soil occurs through apoplast until it reaches endodermis.
Reason: Casparian strips in endodermis are suberized.

153. Assertion: Imbibition is also diffusion.
Reason: Movement of water in above process is along a concentration gradient.

154. Assertion: Pinus seeds can not germinate and established without the presence of mycorrhaizae.
Reason: Mycorrhiza is a symbiotic association of a fungus with a root system.

155. Assertion: Water potential is new term for diffusion pressure deficit.
Reason: Both diffusion pressure deficit and water potential have a positive value.

156. Assertion: Most mineral must enetr the root by active transport.
Reason: The concentration of minerals in the soil is usually lower than the concentration of minerals in roots.

157. Assertion: Plasmolysis will be severe if the process is in the order, limiting → incipient → evident.
Reason: Plasmolysis is endosmosis.

158. Assertion: The more the solute molecules in solution ,the lower (more negative) is the solute potential of solution.
Reason: For asolution at atmospheric pressure, water potential = solute potential

159. Assertion: In apoplast water movement is through mass flow.
Reason: The apoplast does not provide any barrier to water movement.

160. Assertion: Transport saturates in facilitated diffusion.

Reason: Facilitated diffusion occur through protien molecule.

161. **Assertion:** Light is very important factor in transpiration.

Reason: It induces stomatal opening and darkness closing. Therefore, transpiration increases in light decreases in dark.

162. **Assertion:** In rooted palnt, the transport in xylem of water and minerals is essentially multidirectional.

Reason: Organic compound and nutrient undergo unidirectional transport only.

163. **Assertion:** Guttation liquid is found on the margins of leaves of herbaceous plant.

Reason: Hydathodes are found on the margins of herbaceous plant.

164. **Assertion:** Transpiration occurs when stomata are open.

Reason: Transpiration occurs only through stomata.

AIPMT PREVIOUS YEAR QUESTIONS

1. Transport of food material in higher plants takes place through:

[AIPMT MAINS 2010]

(a) Companion cells
(b) Transfusion tissues
(c) Tracheids
(d) Sieve elements

2. Which one of the following structures between two adjacent cells is an effective transport pathway?

[AIPMT PRE 2010]

(a) Plasmodesmata
(b) Plastoquinones
(c) Endoplasmic reticulum
(d) Plasmalemma

3. Function of companion cells is

[AIPMT MAINS 2011]

(a) Providing energy to sieve elements for active transport
(b) Providing water to phloem
(c) Loading of sucrose into sieve elements by passive transport
(d) Loading of sucrose into sieve elements

4. Guttation is the result of

[AIPMT MAINS 2011]

(a) Diffusion
(b) Transpiration
(c) Osmosis
(d) Root pressure

5. Which one of the following is correctly matched?

[AIPMT PRE 2012]

(a) Passive transport of nutrients – ATP
(b) Apoplast – Plasmodesmata
(c) Potassium – Readily immobilisation
(d) Bakane of rice seedlings – F.skoog

6. Which of the following criteria does not pertain to facilitated transport?

[AIPMT 2013]

(a) Requirement of special membrane proteins

(b) High selectivity
(c) Transport saturation
(d) Uphill transport

7. The osmotic expansion of a cell kept in water is chiefly regulated by: [AIPMT 2014]
(a) Mitochondria
(b) Vacuoles
(c) Plastids
(d) Ribosomes

8. Transpiration and root pressure cause water to rise in plants by: [AIPMT 2015]
(a) Pulling it upward
(b) Pulling and pushing it respectively
(c) Pushing it upward
(d) Pushing and pulling it respectively

9. In a ring girdled plant: [AIPMT 2015]
(a) The shoot dies first
(b) The root dies first
(c) The shoot and root dies together
(d) Neither root nor shoot will die

10. A column of water within xylem vessels of tall trees does not break under its weight because of: [RE-AIPMT 2015]
(a) Tensile strength of water
(b) Lignification of xylem vessels
(c) Positive root pressure
(d) Dissolved sugars in water

11. Root pressure develops due to: [RE-AIPMT 2015]
(a) Low osmotic potential in soil
(b) Passive absorption
(c) Increase in transpiration
(d) Active absorption

12. A protoplast is a cell:

Answer Keys

1. (d) 2. (d) 3. (a) 4. (d) 5. (d) 6. (a) 7. (d) 8. (a) 9. (b) 10. (d)
11. (a) 12. (a) 13. (d) 14. (c) 15. (b) 16. (a) 17. (d) 18. (a) 19. (b) 20. (c)
21. (c) 22. (d) 23. (c) 24. (c) 25. (c) 26. (a) 27. (d) 28. (d) 29. (d) 30. (d)
31. (d) 32. (c) 33. (b) 34. (d) 35. (a) 36. (c) 37. (c) 38. (a) 39. (a) 40. (c)
41. (b), (a), (d) 42. (c) 43. (b) 44. (c) 45. (d) 46. (c) 47. (c) 48. (a) 49. (b)
50. (a) 51. (d) 52. (a) 53. (c) 54. (b) 55. (d) 56. (a) 57. (c) 58. (a) 59. (a)
60. (a) 61. (a) 62. (a) 63. (a) 64. (a) 65. (d) 66. (a) 67. (b) 68. (a) 69. (d)
70. (c) 71. (d) 72. (c) 73. (d) 74. (d) 75. (d) 76. (c) 77. (d) 78. (d) 79. (d)
80. (d) 81. (a) 82. (c) 83. (b) 84. (d) 85. (c) 86. (b) 87. (d) 88. (c) 89. (d)
90. (b) 91. (a) 92. (c) 93. (d) 94. (d) 95. (d) 96. (d) 97. (a) 98. (a) 99. (a)
100. (d) 101. (a) 102. (a) 103. (b) 104. (b) 105. (b) 106. (c) 107. (b) 108. (c) 109. (d)
110. (a) 111. (b) 112. (d) 113. (b) 114. (a) 115. (d) 116. (d) 117. (c) 118. (b) 119. (c)
120. (a) 121. (d) 122. (b) 123. (c) 124. (b) 125. (b) 126. (c) 127. (a) 128. (b) 129. (a)
130. (b) 131. (a) 132. (d) 133. (c) 134. (a) 135. (a) 136. (c) 137. (c) 138. (b) 139. (d)
140. (c) 141. (d) 142. (c) 143. (c) 144. (d) 145. (d) 146. (d) 147. (c) 148. (d) 149. (b)
150. (d) 151. (a) 152. (a) 153. (a) 154. (b) 155. (c) 156. (a) 157. (c) 158. (b) 159. (b)
160. (a) 161. (a) 162. (d) 163. (a) 164. (c)

AIPMT Previous Year Questions

1. (d) 2. (a) 3. (d) 4. (d) 5. (c) 6. (d) 7. (b) 8. (b) 9. (b) 10. (a)
11. (d) 12. (c)

CHAPTER

12

Mineral Nutrition

1. In 1860, __________ demonstrated first time hydroponics.
   (a) Van Neil (b) Von Sachs (c) Arnon (d) Lundergarth
2. Hydroponics require
   (a) purified water (b) impure water
   (c) mineral nutrient salt (d) both (a) and (c)
3. Hydroponic is a successfully employed technique for the commercial production of vegetables like
   (a) tomato (b) seedless cucumber
   (c) lettuce (d) all
4. Find the true/false statement from the following:
   (a) Only 50 elements are found in different plants
   (b) In hydroponics, nutrient solution must be adequately aerated to obtain the optimum growth
   (c) Some plant species accumulate selenium
   (d) By hydroponics essential elements were identified and their deficiency symptoms discovered

   (a) FTTT (b) FFTT (c) FTFT (d) FFFT
5. Which one of the following is Arnon's criterion for essentiality of element?
   (a) In the absence of element plant do not complete their life cycle or set the seeds
   (b) Deficiency of element cannot be met by supplying other element
   (c) Element must be directly involved in the metabolism of the plant
   (d) All of the above
6. What indicates A to D in the given figure?

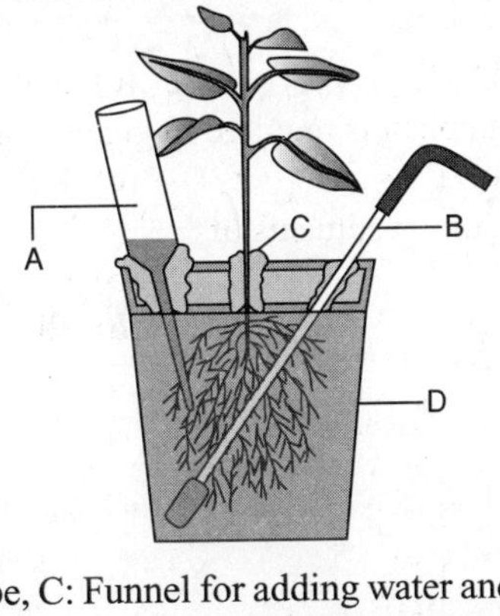

   (a) A: Cotton, B: Aerating tube, C: Funnel for adding water and nutrients, D: Nutrient solution
   (b) A: Funnel for adding water and nutrients, B: Aerating tube, C: Cotton, D: Nutrient solution

(c) A: Nutrient solution, B: Cotton, C: Funnel for adding water and solution, D: Aerating tube
(d) A: Cotton, B: Aerating tube, C: Nutrient solution, D: Funnel for adding water and nutrients

7. By some techniques ____________ are able to detect the mineral at very low concentration.
(a) 10^{-12} gm/ml (b) 10^{-15} gm/ml (c) 10^{-10} gm/ml (d) 10^{-8} gm/ml

8. On which basis nutrients are divided into macro and micro nutrients?
(a) Quantitative requirement (b) Qualitative requirement
(c) Both (d) None

9. Following are macronutrients except
(a) N (b) P (c) S (d) Mn

10. Following are micronutrients except
(a) Zn (b) B (c) Mo (d) Ca

11. Select the total number of macronutrient from the following:
C, H, O, N, P, S, Cu, Zn, B, Cl, Mn, Ni, K, Ca, Mg, Mo
(a) 8 (b) 9 (c) 10 (d) 11

12. C, H, O is mainly obtained from
(a) Soil and H_2O (b) Soil only (c) H_2O and CO_2 (d) CO_2 only

13. What is the number of the absolutely essential elements for growth and metabolism of most plants?
(a) 14 (b) 17 (c) 21 (d) 23

14. Some beneficial element required by higher plants are
(a) Na, Si, Co, Se (b) Na, Si, Os, I (c) Na, Co, Ir, At (d) Na, Si, W, Ag

15. Structural elements of cell are
(a) C, H, O, N (b) N, P, K, Ca (c) Ca, Mg, K (d) Ca, Mg, Fe, O

16. Select the correct match:

Column I		Column II
A. Mg^{2+}	–	1. Chlorophyll
B. P	–	2. ATP
C. Zn	–	3. Alcohol dehydrogenase
D. Mo	–	4. Nitrogenase

(a) A–2, B–1, C–3, D–4 (b) A–1, B–2, C–3, D–4
(c) A–4, B–1, C–2, D–3 (d) A–4, B–3, C–2, D–1

17. Which element play important role in opening and closing of stomata?
(a) P (b) N (c) K (d) Ca

18. In how many broad categories can the essential elements be grouped on the basis of their diverse function?
(a) 1 (b) 2 (c) 3 (d) 4

19. Which essential nutrient in plant is required in greatest amount?
(a) N (b) P (c) K (d) Ca

20. Nitrogen is one of the major constituents of
(a) protein (b) nucleic acid
(c) vitamins and hormones (d) all

21. Select the incorrect match:

Element		Absorbable form
(a) Nitrogen	–	NO_3^-, NO_2^-, NH_4^+,
(b) Sulphur	–	S^{2-}
(c) Iron	–	Fe^{3+}
(d) Boron	–	BO_3^{3-}, $B_4O_7^{2-}$

22. Which is required for all phosphorylation reaction?
(a) N (b) Ca (c) P (d) K

23. Which of the following is the function of potassium?
(1) Cation–anion balance in cell.
(2) Involved in protein synthesis.
(3) Activation of enzyme.
(4) Opening and closing of stomata.
(5) Maintenance of turgidity of cell.
(a) All except 1 (b) All except 1 and 2 (c) All except 3 (d) All

24. Which element is involved in the formation of mitotic spindle?
(a) N (b) P (c) Ca (d) K

25. Following functions are related to which element mainly?
(1) Activate enzyme of photosynthesis and respiration.
(2) Involved in synthesis of DNA and RNA.
(3) Help to maintain structure of ribosome.
(a) Ca (b) Mg (c) S (d) Fe

26. Which of the following group contains sulphur in all members?
(a) Thiamine, ferredoxin, aspartic acid (b) Biotin, coenzyme A, methionine
(c) Methionine, proline, leucine (d) DNA and RNA

27. Which of the following is true about iron?
(a) It is a constituent of ferredoxin and cytochrome
(b) It activates catalase enzyme
(c) It is essential for formation of chlorophyll
(d) All

28. Which element is related to the splitting of water in light reaction of photosynthesis?
(a) Mn (b) Mo (c) Fe (d) B

29. Match the column:

Column I		**Column II**
A. Zinc	–	1. Needed for synthesis of Auxin
B. Copper	–	2. Essential for water splitting reaction
C. Boron	–	3. Pollen germination
D. Molybdenum	–	4. Component of nitrate reductase
E. Chlorine	–	5. Associated with enzyme involved in Redox reaction

(a) A–2, B–3, C–1, D–5, E–4 (b) A–1, B–2, C–3, D–4, E–5
(c) A–1, B–5, C–3, D–4, E–2 (d) A–5, B–4, C–3, D–2, E–1

30. Which element generally activates carboxylase enzyme?
(a) Mo (b) Mn (c) Mg (d) Zn

31. Following functions are related to
(1) Uptake and utilization of calcium
(2) Carbohydrate translocation
(3) Cell elongation and maturation
(4) Membrane functioning
(a) Ca (b) B (c) Mo (d) Zn

32. Element involved in splitting of water is
(a) Mn (b) Ca (c) Cl (d) all

33. Mn induced deficiency of
(a) Fe (b) Mg (c) Ca (d) all
34. Which one of the following statement is incorrect?
(a) The first phase of mineral absorption is the rapid uptake of ions into free or outer space
(b) In the second phase of uptake, ions are slowly taken into inner space the symplast of the cells
(c) Movement of ion is usually called flux
(d) Inward movement of ion outflux and outword movement of ion is called influx
35. Ascent of mineral is mainly due to
(a) xylem (b) phloem (c) pericycle (d) cortex
36. Mineral available to plant is mainly obtained from
(a) decay of other plants (b) decay of other animals
(c) weathering of rocks (d) none
37. Function of soil is to
(a) supply mineral to plant (b) harbour nitrogen fixing bacteria
(c) hold water and supply air to root (d) all
38. Fertilizer contains
(a) micronutrient (b) macronutrient (c) both (d) none
39. Nitrogen is limiting mineral for
(a) natural ecosystem (b) agro ecosystem (c) both (d) none
40. Conversion N_2 to ammonia is known as
(a) nitrogen fixation (b) nitrification (c) denitrification (d) ammonification
41. Lightening and UV radiation can cause a reaction between nitrogen and oxygen and produces
(a) NO (b) NO_2 (c) N_2O (d) All
42. Decomposition of organic nitrogen of dead plants and animals into ammonia is called
(a) Nitrogen fixation (b) Nitrification (c) Denitrification (d) Ammonification
43. What happens to ammonia formed by ammonification?
(a) Some gets volatilized
(b) Most of it gets converted into nitrate by soil bacteria
(c) Some will undergo biological nitrogen fixation
(d) Both (a) and (b)
44. $2NH_3 + 3O_2 \rightarrow 2NO_2^- + 2H^+ + 2H_2O$.
Reaction can be caused by
(1) nitrosomonas. (2) nitrococcus. (3) nitrobacter.
(4) pseudomonas. (5) thiobacillus.
(a) 1 and 5 only (b) 1 and 2 only (c) 4 and 5 only (d) Only 3
45. $2NO_2^- + O_2 \rightarrow 2NO_3^-$.
This step of process nitrification is done by ____________ bacteria.
(a) pseudomonas (b) thiobacillus (c) nitrobacter (d) nitrococcus
46. Nitrifying bacteria are
(a) photoautotroph (b) chemoautotroph (c) heterotrophy (d) all
47. Nitrate present in the soil is also reduced to nitrogen by the process of denitrification it is carried out by
(a) pseudomonas (b) thiobacillus (c) rhizobium (d) both (a) and (b)
48. Reduction of nitrogen to ammonia by living organism is called
(a) nitrification (b) denitrification
(c) biological nitrogen fixation (d) ammonification

49. $N \equiv N \rightarrow NH_3$.
Reaction catalyzed by enzyme:
(a) Isomerase (b) Nitrogenase
(c) Carbonic anhydrase (d) Higase

50. Frankia produced nitrogen by fixing nodule on
(a) lentils (b) garden pea (c) alnus (d) broad bean

51. Which of the following statement is incorrect?
(a) Rhizobium and frankia are free living bacteria of soil
(b) Rhizobium is rod shaped (Bacillus)
(c) Root nodule of pulse are pink due to the presence of leg-hemoglobin
(d) Rhizobium and frankia can fix nitrogen as free living bacteria

52. Leg-hemoglobin means
(a) low grade hemoglobin (b) luminous hemoglobin
(c) leguminous hemoglobin (d) low level hemoglobin

53. Sequential stage for principal stages of nodule formation are
(1) Rhizobia multiply and colonies the surrounding roots.
(2) Rhizobia attached to epidermal and root hair cells.
(3) Root hair curl and bacterial invade root hair.
(4) Initiation of nodule formation in cortex.
(5) Infection thread is produced carrying bacteria to cortex.
(6) Bacteria released from thread into cells and causes their differentiation in specialized nitrogen fixing cells.
(7) Nodule formed establish, a direct vascular connection with the host for exchange of nutrient.
(a) I → VII → II → VI → III → V → IV (b) II → III → IV → I → VII → V → VI
(c) VII → VI → IV → I → III → V → II (d) I → II → III → V → IV → VI → VII

54. Root nodule of leguminous plant contains
(a) nitrogenase (b) leg hemoglobin (c) both (d) none

55. Enzyme nitrogenase is
(a) Mo-Fe protein (b) Mo-Mn protein (c) Mn-Fe protein (d) Cu-Fe protein

56. Which cells are divided for nodule formation?
(a) Inner cortex (b) Pericycle (c) Endodermis (d) Both (a) and (b)

57. For production of 2 mol. NH_3 how much ATP is required in biological nitrogen fixation reaction (i. e. $N_2 \rightarrow 2NH_3$)?
(a) 4 (b) 8 (c) 16 (d) 32

58. Nitrogenase require ____________ condition for its activity.
(a) aerobic (b) anaerobic
(c) ozonised environment (d) CO_2

59. Which of the following is incorrect about nitrogen fixation in nodule?
(a) It is a high energy process
(b) Leg-hemoglobin acts as oxygen scavenger
(c) Mg is required as a cofactor for nitrogenase enzyme
(d) Process use atmospheric nitrogen but not atmospheric hydrogen directly

60. Fats of NH_3 formed during biological nitrogen fixation is
(a) NH_3 protonated to form
(b) NH_4^+ ion formed used for reductive amination
(c) glutamic acid formed under reductive amination undergo transamination
(d) all

61. Which is the main amino acid that is used for transamination?
(a) Tyrosine (b) Proline (c) Glutamic acid (d) Alanine

62. (i) α-ketoglutaric acid $+NH_4^+ + NADPH \xrightarrow{A}$ glumate $+ H_2O +$ NADP
(ii)
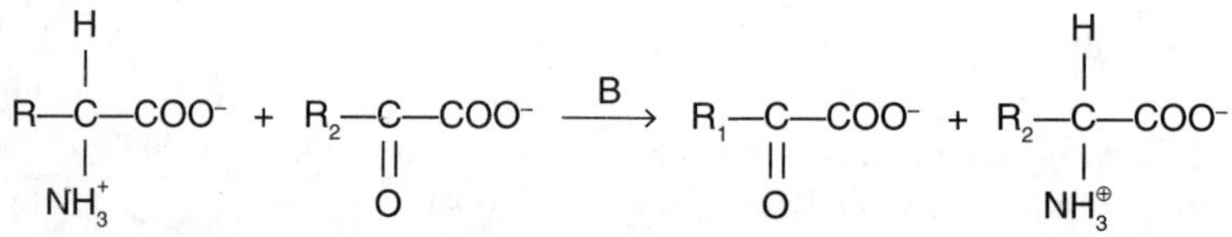
What is A and B put on arrow?
(a) A–Glutamate dehydrogenase, B–Transaminase
(b) A–Transaminase, B–Glutamate dehydrogenase
(c) A–Nitrogenase, B–Transaminase
(d) A–Glumate aminase, B–Dehydrogenase

63. Select the incorrect statement from the following:
(a) The amides–aspargine and glutamine are found in plant as structural part of protein
(b) Amides contain less nitrogen than amino acid
(c) NH_2 radicle transported to other parts via xylem
(d) In soyabean fixed nitrogen is transported as ureides

64. Ureides have
(a) high N/C ratio (b) low N/C ratio (c) any of the above (d) none

65. Which of the following is incorrect about NH_4^+ ion?
(a) Formed by protonation of NH_3
(b) Less toxic so can be accumulated in plant
(c) Used to synthesize amino acid in plant
(d) All

66. Select true and false statement:
(a) Boron deficiency leads to stout axis
(b) Every mineral element that is present in a cell is needed by the cell
(c) Nitrogen as a nutrient element is highly immobile in the plants
(d) It is very easy to establish the essentiality of micronutrients because they are required only in trace quantities
(a) FFFT (b) FFTT (c) TTFF (d) TTTF

67. What is critical concentration?
(a) Concentration of essential element which causes flowering in plant
(b) Concentration of essential element which is easily absorbed by plant
(c) Concentration of essential element below which plant growth is retarded
(d) All

68. Select true and false statement:
(1) Morphological changes which are indicative of certain element deficiencies are known as deficiency symptoms.
(2) For actively mobilized element deficiency symptoms first appear in older tissues.
(3) When element is relatively immobile deficiency symptom first appear in younger tissue.
(4) Mineral nutrition study of plant have great significance to agriculture and horticulture.
(a) FFFT (b) FFTT (c) TTFF (d) TTTT

69. Deficiency symptom of N, K and Mg appears in
(a) young leaf (b) meristematic tissue
(c) young stem (d) senescent leaves

70. Which elements are relatively immobalized?
(a) N and P (b) K and Mg (c) S and Ca (d) N and Mg

71. Deficiency symptom of plants includes
(a) chlorosis and necrosis
(b) stunted plant growth and inhibition of cell division
(c) premature fall of leaves and buds
(d) all

72. Chlorosis is caused due to the deficiency of
(a) N, K, Mg (b) S, Fe, Mn (c) Zn and Me (d) All

73. Necrosis particularly leaf tissue is caused by
(a) Ca and Mg (b) Cu (c) K (d) All

74. Low level of N, K, S, Mo is caused by
(a) chlorosis (b) inhibition of cell division
(c) both (d) none

75. Delay in flowering occurs due to the deficiency of
(a) N (b) S (c) Mo (d) All

76. Technique of growing plants without soil in nutrient solutions is called
(a) parthenogenesis (b) hydroponics (c) aquaculture (d) tissue culture

77. Which of the following element is not essential for plants?
(a) Iron (b) Zinc (c) Potassium (d) Iodine

78. Inorganic nutrients are present in the soil in the form of
(a) molecules (b) atoms
(c) electrically charged ions (d) parasite

79. Tracer elements are
(a) micro elements (b) macro elements
(c) radio isotopes (d) vitamins

80. Death of stem and root tips occur due to the deficiency of
(a) phosphorus (b) calcium
(c) nitrogen (d) carbon

81. Plants requiring two metallic compounds (minerals) for chlorophyll synthesis are
(a) Fe and Ca (b) Fe and Mg
(c) Cu and Ca (d) Ca and K

82. Calcium can effect
(a) permeability of plasma membrane
(b) hydration of colloids
(c) translocation of carbohydrates and amino acids
(d) development of root

83. Which of the following is not absorbed through soil?
(a) Carbon (b) Nitrogen
(c) Potassium (d) All

84. Which of the following is considered to be the elements between macro nutrients and micro nutrients?
(a) Iron (b) Nitrogen
(c) Phosphorus (d) Manganese

85. The major role of phosphorus in plant metabolism is
(a) to generate metabolic energy
(b) to evolve oxygen during photosynthesis
(c) to evolve carbon dioxide during respiration
(d) to create anaerobic conditions

86. Phosphorus is a structural element in
(a) Fat (b) Starch (c) Nucleotide (d) Carbohydrate

87. The most abundent element present in the plants is
(a) Manganese (b) Iron (c) Carbon (d) Nitrogen

88. Photosynthetic photolysis of water takes place in presence of
(a) Mn (b) Cl (c) Both (a) and (b) (d) None

89. Copper is the component of
(a) Cytochrome oxidase (b) Plastocyanin
(c) Both (a) and (b) (d) None

90. Which of the following element is a component of ferredoxin?
(a) Cu (b) Mn (c) Zn (d) Fe

91. Function of zinc is
(a) synthesis of chlorophyll (b) biosynthesis of IAA
(c) closing of stomata (d) oxidation of carbohydrate

92. The process by which minerals are absorbed is
(a) active absorption (b) passive absorption
(c) both (a) and (b) (d) none

93. Active uptake of minerals by roots mainly depends on the
(a) availability of oxygen (b) light
(c) temperature (d) availability of carbon dioxide

94. Identify A–D in the given figure.

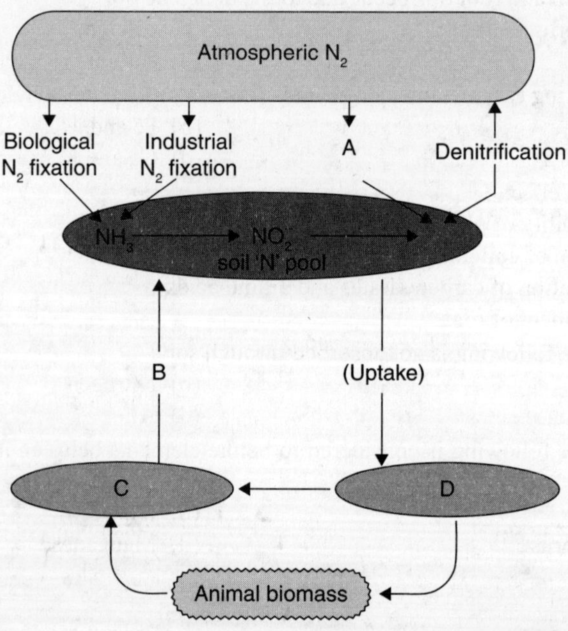

(a) A–Decaying biomass, B–Electrical N2-fixation, C–Plant biomass, D–Ammonification
(b) A–Plant biomass, B–Decaying biomass, C–Ammonification, D–Electrical N2-fixation
(c) A–Electrical N2-fixation, B–Ammonification, C–Decaying biomass, D–Plant biomass
(d) A–Ammonification, B–Plant biomass, C–Electrical N2-fixation, D–Decaying biomass

95. Nitrogen is a component of
(a) Protein (b) Chlorophyll
(c) Nucleic acid (d) All

96. Which one of the following can fix atmospheric nitrogen directly?
(a) Pea (b) Brassica
(c) Castor (d) Petunia

97. Knot like bodies known as 'nodules' found in the roots of groundnut plant are produced by
(a) Azospirillum (b) Azotobacter
(c) Pseudomonas (d) Rhizobium

98. Nitrogen fixation means
(a) N_2 changes in NO_3^- (b) N_2 changes in NH_3
(c) N_2 change into nitrates (d) none

99. Nif genes occur in
(a) Rhizobium (b) Aspergillus
(c) Penicillium (d) Streptococcus

100. Identify A–C in the given figure.

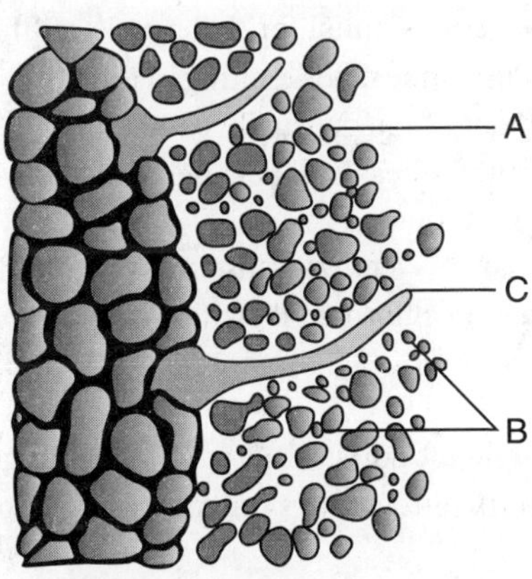

(a) A–Bacteria, B–Root hair, C–Soil particles
(b) A–Root hair, B–Bacteria, C–Soil particles
(c) A–Root hair, B–Soil particles, C–Bacteria
(d) A–Soil particles, B–Bacteria, C–Root hair

101. Which of the following pigments is essential for the nitrogen fixation by leguminous plants?
(a) Anthocyanin
(b) Phycocyanin
(c) Phycoerythrin
(d) Leghaemoglobin

*Read the **assertion** and **reason** carefully to mark the correct option out of the options given below:*

(a) If both the assertion and the reason are true and the reason is a correct explanation of the assertion
(b) If both the assertion and reason are true but the reason is not a correct explanation of the assertion
(c) If the assertion is true but the reason is false
(d) If both the assertion and reason are false

102. **Assertion:** Biological nitrogen fixation is very high energy input process.
Reason: One molecule of ammonia formation require 8 ATP during biological nitrogen fixation.

103. **Assertion:** Leguminous plants are nitrogen fixers.
Reason: Leguminous plants have Rhizobium in their root nodules.

104. **Assertion:** Use of fertilizers greatly enhances crop productivity.
Reason: Irrigation is very important in increasing crop productivity.

105. **Assertion:** Hydroponics is used for solution culture.
Reason: A balanced nutrient solution contains both essential and nonessential elements.

106. **Assertion:** Nitrogen is very essentisl for sustenance of life.
Reason: Plant can not use atmospheric nitrogen directly.

107. **Assertion:** The movement of ion is usually called flux.
Reason: The concentration of essential elements below which the plant growth is retarded is termed as critical concentration.

108. **Assertion:** Iron takes part in electron transport system of mitochondria.
Reason: Iron has no role in chlorophyll synthesis.

109. **Assertion:** Decomposition of organic nitrogen of dead plants and animals into ammonia is called ammonification.
Reason: Nitrate present in the soil is also reduced to nitrogen by the process of denitrification.

110. **Assertion:** Rhizobium fix nitrogen in symbiotic association with root nodules of leguminous plants only.
Reason: Biological nitrogen fixation is anaerobic process.

111. **Assertion:** Nitrogen-fixing bacteria in legume root nodules survive in oxygen-depleted cells of nodules.
Reason: Leghaemoglobin completely removes oxygen from the nodule cells.

112. **Assertion:** Deficiency of sulphur causes chlorosis in plants.
Reason: Sulphur is a constituent of chlorophyll, proteins and nucleic acids.

113. **Assertion:** S and Ca are immobile.
Reason: S and Ca are part of the structural component of cell and hence not easily released.

114. **Assertion:** Boron is required for uptake and utilization of calcium ion.
Reason: Boron is not required for carbohydrate translocation.

115. **Assertion:** Iorn is essential for formation of chlorophyll.
Reason: It activates catalase enzyme.

116. **Assertion:** Calcium is a constituent of middle lamella.
Reason: Calcium is required in mitotic division.

117. **Assertion:** Sulphur is present in two amino acids cysteine and methionine.
Reason: Vitamin (thiamine,biotin,coenzyme-A) and ferredoxin also contain sulphur.

AIPMT PREVIOUS YEAR QUESTIONS

1. Leguminous plants are able to fix atmospheric nitrogen through the process of symbiotic nitrogen fixation. Which one of the following statements is not correct during this process of nitrogen fixation?

[AIPMT MAINS 2010]

(a) Leghaemoglobin scavenges oxygen and is pinkish in colour
(b) Nodules act as sites for nitrogen fixation
(c) The enzyme nitrogen catalyses the conversion of atmospheric N_2 to NH_3
(d) Nitrogenase is insensitive to oxygen

2. Study the cycle shown below and select the option which gives correct word for all the four blanks A, B, C and D.

[AIPMT MAINS 2010]

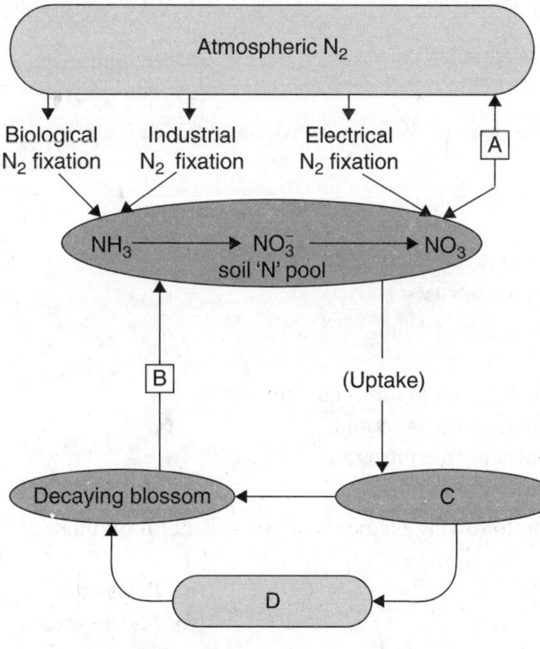

(a) A: Nitrification, B: Ammonification, C: Animals, D: Plants
(b) A: Denitrification, B: Ammonification, C: Plants, D: Animals
(c) A: Nitrification, B: Denitrification, C: Animals, D: Plants
(d) A: Denitrification, B: Nitrification, C: Plants, D: Animals

3. The genetically-modified (GM) brinjal in India has been developed for: [AIPMT PRE 2010]

(a) Insect-resistance (b) Enhancing self life
(c) Enhancing mineral content (d) Drought-resistance

4. An element playing important role in nitrogen fixation is [AIPMT PRE 2010]

(a) Molybdenum (b) Copper
(c) Manganese (d) Zinc

5. Which one of the following is not a micronutrient? [AIPMT PRE 2010]

(a) Molybdenum (b) Magnesium
(c) Zinc (d) Boron

6. The free-living, anaerobic nitrogen-fixer is: [AIPMT PRE 2010]

(a) Beijerinckia (b) Rhodospirillum
(c) Rhizobium (d) Azotobacter

7. The common nitrogen-fixer in paddy fields is: [AIPMT PRE 2010]

(a) Rhizobium (b) Azospirillum
(c) Oscillatoria (d) Frankia

8. Which one of the following is not an essential mineral element for plants while the remaining three are? [AIPMT MAINS 2011]

(a) Iron (b) Manganese
(c) Cadmium (d) Phosphorus

9. The function of leghaemoglobin in the root nodules of legumes is: [AIPMT PRE 2011]

(a) Oxygen removal
(b) Nodule differentiation
(c) Expression of nif gene
(d) Inhibition of nitrogenase activity

10. Nitrifying bacteria [AIPMT PRE 2011]

(a) Convert free nitrogen to nitrogen compounds
(b) Convert proteins into ammonia
(c) Reduce nitrates to free nitrogen
(d) Oxidize ammonia to nitrates

11. Which one of the following elements in plants is not remobilised? [AIPMT PRE 2011]

(a) Calcium (b) Potassium
(c) Sulphur (d) Phosphorus

12. An organism used as a biofertilizer for raising soyabean crop is: [AIPMT PRE 2011]

(a) Azospirillum (b) Rhizobium
(c) Nostoc (d) Azotobacter

13. For its action, nitrogenase requires:

[AIPMT MAINS 2012]

(a) Light (b) Mn^{2+}
(c) Super oxygen radicals (d) High input of energy

14. For its activity, carboxypeptidases requires:

[AIPMT MAINS 2012]

(a) Iron (b) Niacin
(c) Copper (d) Zinc

15. Read the following four statements (A-D):

(A) Both, photophosphorylation and oxidative phosphorylation involve uphill transport of protons across the membrane
(B) In dicot stems, a new cambium originates from cells of pericycle at the time of secondary growth
(C) Stamens in flowers of Gloriosa and Petunia are polyandrous
(D) Symbiotic nitrogen-fixers occur in free- living state also in soil

[AIPMT MAINS 2012]

How many of the above statements are right

(a) Three (b) Four
(c) One (d) Two

16. Best defined function of Manganese in green plants is:

[AIPMT PRE 2012]

(a) Photolysis of water (b) Calvin cycle
(c) Nitrogen fixation (d) Water absorption

17. Which one of the following is wrong statement?

[AIPMT PRE 2012]

(a) Anabaena and Nostoc are capable of fixing nitrogen in free-living state also.
(b) Root nodule forming nitrogen fixers live as aerobes under free-living conditions.
(c) Phosphorus is a constituent of cell membranes, certain nucleic acids and all proteins
(d) Nitrosomonas and Nitrobacter are chemoautotrophs

18. The most abundant intracellular cation is:

[AIPMT PRE 2012]

(a) Na^+ (b) Ca^+
(c) H^+ (d) K^+

19. The first stable product of fixation of atmospheric nitrogen in leguminous plants is:

[AIPMT PRE 2012]

(a) NO_2^- (b) Ammonia
(c) NO_3^- (d) Glutamate

20. Deficiency symptoms of nitrogen and potassium are visible first in:

[AIPMT 2014]

(a) Senescent leaves (b) Young leaves
(c) Roots (d) Buds

21. A few normal seedlings of tomato were kept in a dark room. After a few days they were found to have become white coloured like albinos. Which of the following terms will you use to describe them?

[AIPMT 2014]

(a) Mutated (b) Embolised
(c) Etiolated (d) Defoliated

22. Mineral known to be required in large amounts for plant growth include: [AIPMT 2015]

(a) Phosphorus, potassium, sulphur, calcium
(b) Calcium, magnesium, manganese, copper
(c) Potassium, phosphorus, selenium, boron
(d) Magnesium, sulphur, iron, zinc

23. Which one gives the most valid and recent explanation for stomatal movements? [AIPMT 2015]

(a) Transpiration (b) Potassium influx and efflux
(c) Starch hydrolysis (d) Guard cell photosynthesis

24. The oxygen evolved during photosynthesis comes from water molecules. Which one of the following pairs of elements is involved in this reaction? [RE-AIPMT 2015]

(a) Manganese and Potassium (b) Magnesium and Molybdenum
(c) Magnesium and Chlorine (d) Manganese and Chlorine

25. During biological nitrogen fixation, inactivation of nitrogenase by oxygen poisoning is prevented by: [RE-AIPMT 2015]

(a) Xanthophyll (b) Carotene
(c) Cytochrome (d) Laghaemoglobin

Answer Keys

1. (b)	2. (d)	3. (d)	4. (a)	5. (d)	6. (b)	7. (d)	8. (a)	9. (d)	10. (d)
11. (b)	12. (c)	13. (b)	14. (a)	15. (a)	16. (b)	17. (c)	18. (d)	19. (a)	20. (d)
21. (b)	22. (c)	23. (d)	24. (c)	25. (b)	26. (b)	27. (d)	28. (a)	29. (c)	30. (d)
31. (b)	32. (d)	33. (d)	34. (d)	35. (a)	36. (c)	37. (d)	38. (c)	39. (c)	40. (a)
41. (d)	42. (d)	43. (d)	44. (b)	45. (c)	46. (b)	47. (d)	48. (c)	49. (b)	50. (c)
51. (d)	52. (c)	53. (d)	54. (c)	55. (a)	56. (d)	57. (c)	58. (b)	59. (c)	60. (d)
61. (c)	62. (a)	63. (b)	64. (a)	65. (b)	66. (a)	67. (c)	68. (d)	69. (d)	70. (c)
71. (d)	72. (d)	73. (d)	74. (c)	75. (d)	76. (b)	77. (d)	78. (c)	79. (c)	80. (b)
81. (b)	82. (a)	83. (a)	84. (a)	85. (a)	86. (c)	87. (c)	88. (c)	89. (c)	90. (d)
91. (b)	92. (c)	93. (a)	94. (c)	95. (d)	96. (a)	97. (d)	98. (b)	99. (a)	100. (d)
101. (d)	102. (a)	103. (a)	104. (b)	105. (c)	106. (b)	107. (b)	108. (c)	109. (b)	110.(a)
111. (d)	112. (c)	113. (a)	114. (a)	115. (b)	116. (b)	117. (b)			

AIPMT Previous Year Questions

1. (d)	2. (b)	3. (a)	4. (a)	5. (b)	6. (b)	7. (c)	8. (a)	9. (a)	10. (d)
11. (a)	12. (b)	13. (d)	14. (d)	15. (d)	16. (a)	17. (c)	18. (d)	19. (b)	20. (a)
21. (c)	22. (a)	23. (b)	24. (d)	25. (d)					

CHAPTER

13

Photosynthesis in Higher Plants

1. Photosynthesis is a
   (a) physical process
   (b) chemical process
   (c) physico–chemical process
   (d) physiological process
2. All living forms on earth depend on _________ for energy.
   (a) sun
   (b) hydrothermal vent
   (c) volcanic eruption
   (d) moon
3. During photosynthesis, light energy is use to synthesize
   (a) inorganic compound
   (b) organic compound
   (c) both
   (d) none
4. Photosynthesis is important because
   (a) it is the primary source of all food on earth
   (b) it is responsible for release of O_2
   (c) both
   (d) none
5. Select the incorrect statement from the following:
   (a) All animals including human depends on plant for their food
   (b) The use of energy from sunlight by plants doing photosynthesis is the basis of life of earth
   (c) Green plants carry out photosynthesis
   (d) None of the above
6. Which of the following is required for photosynthesis?
   (a) CO_2
   (b) Chlorophyll
   (c) Light
   (d) All
7. Experiment using two leaves—a variegated leaf or a leaf that was covered with black paper and one that was exposed to light on testing these leaves for starch—shows that photosynthesis occurs only in _________ part of leaf in _________ of sunlight
   (a) non-green, presence
   (b) green, presence
   (c) non-green absence
   (d) green, absence
8. Half leaf experiment proved that _________ required for photosynthesis.
   (a) carbon dioxide
   (b) chlorophyll
   (c) light
   (d) oxygen
9. Which of the following substance is used in half leaf experiment to absorb CO_2?
   (a) HCl
   (b) KOH
   (c) HNO_3
   (d) H_2SO_4
10. _________ in 1770 performed a series of experiments that revealed the essential role of air in growth of green plants.
    (a) Jan Ingenhousz
    (b) Joseph Priestley
    (c) Von Sachs
    (d) Cornelius Van Niel
11. Bell Jar Experiment was performed by
    (a) Jan Ingenhousz
    (b) Joseph Priestley
    (c) Von Sachs
    (d) Cornelius Van Niel

12. 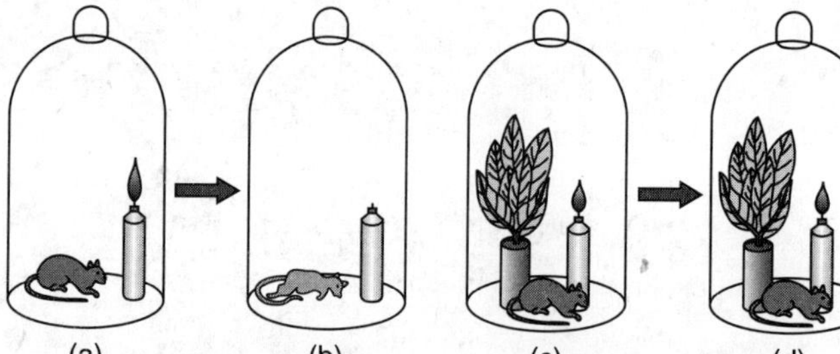

Priestley's experiment

Priestly concluded on the basis of above experiment is that
(a) Burning candle or animal that breathe air, somehow, damage the air
(b) Plants restore to the air, whatever breathing animal and burning candle remove
(c) Both
(d) Light is essential for it

13. Find the method use to light the candle in belljar experiment without disturbing the setup
(a) Removing belljar slowly and light the candle
(b) Creating a hole in bell jar
(c) Using hand len
(d) Through a sudden replacement by another enlightened candle

14. Who proved that light is essential for plant process that purifies foul air by placing priestly and setup once in light and once in dark?
(a) Jan Ingenhousz (b) Joseph Priestley
(c) Von Sachs (d) Cornelius Van Niel

15. ___A___ performed an elegant experiment with an ___B___ plant to show that in bright sunlight, small bubble, were formed around the ___C___ parts, while in dark they do not die.

	A	B	C
(a)	Ingenhousz	Aquatic	Green
(b)	Ingenhousz	Terrestrial	Green
(c)	Priestly	Aquatic	Green
(d)	Priestly	Aquatic	Non-green

16. Which of the following proved that green part could release O_2 by his experiment on an acquatic plant?
(a) Jan Ingenhousz (b) Joseph Priestley
(c) Von Sachs (d) Cornelius Van Niel

17. Stored form of glucose in plant is
(a) inulin (b) sucrose (c) starch (d) glycogen

18. Who provided evidence for the production of glucose when plant grow?
(a) Ian Ingenhousz (b) Joseph Priestley
(c) Von Sachs (d) Cornelius Van Niel

19. Von Sachs studies shows that
(a) green substance in plants is located in special bodies within the plant cell
(b) glucose is made in green paut of plant
(c) glucose is usually stored as starch
(d) all

20. First action spectrum of photosynthesis is described often as an experiment of
(a) Jan Ingenhousz (b) Joseph Priestley (c) Von Sachs (d) Engelmann

21. Which of the following is incorrect about the experiemnt performed by T.W. Engelmann?
(a) Cldophora (a green algae) is used
(b) Suspension of aerobic bacteria is used
(c) Bacteria accumulated mainly in the region of orange and green lifht of the split spectrum
(d) Prism was used to split light into its spectral component

22. A first action spectrum of photosynthesis was described on the basis of experiment performed by T.W. Engelmann on ________ algae.
(a) green (b) red (c) brown (d) all

23. Which of the following pigments resemble the action spectrum produced on the basis of Engelmann experiment?
A. Chl a B. Chl b C. Xanthophyll D. Carotenoids
(a) A and C only (b) A and B only (c) Only A (d) C and D only

24. Who demostrated that photosynthesis is essentially a light-dependent reaction in which hydrogen from a suitable oxidisable compound reduces CO_2 to carbohydrates?
(a) Engelmann (b) Van Sachs (c) C. Van Niel (d) Ingenhousz

25. Van Neil performed the experiment O_2 on
(a) Purple and Green bacteria (b) Green algae
(c) Green plants (d) Fungus

26. Van Neil was a
(a) physicist (b) microbiologist (c) biochemist (d) chemist

27. Which of the following reaction expresses Van Niel reaction for photosynthesis?

(a) $CO_2 + H_2O \xrightarrow{\text{Light}} [CH_2O] + O_2$

(b) $2H_2A + CO_2 \xrightarrow{\text{Light}} 2A + CH_2O + H_2O$

(c) $6CO_2 + 12H_2O \xrightarrow{\text{Light}} C_6H_{12}O_6 + 6H_2O + 6O_2$

(d) $6CO_2 + 6H_2O \xrightarrow{\text{Light}} C_6H_{12}O_6 + 6O_2$

28. What are the probable oxidation production of H_2S in purple and green sulphur bacteria?
(a) Sulphur (b) Sulphate (c) Both (d) None

29. The correct equation of photosynthesis is

(a) $CO_2 + H_2O \xrightarrow{\text{Light}} [CH_2O] + O_2$

(b) $2H_2A + CO_2 \xrightarrow{\text{Light}} 2A + CH_2O + H_2O$

(c) $6CO_2 + 12H_2O \xrightarrow{\text{Light}} C_6H_{12}O_6 + 6H_2O + 6O_2$

(d) $6CO_2 + 6H_2O \xrightarrow{\text{Light}} C_6H_{12}O_6 + 6O_2$

30. By using a ________ isotope it can be proved that O_2 is released from water during photosynthesis
(a) radioactive (b) heavy (c) both (d) none

31. Photosynthesis is a
(a) single-step process (b) two-step process
(c) three-step process (d) multi-step process

32. Photosynthesis occurs in
(a) green leaf (b) green stem (c) guard cells (d) all

33. Within chloroplast, membranous system is made up of
(a) grana (b) stroma lamellae (c) stroma (d) Both (a) and (b)

34. Calvin cycle is termed as dark reaction because it
(a) is not dependent on light for CO_2 fixation in stroma
(b) occurs in dark
(c) is by convention only
(d) requires light

35. Where does light reaction occur in chloroplast?
(a) Membrane system (grana) (b) Stroma
(c) Both (d) None

36. Identify A–H in the given figure.

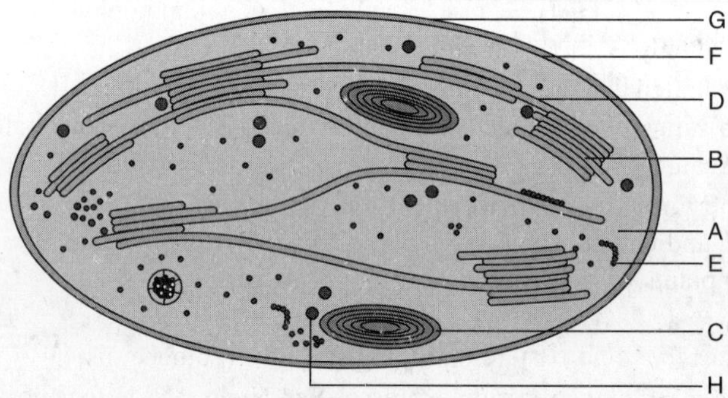

(a) A–Stroma, B–Grana, C–Starch granule, D–Stromal lamella, E–Ribosomes, F–Inner membrane, G–Outer membrane, H–Lipid droplet
(b) A–Lipid droplet, B–Stroma, C–Ribosomes, D–Outer membrane, E–Grana, F–Stromal lamella, G–Starch granule, H–Inner membrane
(c) A–Starch granule, B–Ribosomes, C–Outer membrane, D–Lipid droplet, E–Grana, F–Stroma, G–Stromal lamella, H–Inner membrane
(d) A–Inner membrane, B–Outer membrane, C–Stroma, D–Stromal lamella, E–Ribosomes, F–Grana, G–Lipid droplet, H–Starch granule

37. Which of the following is correct about light reaction?
(a) light is required (b) ATP is produce during reaction
(c) NADPH is produced during reaction (d) all

38. Find out the incorrect statement from the following:
(a) Dark reaction depends on product formed by light reaction
(b) In stroma, enzymatic reactions incorporates CO_2 into the plant leading to synthesis of sugar
(c) Purple and green sulphur bacteria use H_2S as hydrogen donar
(d) There is no division of labour in chloroplast

39. Match the column:

	Pigment			Colour (in chromatogram)
A.	Chl a	–	i)	Bright or blue green
B.	Chl b	–	ii)	Yellow
C.	Xanthophylls	–	iii)	Yellow–Green
D.	Carotenoids	–	iv)	Yellow to yellow–orange

(a) A–i, B–ii, C–iii, D–iv (b) A–i, B–iii, C–ii, D–iv
(c) A–ii, B–i, C–iii, D–iv (d) A–iii, B–ii, C–i, D–iv

40. Chief pigment associated with photosynthesis is
(a) Chl b (b) Chl a (c) Xanthophyll (d) Carotenoid

41. Which light is maximum absorb by Chl 'a'?
(a) Yellow and Green (b) Red and Blue
(c) Yellow and Orange (d) Yellow and Red

42. Which light shows higher rate of photosynthesis?
(a) Yellow and Green (b) Red and Blue
(c) Yellow and Orange (d) Yellow and Red

43. Light reaction and photochemical phase include
(a) light absorption (b) water splitting and release of oxygen
(c) ATP and NADPH formation (d) all

44. Which of the following is incorrect about photosystem?
(a) There are two photosystem (PSI and PSII)
(b) PSI and PSII are named in sequence of their discovery
(c) LHC is made up of hundred of pigment molecules which are bounded proteins
(d) Each photosystem has all the pigments (Except one molecule of chlorophyll 'b')

45. Select the correct sequence of electron transfer in Z-scheme of light reaction:
(a) e^- Acceptor → ETS (made of cytochrome) → PSII → $NADP^+$ → PSI → e^- Acceptor
(b) PSII → e^- Acceptor → ETS (made of cytochrome) → PSI → e^- Acceptor → $NADP^+$
(c) ETS (made of cytochrome) → PSI → e^- Acceptor → PSII → e^- Acceptor → $NADP^+$
(d) e^- Acceptor → PSI → PSII → e^- Acceptor → ETS (made of cytochrome) → $NADP^+$

46. In Z-scheme, Z-shape is formed when
(a) carriers are placed uphill
(b) carriers are placed downhill
(c) carriers are placed in sequence on a redox potential scale
(d) none of the above

47. Where water splitting complex associated with PSII is situated?
(a) Inner side of chloroplast outer membrane
(b) Inner side of thylakoid membrane
(c) Outer side of thylakoid membrane
(d) Inner side of chloroplast outer membrane

48. Where are the protons and O_2 formed likely to be released?
(a) Lumen of thylakoid (b) Outside of thylakoid membrane
(c) In stroma (d) None

49. Phosphorylation occurs in
(a) mitochondria (b) chloroplast (c) cytoplasm (d) all

50. Oxidative phosphorylation occurs in
(a) mitochondria (b) chloroplast (c) cytoplasm (d) all

51. Place where cyclic flaw of electrons occur:
(a) Thylakoid of grana (b) Stroma (c) Stroma lamellae (d) All

52. Stroma lamellae lacks all except
(a) PSII (b) NADP reductase
(c) PSI (d) water splitting complex

53. Which of the following is incorrect about cyclic photophosphorylation?
    (a) Only PSI involved
    (b) It occurs when only light of wavelength beyond 680 nm is available for excitation
    (c) Only synthesis of ATP occurs
    (d) Synthesis of NADPH + H^+ occurs
54. What is the processes that creates proton gradient across thylakoid membrane?
    (a) Splitting of water molecule on inner side of membrane (towards lumen)
    (b) H^+ carrier transport H^+ ion from stroma to lumen
    (c) NADH reductase removes H+ ion from stroma for reduction of $NADP^+$
    (d) All
55. During light reaction
    (a) pH of stroma ↓es (b) pH of lumen ↑es
    (c) pH of lumen ↓es (d) pH of stroma has no effect
56. Which acts as a transmembrane channel?
    (a) F_0 of ATPase (b) F_1 of ATPase (c) both (d) none
57. Chemiosmosis requires
    (a) membrane (b) proton pump (c) proton gradient (d) all
58. Which type of phosphorylation takes place in photosynthesis?
    (a) Cyclic (b) Non-cyclic
    (c) Both (a) and (b) (d) None of the above
59. Unidirectional flow of electrons in photophosphorylation takes place in
    (a) cyclic (b) non-cyclic (c) pseudocyclic (d) all
60. In light reaction of photosynthesis, chlorophyll is subjected to
    (a) destruction (b) permanent reduction
    (c) oxidation and reduction (d) neutralization
61. Photosynthetic pigments in chloroplast are embedded in membrane of
    (a) thylakoids (b) photoglobin
    (c) matrix (d) envelope of chloroplast
62. Identify A–D in the given figure.

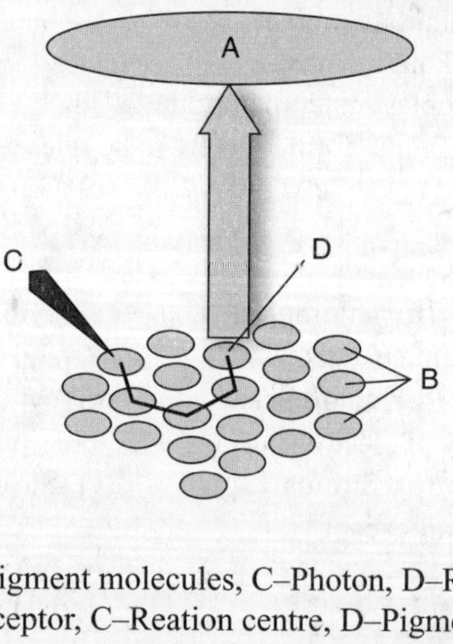

    (a) A–Primary acceptor, B–Pigment molecules, C–Photon, D–Reaction centre
    (b) A–Photon, B–Primary acceptor, C–Reation centre, D–Pigment molecules

(c) A–Pigment molecules, B–Primary acceptor, C–Photon, D–Reaction centre
(d) A–Reaction centre, B–Primary acceptor, C–Pigment molecules, D–Photon

63. Which of the following wavelength occurs in red part of the spectrum?
(a) 470 nm (b) 390 nm (c) 680 nm (d) 830 nm

64. The process for which manganese and chloride ions are required in
(a) photolysis of water
(b) for transfer of H^+ ion to NADP
(c) for transfer of charge of hydroxyl ion to chlorophyll
(d) none of the above

65. What is the absorption maxima of P-700?
(a) 700 Å (b) 683 nm (c) 700 cm (d) 700 nm

66. $NADPH_2$ is generated through
(a) glycolysis (b) Photosystem-I
(c) Photosystem-II (d) anaerobic respiration

67. Identify A–D in the given figure.

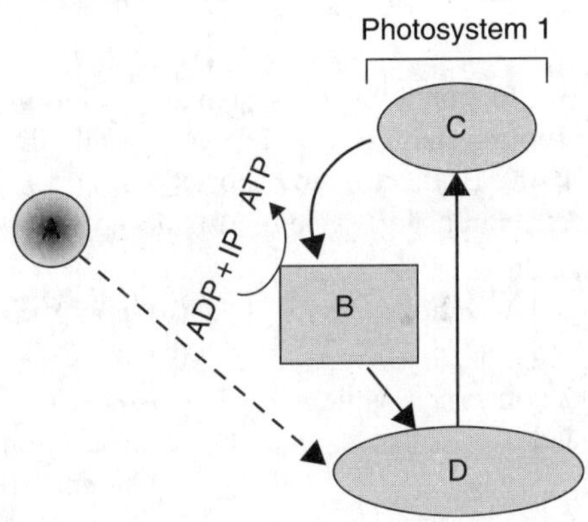

(a) A–e^- acceptor, B–Light, C–Chlorophyll P700, D–Electron transport system
(b) A–Light, B–Electron transport system, C–e^- acceptor, D–Chlorophyll P700
(c) A–Electron transport system, B–e^- acceptor, C–Chlorophyll P700, D–Light
(d) A–Chlorophyll P700, B–Electron transport system, C–Light, D–e^- acceptor

68. Quantasomes are present in
(a) pigment system-I (b) pigment system-II
(c) both (a) and (b) (d) none

69. Which of the chlorophyll type ejects the electron during photophosphorylation?
(a) Chlorophyll 'b' (b) Chlorophyll 'a'
(c) Chlorophyll 'a' and 'b' (d) Xanthophyll

70. In cyclic photophosphorylation which one of the following is formed?
(a) ATP (b) NADP and ATP
(c) $NADH_2$ and O_2 (d) $NADPH_2$, ATP and O_2

71. Where does the primary photochemical reaction occur in chloroplast/Where does the light reaction of photosynthesis takes place?
(a) Stroma (b) Edoplasmic reticulum
(c) Quantasome or thylakoids (Grana) (d) Inner membrane of chloroplast

72. The trapping centre of light energy in photosystem-I is
(a) P-660 (b) P-680 (c) P-700 (d) P-720

73. What indicates A–D in the given figure?

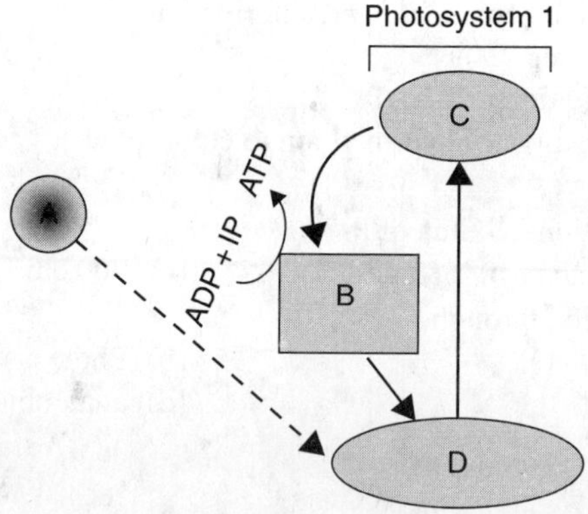

(a) A–e^- acceptor, B–Electron transport system, C–Chlorophyll P700, D–Light
(b) A–Electron transport system, B–e^- acceptor, C–Light, D–Chlorophyll P700
(c) A–Chlorophyll P700, B–Electron transport system, C–Light, D–e^- acceptor
(d) A–Light, B–Electron transport system, C–e^- acceptor, D–Chlorophyll P700

74. Pigment system–I conducts
(a) cyclic photophosphorylation (b) non-cyclic photophosphorylation
(c) both (a) and (b) (d) none

75. Pigment system–II is concerned with
(a) photolysis of water (b) reduction of CO_2
(c) flowering (d) none

76. Photophosphorylation is a process in which
(a) light energy is converted into chemical energy in the form of ATP
(b) NADP is formed
(c) chemical energy is used to produce ATP
(d) CO_2 is reduced to carbohydrate

77. The reaction centre for PS-I and PS-II are
(a) P_{700} and P_{680} respectively (b) P_{680} and P_{700} respectively
(c) P_{580} and P_{700} respectively (d) P_{700} and P_{580} respectively

78. Results of light reaction is/are
(a) only ATP (b) only $NADPH_2$
(c) ATP and $NADPH_2$ (d) only FAD

79. Biosynthetic phase of life use all except ________ that is produced in photochemical phase.
(a) ATP (b) NADPH (c) O_2 (d) None

80. If light is available for a given duration and than again made unavailable, the biosynthetic process will
(a) continue for long duration (b) continue for unlimited time
(c) continue for short duration (d) will stop immediately

81. Which of the following is correct about biosynthetic phase?
(a) C_{14} isotope is used to find out this pathway
(b) Calvin worked on this pathway
(c) Melvin Calvin use photosynthetic algae for this pathway
(d) All

82. Similarity between C_3 and C_4 pathway:
(a) Both are equally efficient
(b) Organic acid is the formed as the first product of CO_2 fixation
(c) Both require one type of cell to occur
(d) Both takes place in all the plants

83. Which pathway takes place in all photosynthetic plant?
(a) C_3 (b) C_4 (c) Both (d) None

84. For easy understanding, Calvin cycle is divided into how many stages?
(a) 1 (b) 2 (c) 3 (d) 4

85. Calvin cycle include
(a) carboxylation (b) reduction
(c) regeneration of RuBP (d) all

86. Which process of Calvin cycle requires RuBP?
(a) Carboxylation (b) Reduction (c) Regeneration (d) None

87. Reduction process of Calvin cycle requires how many ATP and NADPH for reduction of one molecule of CO_2?
(a) 2 mole ATP and 3 mole NADPH (b) 2 mole ATP and 2 mole NADPH
(c) 1 mole ATP and 2 mole NADPH (d) 3 mole ATP and 2 mole NADPH

88. How many mols of ATP is required to regenerate one mol of RuBP?
(a) 1 (b) 2 (c) 3 (d) 4

89. First stable product of Calvin cycle has
(a) 2 carbon atoms (b) 3 carbon atoms (c) 4 carbon atoms (d) 6 carbon atoms

90. In dark reaction, first reaction is the
(a) carboxylation (b) decarboxylation (c) dehydrogenation (d) deamidation

91. In C_4 plants, CO_2 combines with PEP in presence of
(a) PEP carboxylase (b) RuBP carboxylase (c) RuBP oxygenase (d) hydrogenase

92. Dark reaction of photosynthesis is called so because it
(a) can also occur in dark (b) does not require light energy
(c) cannot occur during day time (d) occurs more rapidly at night

93. The initial enzyme of Calvin cycle is
(a) ribulose 1, 5 diphosphate carboxylase (b) triose phosphate dehydrogenase
(c) phosphopentokinase (d) cytochrome oxidase

94. During photosynthesis, when PGA is changed into phosphoglyceraldehyde, which of the following reaction occurs?
(a) oxidation (b) reduction (c) electrolysis (d) hydrolysis

95. Ribulose diphosphate carboxylase enzyme catalyses the carboxylation reaction between
(a) Oxaloacetic acid and acetyl CoA
(b) CO_2 and ribulose 1, 5 diphosphate
(c) Ribulose diphosphate and phosphoglyceraldehyde
(d) PGA and dihydroxy acetone phosphate

96. Calvin cycle occurs in
(a) chloroplasts (b) cytoplasm (c) mitochondria (d) glyoxisomes

97. In C_3 plants, the first stable product of photosynthesis during dark reaction is
(a) 3-phosphoglyceric acid (b) phosphoglyceraldehyde
(c) maleic acid (d) oxaloacetic acid

98. How many Calvin cycle form one hexose molecule?
(a) 2 (b) 6 (c) 4 (d) 8

99. In which plant Calvin experimented the radioactive isotopy to discover the stable product of C_3 cycle?
(a) Chlorella (b) Cycas (c) Carrot (d) Tobacco

100. Mesophyll chloroplast of which plant alone is capable of synthesising starch or sucrose?
(a) C_3 plant (b) C_4 plant (c) both (a) and (b) (d) Neither C_3 nor C_4

101. The enzymes of dark reaction in C_4 plants are found in
(a) bundle sheath chloroplast (b) mesophyll chloroplast
(c) both (a) and (b) (d) none

102. In C_4 plants, mesophyll cells are connected with bundle sheath cells with the help of
(a) Cytoplasmic connection (b) Special connecting tissues
(c) Plasmodesmata (d) Connection is not essential

103. In case of C_4 pathway, CO_2 combines with
(a) PGA (b) PEP
(c) RuDP (d) RMP

104. Which one is a C_4 plant?
(a) Papaya (b) Pea (c) Potato (d) Maize

105. C_4 plants are also known as
(a) Hatch and Slack type (b) Calvin type
(c) Calvin and Bassham type (d) Emerson type

106. In C_4 plants, Calvin cycle occurs in
(a) stroma of bundle sheath chloroplast
(b) mesophyll chloroplast
(c) grana of bundle sheath chloroplast
(d) does not occur as CO_2 is fixed mainly by PEP and no CO_2 is left for the Calvin cycle

107. Tropical plant like sugarcane show high efficiency of CO_2 fixation because of
(a) Calvin cycle (b) Hatch and Slack cycle
(c) EMP pathway (d) TCA cycle

108. Which of the following cycle shows oxaloacetic acid as first stable product?
(a) Calvin cycle (b) Hatch and Slack cycle
(c) C_2 cycle (d) None

109. Kranz type of anatomy is found in
(a) C_2 plants (b) C_3 plants (c) C_4 plants (d) CAM plants

110. C_4 plants are adapted to
(a) hot and dry climate (b) temperate climate
(c) cold and dry climate (d) hot and humid climate

111. Which one of the following is wrong in relation to photorespiration?
(a) It is a characteristic of C_3 plants (b) It occurs in chloroplasts
(c) It occurs in day time only (d) It is a characteristic of C_4 plants

112. How many types of photosynthetic cells occur in C_4 plant?
(a) One type (b) Two types (c) Four types (d) Eight types

113. Which of the following cells of C_4 plants are prominently loaded with starch?
(a) Epidermal cells (b) Mesophyll cells
(c) Bundle sheath cells (d) All

114. Number of carboxylation in C_4 cycle is/are
(a) 1 (b) 2 (c) 5 (d) 3

115. Photorespiration takes place in
(a) chloroplast, mitochondria (b) mitochondria, peroxisome
(c) chloroplasts, peroxisome, mitochondria (d) chloroplasts, cytoplasm, mitochondria

116. Photorespiration is called
(a) C_2 cycle (b) C_3 cycle (c) C_4 cycle (d) none

117. The first reaction in photorespiraton is
(a) carboxylation (b) decarboxylation (c) oxygenation (d) phosphorylation

118. C_4 plant is characterized by
(a) high tolerance to temperature (b) lacks process of photorespiration
(c) greater productivity of biomass (d) all

119. Bundle sheath cells having following characters except
(a) large in size
(b) large number of chloroplast
(c) thick wall impervious to gaseous exchange
(d) with intercellular spaces

120. Primary CO_2 acceptor in C_4 plant occurs in
(a) inner layer cells of bundle sheath (b) outer layer cells of bundle sheath
(c) mesophyll cells (d) none

121. Bundle sheath cells are rich in
(a) RubisCO (b) PEP case (c) both (d) none

122. Which of the following is correct about photorespiration?
(a) Wasteful process (b) ATP is utilized (c) Release of CO_2 (d) All

123. During photorespiration
(a) RubisCO binds with O_2
(b) phosphoglycerate and phosphoglycolate is formed
(c) sugar is not synthesized
(d) all

124. Photorespiration does not takes place in C_4 plant because
(a) O_2 is not released in C_4 plant during photosynthesis
(b) intracellular concentration of CO_2 is high in bundle sheath ensure RubisCO function as carboxylase
(c) they are found in cold environment
(d) stomata in them open in night

125. External factor affecting photosynthesis are
(a) sunlight and temperature (b) CO_2 concentration
(c) water (d) all

126. Internal factor affecting photosynthesis are
(a) number and size of leaf
(b) age of leaf and orientation
(c) internal CO_2 conc. and amount of chlorophyll
(d) all

127. Internal factor of plant depends on
(a) growth of plant (b) genetic predisposition
(c) both (d) none

128. Which is a limiting factor?
(a) Green leaf (b) Optimal light (c) Optimal CO_2 (d) Low temperature

129. Photosynthesis is affected by
(a) quality of light (b) intensity of light (c) duration of light (d) all

130. Light saturation occurs at _______ % of the fall sunlight.
(a) 2% (b) 5% (c) 10% (d) 20%

131. Light may be a limiting factor for
(a) plants in dense forest (b) plant in temperate forest
(c) plant in grassland (d) all

132. What is the relationship between CO_2 fixation and incident light at low intensities?
(a) Linear (b) Parabola (c) Hyperbola (d) None

133. Select the incorrect statement from the following:
(a) At high intensities, both C_3 and C_4 plants shows increase in rate of photosynthesis by increasing CO_2 concentration
(b) C_4 plants shows saturation at 360 μl/L
(c) C_3 plant shows saturation beyond 450 μl/L
(d) Productivity of tomatoes and ball papers can't be increased by enriching environment by CO_2

134. Select the incorrect statement from the following:
(a) Dark reaction is more sensitive to temperature
(b) Light reaction is less sensitive to temperature
(c) C_4 plant respond to higher temperature and C_3 plant have lower optimum temperature
(d) Tropical plant have lower optimum temperature for photosynthesis

135. Water stress leads to
(a) closing of stomata (b) wilting of leaves
(c) reduced activity of leaf (d) all

136. Which factor affect indirectly to process of photosynthesis?
(a) Light (b) Temperature
(c) CO_2 concentration (d) Water

137. Photosynthesis takes place
(a) only in sunlight
(b) only in yellow light
(c) in the visible light obtained from any source
(d) only in very high intensity of light

138. Photo-oxidation of chlorophyll is called
(a) intensification (b) chlorosis
(c) solarization (d) defoliation

139. Which one of the following is not a limiting factor for photosynthesis?
(a) Oxygen (b) Carbon dioxide
(c) Chlorophyll (d) Light

140. If a plant is kept in 300ppm CO_2 concentration, what will happen to it?
(a) plant will die soon
(b) plant will grow but will not die
(c) plant will show normal photosynthesis
(d) respiration will be greatly decreased

141. What will be the effect of intermittent light on photosynthesis?
(a) It will increase
(b) It will decrease
(c) Nothing will happen
(d) Process will stop

142. The diagram below shows three plants with identical leaf surface areas:

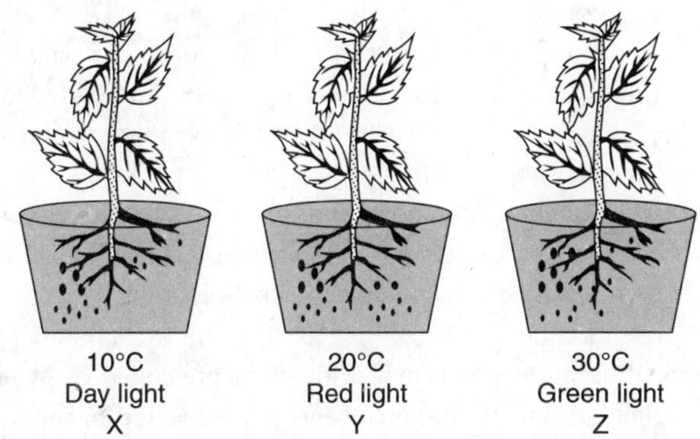

Assuming all other conditions were identical for all three plants, which of the plants would likely to photosynthesize slowest and fastest.
(a) Y slowest, Z fastest
(b) Z slowest, X fastest
(c) X slowest, Z fastest
(d) Z slowest, Y fastest

143. Main factor which limits the rate of photosynthesis on a clear day is
(a) chlorophyll (b) light (c) CO_2 (d) water

144. Blackman's law of limiting factor is applied to
(a) growth (b) respiration
(c) transpiration (d) photosynthesis

145. Which factor is not limited to normal conditions for photosynthesis?
(a) Air (b) CO_2
(c) Water (d) Chlorophyll

146. The first product of CO_2 fixation in Hatch and Slack (C_4) cycle in plants is formation of
(a) oxaloacetate by carboxylation of phosphoenol pyruvate (PEP) in bundle sheath cells
(b) phosphoglyceric acid in mesophyll cells
(c) bundle sheath cells
(d) oxaloacetate by carboxylation of phosphoenol pyruvate (PEP) in the mesophyll cells

Read the **assertion** *and* **reason** *carefully to mark the correct option out of the options given below:*

(a) If both the assertion and the reason are true and the reason is a correct explanation of the assertion
(b) If both the assertion and reason are true but the reason is not a correct explanation of the assertion
(c) If the assertion is true but the reason is false
(d) If both the assertion and reason are false

147. **Assertion:** C_4 pathway of CO_2 fixation is found in some tropical plants.
Reason: In this pathway CO_2 is fixed by 3C compound

148. **Assertion:** Six molecules of CO_2 and twelve molecules of $NADPH^+ + H^+$ and 18 ATP are used to form one hexose molecule.
Reason: Light reaction results in formation of ATP and $NADPH_2$ and oxygen

149. **Assertion:** The first CO_2 fixation product was a C – organic compound.
Reason: Use of radioactive C^{14} in algal photosynthesis studied led to this discovery.

150. **Assertion:** There is a decrease in photosynthesis, if the photosynthetic cells are illuminated by light of P_{680} nm or more wavelength.
Reason: In red drop phenomenon the rate of photosynthesis decreases.

151. **Assertion:** CAM plants lack structural compartmentation of leaf, as found in C_4 plants.
Reason: Stomata of CAM plants are open during the night.

152. **Assertion:** Plants utilizing first RuBP in CO_2 fixations are called C_3 plants.
Reason: Plants utilizing first PEP in CO_2 fixations are called C_2 plants.

153. **Assertion:** Cyclic pathway of photosynthesis first appeared in some eubacterial species.
Reason: Oxygen started accumulating in the atmosphere after the non-cyclic pathway of photosynthesis evolved.

154. **Assertion:** The stromal thylakoids are rich in both PS I and PS II.
Reason: The granal membranes are rich in ATP synthetase.

155. **Assertion:** Cyclic photophosphorylation synthesizes NADPH.
Reason: NADPH synthesise in cyclic photophosphorylation is not associated with ATP formation.

156. **Assertion:** Oxidative phosphorylation requires oxygen.
Reason: Oxidative photophosphorylation occurs in chloroplast.

157. **Assertion:** Each molecule of ribulose-1, 5-bisphosphate fixes one molecule of CO_2.
Reason: Three molecules of NADPH and two ATP are required for fixation of one molecule of CO_2.

158. **Assertion:** Regeneration of CO_2 acceptor molecule RuBP is crucial if the cycle is to continue uninterrupted.
Reason: The regeneration steps require one ATP for phosphorylation to form RuBP.

159. **Assertion:** C_4 photosynthetic pathway is more efficient than the C_3 pathway.
Reason: Photorespiration is suppressed in C_4 plants.

AIPMT PREVIOUS YEAR QUESTIONS

1. Read the following four statements. (i), (ii), (iii) and (iv) and select the right option having both correct statements.

   [AIPMT MAINS 2010]

   Statements:

   (1) Z scheme of light reaction takes place in presence of PS I only
   (2) Only PS I is functional in cyclic photophosphorylation.
   (3) Cyclic photophosphorylation results into synthesis of ATP and $NADPH_2$
   (4) Stromal lamellae lack PS II as well as NADP.

   (a) (2) & (4) (b) (1) & (2)
   (c) (2) & (3) (d) (3) & (4)

2. Study the pathway given below:

   [AIPMT MAINS 2010]

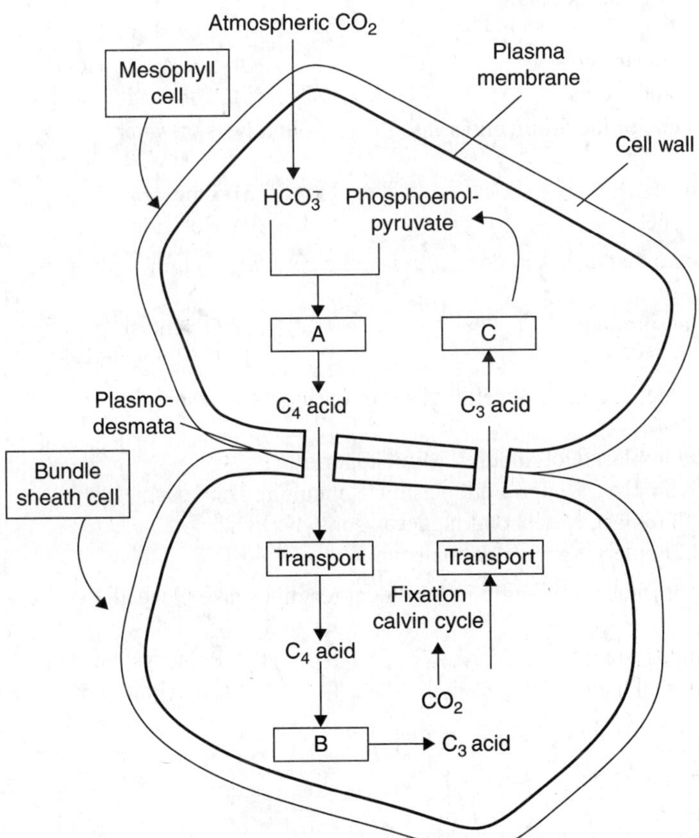

In which of the following options, correct words for all the three blanks A, B and C are indicated?
(a) A: Decarboxylation, B: Reduction, C: Regeneration
(b) A: Fixation, B: Transamination, C: Regeneration
(c) A: Fixation, B: Decarboxylation, C: Regeneration
(d) A: Carboxylation, B: Decarboxylation, C: Reduction

3. PGA as the first CO_2 fixation product was discovered in photosynthesis of: [AIPMT PRE 2010]
(a) Bryophyte (b) Gymnosperm
(c) Angiosperm (d) Alga

4. C_4 plants are more efficient in photosynthesis than C_3 plants due to: [AIPMT PRE 2010]
(a) Higher leaf area
(b) Presence of larger number of chloroplasts in the leaf cells
(c) Presence of thin cuticle
(d) Lower rate of photorespiration

5. CAM helps the plants in: [AIPMT PRE 2011]
(a) Secondary growth (b) Disease resistance
(c) Reproduction (d) Conserving water

6. Which one of the following is essential for photolysis of water? [AIPMT MAINS 2011]
(a) Manganese (b) Zinc
(c) Copper (d) Boron

7. A process that makes important difference between C_3 and C_4 plants is: [AIPMT PRE 2012]
(a) Transpiration (b) Glycolysis
(c) Photosynthesis (d) Photorespiration

8. The correct sequence of cell organelles during photorespiration is: [AIPMT PRE 2012]
(a) Chloroplast, Golgibodies, Mitochondria
(b) Chloroplast, Rough Endoplasmic Reticulum, Dictyosomes
(c) Chloroplast, Mitochondria, Peroxisome
(d) Chloroplast, Vacuole, Peroxisome.

9. In photosynthesis, the light-independent reactions take place at: [RE-AIPMT 2015]
(a) Photosystem I (b) Photosystem II
(c) Stromal matrix (d) Thylakoid lumen

Answer Keys

1. (c)	2. (a)	3. (b)	4. (c)	5. (d)	6. (d)	7. (b)	8. (a)	9. (b)	10. (b)
11. (b)	12. (c)	13. (c)	14. (a)	15. (a)	16. (a)	17. (c)	18. (c)	19. (d)	20. (d)
21. (c)	22. (a)	23. (b)	24. (c)	25. (a)	26. (b)	27. (b)	28. (c)	29. (c)	30. (a)
31. (d)	32. (d)	33. (d)	34. (c)	35. (a)	36. (a)	37. (d)	38. (d)	39. (b)	40. (b)
41. (b)	42. (b)	43. (d)	44. (d)	45. (b)	46. (c)	47. (b)	48. (a)	49. (b)	50. (a)
51. (c)	52. (c)	53. (d)	54. (d)	55. (c)	56. (a)	57. (d)	58. (c)	59. (b)	60. (b)
61. (a)	62. (a)	63. (c)	64. (a)	65. (d)	66. (b)	67. (b)	68. (c)	69. (b)	70. (a)
71. (c)	72. (c)	73. (d)	74. (c)	75. (a)	76. (a)	77. (a)	78. (c)	79. (c)	80. (c)
81. (d)	82. (b)	83. (a)	84. (c)	85. (d)	86. (a)	87. (b)	88. (a)	89. (b)	90. (a)
91. (a)	92. (b)	93. (a)	94. (b)	95. (b)	96. (a)	97. (a)	98. (b)	99. (a)	100. (a)
101. (c)	102. (c)	103. (b)	104. (d)	105. (a)	106. (a)	107. (b)	108. (b)	109. (c)	110. (a)
111. (d)	112. (b)	113. (c)	114. (b)	115. (c)	116. (a)	117. (c)	118. (d)	119. (d)	120. (c)
121. (a)	122. (d)	123. (d)	124. (b)	125. (d)	126. (d)	127. (c)	128. (d)	129. (d)	130. (c)
131. (a)	132. (a)	133. (d)	134. (d)	135. (d)	136. (d)	137. (c)	138. (c)	139. (a)	140. (c)
141. (a)	142. (d)	143. (c)	144. (d)	145. (d)	146. (d)	147. (b)	148. (b)	149. (a)	150. (b)
151. (b)	152. (c)	153. (b)	154. (d)	155. (d)	156. (c)	157. (c)	158. (b)	159. (a)	

AIPMT Previous Year Questions

1. (a)	2. (c)	3. (d)	4. (d)	5. (d)	6. (a)	7. (d)	8. (c)	9. (c)

CHAPTER

14

Respiration in Plants

1. Partial oxidation of glucose without the help of oxygen into pyruvic acid is known as
   (a) glycolysis (b) Kreb's cycle (c) ETS (d) all
2. Scheme of glycolysis is given by
   (a) Embden (b) Meyerhof (c) Parnas (d) All
3. Which of the following is correct about glycolysis (EMP pathway)?
   (a) It is a common path for aerobic and anaerobic respiration
   (b) It occurs in cytoplasm
   (c) O_2 is not required for process
   (d) All
4. Glycolysis occur in how many controlled steps
   (a) 1 (b) 5 (c) 10 (d) 15
5. In plant the end product of photosynthesis is
   (a) sucrose (b) starch (c) glycogen (d) glucose
6. Sucrose is converted to glucose and fructose by enzyme:
   (a) Maltase (b) Invertase (c) Lactase (d) Hexokinase
7. Glucose → Glu-6-phosphate occur due to enzyme
   (a) Hexokinase (b) Oxidase (c) Hydrolase (d) Lysase
8. Common to all living organism is
   (a) Kreb's cycle (b) EMP pathway (c) ETC (d) All
9. 1 molecule of glucose on glycolysis produces
   (a) 2 molecule of pyruvic acid (b) 1 molecule of pyruvic acid
   (c) 2 molecule of CO_2 (d) 2 molecule of O_2
10. Which of the following is a energy yielding process?
    (a) 2-phosphoglycerate to 2-phosphoenol pyruvate
    (b) Frutose to Fructose-6-phosphate
    (c) Phosphoenol pyruvic acid to pyruvic acid
    (d) Frutose 1, 6-biphosphate to PGAL and DHAP
11. Yeast poisons themselves to death when alcohol concentration reaches to ________ in alcoholic fermentation.
    (a) 2% (b) 10% (c) 13% (d) 20%
12. Lactic acid fermentation occurs in
    (a) some bacteria (b) muscle cell under anaerobic condition
    (c) both (a) and (b) (d) aerobic condition

13. How much % of energy released in fermentation?
(a) < 1% (b) < 7% (c) > 10% (d) > 20%

14. Which of the following relation shows substrate level phosphorylation?
(a) Citric acid → α-ketoglutaric acid
(b) Malic acid → oxalo-acetic acid
(c) α-ketoglutaric acid → Succinyl Co A
(d) Succinyl-Co A → Succinic acid

15. Which of the following is a '5C' compound?
(a) Oxaloacetic acid (b) Citric acid
(c) α-ketoglutaric acid (d) Succinic acid

16. At how many places in Kreb's cycle NADH + H^+ is formed?
(a) 1 (b) 2 (c) 3 (d) 4

17. At how many places in Kreb's cycle $FADH_2$ is formed?
(a) 1 (b) 2 (c) 3 (d) 4

18. ETS is present in
(a) stroma
(b) matrix of mitochondria of mitochondria
(c) inner membrane of mitochondria
(d) outer membrane of mitochondria

19. Match the column:

Column I		Column II
A. NADH dehydrogenase	–	1. Complex IV
B. Cytochrome bc_1	–	2. Complex III
C. Cytochrome aa_3	–	3. Complex I
D. ATP synthase	–	4. Complex V

(a) A–1, B–2, C–3, D–4 (b) A–3, B–2, C–1, D–4
(c) A–4, B–1, C–3, D–2 (d) A–1, B–4, C–2, D–3

20. Ubiquinone transfer its electron to
(a) Complex II (b) Complex I (c) Cytochrome c (d) Matrix

21. Which of the following is correct about cytochrome?
(a) Small protein attach to outer surface of inner membrane of mitochondria
(b) Act as mobile carrier
(c) Transfer electron between complex III and IV
(d) All

22. 1 molecule of NADH gives rise to ________ molecules of ATP, while 1 molecule of $FADH_2$ gives ________ molecule of ATP
(a) 3, 2 (b) 2, 3 (c) 2, 2 (d) 3, 3

23. O_2 acts as
(a) terminal hydrogen acceptor (b) Terminal electron acceptor
(c) both (d) none

24. Which type of phosphorylation occurs in mitochondria?
(a) Oxidative phosphorylation (b) Substrate level phosphorylation
(c) Photophosphorylation (d) Both (a) and (b)

25. When $12H^+$ pass through F_0-F_1 particle, how many ATPs are produced?
(a) 6 ATP (b) 4 ATP (c) 8 ATP (d) 10 ATP

26. Identify A, B, C and D in the given figure.

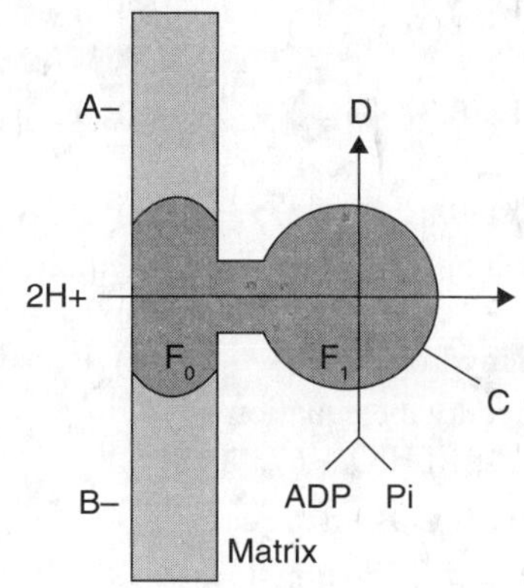

(a) A–Outer side, B–Inner mitochondrial membrane, C–Inner membranepart, D–ATP
(b) A–Inner membrane part, B–Outer side, C–Inner mitochondrial membrane, D–ATP
(c) A–ATP, B–Inner membrane part, C–Outer side, D–Innet mitochondria membrane
(d) A–Inner mitochondrial membrane, B–ATP, C–Outer side, D–Inner membrane part

27. To form respiratory balance sheet, calculations can be made on certain assumptions like:
(a) There is sequential pathway functioning like glycolysis, TCA cycle and ETS following one often another
(b) NADH formed in glycolysis transferred to mitochondria and undergoes oxidative phosphorylation
(c) None of the intermediates in pathway are utilized to synthesize any other compound and glucose is being respired—no other alternative substrate are entering in the pathway at any of the intermediary stages
(d) All

28. How many molecules of ATP are produce by oxidation of 1 molecule of glucose?
(a) 30 (b) 36 (c) 4 (d) 40

29. Which of the following is incorrect about fermentation?
(a) It account for partial breakdown of glucose
(b) Net gain is only 2 ATP
(c) NADH to NAD^+ formation reaction is vigorous
(d) It occur in cytoplasm

30. Respiratory pathway is best defined as
(a) catabolic pathway (b) anabolic pathway
(c) amphibolic pathway (d) none

31. Glycerol enters the respiratory pathway at
(a) Glu-6–phosphate (b) PGA (c) PGAL (d) PEP

32. Amino acid enters in respiratory pathway at
(a) Kreb's cycle (b) Pyruvate
(c) Acetyl CoA (d) any of the above

33. Fatty acid for entry into Kreb's cycle degraded to
(a) Pyruvate (b) Citric acid (c) Acetyl CoA (d) PGA

34. RQ for tripalmitin is
(a) 0.8 (b) 0.7 (c) 0.9 (d) 0.5

35. RQ for protein is
(a) 0.8 (b) 0.7 (c) 0.9 (d) 0.5

36. RQ for carbohydrate is
(a) 0.7 (b) 0.9 (c) 1 (d) 0.4

37. Conversion of pyruvic acid into ethyl alcohol is facilitated by
(a) Carboxylase (b) Dehydrogenase
(c) Decarboxylase and dehydrogenase (d) Phosphatase

38. Fermentation is represented by the equation
(a) $C_6H_{12}O_6 + 6O_2 \rightarrow 6CO_2 + 6H_2O + 673$ k cal
(b) $C_6H_{12}O_6 \rightarrow 2C_2H_5OH + 2CO_2 + 18$ k cal
(c) $6CO_2 + 12H_2O \xrightarrow[\text{Chlorophyll}]{\text{Light}} C_6H_{12}O_6 + 6H_2O + 6O_2$
(d) $6CO_2 + 6H_2O \rightarrow C_6H_{12}O_6 + 6O_2$

39. Anaerobic respiration takes place in the
(a) mitochondria (b) cytoplasm (c) lysosomes (d) ER

40. What is the total gain of energy during anaerobic respiration?
(a) One molecule of ATP (b) Two molecules of ATP
(c) Four molecules of ATP (d) Eight molecules of ATP

41. Cyanide resistant pathway is
(a) anaerobic respiration (b) aerobic respiration
(c) both (a) and (b) (d) none

42. Energy accumulating in ATP is
(a) disulphide bond (b) hydrogen bonds
(c) high energy phosphate bond (d) Ester bond

43. In plants, respiration takes place
(a) only in leaves during night (b) only in leaves during day
(c) in all living cells (d) none

44. In both aerobic and anaerobic respiration which same product is formed?
(a) Lactic acid (b) Pyruvic acid (c) Citric acid (d) Organic acid

45. Which of the following is reverse of photosynthesis?
(a) Respiration (b) Protein synthesis (c) Fat synthesis (d) All

46. The process of phosphorylation takes place in
(a) glycolysis (b) Kreb's cycle (c) HMP pathway (d) all

47. Match the given below organelles with their function:

Column I		Column II
A. Kreb's cycle	–	1. Stalked particles of mitochondria
B. Photorespiration	–	2. Cytoplasm
C. Oxidative phosphorylation	–	3. Peroxisomes
D. Glycolysis	–	4. Inner surface of membrane of mitochondria

(a) A–2, B–3, C–4, D–1 (b) A–1, B–2, C–3, D–4
(c) A–4, B–3, C–1, D–2 (d) A–3, B–2, C–4, D–1

48. Match the name of scientist with his work:

Column I		Column II
A. PPP (Pentose Phosphate Pathway)	–	1. Kuhne
B. Demonstration of fermentation	–	2. Kreb's
C. TCA cycle	–	3. Warburg–Dickens
D. Glycolysis	–	4. Embden Mayerhof Parnas

(a) A–1, B–2, C–3, D–4 (b) A–2, B–4, C–3, D–1
(c) A–1, B–2, C–4, D–3 (d) A–3, B–1, C–2, D–4

49. Match the correct answers with type of respiration and respiratory substrates:

Column I		Column II
A. Respiration	–	1. Proteins
B. Floating respiration	–	2. Starch
C. Cytoplasmic respiration	–	3. Carbohydrates
D. Protoplasmic respiration	–	4. Lactose

(a) A–3, B–2, C–1, D–4 (b) A–2, B–3, C–4, D–1
(c) A–1, B–2, C–3, D–4 (d) A–2, B–4, C–1, D–3

50. The energy yield as a result of total oxidation of one glucose molecule during cellular respiration is to convert
(a) 34 molecules of ADP into 34 molecules of ATP
(b) 30 molecules of ADP into 30 molecules of ATP
(c) 36 molecules of ADP into 36 molecules of ATP
(d) 32 molecules of ADP into 32 molecules of ATP

51. The connecting link among glycolysis, Kreb's cycle and beta-oxidation of fatty acid is
(a) pyruvic acid (b) acetyl CoA (c) acetaldehyde (d) citric acid

52. Which of the following is the source of respiration?
(a) Stored food (b) RNA (c) DNA (d) ATP

53. From substrate level, phosphorylation ATP are produced
(a) 2 (b) 6 (c) 10 (d) 8

54. Select the incorrect statement:
(a) Plants have no special system for breathing or gaseous exchange
(b) Acetyl co-A enter in TCA cycle running in matrix of mitochondria
(c) The RQ depends upon the type of respirarory substance used during respiration
(d) In fermentation complete oxidation of glucose occur in some bacteria

55. The aerobic respiration yields
(a) $8NADH_2$, $2FADH_2$, 2ATP (b) $10NADH_2$, $2FADH_2$, 38ATP
(c) $12NADH_2$, 30ATP, H_2O (d) $10NADH_2$, $2FADH_2$, 2GTP, 2ATP

56. How many ATP are used/required in glycolysis or for complete phosphorylation of a glucose molecule?
(a) 4 (b) 2 (c) 6 (d) 8

57. Identify A–E in the given figure.

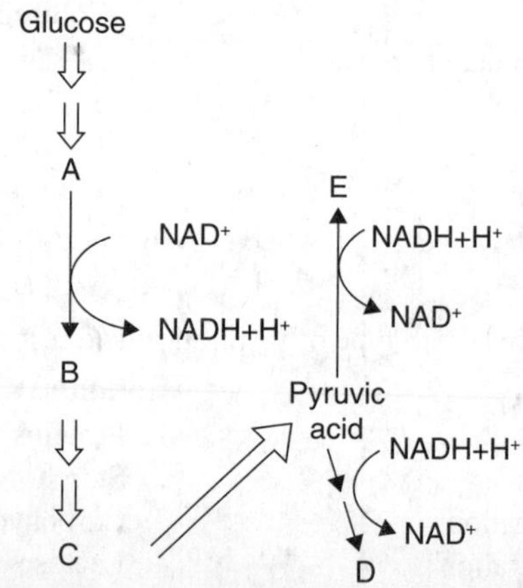

(a) A–Phosphoenol Pyruvic acid, B–Lactic acid, C–3-Phosphoglyceric acid, D–Ethanol + CO_2, E–Glyceraldehyde 3-Phosphate
(b) A–Glyceraldehyde 3-Phosphate, B–3-Phosphoglyceric acid, C–Phosphoenol Pyruvic acid, D–Ethanol + CO_2, E–Lactic acid
(c) A–Lactic acid, B–Ethanol + CO_2, C–Glyceraldehyde 3-Phosphate, D–Phosphoenol Pyruvic acid, E–3-Phosphoglyceric acid
(d) A–3-Phosphoglyceric acid, B–Phosphoenol Pyruvic acid, C–Lactic acid, D–Glyceraldehyde 3-Phosphate, E–Ethanol + CO_2

58. Isomerization takes place in
(a) glycolysis (b) Kreb's cycle
(c) oxidative phosphorylation (d) none

59. In cellular respiration, O_2 is used as a final receptor of
(a) ATP and NADH (b) H and e- (c) Fe (d) Cytochrome

60. First stage in respiration is
(a) aerobic oxidation of pyruvic acid (b) liberation of CO_2
(c) glycolysis (d) electron transport system

61. Besides the net gain of 2 ATP molecules in glycolysis which other molecules are simultaneously formed
(a) $FADH_2$ (b) $NADPH_2$ (c) $NADH_2$ (d) $FAMH_2$

62. Total ATP production during EMP pathway is
(a) 24 ATP molecules (b) 8 ATP molecules
(c) 38 ATP molecules (d) 6 ATP molecules

63. Glycolysis takes place in
(a) mitochondria (b) cytoplasm
(c) both mitochondria and cytoplasm (d) vacuole

64. Pyruvate (pyruvic acid) dehydrogenase is used in converting
(a) pyruvate to glucose (b) glucose to pyruvate
(c) pyruvic acid to lactic acid (d) pyruvate (pyruvic acid) to acetyl CoA

65. The number of molecules of pyruvic acid formed from one molecule of glucose at the end of glycolysis is
(a) 1 (b) 2 (c) 3 (d) 4

66. What is the other name of glycolysis?
(a) EMP pathway (b) TCA pathway
(c) HMS pathway (d) None
67. The common phase between aerobic and anaerobic respiration is called
(a) Tricarboxylic acid cycle (b) Oxidative phosphorylation
(c) Embden, Meyerhoff, Parnas cycle (d) Kreb's cycle
68. The oxidation of one $NADH_2$ yields
(a) 18 ATP (b) 6 ATP (c) 3 ATP (d) 2 ATP
69. The end product of glycolysis is
(a) acetyl Co-A (b) citric acid (c) pyruvic acid (d) fumaric acid
70. Which one of the following is the first step of glycolysis?
(a) Breakdown of glucose (b) Phosphorylation of glucose
(c) Conversion of glucose into fructose (d) Dehydrogenation of glucose
71. Which of the following is the correct sequence of glycolysis?
(a) G 6–P → PEP → 3–PGAL → 3–PGA
(b) G 6–P → 3–PGAL → 3–PGA → PEP
(c) G 6–P → PEP → 3–PGA → 3–PGAL
(d) G 6–P → 3–PGA → 3–PGAL → PEP
72. Which intermediate compound is involved in the synthesis of amino acids?
(a) Malic acid (b) Citric acid
(c) α-ketogluteric acid (d) Isocitric acid
73. In ATP molecule energy is stored in
(a) chemical bonds (b) hydrogen bonds
(c) carbon bonds (d) pyrophosphate bonds
74. What indicated A–F in the given figure?

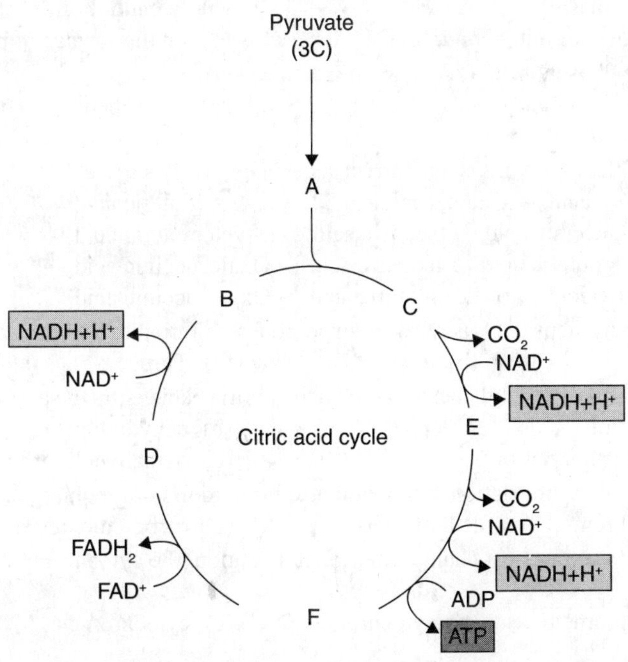

(a) A–Oxaloacetic acid (4C), B–Malic acid (4C), C–Succinic acid (4C), D–Acetyl coenzyme A (2C), E–Citric acid (6C), F–α-ketoglutaric acid
(b) A–α-ketoglutaric acid, B–Citric acid (6C), C:Oxaloacetic acid (4C), D–Succinic acid (4C), E–Acetyl coenzyme A (2C), F–Malic acid (4C)
(c) A–Acetyl coenzyme A (2C), B–Oxaloacetic acid (4C), C–Citric acid (6C), D–Malic acid (4C), E–α-ketoglutaric acid, F–Succinic acid (4C)
(d) A–Succinic acid (4C), B–Acetyl coenzyme A (2C), C–Malic acid, D–α-ketoglutaric acid, E–Citric acid (6C), F–Oxaloacetic acid (4C)

75. Kreb's cycle is termed as the aerobic phase of respiration because
(a) it consumes oxygen
(b) oxygen acts as a catalyst
(c) aerobic conditions are essential for the continued operation of electron transport system
(d) all

76. Between which of the following stages, GTP is formed by substrate level phosphorylation?
(a) Succinate to fumarate (b) Ketoglutarate to succinate
(c) Oxalosuccinate to glutarate (d) Fumarate to malate

77. How many molecules of ATP are produced per molecule of $FADH_2$ oxidised?
(a) One (b) Two (c) Three (d) Four

78. A molecule of ATP is formed when electron passes from
(a) Cyt c to Cyt a (b) Cyt a to Cyt c (c) Cyt b to Cyt c_1 (d) Cyt c to Cyt b

79. Kreb's cycle is also known as
(a) glyoxylate cycle (b) EMP pathway (c) citric acid cycle (d) glycolate cycle

80. Link between glycolysis and Kreb's cycle is
(a) citric acid (b) acetyl CoA (c) succinic acid (d) oxaloacetic acid

81. The reaction of Kreb's cycle take place
(a) in cytoplasm (b) in endoplasmic reticulum
(c) in matrix of mitochondria (d) on the surface of mitochondrion

82. Oxidative phosphorylation occurs in the
(a) outer membrane of mitochondria (b) inner membrane of mitochondria
(c) stroma of chloroplast (d) grana of chloroplast

83. Which of the following is the correct sequence in Kreb's cycle?
(a) Isocitric acid → Oxalosuccinic acid → α–ketogluteric acid
(b) Oxalosuccinic acid → Isocitric acid → α–ketogluteric acid
(c) α–ketogluteric acid → Isocitric acid → Oxalosuccinic acid
(d) Isocitric acid → α–ketogluteric acid → Oxalosuccinic acid

84. In how many steps, CO_2 is released in aerobic respiration of pyruvic acid?
(a) One (b) Six (c) Three (d) Twelve

85. The formation of acetyl coenzyme–A from pyruvic acid is the result of its
(a) reduction (b) dehydration
(c) dephosphorylation (d) oxidative decarboxylation

86. Oxidative phosphorylation and photophosphorylation both require the electron carrier
(a) cytochrome (b) oxygen (c) carbon dioxide (d) water

87. In an electron transport chain, in terminal oxidation, the cytochrome which donates electrons to O_2 is
(a) cytochrome b (b) cytochrome c (c) cytochrome a_3 (d) cytochrome a

88. The last or terminal cytochrome in respiratory chain is
(a) Cyt b (b) Cyt a_3 (c) Cyt a (d) Cyt c

89. The correct sequence of electron acceptor in ATP synthesis is
(a) Cyt a a_3 b c (b) Cyt b c a a_3 (c) Cyt b c a_3 a (d) Cyt c b a a_3

90. In Kreb's cycle, the FAD precipitates as electron acceptor during the conversion of
(a) Succinyl CoA to succinic acid (b) α-ketoglutarate to succinyli CoA
(c) Fumaric acid to maleic acid (d) Succinic acid to fumaric acid

91. RQ for glucose is
(a) 1 (b) 0.5 (c) 2 (d) 0.05

92. With which of the following fatty acid value of RQ is one?
(a) Acetic acid (b) Oleic acid (c) Stearic acid (d) Palmitic acid

93. RQ is defined as
(a) Ratio between CO_2 liberated and O_2 taken
(b) Volume of oxygen taken
(c) Volume of carbon dioxide liberated
(d) Ratio between oxygen taken and fat utilized

94. RQ of fatty substances is generally
(a) unity (b) less than one (c) greater than one (d) zero

95. RQ of sprouting potato tubers will be
(a) 1 (b) < 1 (c) > 1 (d) 0

96. RQ in anaerobic respiration is
(a) 0 (b) $\propto$ (c) 1 (d) > 1

97. What indicates A–E in the given figure?

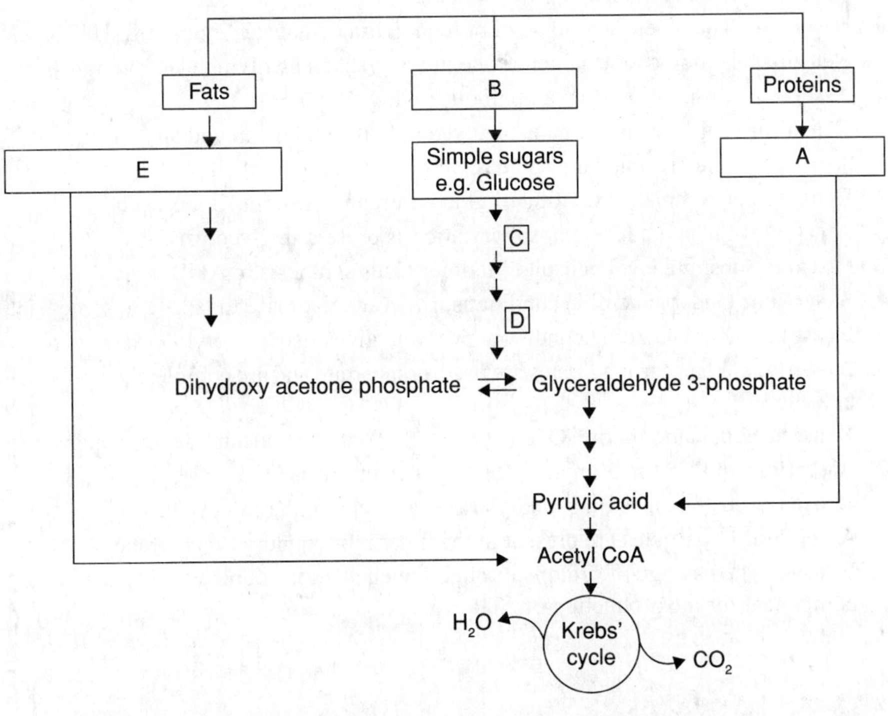

(a) A–Glucose 6-phosphate, B–Fatty acids and glycerol, C–Carbohydrate, D–Amino acid, E–Fructose 1, 6-bisphosphate
(b) A–Fatty acids and glycerol, B–Glucose 6-phosphate, C–Amino acid, D–Carbohydrates, E–Fructose 1, 6-bisphosphate
(c) A–Fructose 1, 6-bisphosphate, B–Amino acid, C–Glucose 6-phosphate, D–Fatty acids and glycerol, E–Carbohydrate
(d) A–Amino acid, B–Carbohydrate, C–Glucose 6-phosphate, D–Fructose 1, 6-bisphosphate, E–Fatty acids and glycerol

Read the ***assertion*** *and* ***reason*** *carefully to mark the correct option out of the options given below:*

(a) If both the assertion and the reason are true and the reason is a correct explanation of the assertion
(b) If both the assertion and reason are true but the reason is not a correct explanation of the assertion
(c) If the assertion is true but the reason is false
(d) If both the assertion and reason are false

98. **Assertion:** Glycolysis occurs in cytoplasm.
Reason: Enzymes for glycolysis are found in cytoplasm.

99. **Assertion:** Power house of cell is mitochondria.
Reason: ATP is produced in mitochondria.

100. **Assertion:** The inner membrane of mitochondria contains enzymes of Kreb's cycle
Reason: The mitochondrial matrix contains systems involving electron transport.

101. **Assertion:** Respiration is an amphibolic pathway.
Reason: Respiratory pathway is involved in both catabolism and anabolism.

102. **Assertion:** The breakdown of glucose to pyruvic acid is called glycolysis.
Reason: For complete oxidation of glucose organism adopt Kreb's cycle.

103. **Assertion:** Substrate level phosphorylation is present in glycolysis.
Reason: Substrate level phosphorylation causes synthesis of ATP.

104. **Assertion:** Under anaerobic conditions, pyruvate gives rise to lactate in some bacteria.
Reason: Under anaerobic condition, pyruvate gives rise to acetyl CoA.

105. **Assertion:** When carbohydrates are used as substrate and are completely oxidised, the RQ will be 1.
Reason: Equal amount of CO_2 and O_2 are evolved and consumed during above process.

106. **Assertion:** In ETS the ultimate acceptor of electrons is O_2.
Reason: Substrate level phosphorylation also occur in Kreb's cycle.

107. **Assertion:** F_1 particles are present in the inner mitochondrial membrane.
Reason: The passage of protons through the channel is coupled to the catalytic site of the F_1 component for the production of ATP.

AIPMT PREVIOUS YEAR QUESTIONS

1. The energy-releasing metabolic process in which substrate is oxidised without an external electron acceptor is called

[AIPMT PRE 2010]

(a) Glycolysis (b) Fermentation
(c) Aerobic respiration (d) Photorespiration

2. The three boxes in this diagram represent the three major biosynthetic pathways in aerobic respiration. Arrows represent net reactions or products.

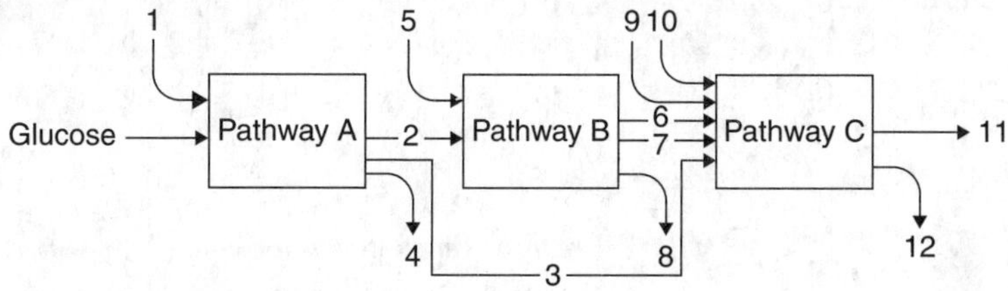

Arrows numbered 4, 8 and 12 can all be: [AIPMT 2013]

(a) NADH (b) ATP (c) H_2O (d) FAD^+ or $FADH_2$

3. Which of the metabolites is common to respiration mediated breakdown of fats, carbohydrates and proteins?

[AIPMT 2013]

(a) Glucose - 6 - phosphate (b) Fructose 1, 6 – bisphosphate
(c) Pyruvic acid (d) Acetyl CoA

4. In which one of the following processes CO_2 is not released?

[AIPMT 2014]

(a) Aerobic respiration in plants (b) Aerobic respiration in animals
(c) Alcoholic fermentation (d) Lactate fermentation

5. Cytochromes are found in:

[AIPMT 2015]

(a) Matrix of mitochondria (b) Outer wall of mitochondria
(c) Cristae of mitochondria (d) Lysosomes

Answer Keys

1. (a)	2. (d)	3. (d)	4. (c)	5. (a)	6. (b)	7. (a)	8. (b)	9. (a)	10. (c)
11. (c)	12. (c)	13. (b)	14. (d)	15. (c)	16. (c)	17. (a)	18. (c)	19. (b)	20. (c)
21. (d)	22. (a)	23. (c)	24. (d)	25. (a)	26. (a)	27. (d)	28. (b)	29. (c)	30. (c)
31. (c)	32. (d)	33. (c)	34. (b)	35. (c)	36. (c)	37. (c)	38. (b)	39. (b)	40. (b)
41. (a)	42. (c)	43. (c)	44. (b)	45. (a)	46. (d)	47. (c)	48. (d)	49. (b)	50. (c)
51. (b)	52. (a)	53. (b)	54. (d)	55. (b)	56. (b)	57. (b)	58. (a)	59. (b)	60. (c)
61. (c)	62. (b)	63. (b)	64. (d)	65. (b)	66. (a)	67. (c)	68. (c)	69. (c)	70. (b)
71. (b)	72. (c)	73. (d)	74. (c)	75. (c)	76. (b)	77. (b)	78. (c)	79. (c)	80. (b)
81. (c)	82. (b)	83. (a)	84. (c)	85. (d)	86. (a)	87. (c)	88. (b)	89. (b)	90. (d)
91. (a)	92. (a)	93. (a)	94. (b)	95. (a)	96. (b)	97. (d)	98. (a)	99. (a)	100. (d)
101. (a)	102. (b)	103. (b)	104. (c)	105. (a)	106. (b)	107. (b)			

AIPMT Previous Year Questions

1. (b)	2. (b)	3. (d)	4. (d)	5. (c)

CHAPTER

15

Plant Growth and Development

1. What occurs due to plant growth and development?
(a) Leaves, flowers, fruits etc. arise in orderly pattern
(b) Increase in girth
(c) Falling of leaves and fruits
(d) All

2. Development consists of
(a) growth (b) differentiation (c) both (d) None

3. Which of the following is correct about the development of a mature plant from a zygote?
(a) Follows a precise and ordered succession of events
(b) Only differentiation occurs
(c) Occurs due to environmental effect only
(d) None

4. What kinds of factors govern a plant's developmental process?
(a) Intrinsic factors (b) Extrinsic factors (c) Both (d) None

5. All cells of the plants are descendents of
(a) Zygote (b) Seeds (c) gametes (d) Both (b) and (c)

6. Appearance and fall of fruits occurs due to
(a) hormonal influence (b) growth and development
(c) differentiation (d) Both (a) and (b)

7. Which is one of the most fundamental and conspicuous characteristic of living being?
(a) Development (b) Differentiation (c) Maturation (d) Growth

8. What is an irreversible permanent increase in size of an organ or its part or even of an individual cell?
(a) Development (b) Differentiation (c) Growth (d) Maturation

9. Growth is accompanied by
(a) Anabolism (b) Catabolism (c) Both (d) None

10. Metabolism occurs on the expense of
(a) nutrition (b) water (c) energy (d) hormones

11. If expansion of leaf occurs, it is known as
(a) swelling (b) imbibitions (c) differentiation (d) growth

12. Why the growth of a plant is unique?
(a) The plant retains the capacity of unlimited growth
(b) The plant can regenerate the same characters

(c) There is no change in offspring's characters
(d) None

13. The unique ability to retain the capacity of growth in plants is due to presence of
(a) lifetime differentiation
(b) activator hormones
(c) chlorophyll to utilize energy lifetime
(d) meristems at certain locations

14. What is the special feature of meristem?
(a) Its present in every tissue (b) Its capacity to divide
(c) Its capacity to self perpetuate (d) Both (b) and (c)

15. Cells that further make up the plant body ________.
(a) loose capacity to divide (b) loose capacity to grow
(c) loose capacity to differentiate (d) None

16. Continued growth due to activity of meristem is which type of growth?
(a) Closed growth (b) Intranets growth (c) Both (a) and (b) (d) Open growth

17. Meristems are found in
(a) root apex (b) shoot apex (c) both (d) none

18. Meristems are responsible for ________
(a) secondary growth (b) primary growth (c) both (d) none

19. What is the contribution of meristem in growth of plant?
(a) Elongation along the axis
(b) Differentiation
(c) Both (a) and (b)
(d) None

20. Secondary growth of plant occurs due to ________
(a) lateral meristems (b) vascular cambium
(c) cork cambium (d) all

21. At cellular level, growth is an
(a) increase in cytoplasm (b) increase in size
(c) increase in nuclear size (d) increase in protoplasm

22. Which of the following is not the parameter for measuring growth?
(a) Wet weight (b) Dry weight (c) Volume (d) Cell member

23. One single maize root apical meristem can give rise to how many cells per hour?
(a) 17500 (b) >17500 (c) <17500 (d) None

24. By how many times, cells of watermelon increase in size?
(a) 3,15,000 (b) 3,50,000 (c) 3,25,000 (d) 3,17,000

25. In question 23 and 24 respectively growth can be expressed as increase in cell.
(a) Size, number (b) Volume, size (c) number, size (d) Size, volume

26. Growth of pollen tube is measured in terms of
(a) weight (b) width (c) volume (d) length

27. Growth of a dorsiventral leaf can be measured in terms of ________
(a) length (b) width (c) volume of cells (d) surface area

28. Which of the following are phases of growth?
(a) Meristemation (b) Elongation (c) Maturation (d) All

29. Identify A, B, C, D and E in the given figure.

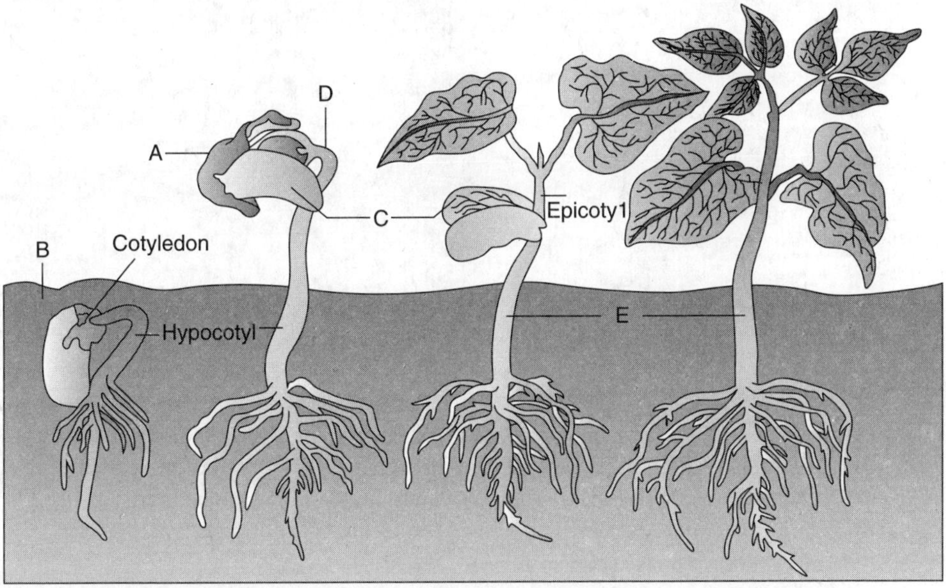

(a) A–Epicotyl hook, B–Soil line, C–Cotyledons, D–Hypocotyl, E–Seed coat
(b) A–Soil line, B–Seed coat, C–Hypocotyl, D–Epicotyl hook, E–Cotyledons
(c) A–Seed coat, B–Soil line, C–Cotyledons, D–Epicotyl hook, E–Hypocotyl
(d) A–Hypocotyl, B–Seed coat, C–Epicotyl hook, D–Cotyledons, E–Soil line

30. Which of the following represent meristematic phase of growth?
(a) Root apex (b) Shoot apex (c) Both (d) None

31. Which of the following are characteristics of the cells in meristematic region?
(a) Rich in protoplasm (b) Large nuclei
(c) Thin plasma membrane (d) Both (a) and (b)

32. Which of the following is not the characteristics of cell wall of meristematic cells?
(a) Primary in nature (b) Cellulosic
(c) Abundant plasmodesmata (d) None

33. Where can we find cells representing phases of elongation?
(a) Root Apex (b) Shoot Apex
(c) Cells proximal to both (d) All

34. Which of the following is not the characteristic of the cells in elongation phase?
(a) Cell enlargement (b) New cell wall deposition
(c) Decrease in volume (d) Both (a) and (b)

35. Cells proximal to phase of elongation show ________.
(a) meristematic phase (b) maturative phase
(c) elongation phase (d) all

36. What is A, B and C in the given figure?

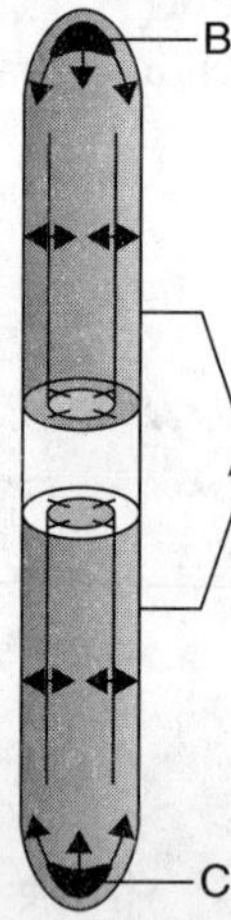

(a) A–Shoot apical meristem, B–Root apical meristem, C–Vascular cambium
(b) A–Vascular cambium, B–Root apical meristem, C–Shoot apical meristem
(c) A–Root apical meristem, B–Vascular cambium, C–Shoot apical meristem
(d) A–Vascular cambium, B–Shoot apical meristem, C–Root apical meristem

37. Cells of maturative phase show
(a) thickening of walls (b) protoplasmic modification
(c) both (d) none

38. Increased growth per unit time is called
(a) growth rate (b) growth speed (c) both (d) none

39. The growth rate shows an increase that can be
(a) mathematical (b) arithmetic (c) geometrical (d) both (b) and (c)

40. In arithmetic growth, other than daughter cells, what happens to the other cells?
(a) They undergo maturation
(b) They undergo differentiation
(c) Both (a) and (b)
(d) They undergo continuous cell division

41. Examples of arithmetic growth is/are
(a) root elongation (b) increase in girth (c) both (d) none

42. Slow initial growth is called
(a) log phase (b) lag phase (c) exponential phase (d) none

43. Rapidly increase in growth after show initial period is called
(a) log phase (b) leg phase (c) both (d) none

44. What is the speciality of the cells after mitotic cell division in geometric growth?
(a) Thickened cell wall (b) Occurring of well organised growth
(c) Retaining the ability to divide (d) None

45. Stationary phase occurs due to
(a) Increase in distance (b) Limited nutrient supply
(c) Thickening of cell wall (d) None

46. Geometrical growth graphically shows
(a) linear curve (b) sigmoid curve (c) both one by one (d) straight line

47. Living organism growing in a natural environment can be found graphically by presence of
(a) sigmoid curve (b) linear curve (c) straight line (d) all

48. Sigmoid curve is typical for which components of plant body?
(a) Cells (b) tissue (c) Organs (d) All

49. Exponential growth can be expressed as
(a) $W_1 = W_0 e^{rt}$ (b) $W_0 = W_1 e^{rt}$ (c) $W_1 = W_0 e^{\Delta rt}$ (d) None

50. In the expression of exponential growth 'e' stands for (Question number 50-52 with respect to equation in question number 49)
(a) exponential growth rate (b) base of natural log
(c) relative growth rate (d) change in size

51. In expression of exponential growth 'r' is referred to as
(a) growth rate (b) efficiency index
(c) both (d) relative growth rate

52. Final size i.e., W_1 depends principally on
(a) W_0 (b) r (c) t (d) e

53. Quantitative comparisons can be made by
(a) absolute growth rate (b) relative growth rate
(c) both (d) none

54. Measurement and comparison of total growth per unit time is called
(a) absolute growth rate (b) relative growth rate
(c) both (d) none

55. The growth of the given system per unit time is expressed on a common basis or per unit initial parameter is known as
(a) absolute growth rate (b) relative growth rate
(c) both (d) none

56. Which of the following are not essential elements for growth?
(a) Water (b) Oxygen (c) Both (d) None

57. Cell enlargement requires mainly
(a) oxygen (b) water (c) nutrients (d) none

58. Extension of growth is supported by
(a) oxygen (b) turgidity (c) osmosis (d) imbibitions

59. Plant growth and further development is intimately linked to
(a) oxygen requirement (b) maintains temperature
(c) water status (d) none

60. How does water help enzymatic activities needed for growth?
(a) Water maintains pH (b) Water maintains temperature
(c) Water provides ions (d) Water provides medium

61. What helps in releasing metabolic energy essential for growth activities?
(a) Oxygen (b) Water (c) Nutrients (d) None

62. What are required for synthesis of protoplasm and act as source of energy?
(a) Oxygen (b) Micronutrients (c) Macronutrients (d) Both (b) and (c)

63. What can affect phases/stages of growth?
(a) temperature (b) light (c) gravity (d) all

64. The process of derivation of cells from meristems and maturation to perform specific function is known as ________
(a) regeneration (b) dedifferentiation (c) dedifferentiation (d) differentiation

65. During differentiation, what kind of changes take place?
(a) Structural (b) Functional (c) Both (d) None

66. What changes would occur in a cell to form a treachery element?
(a) Loose their protoplasm
(b) Strong, elastic, lignocelluloses secondary cell wale
(c) Both
(d) None

67. What is the phenomenon of de-differentiation?
(a) Regaining the capacity to divide (b) Loosing the capacity to divide
(c) Loosing capacity to divide after regaining (d) All

68. What is re-differentiation?
(a) regaining the capacity to divide
(b) loosing the capacity to divide
(c) loosing the capacity to divide after regaining
(d) all

69. Identify A, B, C and D in the given figure.

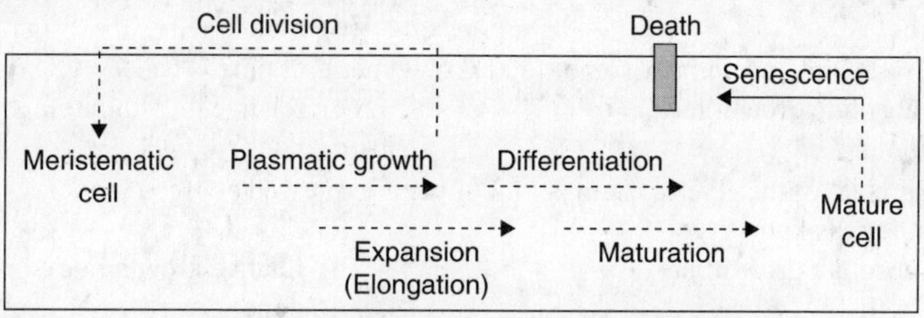

Sequence of developmental process in a plant cell.

(a) A–Cell division, B–Senescence, C–Plasmatic growth, D–Mature cell
(b) A–Meristematic cell, B–Plasmatic growth, C–Maturation, D–Senescence
(c) A–Mature cell, B–Maturation, C–Senescence, D–Meristematic cell
(d) A–Maturation, B–Cell division, C–Meristematic cell, D–Differentiation

70. What kind of differentiation is seen in plants?
(a) Open (b) close (c) primary (d) all

71. Identify the part of A, B and C in this figure.

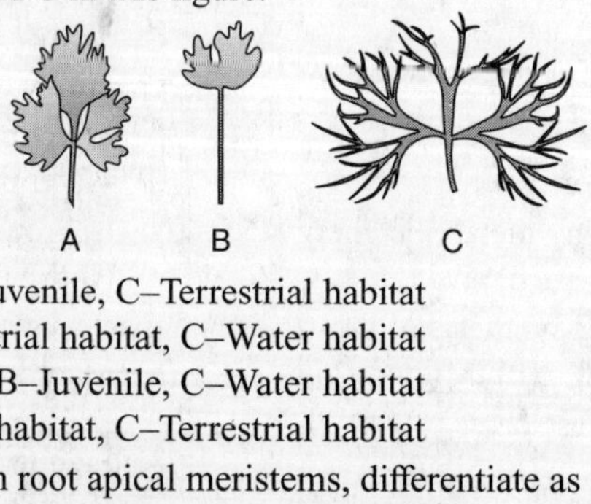

(a) A–Water habitat, B–Juvenile, C–Terrestrial habitat
(b) A–Juvenile, B–Terrestrial habitat, C–Water habitat
(c) A–Terrestrial habitat, B–Juvenile, C–Water habitat
(d) A–Juvenile, B–Water habitat, C–Terrestrial habitat

72. Cells positioned away from root apical meristems, differentiate as
(a) Epidermis (b) Root cap (c) Both (d) None

73. All those changes which an organism goes through during its life cycle from germination of the seed to senescence is termed as
(a) growth (b) differentiation (c) development (d) none

74. On whose response plasts follow different pathways to form different kind of structures?
(a) Environment (b) Phases of life (c) Both (d) None

75. The ability of plants to follow different pathways in response to environment or phases of life to form different kind of structures is called?
(a) Adaptation (b) differentiation (c) maturation (d) Plasticity

76. In which of the following plant the leaves of juvenile plant are different in shape than those in mature plants?
(a) Cotton (b) coriander (c) larkspur (d) all

77. Leaves of which plant show environmental heterophylly?
(a) Cotton (b) coriander (c) larkspur (d) Buttercup

78. The phenomenon of environmental heterophyll is also called
(a) Adaptation (b) Maturation (c) Plasticity (d) growth

79. What is the sum of growth and differentiation?
(a) plasticity (b) development (c) maturation (d) all

80. Development in plants is mainly controlled by ________
(a) intrinsic factor (b) extrinsic factor (c) both (d) none

81. Intrinsic factor for plant development includes
(a) Intercellular (b) Intracellular (c) Both (d) None

82. Intercellular in the former of plant development means ________
(a) chemical regulators (b) genetic
(c) both (d) none

83. Intracellular in the former of plant development means ________
(a) chemical regulators (b) genetic
(c) both (d) none

84. Extrinsic sector for plant development includes ________
(a) light (b) temperature (c) water (d) all

85. Nutrition is included in which phase of plant development?
(a) Former (b) Latter (c) Both (d) None

86. Oxygen is exchanged in which phase of plant development?
(a) Former (b) Latter (c) Both (d) None

87. Which of the following is not a characteristic of a PGR?
(a) They are large
(b) Simple molecules
(c) They are of diverse chemical composition
(d) None

88. Match the following for PGR.

Column I		**Column II**
A. IAA	–	i. Caretenoids
B. Kinetin	–	ii. Terpenes
C. ABA	–	iii. Indole compounds
D. GA_3	–	iv. Adenine derivatives

(a) (A–iii) (B–iv) (C–i) (D–ii) (b) (A–i) (B–iii) (C–ii) (D–iv)
(c) (A–iv) (B–ii) (C–iii) (D–i) (d) (A–ii) (B–i) (C–iv) (D–iii)

89. N^6–Furfurylavmino purine is which derivative?
(a) In dole compounds (b) Adenine
(c) Terpenes (d) carotenoids

90. How many of the following are phytohormones?
ABA, C_2H_4, IAA, GA_3, ABA
(a) 2 (b) 3 (c) 4 (d) 5

91. Which of the following is not a plant growth promoter?
(a) Auxins (b) Gibberellins (c) Ethylene (d) Abscisic acid

92. Who initiated the discovery of plant growth hormones?
(a) Charles Darwin (b) Francis Darwin (c) both (d) none

93. According to Charles Darwin, which plant would help in the discovery of PGH?
(a) Larkspur (b) Buttercup (c) Canary grass (d) All

94. Coleoptiles responded to ________
(a) light (b) water (c) touch (d) all

95. As a response to stimuli the coleoptiles caused ________
(a) bending (b) flowering (c) budding (d) all

96. Auxins are discovered by
(a) Charles Darwin (b) Francis Darwin
(c) F. W. Went (d) Both (a) and (b)

97. Gabriella fujikuroi caused what disease in rice plants?
(a) Foolish seeding (b) Bikaner (c) Both (d) None

98. Who repotted that the symptoms reappeared in uninfected plants treated with sterile filtrate of giberella fungus?
(a) E. Kurosaeva (b) F. Skoog (c) Both (d) None

99. Callus from which plant was observed by miller?
(a) Tomato (b) Tobacco (c) Rice plant (d) None

100. Addition of what to auxins in nutrients medium cause proliferation of callus?
(a) DNA (b) Yeast extract (c) Coconut milk (d) All

101. Who crystallized cytokinin?
(a) Skoog and miller (b) Charles Darwin (c) Both (a) and (b) (d) F. W. Went

102. Skoog and miller termed cytokinin as
(a) Cytokines is (b) kinetin (c) Both (d) None

103. Which three different kinds of inhibitors were found in mid-1960s?
(a) Inhibitor–A, Abscission–II and dorm in
(b) Inhibitor–B, Abscission–II and dorm in
(c) Inhibitor–A, Abscission–III and dorm in
(d) Inhibitor–B, Abscission–III and dorm in

104. All individually found inhibitors in mid-1960s were later named
(a) Giber relic acid (b) Auxin (c) Abscissic acid (d) None

105. The volatile substance causing ripening of unripened bananas?
(a) Abscissic acid (b) Auxin (c) Ethylene (d) Terpenes

106. The only gaseous PGR is ________
(a) IBA (b) Kinetin (c) Terpenes (d) Ethylene

107. The Greek meaning of 'Auxein' is ________
(a) to flower (b) to seed (c) to grow (d) to enlarge

108. Auxin was first isolated from ________
(a) frog's wine (b) Zeatin (c) human wine (d) none

109. The name 'Auxin' was given to which chemical?
(a) Indole–3–acetic acid (b) Indole–6–acetic acid
(c) Indole–3–butyric acid (d) Indole–6–butyric acid

110. How many of the following auxins are obtained from plants?
IAA, IBA, NAA, 2, 4–D
(a) 1 (b) 2 (c) 3 (d) 4

111. NAA stands for ________.
(a) Nitro–acetic acid (b) Nitro aceto acetate
(c) Naphthalene acetic acid (d) Naphthaloaceto acetic acid

112. 2, 4–D stands for ________
(a) 2, 4–Dichlorophenoxy acetate (b) 2, 4–Dextrophenoxy acetate
(c) 2, 4–Diphosphenoxy acetate (d) 2, 4–Dichloromethoxy acetate

113. Synthetic auxins are extesively used in
(a) agriculture (b) horticulture (c) both (d) none

114. Natural auxins are extensively used in
(a) agriculture (b) horticulture (c) both (d) none

115. Which effect of auxin is applied worldwide for plant propagation?
(a) Apical dominance (b) Herbicidal action
(c) Initiate rooting in stem cutting (d) None

116. Auxins promote flowering in
(a) tomatoes (b) pineapples (c) oranges (d) none

117. What prevents fruit and leaf to drop in early?
(a) ABA (b) IAA (c) NAA (d) Both (b) and (c)

118. What promotes abscission of older mature leaf?
(a) Abscisic acid (b) Auxin (c) ehtylene (d) Cytokinins

119. In most higher plants, the growing apical bud inhibits growth of lateral bud. This phenomena is called
(a) Apical tolerance (b) Axial intolerance
(c) Apical ordinance (d) Apical dominance

120. What can help removing apical dominance?
(a) Removal of shoot tips (b) provide plant with a lot of auxin
(c) Both (d) None

121. The process of removal of shoot tip to avoid apical dominance is called ________
(a) Apexotomy (b) Decapitation (c) Both (d) Capitation

122. Decapitation is widely used for
(a) tea plantation. (b) hedge-making. (c) both. (d) none.

123. Which of the following PGR can induce parthenocarpy?
(a) IBA (b) 2, 4–D (c) Terpenes (d) Kinetin

124. Auxins induce parthenocarpy in which plants?
(a) Tomato (b) Pineapple (c) Apple (d) All

125. Which of the following PGR is widely used as herbicide?
(a) Auxin (b) Gibberiellic acid (c) Cytokinins (d) All

126. Which of the following PGR is widely used to kill dicotyledonous weeds?
(a) IAA (b) NAA (c) 2, 4–D (d) ABA

127. 2, 4–D does not show herbicidal action on
(a) chicory ledones (b) monocoty ledonous
(c) mature dicotyledonous (d) mature monocotyledonous

128. Auxin 2, 4–D used for what?
(a) To remove weeds from farms by formers.
(b) To remove weeds from lawn by gardeners
(c) To induce flowering in horticulture
(d) All

129. Auxin helps in what?
(a) Controlling phloem differentiation (b) Controlling xylem differentiation
(c) Cell division (d) Both (b) and (c)

130. How many varieties of Gibberellins reported from widely different verity of organisms?
(a) 100 (b) 120 (c) 145 (d) 140

131. Different types of Gibberellins is reported from what kind of organisms?
(a) fungi (b) higher plants (c) both (d) none

132. Which of the following was first reported gibberellins to be discovered?
(a) GA_1 (b) GA_2 (c) GA_3 (d) GA_4

133. What is the chemical natural of all the GAs?
(a) Basic (b) Acidic (c) Neutral (d) Slightly basic

134. Gibberellins bring about what kind of change in plants?
(a) Morphological (b) Physiological (c) Genetical (d) None

135. Which ability of gibberellins is used to increase the length of grape stalks?
(a) ability to increase apically (b) ability to increase in length of axis
(c) ability to avoid apical dominance (d) all

136. How does gibberellins not chance quality of an apple?
(a) Make it sweeter (b) Elongate it in size (c) Improve its shape (d) All

137. How can Gibberellins help to extend the market period?
(a) It delays senescence (b) Increases ripening period
(c) Increases flowering time (d) All

138. In the form of sugar, sugarcane stores what?
(a) Proteins (b) Carbohydrates (c) Glycoproteins (d) None

139. On spraying Gibberellins on sugarcane crops what major change will it bring?
(a) Increase sweetness (b) Increase length of stem
(c) Increase root strength (d) All

140. Spraying of Gibberellins over sugarcane can increase the yield by how much?
(a) 20 tonnes/acre (b) 20 kg/acre
(c) 20 quintet/acre (d) None

141. What change does it bring in juvenile conifers when sprayed with GAs?
(a) hastens maturity period (b) hastens germination period
(c) hastens dormancy period (d) None

142. Spraying of GAs on juvenile conifers causes
(a) early flowering (b) early germination
(c) early seed production (d) all

143. Cytokinins have specific effects on
(a) cytokinosis (b) cytokinesis (c) cytoketosis (d) cytolysis

144. In what form cytokinins were discovered?
(a) Terpenes (b) Toluenes (c) Kinetin (d) None

145. Gibberellins promoters bolting in which plants?
(a) Beet (b) Cabbage (c) Both (d) None

146. Kinetin is ________
(a) Cytokinins (b) Modified form of adenine
(c) Purine (d) All

147. Kinetin was first discovered from
(a) corn-kernels (b) autoclaved herring sperm DNA
(c) coconut milk (d) all

148. Naturally kinetin occurs in
(a) coconut milk (b) pineapple (c) corn (d) none

149. Naturally available cytokinin—like substance is
(a) kinetin (b) zeatin (c) both (d) none

150. Zeatin was isolated from what?
(a) corn-kernels (b) coconut milk (c) both (d) none

151. Where are natural cytokinins synthesized?
(a) Areas of rapid cell division (b) Areas undergoing differentiation
(c) Both (d) None

152. Where are natural cytokinins synthesized?
(a) Root apices (b) Young fruits
(c) Developing shoot buds (d) All

153. How many of the following PGR help to overcome apical dominance?
Auxins, Gibberellins, Cytokinins, Ethylene
(a) 1 (b) 2 (c) 3 (d) 4

154. How many of the following PGRs help in delay of senescence?
Auxins, Gibberellins, Cytokinins, Ethylene
(a) 1 (b) 2 (c) 3 (d) 4

155. A plant tissue is undergoing senescence, which PGR would be found in it?
(a) Auxins (b) Gibberellins (c) Cytokinins (d) Ethylene

156. Large amounts of ethylene is synthesized in
(a) Ripening fruit (b) Newly grown leaf
(c) Apex (d) Axial bud

157. What are the influences of ethylene on plants?
(a) horizontal growth of seedlings (b) swelling of the axis
(c) apical hook formation in dicot seedling (d) all

158. What is the of ethylene effect on plant organs, especially leaves and flowers?
(a) promotes abscission (b) promotes senescence
(c) both (d) none

159. What is the effect of ethylene on ripening fruit?
(a) increases rate of growth (b) increase in rate of respiration
(c) both (d) none

160. Rise is rate of respiration is called
(a) respiratory climax (b) respiratory rise
(c) respiratory climactic (d) none

161. Which of the following PGR is used to break seed and bud dormancy?
(a) Auxins (b) Gibberellins (c) Cytokinins (d) Ethylene

162. Ethylene initiates germination in which seed?
(a) Mustard (b) Peanut (c) Both (d) None

163. Sprouting of potato tubers is initiated by which of the following PGR?
(a) Cytokinin (b) Ethylene (c) Both (d) None

164. How does ethylene help plants to increase their absorption surface?
(a) promote growth of root (b) promote formation of root hair
(c) both (d) none

165. Ethylene is used to initiate flowering and for synchronizing fruit set in which fruit?
(a) Apple (b) Pineapple (c) Banana (d) All

166. Ethylene induces flowering in which fruit?
(a) Mango (b) Apple (c) Pineapple (d) All

167. Which of the following is the most widely used PGR in agriculture?
(a) IAA (b) ABA (c) GA_3 (d) Ethylene

168. Which of the following is a characteristic of ethephon?
(a) readily absorbed (b) transported within the plant
(c) releases ethylene slowly (d) all

169. Ethephon hastens fruit ripening in
(a) Mango (b) Tomato (c) Apple (d) Both (b) and (c)

170. Ethephon accelerates abscission in flowers and fruits like
(a) Cherry (b) Walnut (c) Cotton (d) All

171. How does ethephon increase the yield of cucumber?
(a) promote senescence (b) promotes female flowers
(c) promotes male flowers (d) both (a) and (b)

172. For which role ABA was discovered?
(a) Abscission (b) Dormancy (c) Both (a) and (b) (d) Ripening fruits

173. What are the actions of ABA?
(a) General plant growth inhibitor (b) Inhibitor of plant metabolism
(c) Stimulates closure of stomata in epidermis (d) All

174. Why is ABA called stress hormone
(a) Removes various stresses from plant
(b) Increase tolerance of plant to various kind of stresses
(c) Both (a) and (b)
(d) None

175. ABA plays an important role in all except
(a) Seed development (b) Maturation (c) Dormancy (d) Germination

176. What is/are the factors that are unfavorable growth of seeds?
(a) Desiccation (b) Air (c) Carbon dioxide (d) All

177. ABA is antagonist to
(a) IBA (b) IAA (c) GA_2 (d) All

178. All are types of roles played by PGR except
(a) Individualistic (b) Synergistic (c) Both (a) and (b) (d) None

179. Which of the following events are controlled by extrinsic factors via PGR?
(a) Vernalisation (b) Flowering (c) Dormancy (d) All

180. All are extrinsic factors for growth and development except
(a) Temperature (b) Light (c) Both (a) and (b) (d) Nutrition

181. What kind of plants require the exposure to light for a period exceeding a well defined critical duration?
(a) Short day plants (b) Day-neutral plants
(c) Long day plants (d) None

182. What kind of plants require the exposure to light for a period less than critical duration?
(a) Short day plants (b) Day-neutral plants
(c) Long day plants (d) None

183. Plants with no such correlation between exposure to light duration and induction of flower response are called
(a) Long day plant (b) Day-neutral plants
(c) Short day plant (d) None

184. What is more important of these?
(a) Light period (b) Dark period
(c) Both (a) and (b) (d) None

185. According to Hypothesis, which substances are responsible for photoperiodism?
(a) Hormonal substance (b) Abcissic acid
(c) Gibberellins (d) All

186. When flowering is either quantitatively or qualitatively dependent or exposure to low temperature it is called ____ phenomenon
(a) Photoperiodism (b) Thermoperiodism
(c) Vernalisation (d) Dormancy

187. Which of the plants don't have winter and spring varieties?
(a) Wheat (b) Rice (c) Barley (d) Rye

188. When are winter varieties planted?
(a) Spring (b) Winter (c) Autumn (d) All

189. When is the harvesting of winter varieties done?
(a) Spring (b) Winter (c) Mid-summer (d) Autumn

190. Biennials are what kind of plants
(a) Dicarpous (b) Monocarpic (c) Polycarpic (d) None

191. Which of the following are common biennials?
(a) Carrots (b) Cabbages (c) Sugarbeet (d) All

192. Cold treatment to biennial plants will stimulate what kind of response?
(a) Photo hastens (b) Photoropism (c) Photoperiodism (d) All

*Read the **assertion** and **reason** carefully to mark the correct option out of the options given below:*

(a) If both the assertion and the reason are true and the reason is a correct explanation of the assertion
(b) If both the assertion and reason are true but the reason is not a correct explanation of the assertion
(c) If the assertion is true but the reason is false
(d) If both the assertion and reason are false

193. **Assertion:** Plant retain the capacity for unlimited growth throughout their life.
Reason: This ability of the plants is due to the presence of meristem at certain location of body.

194. **Assertion:** A sigmoid curve is a characterstic of living organism growing in a natural environment.
Reason: Sigmoid curve is S – shape curve.

195. **Assertion:** Auxin induce parthenocarpy in tomatoes.
Reason: 2,4 –D used as herbicides.

196. **Assertion:** GA increase yield in sugarcane.
Reason: GA causes increase in length of sugarcane stem.

197. **Assertion:** Cytokinin delays leaf senescence.
Reason: Cytokinin promotes nutrient mobilisation.

198. **Assertion:** ABA increases the tolerance of plant to various kinds of stresses.
Reason: ABA stimulates the closure of stomata in the epidermis

199. **Assertion:** Ethylene increase yield in cucumber.
Reason: Ethylene promotes female flower in cucumber.

200. **Assertion:** Ethylene is a simple liquid PGR.
Reason: Etylene inhibits sprouting of potato tuber.

201. **Assertion:** The pigment which causes photoperiodic stimulus is called phytochrome.
Reason: Chemically phytochrome is a starch and lipid.

202. **Assertion:** Floral initiation is done by hormonal substance.
Reason: Hormonal substance is translocated from flowers to leaves.

203. **Assertion:** Vernalisation refers specially to the promotion of flowering by a period of low temprature.
Reason: Vernalisation also seen in biennial plants.

204. **Assertion:** Auxins have been used extensively in agriculture and horticulture.
Reason: They help to initiate rooting in stem cuttings.

205. **Assertion:** A plant hormone is a growth regulator.
Reason: Growth regulators promote or inhibit the growth.

AIPMT PREVIOUS YEAR QUESTIONS

1. One of the commonly used plant growth hormone in tea plantation is: [AIPMT MAINS 2010]
(a) Ethylene (b) Abscisic acid
(c) Zeatin (d) Indole-3-acetic acid

2. Root development is promoted by: [AIPMT MAINS 2010]
(a) Abscisic acid (b) Auxin
(c) Gibberellins (d) Ethylene

3. Phototropic curvature is the result of uneven distribution of [AIPMT PRE 2010]
(a) Gibberellin (b) Phytochrome
(c) Cytokinins (d) Auxin

4. Photoperiodism was first characterised in: [AIPMT PRE 2010]
   (a) Tobacco (b) Potato
   (c) Tomato (d) Cotton
5. Through their effect on plant growth regulators, what do the temperature and light control in the plants? [AIPMT MAINS 2012]
   (a) Flowering (b) Closure of stomata
   (c) Fruit elongation (d) Apical dominance
6. Vernalisation stimulates flowering in: [AIPMT MAINS 2012]
   (a) Turmeric (b) Carrot
   (c) Ginger (d) Zamikand
7. Which one of the following generally acts as an antagonist to gibberellins? [AIPMT MAINS 2012]
   (a) Ethylene (b) ABA
   (c) IAA (d) Zeatin
8. During seed germination its stored food is mobilized by: [AIPMT 2013]
   (a) Ethylene (b) Cytokinin
   (c) ABA (d) Gibberellin
9. Dr. F. Went noted that if coleoptiles tips were removed and placed on agar for one hour, the agar would produce a bending when placed on one side of freshly cut coleoptile stumps. Of what significance is this experiment? [AIPMT 2014]
   (a) It made possible the isolation and exact identification of auxin
   (b) It is the basis for quantitative determination of small amounts of growth – promoting substances
   (c) It supports the hypothesis that IAA is auxin
   (d) It demonstrated polar movement of auxins
10. Which one of the following growth regulators is known as 'stress hormone'? [AIPMT 2014]
    (a) Abscissic acid (b) Ethylene
    (c) GA3 (d) Indole acetic acid
11. What causes a green plant exposed to the light on only one side, to bend toward the source of light as it grows? [AIPMT 2015]
    (a) Green plants need right to perform photosynthesis.
    (b) Green plants seek light because they are phototropic.
    (c) Light stimulates plant cells on the lighted side to grow faster
    (d) Auxin accumulates on the shaded side, stimulating greater cell elongation there
12. Typical growth curve in plants is: [AIPMT 2015]
    (a) Sigmoid (b) Linear
    (c) Stair – steps shaped (d) Parabolic

13. Which of the following enhances or induces fusion of protoplast? [AIPMT 2015]

(a) Sodium chloride and potassium chloride
(b) Polyethylene glycol and sodium nitrate
(c) IAA and kinetin
(d) IAA and gibberellins

14. Auxin can be bioassayed by: [RE-AIPMT 2015]

(a) Hydroponics
(b) Potometer
(c) Lettuce hypocotyl elongation
(d) Avena coleoptile curvature

Answer Keys

1. (d)	2. (c)	3. (a)	4. (c)	5. (a)	6. (d)	7. (d)	8. (c)	9. (c)	10. (c)
11. (d)	12. (a)	13. (d)	14. (d)	15. (a)	16. (d)	17. (c)	18. (c)	19. (a)	20. (d)
21. (d)	22. (a)	23. (b)	24. (b)	25. (c)	26. (d)	27. (d)	28. (d)	29. (c)	30. (c)
31. (d)	32. (d)	33. (c)	34. (c)	35. (b)	36. (d)	37. (c)	38. (a)	39. (d)	40. (c)
41. (a)	42. (b)	43. (a)	44. (c)	45. (b)	46. (b)	47. (a)	48. (d)	49. (a)	50. (b)
51. (c)	52. (a)	53. (c)	54. (a)	55. (b)	56. (d)	57. (b)	58. (b)	59. (c)	60. (d)
61. (a)	62. (d)	63. (d)	64. (d)	65. (c)	66. (c)	67. (a)	68. (c)	69. (b)	70. (a)
71. (c)	72. (b)	73. (c)	74. (c)	75. (d)	76. (d)	77. (d)	78. (c)	79. (b)	80. (c)
81. (c)	82. (a)	83. (b)	84. (d)	85. (b)	86. (a)	87. (a)	88. (a)	89. (b)	90. (d)
91. (d)	92. (c)	93. (c)	94. (a)	95. (a)	96. (c)	97. (c)	98. (a)	99. (b)	100. (d)
101. (a)	102. (b)	103. (b)	104. (c)	105. (c)	106. (d)	107. (c)	108. (c)	109. (a)	110. (b)
111. (c)	112. (a)	113. (c)	114. (c)	115. (c)	116. (b)	117. (d)	118. (b)	119. (d)	120. (a)
121. (b)	122. (c)	123. (b)	124. (a)	125. (a)	126. (c)	127. (b)	128. (b)	129. (d)	130. (a)
131. (c)	132. (c)	133. (b)	134. (b)	135. (b)	136. (a)	137. (a)	138. (b)	139. (b)	140. (a)
141. (a)	142. (c)	143. (b)	144. (c)	145. (c)	146. (d)	147. (b)	148. (d)	149. (c)	150. (c)
151. (a)	152. (d)	153. (b)	154. (b)	155. (d)	156. (a)	157. (d)	158. (c)	159. (b)	160. (c)
161. (d)	162. (b)	163. (b)	164. (c)	165. (b)	166. (a)	167. (d)	168. (d)	169. (d)	170. (d)
171. (b)	172. (c)	173. (d)	174. (b)	175. (d)	176. (a)	177. (c)	178. (d)	179. (d)	180. (d)
181. (c)	182. (a)	183. (b)	184. (d)	185. (a)	186. (c)	187. (b)	188. (c)	189. (c)	190. (b)
191. (d)	192. (c)	193. (a)	194. (b)	195. (b)	196. (a)	197. (a)	198. (a)	199. (a)	200. (d)
201. (c)	202. (c)	203. (b)	204. (b)	205. (a)					

AIPMT Previous Year Questions

1. (c)	2. (b)	3. (d)	4. (a)	5. (a)	6. (b)	7. (b)	8. (d)	9. (b)	10. (a)
11. (d)	12. (a)	13. (b)	14. (d)						

Unit V

Human Physiology

Unit V includes human physiology. This unit includes topics which fascinates all biology students. In this section you need to focus on anatomy and physiology of organ system. Concentrate on data related to various organ systems like heart rate respiratory rate, cardiac output, and the amount of urea excreted in 24 hrs. Special emphasis is given to nervous and endocrine system. Since the last two years, diagram-based questions are frequently asked from this unit, so do carefully study the diagram-based questions given in this book. This unit comprises an equivalent of 10–14 questions in AIPMT paper.

CHAPTER 16

Digestion and Absorption

1. The process of conversion of complex food substances to simple absorbable forms is called
   (a) Egestion (b) Digestion (c) Ingestion (d) Assimilation
2. The major components of our food are
   (a) Carbohydrates (b) Proteins (c) Fats (d) All
3. Which of the following substances do not get digested in our digestive system?
   (a) Carbohydrates (b) Proteins and fats
   (c) Vitamins and minerals (d) All
4. Which of the following are important for our body but required in less amount?
   (a) Vitamins and minerals (b) Proteins
   (c) Fats (d) Carbohydrates
5. Which of the following is a function of food?
   (a) Providing energy to the body
   (b) Providing organic materials for growth and repair of tissues
   (c) Providing organic materials for repair of tissues
   (d) All
6. Digestion in our body takes place by means of
   (a) Biochemical method (b) Mechanical method
   (c) Both of the above (d) Chemical method
7. Which of the following molecules are not utilized by our body in their original form?
   (a) All biomacromolecule
   (b) All biomicromolecule
   (c) Biomolecules having molecular weight less than 1000 dalton
   (d) All
8. Human digestive system consists of
   (a) alimentary canal (b) associated glands
   (c) both of the above (d) gastrointestinal tract only
9. The role of water in our body is to
   (a) act as medium for transport of substances
   (b) provide medium for all metabolic reactions
   (c) prevent dehydration of body
   (d) all
10. The anterior opening of alimentary canal is
    (a) anus (b) mouth (c) vestibule (d) pupil
11. The posterior opening of alimentary canal is
    (a) anus (b) mouth (c) vestibule (d) pupil

12. Teeth of human are
(a) thecodont (b) diphyodont (c) heterodont (d) all

13. If tooth is embedded in a socket of jaw bone than it is known as
(a) thecodont (b) diphyodont (c) heterodont (d) all

14. Marasmus is found in
(a) infant (b) adult (c) old age person (d) all

15. In majority of mammals, including human, two sets of teeth get formed during their life time. These teeth are called
(a) thecodont (b) hetrodont (c) diphyodont (d) lophodont

16. An adult human has 32 permanent teeth which are of four different types and are called
(a) thecodont (b) heterodont (c) diphyodont (d) lophodont

17. Arrangement of teeth in each half of the upper and lower jaw in the order I, C, PM, M is represented by
(a) Dental formula (b) Odontology (c) Dentology (d) Enamel

18. The dental formula of human is
(a) $\frac{0033}{3133}$ (b) $\frac{1003}{1003}$ (c) $\frac{2123}{2123}$ (d) $\frac{3131}{3121}$

19. Identify A, B, C, D and E in the given figure.

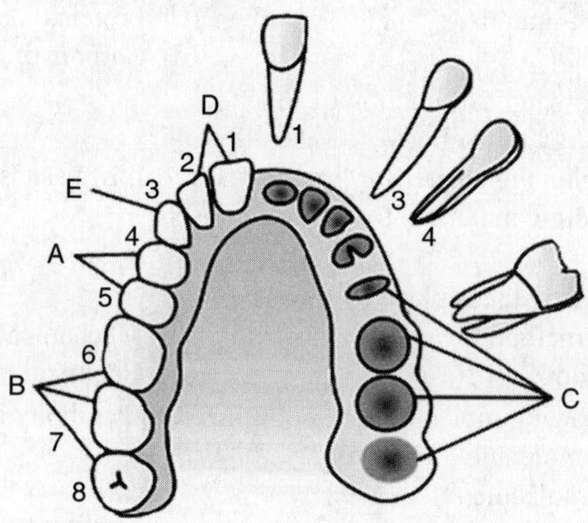

(a) A–Molars, B–Incisor, C–Premolars, D–Canine, E–Socket of jaw
(b) A–Premolars, B–Socket of jaw, C–Canine, D–Molars, E–Incisor
(c) A–Premolars, B Molars, C–Socket of jaw, D–Incisor, E–Canine
(d) A–Socket of jaw, B–Canine, C–Premolars, D–Molars, E–Incisor

20. Dental formula is given to show
(a) the structure of molars
(b) number and types of teeth in both jaws
(c) homodont condition
(d) diphyodont condition

21. Dental formula of human being is
(a) I_2, C_2, P_1, M_3 (b) I_2, C_1, P_2, M_3 (c) I_3, C_1, P_2, M_2 (d) I_2, C_2, P_3, M_1

22. The hardest substance in vertebrate body is
(a) Keratin (b) Dentine (c) Chondrin (d) Enamel

23. Select the incorrect statement among the following about human tongue.
(a) The human tongue has freely movable muscular organ
(b) It is attached to the floor of the oral cavity by the frenulum
(c) The upper surface of the tongue has small projections called papillae
(d) All papillae of human tongue bear taste buds

24. The tongue is attached to the floor of oral/buccal cavity by
(a) epiglottis (b) frenulum (c) gubernaculums (d) mesentery

25. Which of the following acts as a common passage for food and air?
(a) Larynx (b) Pharynx (c) Oesophagus (d) Glottis

26. A cartilaginous flap called __________ prevents the entry of food into the glottis (opening of the wind pipe) during swallowing.
(a) Capsule (b) Epiglottis (c) Glottis (d) Gullet

27. Select the total number of correct statement from the following:
A. The esophagus and the trachea (wind pipe) open into the pharynx
B The hard chewing surface of the teeth, made up of dentine, helps in the mastication of food.
C. The oral cavity leads into a long pharynx which serves as a common passage for food and air
D. The tongue is a freely movable muscular organ attached to the roof of the oral cavity by the frenulum
(a) 1 (b) 2 (c) 3 (d) 4

28. Stomach is divided into how many major parts?
(a) 1 (b) 2 (c) 3 (d) 4

29. Which part of stomach opens into the first part of small intestine?
(a) Cardiac (b) Fundic (c) Pyloric (d) Any of the above

30. Which of the following is a highly-coiled part of small intestine?
(a) Duodenum (b) Jejunum (c) Ileum (d) All

31. Identify A–E in the given figure.

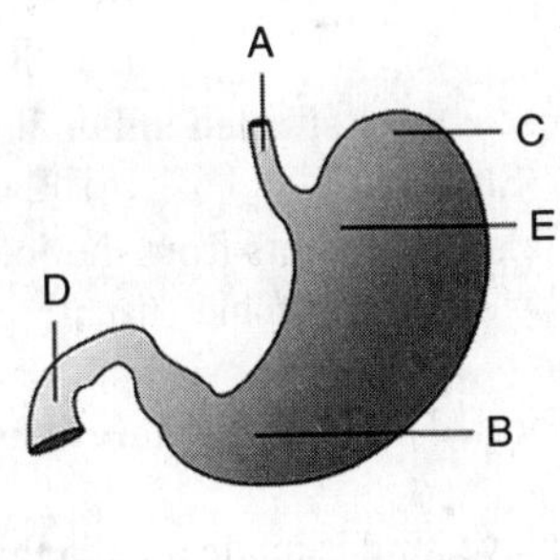

(a) A–Oesophagus, B–Pyloric, C–Fundus, D–Superior portion of duodenum, E–Cardiac
(b) A–Pyloric, B–Cardiac, C–Fundus, D–Oesophagus, E–Superior protein of duodenum
(c) A–Superior protein of duodenum, B–Oesophagus, C–Cardiac, D–Fundus, E–Pyloric
(d) A–Oesophagus, B–Fundus, C–Pyloric, D–Superior protein of duodenum, E–Cardiac

32. A muscular sphincter that regulates the opening of oesophagus into stomach is
(a) Pyloric sphincter (b) Gastroesophageal sphincter
(c) Sphincter of Oddi (d) Cervical sphincter

33. Select the incorrect from the following.
(a) J-shape–stomach
(b) U-shape–duodenum
(c) Bean-shape–kidney
(d) O-shape–vasa recta

34. A muscular sphincter that regulates the opening of stomach into duodenum is
(a) Pyloric sphincter
(b) Gastroesophageal sphincter
(c) Sphincter of Oddi
(d) Cervical sphincter

35. Large intestine consists of
(a) Caecum (b) Colon (c) Rectum (d) All

36. A part of large intestine which is a blind sac and harbor some symbiotic micro organism is
(a) Colon (b) Caecum (c) Rectum (d) Ileum

37. Colon is divided into
(a) Ascending colon
(b) Descending colon
(c) Transverse colon
(d) All

38. Which of the following is true about appendix?
(a) Narrow finger-like tubular projection
(b) Arises from the caecum
(c) Vestigial organ
(d) All

39. The wall of alimentary canal from oesophagus to rectum possesses how many histological layers?
(a) 1 (b) 2 (c) 3 (d) 4

40. The following histological layers are present in wall of human alimentary canal from esophagus to rectum.
A. Serosa
B. Bowman's layer
C. Muscularis
D. Sub-mucosa
E. Mucosa
F. Ganglion layer
(a) A,B,C,D (b) B,C,D,E (c) A,B,D,F (d) A,C,D,E

41. Which of the following is the outermost histological layer of alimentary canal?
(a) Serosa (thin mesothelium)
(b) Mucosa
(c) Sub mucosa
(d) Muscularis

42. Where does the oblique muscle layer situated in human alimentary canal?
(a) Esophagus (b) Stomach (c) Large intestine (d) Small intestine

43. Select the total number of false statements from the following.
A. Muscularis is formed by smooth muscles usually arranged into an inner circular and an outer longitudinal layer.
B. Submucosal layer is formed of loose connective tissues containing nerves, blood and lymph vessels
C. Serosa is the outermost layer and is made up of a thin mesothelium (epithelium of visceral organs) with some connective tissues.
D. The innermost layer lining the lumen of the alimentary canal is the mucosa.
E. Mucosal epithelium has goblet cells which secrete mucus that help in lubrication.
(a) 3 (b) 4 (c) 5 (d) All are true

44. Mucosal layer that forms irregular folds in the stomach is called
(a) Rugae (b) Villi (c) Microvilli (d) Papilla

45. Mucosal layer that forms small finger like projections in intestine is called
(a) Villi (b) Microvilli (c) Crypts (d) Papilla

46. Mucosal layer that forms depressions in between villi in intestine is called
(a) Villi (b) Microvilli (c) Crypts (d) Papilla

47. In the wall of alimentary canal which are/is true sequence from outer to inner?
(a) Serosa, longitudinal muscle, mucosa, sub mucosa
(b) Mucosa, serosa, long muscle
(c) Serosa, long muscle, circular, sub-mucosa, mucosa
(d) Serosa, long muscle, sub-mucosa, mucosa

48. The narrow distal end of stomach is called
(a) Cardiac (b) Duodenum (c) Pharynx (d) Pylorus

49. Intestinal villi are mainly concerned with
(a) Assimilation (b) Secretion (c) Ultrafilteration (d) Absorption

50. Pylorus is situated at the junction of
(a) oesophagus and stomach (b) stomach and duodenum
(c) duodenum and ileum (d) ileum and rectum

51. Brush bordered epithelium is found in
(a) trachea (b) stomach (c) small intestine (d) fallopian tube

52. Vermiform appendix is a part of
(a) alimentary canal (b) nervous system
(c) vascular system (d) reproductive system

53. Crypt of Lieberkuhn is an example for
(a) simple tubular gland (b) coiled tubular gland
(c) compound alveolar gland (d) compound tubular gland

54. Serosa is made up of
(a) mesothelium (b) some connective tissue
(c) both (d) none

55. In duodenum, glands are present in
(a) mucosa (b) sub-mucosa (c) muscular layer (d) both (a) and (b)

56. Which is responsible for the increase in surface area of small intestine?
(a) Villi (b) Microvilli (c) both (d) Bigger lumen

57. Which of the following is true about villi?
(a) They are small finger like folding in small intestine
(b) They are supplied with network of capillaries
(c) They are supplied with large lymph vessel called lacteals
(d) All

58. Goblet cells are an example of
(a) multicellular gland (b) unicellular gland
(c) alveolar gland (d) tubular gland

59. Select the incorrect statement from the following.
(a) Mucosal epithelium has goblet cells which secrete mucous that help in lubrication.
(b) Mucosa form gastric gland in stomach and crypts of Lieberkuhn in Intestine.
(c) All the four histological layers shows modification in different parts of alimentary canal.
(d) Muscularis layer is formed by outer circular and inner longitudinal muscle layer.

60. Which of the following are digestive glands associated with alimentary canal?
(a) Salivary gland (b) Liver
(c) Pancreas (d) All

61. How many salivary glands are present in the human body?
(a) 3 (b) 4 (c) 5 (d) 6

62. The following are salivary glands except
(a) Parotid (b) Sub-maxillary/sub-mandibular
(c) Sub-lingual (d) Brunner gland

63. Gland which is situated below tongue is
(a) parotid (b) sub-maxillary (c) sub-lingual (d) sub-mandibular

64. Select the incorrect match:

Position		Gland
(a) Cheeks	–	Parotid
(b) Lower jaw	–	Sub-maxillary/sub-mandibular
(c) Below tongue	–	Sub-lingual
(d) Pineal gland	–	Dorsal side of mid brain

65. Which is the largest gland of our body?
(a) Parotid (b) Pancrease (c) Liver (d) Adrenal

66. What is the approximate weight of the liver of an adult human?
(a) 1.2–1.5 kg (b) 2.5–3.5 kg
(c) 0.5–1.0 kg (d) 200 gms

67. Liver is situated in
(a) thoracic cavity (b) abdominal Cavity
(c) pelvic cavity (d) cranial cavity

68. Liver is majorly divided into how many lobes?
(a) 1 (b) 2 (c) 3 (d) 4

69. Each lobule in liver is covered by a thin connective tissue sheath called
(a) Hepatic Fascia (b) Glisson's Capsule
(c) Falcicorm ligament (d) Coronary ligament

70. Structural and functional unit of liver is
(a) Cystic duct (b) Hepatocyte (c) Hepatic lobules (d) Kupffer cells

71. Function of gall bladder is
(a) Storage of bile (b) Concentration of bile
(c) Both (a) and (b) (d) Formation of bile

72. Common bile duct is formed by the joining of
(a) Hepatic ducts (b) Cystic duct (c) Duct of Wirsung (d) Both (a) and (b)

73. Cystic duct is located in
(a) Urinary bladder (b) Gall Bladder (c) Liver (d) Pancreas

74. Bile is secreted by
(a) Glisson's Capsule (b) Gall bladder (c) Hepatic Cells (d) Kupffer cells

75. The bile duct and pancreatic duct open together into the duodenum as hepato-pancreatic duct which is guarded by sphincter called
(a) Sphincter of Boyden (b) Hepato pancreatic ampulla
(c) Sphincter of Oddi (d) Cardiac Sphincter

76. Pancreas secretes
(a) insulin (b) glucagon (c) enzymes (d) all

77. Identify A–F in the given figure.

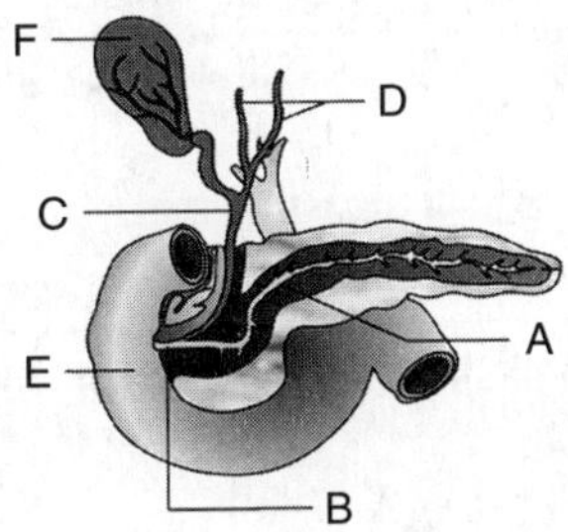

(a) A–Common bile duct, B–Gall bladder, C–Pancreatic duct, D–Duodenum, E–Hepato-pancreatic duct, F–Ducts from liver
(b) A–Pancreatic duct, B–Hepato-pancreatic duct, C–Common bile duct, D–Ducts from liver, E–Duodenum, F–Gall bladder
(c) A–Hepato-pancreatic duct, B–Ducts from liver, C–Pancreatic duct, D–Gall bladder, E–Duodenum, F–Common bile duct
(d) A–Gall bladder, B–Common bile duct, C–Duodenum, D–Pancreatic duct, E–Hepato-pancreatic duct, F–Ducts from liver

78. All are secretion of pancreas, except
(a) insulin (b) glucagon
(c) chymoptrypsinogen (d) enterokinase

79. Mixed Gland (endocrine + exocrine) from the following is
(a) liver (b) parotid (c) pancreas (d) adrenal

80. Major function performed by buccal cavity is
(a) mastication of food (b) facilitation of swallowing
(c) both (d) none

81. The bolus formed in buccal cavity conveyed into pharynx and then esophagus by the process called
(a) peristalsis (b) emesis
(c) deglutination/swallowing (d) dysglutination

82. Mucus in saliva helps in lubricating and adhering the masticate food particle into a ____________ in buccal cavity
(a) chyme (b) chyle (c) bolus (d) any of the above

83. Saliva contains
(a) Salivary amylase / Ptyalin (b) Electrolyte (Na^+, K^+ ,Cl^-, HCO^{3-} etc.)
(c) Lysozyme (d) All

84. Lysozyme
(a) Anti viral agent (b) Anti-bacterial agent
(c) Acts on lipid (d) Acts on carbohydrates

85. Lysozyme
(a) Cellular barrier (b) Cytokine barrier
(c) Physiological barrier (d) Physical barrier

86. How much % of starch is hydrolyzed in mouth?
(a) 30 (b) 50 (c) 70 (d) 90

87. Optimum pH for salivary enzyme is
(a) 6.2 (b) 5.8 (c) 6.8 (d) 8.8

88. Salivary amylase acts on
(a) slightly basic pH (b) highly acidic pH
(c) slightly acidic pH (d) highly basic pH

89. Starch $\xrightarrow[\text{pH 6.8}]{\text{Salivery amylase}}$ Ⓐ. A is
(a) Sucrose (b) Galactose (c) Maltose (d) Glucose

90. Starch $\xrightarrow[\text{pH 6.8}]{\text{Salivery amylase}}$ Ⓐ. A is
(a) Monosaccharide (b) Polysaccharides
(c) Disaccharide (d) Amylopectin

91. Gastric glands are situated in
(a) Sub-mucosa (b) Mucosa (c) Muscularis (d) Serosa

92. Match the column:

A		B
A. Mucus neck cells	–	1. HCl
B. Peptic or Chief cells	–	2. Intrinsic factor
C. Parietal / Oxyntic cells	–	3. Pepsinogen
		4. Mucus

(a) A → 4, B → 3, C → 1, 2 (b) A → 1, 4, B → 2, C → 2
(c) A → 4, B → 1, 3, C → 2 (d) A → 4, B → 2, 3, C → 1

93. Which is required for absorption of Vit B_{12}?
(a) HCl (b) Pepsin (c) Intrinsic factor (d) Amylase

94. The stomach stores food for
(a) 1 hr (b) 2–3hr (c) 4–5 hrs (d) 30 min

95. Digestion of carbohydrates starts from
(a) buccal cavity (b) stomach (c) small intestine (d) large intestine

96. Select the total number of true statement from the following.
A. In stomach bolus is converted to chyme
B. Chief cells secrets intrinsic factor required for absorption of Vit B_{12}
C. Pepsinogen $\xrightarrow{\text{HCl}}$ pepsin
D. Pepsin converts protein into amino acids.
(a) 1 (b) 2 (c) 3 (d) 4

97. Protection of mucosal epithelium from highly conc. HCl in stomach is performed by
A. HCO_3- Ion
B. Mucus
C. Pepsin
D. Intrinsic factor
(a) A and C only (b) B only (c) A and B only (d) A, B and C only

98. Optimal pH for pepsin is
(a) 6.8 (b) 1.8 (c) 3.8 (d) 6.0

99. Which of the following is incorrect about gastric juice?
(a) Gastric juice of an infant contain Rennin
(b) Small amount of lipase is present
(c) Gastric juice is secreted by gastric glands
(d) Rennin doesn't help in digestion of milk protein present in gastric juice of infant.

100. Which of the following is released in small intestine?
(a) Bile juice (b) Pancreatic juice (c) Intestinal juice (d) All

101. Bile and pancreatic juice is released in small intestine by
(a) Cystic duct (b) Bile duct
(c) Pancreatic duct (d) Hepatic–pancreatic duct

102. Select from the following the total number of enzyme secreted by the pancrease.
Trypsinogen, Amylase, **Lipase, Pepsinogen, Prorennin, Maltase, Sucrase, Chymotrypsinogen, Procarboxypeptidase, Nucleases.**
(a) 4 (b) 5 (c) 6 (d) 7

103. Trypsinogen is activated by
(a) Enterokinase (b) chymotrypsin (c) Rennin (d) Acidic pH

104. Which enzyme activates other enzymes in pancreatic juice?
(a) Enterokinase (b) chymotrypsin (c) Trypsin (d) lipase

105. Enterokinase is secreted by
(a) mouth (b) stomach (c) small intestine (d) large intestine

106. Bile juice contains all except
(a) Bilirubin and bili-verdin (b) Bile salts and cholesterol
(c) Phospholipids (d) Enzymes

107. Which of the following is incorrect about bile?
(a) It contains bilirubin and biliverdin which is waste product.
(b) Bile salts in it help in emulsification of fats.
(c) Bile also activates lipases
(d) Bile contain digestive enzyme

108. Intestinal juice or succus entericus is formed by the secretion of
(a) goblet cells
(b) brush border cells lining mucosa
(c) both
(d) none

109. Enzymes like dipeptidases, lipases, nucleosidases, nucleotidases, maltase and sucrase are present in
(a) bile juice (b) gastric juice
(c) pancreatic juice (d) succus entericus

110. Brunner's gland
(a) is situated in mucosal layer (b) is present in sub-mucosal layer
(c) secretes HCI (d) helps in activation of gastric enzyme

111. Select the incorrect from the following:

(a) $\left.\begin{array}{l}\text{Proteins}\\ \text{peptones}\\ \text{proteoses}\end{array}\right\} \xrightarrow[\text{Carboxypeptidase}]{\text{Trypsin/Chymotrypsin}} \text{Dipeptides}$

(b) Starch $\xrightarrow{\text{Amylase}}$ disaccharides

(c) Fats $\xrightarrow{\text{lipases}}$ Diglycerides $\rightarrow$ Monoglycerides

(d) Nucleotides $\xrightarrow{\text{Nuclease}}$ Nucleosides

112. Select the incorrect statement from the following:
(a) Succus entericus act on end products produced by pancreatic enzyme
(b) Final steps of digestion occur far away from the mucosal epithelial cells of the intestine
(c) The breakdown of bio macromolecule generally occurs in the duodenum region of small intestine
(d) Simple substance forms after digestion is absorbed mainly by jejunum and ileum.

113. Action of which enzyme produces glucose?
(a) Maltase (b) Lactase (c) Sucrase (d) All

114. Action of which enzyme produces only glucose?
(a) Maltase (b) Lactase (c) Sucrase (d) All

115. Where we use term feaces for undigested and unabsorbed food particle in alimentary canal.
(a) Jejunum (b) Colon (c) Rectum (d) End of ileum

116. Where faecal matters are temporarily stored till defecation?
(a) Colon (b) Caecum (c) Ileum (d) Rectum

117. The activities of gastrointestinal are under
(a) neural control only
(b) hormonal control only
(c) neither hormonal nor neural control
(d) neural and hormonal control

118. The muscular activities of different parts of alimentary canal also be regulated by
(a) local neural control (b) CNS neural control
(c) both (d) none

119. Absorption is a process by which the end product of digestion pass through the intestinal mucosa into ______
(a) blood/lymph (b) liver (c) CSF (d) heart

120. Secretion of saliva can be stimulated by
(a) sight of food (b) smell of food
(c) presence of food in oral cavity (d) all

121. In addition to controlling the neurons, hormones also influence the
(a) gastric secretions
(b) intestinal secretions
(c) muscular activities of different parts of alimentary canal
(d) all

122. Hormonal control of the secretion of digestive juice is carried out by local ______, produced by __________ and _____ mucosa.
(a) Neurotransmitters, liver, pancreas
(b) Hormones, Liver, pancreas
(c) hormones, Gastric, intestinal
(d) Neurotransmitters, gastric, intestinal

123. Absorption of digested food is carried out by
(a) passive method (b) active transport
(c) facilitated transport (d) all

124. Glucose and amino acids are absorbed in the intestine by
(a) active transport (b) passive transport
(c) selective absorption (d) osmosis

125. Which of the following statements is incorrect?
A. Absorption of simple sugar, alcohol, some water and medicines take place in stomach
B. Maximum water absorption occurs in small intestine
C. Small intestine is the major site of digestion and absorption of food
D. Fatty acid and glycerol are absorbed by lacteals
E. Nothing is absorbed in mouth and large intestine
(a) A, D, and E only (b) D and E only (c) D only (d) B and C only

126. Fructose and some amino acids are absorbed by
(a) active transport (b) diffusion
(c) facilitated transport (d) osmosis

127. A small amount of monosaccharide like glucose, amino acids and some electrolytes like chloride ions are generally absorbed by
(a) active transport (b) simple diffusion
(c) facilitated transport (d) osmosis

128. Carrier ions generally used for facilitated transport of fructose and some amino acids
(a) Ca^{2+} (b) Cl^{-} (c) K^{+} (d) Na^{+}

129. Amino acids, monosaccharide, electrolytes like Na^{+} are mainly absorbed by
(a) osmosis (b) passive transport
(c) facilitated transport (d) active transport

130. Which of the following statement is wrong about Chylomicrons?
A. Chylomicrons are produced in the epithelial cells of small intestinal
B. It contain triglycerides, cholesterol and phospholipids
C. It is protein coated small vesicles
D. Chylomicrons released from the epithelial cell into lacteals
(a) A and D only (b) B and C only
(c) All (d) None

131. Chylomicrons are concerned with the
(a) digestion of fats (b) absorption of proteins
(c) digestion of protein (d) absorption of fats

132. The absorbed substances finally reach the tissues which utilize them for their activities. This process is called
(a) assimilation (b) emulsification (c) catabolism (d) digestion

133. Vomit center is situated at
(a) pons (b) mid-brain (c) cerebellum (d) medulla

134. Defecation
(a) is a voluntary process
(b) is carried out by a mass peristaltic movement
(c) both
(d) is otherwise known as ingestion

135. Which of the following statements is incorrect?
(a) Faecal accumulation in the rectum initiates a neural reflex causing an urge for its removal
(b) Reflex of vomiting is controlled by medulla
(c) Irregular bowel movements cause constipation
(d) In diarrhea absorption of food is increased

136. Marasmus is characterised by
(a) thinning of limbs
(b) skin become dry, thin and wrinkled
(c) decrease growth rate
(d) all

137. Maximum absorption of digested food takes place in
(a) mouth (b) stomach
(c) small intestine (d) large intestine

138. Absorption of simple sugar, water and alcohol takes place in
(a) mouth (b) stomach
(c) small intestine (d) large intestine

139. Mouth can absorb
(a) fatty acid (b) certain drugs (c) alcohol (d) all

140. Jaundice occur due to increase level of
(a) $CaCO_3$ (b) HCO_3 (c) Bile pigments (d) CO_2

141. Following are parasite of intestine
(a) tapeworm and Roundworm (b) thread worm and Hook worm
(c) pinworm (d) all

142. Jaundice is a disorder of
(a) Excretory system (b) Skin and eyes
(c) Digestive system (d) Circulatory system

143. The cause(s) of indigestion is/are
(a) Inadequate enzymes secretion
(b) Anxiety
(c) Food poisoning, over eating and spicy food
(d) All

144. The abnormal frequent bowel movement and increased liquidity of faecal discharge is known as
(a) constipation (b) vomiting
(c) diarrhoea (d) indigestion

145. Swelling of gut is the most common ailment due to
(a) bacterial infections
(b) viral infections
(c) infection of intestinal parasites (e.g. different types of worms)
(d) all

146. Which of the following is correct about vomiting?
(a) Ejection of stomach content through mouth
(b) It is a reflex action.
(c) A feeling of nausea precedes vomiting
(d) All

147. One gram of fat produces
(a) 4.1 kcal of chemical energy
(b) 9.45 kcal of chemical energy
(c) 7.0 kcal of chemical energy
(d) 5.0 kcal of chemical energy

148. The amount of heat liberated from the complete combustion of 1 gm of food in a bomb calorimeter is known as its______________
(a) gross caloric value (b) gross energy value
(c) physiological value (d) both (a) and (b)

*Read the **assertion** and **reason** carefully to mark the correct option out of the options given below:*

(a) If both the assertion and the reason are true and the reason is a correct explanation of the assertion
(b) If both the assertion and reason are true but the reason is not a correct explanation of the assertion
(c) If the assertion is true but the reason is false
(d) If both the assertion and reason are false

149. **Assertion:** Process of conversion of complex food substances to simple absorbable forms is called digestion.
Reason: Biomacromolecules in food can not be utilized by our body in their original form.

150. **Assertion:** Tounge contain receptor for taste.
Reason: The upper surface of the tounge has small projections called papillae, all of which bear taste buds which act as receptor for taste

151. **Assertion:** Large intestine also shows the presence of villi like small intestine.
Reason: Absorption of most substance takes place in large intestine.

152. **Assertion:** Lipases of bile help in the emulsification of fats.
Reason: Lipases can break large fat droplets into smaller ones.

153. **Assertion:** Presence of HCl in stomach is necessary for the process of digestion.
Reason: HCl kills and inhibits the growth of bacteria in the stomach.

154. **Assertion:** Facilitated diffusion is more rapid than simple diffusion.
Reason: Facilitated diffusion involves expenditure of energy unlike simple diffusion.

155. **Assertion:** Mucosal epithelium secretion helps in lubrication.
Reason: Mucosal epithelium has goblet cells which secretes mucus.

156. Assertion: The vermiform appendix which is vestigeal organ arises from ileum.
Reason: Appendix is small blind sac which hosts some non symbiotic bacteria.

157. Assertion: Pancrease is a compound organ.
Reason: Pancrease contain both exocrine and endocrine tissues.

158. Assertion: The chemical process of digestion is initiated in the oral cavity.
Reason: Saliva contain hydrolytic enzyme salivary amylase.

159. Assertion: Jaundice is yellowish discoloration of eye and skin.
Reason: It occurs due to deposition of bile pigments.

160. Assertion: Faeces are retained with in rectum in costipation.
Reason: Bowel movement are regular in costipation.

AIPMT PREVIOUS YEAR QUESTIONS

1. If for some reason the parietal cells of the gut epithelium become partially non-functional, what is likely to happen?

[AIPMT MAINS 2010]

(a) The pancreatic enzymes and specially the trypsin and lipase will not work efficiently
(b) The pH of stomach will fall abruptly
(c) Steapsin will be more effective
(d) Proteins will not adequately hydrolysed by pepsin into proteoses and peptones

2. Jaundice is a disorder of:

[AIPMT MAINS 2010]

(a) Excretory system
(b) Skin and eyes
(c) Digestive system
(d) Circulatory system

3. Carrier ions like Na^+ facilitate the absorption of substance like

[AIPMT PRE 2010]

(a) Amino acids and glucose
(b) Glucose and fatty acids
(c) Fatty acids and glycerol
(d) Fructose and some amino acids

4. Which of the following enzymes carries out the initial step in the digestion of milk in humans?

[AIPMT PRE 2011]

(a) Rennin
(b) Lipase
(c) Trypsin
(d) Pepsin

5. One of the constituents of the pancreatic juice which is poured into the duodenum in humans is

[AIPMT MAINS 2011]

(a) Trypsinogen
(b) Chymotrypsin
(c) Trypsin
(d) Enterokinase

6. Which one of the following correctly represents the normal adult human dental formula?

[AIPMT MAINS 2011]

(a) $\frac{3}{3}, \frac{1}{1}, \frac{3}{2}, \frac{1}{1}$
(b) $\frac{2}{2}, \frac{1}{1}, \frac{3}{2}, \frac{3}{3}$
(c) $\frac{2}{2}, \frac{1}{1}, \frac{2}{2}, \frac{3}{3}$
(d) $\frac{3}{3}, \frac{1}{1}, \frac{3}{3}, \frac{3}{3}$

7. Where do certain symbiotic microorganisms normally occur in human body?

[AIPMT MAINS 2012]

(a) Oral lining and tongue surface
(b) Vermiform appendix and rectum
(c) Duodenum
(d) Caecum

8. Anxiety and eating spicy food together otherwise normal human, may lead to:

[AIPMT PRE 2012]

(a) Indigestion (b) Jaundice
(c) Diarrhoea (d) Vomiting

9. Select the correct match of the digested products in humans given in column I with their absorption site and mechanism in column II.

[AIPMT 2013]

Column-I	Column-II
(a) Glycine, glucose	Small intestine and active absorption
(b) Fructose, Na^+	Small intestine and passive absorption
(c) Glycerol and fatty acids	Duodenum, move as chilomicrons
(d) Cholesterol and maltose	Large intestine and active absorption

10. The initial step in the digestion of milk in humans is carried out by

[AIPMT 2014]

(a) Lipase (b) Trypsin
(c) Rennin (d) Pepsin

11. Fructose is absorbed into the blood through mucosa cells of intestine by the process called

[AIPMT 2014]

(a) Active transport (b) Facilitated transport
(c) Simple diffusion (d) Co – transport mechanism

12. The primary dentition in human differs from permanent dentition in not having one of the following type of teeth

[AIPMT 2015]

(a) Premolars (b) Molars
(c) Incisors (d) Canine

13. The enzyme that is not present in succus entericus is:

[AIPMT 2015]

(a) Nucleases (b) Nucleosidase
(c) Lipase (d) Maltase

14. Which of the following statement is not incorrect?

[AIPMT 2015]

(a) Brunner's glands are present in the submucosa of stomach and secrete pepsinogen
(b) Goblet cells are present in the mucosa of intestine and secrete mucus
(c) Oxyntic cells are present in the mucosa if stomach and secrete HCI
(d) Acini are present in the pancreas and secrete Carboxypeptidase.

15. Gastric juice of infants contains:

[AIPMT 2015]

(a) maltase, pepsinogen, rennin (b) nuclease, pepsinogen, lipase
(c) pepsinogen, lipase, rennin (d) amylase, rennin, pepsinogen

16. The primary dentition in human differs from permanent dentition in not having one of the following type of teeth

[RE-AIPMT 2015]

(a) Premolars (b) Molars
(c) Incisors (d) Canine

17. The enzyme that is not present in succus entericus is:

[RE-AIPMT 2015]

(a) Nucleases (b) Nucleosidase
(c) Lipase (d) Maltase

Answer Keys

1. (b)	2. (d)	3. (c)	4. (a)	5. (d)	6. (c)	7. (a)	8. (c)	9. (d)	10. (b)
11. (a)	12. (d)	13. (a)	14. (a)	15. (c)	16. (b)	17. (a)	18. (c)	19. (c)	20. (b)
21. (b)	22. (d)	23. (d)	24. (b)	25. (b)	26. (b)	27. (a)	28. (c)	29. (c)	30. (c)
31. (a)	32. (b)	33. (d)	34. (a)	35. (d)	36. (b)	37. (d)	38. (d)	39. (d)	40. (d)
41. (a)	42. (b)	43. (d)	44. (a)	45. (a)	46. (c)	47. (c)	48. (d)	49. (d)	50. (b)
51. (c)	52. (a)	53. (a)	54. (c)	55. (d)	56. (c)	57. (d)	58. (b)	59. (d)	60. (d)
61. (d)	62. (d)	63. (c)	64. (d)	65. (c)	66. (a)	67. (b)	68. (b)	69. (b)	70. (c)
71. (c)	72. (d)	73. (b)	74. (c)	75. (c)	76. (d)	77. (b)	78. (d)	79. (c)	80. (c)
81. (c)	82. (c)	83. (d)	84. (b)	85. (c)	86. (a)	87. (c)	88. (c)	89. (c)	90. (c)
91. (b)	92. (a)	93. (c)	94. (c)	95. (a)	96. (b)	97. (c)	98. (b)	99. (d)	100. (d)
101. (d)	102. (c)	103. (a)	104. (c)	105. (c)	106. (d)	107. (d)	108. (c)	109. (d)	110. (b)
111. (d)	112. (b)	113. (d)	114. (a)	115. (d)	116. (d)	117. (d)	118. (c)	119. (a)	120. (d)
121. (d)	122. (c)	123. (d)	124. (a)	125. (b)	126. (c)	127. (b)	128. (d)	129. (d)	130. (d)
131. (d)	132. (a)	133. (d)	134. (c)	135. (d)	136. (d)	137. (c)	138. (b)	139. (b)	140. (c)
141. (d)	132. (c)	143. (d)	144. (c)	145. (d)	146. (d)	147. (b)	148. (d)	149. (b)	150. (c)
151. (d)	152. (d)	153. (b)	154. (c)	155. (a)	156. (d)	157. (a)	158. (a)	159. (a)	160. (c)

AIPMT Previous Year Questions

1. (d)	2. (c)	3. (d)	4. (a)	5. (a)	6. (c)	7. (d)	8. (a)	9. (a)	10. (c)
11. (b)	12. (a)	13. (a)	14. (a)	15. (c)	16. (a)	17. (a)			

CHAPTER

17

Breathing and Exchange of Gases

1. The process of exchange of O_2 from the atmosphere with CO_2 produced by the cell is called
   (a) cellular respiration (b) breathing
   (c) ventilation (d) perfusion
2. The harmful gas produced by catabolic reaction in our body is
   (a) oxygen (b) carbondioxide
   (c) phosphine (d) ozone
3. Oxygen (O_2) is utilized by the organisms to __________ break down nutrient molecules like glucose and to derive energy for performing various activities.
   (a) directly (b) indirectly (c) incompletely (d) any of the these
4. Mechanisms of breathing vary among different groups of animals depending mainly on their ________ and _________.
   (a) habitats (b) levels of organization
   (c) both (a) and (b) (d) None
5. In which of the following, gaseous exchange between O_2 and CO_2 occurs through the entire body surface?
   (a) Sponges (b) Flatworms (c) Coelenterates (d) All
6. Select the total number of organism from the following which respire through their body surface.
   Sycon, Spongilla, Admsia, Taenia, Laccifer, Pila, Antedon, Gorgonia, Jelly fish
   (a) 4 (b) 5 (c) 6 (d) 8
7. In which of the following skin serves as an accessory organ of respiration?
   (a) Rabbit (b) Frog (c) Lizards (d) Birds
8. Match the following:

Animals		**Respiratory Organs**
A. Earthworms	–	1. Lungs
B. Aquatic arthropods/Molluscs	–	2. Tracheal tubes
C. Insects	–	3. Gills
D. Birds/ Reptiles/Mammals	–	4. Moist cuticle
E. Fishes		

   (a) A–2, B and C–3, D–2, E–4 (b) A–4, B and E–3, C–2, D–1
   (c) A–4, B and D–3, D–1, E–2 (d) A–3, B and D–1, C–2, E–4
9. Amphibians, e.g. frogs respire through
   (a) moist skin (b) lungs (c) Buccopharyhgeal cavity (d) All

10. The adult frog does not respire through
(a) buccopharyngeal cavity
(b) gills
(c) skin
(d) lungs

11. Which is the correct sequence of the air passage in man?
(a) Nasal cavity → pharynx → trachea → larynx → bronchi → bronchioles → alveoli
(b) Nasal cavity → pharynx → larynx → trachea → bronchi → bronchioles → alveoli
(c) Nasal cavity → larynx → pharynx → trachea → bronchi → bronchioles → alveoli
(d) Nasal cavity → larynx → bronchi → pharynx → trachea → bronchioles → alveoli

12. In mammal, voice is produced by
(a) Bronchus
(b) Syrinx
(c) Larynx
(d) Inhalation and exhalation

13. Vocal cords occur in
(a) Pharynx
(b) Larynx
(c) Glottis
(d) Bronchial tube

14. Trachea divides into right and left primary bronchi at _________ the thoracic vertebra.
(a) 4 (b) 5 (c) 6 (d) 9

15. Opening of larynx into pharynx is guarded by
(a) Syrinx (b) Epiglottis (c) Tracheal valves (d) All

16. Glottis is a passage for
(a) food
(b) air
(c) both
(d) none

17. Glottis is an opening in the floor of
(a) mouth (b) trachea (c) pharynx (d) diaphragm

18. Which one protects the lungs?
(a) Ribs
(b) Vertebral column
(c) Sternum
(d) All

19. Which one has the smallest diameter?
(a) Right bronchus
(b) Left bronchus
(c) Secondary bronchiole
(d) Respiratory bronchiole

20. Lining of trachea is made of
(a) Simple squamous epithelium
(b) Simple cuboidal epithelium
(c) Pseudostratified epithelium
(d) Stratified cuboidal epithelium

21. Each terminal bronchiole gives rise to a number of very thin, irregular-walled and vascularized bag-like structures called
(a) alveoli
(b) respiratory bronchioles
(c) pleura
(d) follicles

22. Epiglottis is made up of
(a) fibrous cartilage
(b) hyaline cartilage
(c) elastic cartilage
(d) calcified cartilage

23. Covering of the lungs is called
(a) Perichondrium
(b) Pleural membrane
(c) Pericardium
(d) Peritoneum

24. Read the following statements:
A. It is double layered and covers and lungs
B. Outer layer is in contact with thoracic wall
C. Fluid is present between these layers
D. Inner layer is in contact with lungs

The above features refer to
(a) pericardium (b) peritoneum
(c) perichondrium (d) pleura

25. The part starting with the external nostrils up to the terminal bronchioles constitute the
(a) respiratory of respiratory system (b) exchange part of respiratory system
(c) expiratory part (d) conducting part of respiratory system

26. Respiratory or exchange part of the respiratory system consists of
(a) all bronchi
(b) all bronchioles
(c) all bronchi and terminal bronchioles
(d) alveoli and their ducts

27. Sites of gaseous exchange in lungs are
(a) alveoli (b) bronchi (c) bronchioles (d) pleura

28. Pleura is double membrane sac which envelops
(a) Kidneys (b) Brain (c) Lungs (d) Nasal passage

29. Following are functions of conducting part of the respiratory system
(a) removal of foreign particles from incoming air
(b) humidifies incoming air
(c) bring the temperature of incoming air to body temperature
(d) all

30. __________ is the site of actual diffusion of O_2 and CO_2 between blood and atmospheric air.
(a) All bronchi
(b) All bronchioles
(c) All bronchi and terminal bronchioles
(d) Alveoli and their ducts

31. Even when air being absent, human trachea does not collapse due to the presence of
(a) bony rings (b) turgid pressure
(c) chitinous rings (d) cartilaginous rings

32. The chambers formed dorsally by the vertebral column, ventrally by sternum, laterally by ribs and on the lower side by dome-shaped diaphragm is
(a) abdominal chamber (b) cranial chamber
(c) pelvic chamber (d) thoracic chamber

33. Select the incorrect statement from the following:
(a) Pleural fluid reduces friction on the lung surface
(b) The anatomical setup of lungs in thorax is such that any change in the volume of the thoracic cavity will be reflected in the lung (pulmonary) cavity. Such an arrangement is essential for breathing, as we cannot directly alter the pulmonary volume
(c) The tracheae, primary, secondary and tertiary bronchi, and initial bronchioles are supported by complete cartilaginous rings.
(d) During swallowing glottis can be covered by a thin elastic cartilaginous flap called epiglottis to prevent the entry of food into the larynx.

34. During inspiration
(a) Diaphragm and external intercostals muscle relax
(b) Diaphragm and internal intercostals muscles relax
(c) Diaphragm and external intercostals muscles contract
(d) Diaphragm and internal intercostals muscles contract

35. During inspiration, the diaphragm
   (a) relaxes to become dome-shaped
   (b) contracts and flattens
   (c) expands
   (d) shows no change

36. Expiration involves
   (a) Relaxation of diaphragm and intercostals muscles
   (b) Contraction of diaphragm and intercostals muscles
   (c) Contraction of diaphragm muscles
   (d) Contraction of intercostals muscles

37. Which two of the following changes (a – d) usually tend to occur in plain dwellers when they move to higher altitudes (3500 m or more)
   (i) Increase in red blood cell size
   (ii) Increase in red blood cell production
   (iii) Increase in breathing rate
   (iv) Increase in thrombocyte count
   (a) both (iii) and (iv) (b) both (i) and (iv) (c) both (iii) and (i) (d) both (ii) and (iii)

38. In alveolar air, partial pressure of CO_2 is:
   (a) 40 mm Hg
   (b) 44 mm Hg
   (c) 46 mm Hg
   (d) 42 mm Hg

39. Arrange the following steps of respiration properly:
   1. Breathing or pulmonary ventilation by which atmospheric air is drawn in and CO_2 rich alveolar air is released out
   2. Diffusion of gases (O_2 and CO_2) across alveolar membrane
   3. Transport of gases by the blood
   4. Diffusion of O_2 and CO_2 between blood and tissues
   5. Utilization of O_2, by the cells for catabolic reactions and resultant release of CO_2
   (a) 1,2,3,4,5 (b) 1,3,2,5,4 (c) 5,4,3,1,2 (d) 3,4,5,2,1

40. Expiratory muscles contract at the time of
   (a) Deep inspiration
   (b) Normal inspiration and expiration
   (c) Forceful expiration
   (d) Muscular expansion of lungs

41. Which of the following statements is correct?
   (a) Inspiration is an active process
   (b) Inspiration is a passive process
   (c) Expiration is an active process
   (d) Both expiration and inspiration are passive processes

42. Gaseous exchange between blood and alveolar air across respiratory membrane occurs by:
   (a) osmosis
   (b) diffusion
   (c) active transport
   (d) phagocytosis

43. On an average, a healthy human breathes how many times/minute
   (a) 20–40 (b) 72–75 (c) 3–5 (d) 12–16

44. We can increase the strength of inspiration and expiration by the help of additional muscle in
   (a) Abdomen (b) Neck (c) Pelvis (d) Head

45. Match the following:

1. Tidal volume	–	A. Tidal volume and inspiratory reserve volume and expiratory reserve volume
2. Inspiratory reserve volume	–	B. Additional volume of air a person can inspire by a forcible inspiration
3. Expiratory reserve volume	–	C. Volume of air remaining in the lungs even after a forcible expiration

4. Residual volume	–	D.	Tidal volume and inspiratory reserve volume
5. Inspiratory reserve capacity	–	E.	Volume of air inspirited or expired during a normal respiration
6. Vital capacity	–	F.	Vital capacity + residual volume
7. Total lung capacity	–	G.	Additional volume of air a person can expire by a forcible expiration

(a) 1–E, 2–C, 3–B, 4–G, 5–D, 6–A, 7–F
(b) 1–E, 2–G, 3–B, 4–C, 5–A, 6–D, 7–F
(c) 1–E, 2–C, 3–G, 4–B, 5–D, 6–A, 7–F
(d) 1–E, 2–B, 3–G, 4–C, 5–D, 6–A, 7–F

46. Match the following:

1. Tidal Volume	–	A.	2500–3000 ml of air
2. Inspiratory reserve volume	–	B.	1000–1100 ml of air
3. Expiratory reserve volume	–	C.	500 ml of air
4. Residual volume	–	D.	3500–4600 ml of air
5. Vital capacity	–	E.	1100–1200 ml of air

(a) 1–C, 2–D, 3–B, 4–A, 5–E
(b) 1–C, 2–A, 3–B, 4–E, 5–D
(c) 1–C, 2–A, 3–D, 4–E, 5–B
(d) 1–E, 2–A, 3–B, 4–E, 5–D

47. Total lung capacity is equal to
(a) ERV + TV
(b) IRV+ TV
(c) VC + RV
(d) ERV + TV + IRV

48. Vital capacity is equal to
(a) ERV + TV
(b) IRV+ TV
(c) VC + RV
(d) ERV + TV + IRV

49. EC (expiratory capacity) is equal to
(a) ERV + TV
(b) IRV+ TV
(c) VC + RV
(d) ERV + TV + IRV

50. IC (Inspiratory capacity) is equal to
(a) ERV + TV
(b) IRV+ TV
(c) VC + RV
(d) ERV + TV + IRV

51. Arrange the following in order of increasing volume
1. Tidal volume
2. Residual volume
3. Expiratory reserve volume
4. Inspiratory reserve volume

(a) 1< 2<3<4 (b) 1<4<3<2 (c) 1<3<2<4 (d) 1<4<2<3

52. The largest quantity of air that can be expired after a maximum inspiratory effort is
(a) residual volume
(b) tidal volume
(c) vital capacity
(d) total lung volume

53. The vital capacity of adult human lungs is equal to
(a) the maximum volume of air a person can breathe out after a forced inspiration
(b) the maximum volume of air a person can breathe in after a forced expiration
(c) ERV + TV + IRV
(d) all

54. Functional residual capacity can be represented as
(a) TV + ERV (b) ERV + RV (c) RV + IRV (d) ERV + TV + IRV

55. The volume of air involved in breathing movements can be estimated by using a ________ which helps in clinical assessment of pulmonary functions
(a) osmometer (b) potometer
(c) spirometer (d) sphygmomanometer

56. A spirometer cannot be used to measure
(a) IC (b) RV (c) ERV (d) IRV

57. Inspiratory air in lungs ultimately reaches
(a) trachea (b) alveoli (c) bronchi (d) bronchioles

58. Which is not true?
(a) pCO_2 of deoxygenated blood is 95 mm Hg
(b) pCO_2 of alveolar air is 40 mm Hg
(c) pO_2 alveolar air is 104 mm Hg
(d) pO_2 of oxygenated blood is 95 mm Hg
(e) pO_2 of deoxygenated blood is 40 mm Hg

59. Which of the following factors affect the rate of diffusion of gases?
(a) Partial pressure/concentration gradient of diffusing gases
(b) Solubility of gases
(c) Thickness of diffusion membrane
(d) All

60. Lung alveoli of mammals have a thin wall composed of
(a) simple cuboidal epithelium (b) simple squamous epithelium
(c) stratified cuboidal epithelium (d) stratified squamous epithelium

61. The mode of respiration in rabbit is
(a) cutaneous (b) mucosal (c) tracheal (d) pulmonary

62. Respiratory diffusion membrane is majorly made of ________ layers
(a) 2 (b) 3 (c) 4 (d) 5

63. The solubility of CO_2 is ________ times higher than that of O_2
(a) 10–15 (b) 20–25 (c) 30–35 times (d) 210 times

64. What is the value of [PO_2 (in deoxygenated blood) minus PCO_2 (in deoxygenated blood)]?
(a) 5 (b) –5 (c) 45 (d) 40

65. Select the incorrect statement from the following:
(a) Diffusion of O_2 occurs from alveoli to tissue
(b) Diffusion of CO_2 occurs from tissue to alveoli
(c) Amount of CO_2 diffuse through membrane is higher than that of O_2
(d) Partial pressure of O_2 is higher in pulmonary artery than that of pulmonary vein.

66. Total thickness of respiratory diffusion membrane is
(a) less than fm (b) less than micro meter.
(c) much less than mm (d) less than nm.

67. Diffusion membrane is made up of
(a) thin squamous epithelium of alveoli
(b) endothelium of alveolar capillaries
(c) basement membrane between the two layers
(d) all

68. Partial pressures (in mmHg) of O_2 in atmospheric air, alveoli, deoxygenated blood, oxygenated blood and tissues are
(a) 159,104,40,95,40 (b) 104,40,40,95,159
(c) 0.3,40,45,40,45 (d) 159,104,45,95,40

69. Partial pressure (in mmHg) of CO_2 in atmospheric air, alveoli, deoxygenated blood, oxygenated blood and tissues are
(a) 159,104,40,95,40 (b) 104,40,40,95,159
(c) 0.3,40,45,40,45 (d) 159,104,45,95,40

70. Total percentage of O_2 transported by hemoglobin or RBC is
(a) 3% (b) 97% (c) 70% (d) 7%

71. Besides RBC blood plasma also carries O_2 in dissolved state. The percentage is
(a) 3% (b) 97% (c) 70% (d) 7%

72. CO_2 is transported
(a) by RBC (b) as bicarbonates
(c) in dissolved state through plasma (d) all

73. Blood entering the lung is rich in
(a) Oxygen (b) Carbon dioxide (c) Urea (d) More RBCs

74. The majority of CO_2 is transported as
(a) carbonates (b) bicarbonates
(c) carbaminohaemoglobin (d) dissolved state in blood

75. Oxygen is transported in blood mainly by
(a) Blood plasma (b) Leucocytes (c) Thrombocytes (d) Erythrocytes

76. Blood transport of occurs CO_2 in three forms. The correct percentages of CO_2 in these forms are

As Carbaminohaemoglobin in RBC	As bicarbonates	Dissolved form in plasma
(a) 20–25 %	70%	7%
(b) 7%	20–25%	70%
(c) 20–25%	7%	70%
(d) 70%	20–25%	7%

77. Each molecule of hemoglobin can carry at the maximum _______ molecules of O_2
(a) 1 (b) 2 (c) 3 (d) 4

78. Under a given oxygen concentration in blood, dissociation of oxyhaemoglobin will increase if
(a) pH of blood falls (b) pH of blood rises
(c) CO_2 concentration in blood falls (d) Free fatty acid concentration in blood falls

79. The blood coming out of lungs is richer than that one entering into lungs in
(a) CO_2 (b) O_2 (c) Both (d) None

80. When partial pressure of CO_2 (pCO_2) rises, the oxygen dissociation curve of hemoglobin at 37°C will
(a) shift towards right (b) shift towards left
(c) become irregular (d) remain unchanged

81. Dissociation curve is connected with
(a) Myoglobin (b) CO (c) O_2 (d) oxyhaemoglobin

82. A large proportion of oxygen is left unused in the human blood even after uptake by the body tissue. This oxygen
(a) Is enough to keep oxyhaemoglobin saturation at 96%
(b) Helps in releasing more oxygen to epithelial tissues
(c) Acts as reserve during muscular exercise
(d) Raise pCO_2 of blood to 75 mm Hg

83. Oxygen dissociation curve is
(a) parabola (b) sigmoid (c) hyperbola (d) straight line

84. Binding of oxygen with hemoglobin can be affected by
(a) pCO_2 (b) H+ conc (c) Temperature (d) All

85. Amount of O_2 normally carried by 100 ml, of pure blood
(a) 10 ml (b) 20 ml (c) 5 ml (d) 4 ml

86. How much oxygen is delivered to tissue by 100 ml of oxygenated blood under normal physiological condition?
(a) 10 ml (b) 20 ml (c) 5 ml (d) 4 ml

87. How much carbon dioxide is delivered to alveoli by 100 ml of deoxygenated blood under normal physiological condition?
(a) 10 ml (b) 20 ml (c) 5 ml (d) 4 ml

88. Oxygen binding to haemoglobin is
(a) Directly proportional to CO_2 concentration
(b) Directly proportional to CO concentration
(c) Inversely proportional to CO_2 concentration
(d) Independent of CO concentration

89. The most characteristic feature of haemoglobin is
(a) its red colour
(b) presence of iron
(c) its ability to combine reversibly with oxygen
(d) presence of basic protein globin

90. Factors at tissue level favours dissociation of oxygen from oxyhemoglobin
(a) low pO_2, low pCO_2, high H^+, low temperature
(b) high pO_2, high pCO_2, low H^+, high temperature
(c) low pO_2, high pCO_2, high H^+, high temperature
(d) low pO_2, high pCO_2, high H^+, low temperature

91. CO_2 dissociates from Carbaminohaemoglobin when
(a) low PO_2, low PCO_2 (b) high PO_2, high PCO_2
(c) low PO_2, high PCO_2 (d) high PO_2, low PCO_2

92. Dissociation of oxyhaemoglobin can be promoted by
(a) Low pCO_2 (b) High pCO_2
(c) Low body temperature (d) High blood pH

93. Enzyme essential for transport of CO_2 as bicarbonate in blood is:
(a) Carboxypeptidase (b) Succinic dehydrogenase
(c) Carbonic anhydrase (d) Thrombokinase
(e) Lactase

94. What is correct about human respiration?
(a) About 90% of CO_2 is carried by haemoglobin as carbaminohaemoglobin
(b) Neural signals from pneumotaxic centre of pons can increase duration of inspiration
(c) Workers in grinding and stone breaking industries may suffer from lung fibrosis
(d) Cigarette smoking leads to inflammation of bronchi

95. Choose the right sequential phenomena during passage of CO_2 from blood to tissues:
(P) Absorption of CO_2 by blood.
(Q) Reaction of CO_2 with water forming H_2CO_3 inside RBCs and then and HCO_3^- and H^+ ions.
(R) Reaction of CO_2 with water forming H_2CO_3 inside plasma followed by conversion into H^+ and HCO_3^- ions.

(S) Combination of H^+ with haeme part of HbO_2 to release O_2.
(T) Combination of HCO_3 with haeme part of HbO_2 to form reduced haemoglobin and release of O_2.

(a) P, R, S (b) P, Q, T (c) P, Q, S (d) P, R, T

96. The transport of CO_2 by the blood in primarily dependent on the
(a) solubility of CO_2 in blood
(b) presence of carbonic anhydrase in RBCs
(c) ability of hemoglobin to bind and transport CO_2
(d) ability of other blood proteins

97. Pick the correct statement:
(a) Contraction of internal intercostals muscles lifts up the ribs and sternum
(b) RBCs transport oxygen only
(c) Thoracic cavity is anatomically an air tight chamber
(d) Healthy man can inspire approximately 500 mL of air per minute
(e) During expiration the interpleural pressure is slightly below the surrounding atmospheric pressure

98. Respiratory rhythm centre is present in which part of brain?
(a) Pons (b) Medulla oblongata
(c) Cerebrum (d) Cerebellum

99. Pneumotaxic centre is present in
(a) pons (b) medulla oblongata
(c) cerebrum (d) cerebellum

100. Human beings have a significant ability to maintain and moderate the respiratory rhythm to suit the demands of the body tissues. This is done by
(a) endocrine system (b) neural system
(c) excretory system (d) all

101. A (1) _________ sensitive area is situated adjacent to the rhythm centre which is highly sensitive to _________ (2) _and _ (3) _________ ions
(a) (1)–thermo, (2)–CO_2, (3)–hydroxide (b) (1)–chemo, (2)–O_2, (3)–hydroxide
(c) (1)–thigmo, (2)–O_2, (3)–hydrogen (d) (1)–chemo, (2)–CO_2, (3)–hydrogen

102. All of the following factors play role in the regulation of respiratory rhythm except
(a) CO_2 (b) H^+ conc (c) O_2 (d) None of the above

103. Select the incorrect statement from the following:
(a) Neural signal from Pneumotaxic centre can reduce the duration of inspiration
(b) The role of oxygen in the regulation of respiratory rhythm is quite significant
(c) RBCs contain a very high concentration of the enzyme, carbonic anhydrase and minute quantities of the same is present in the plasma too
(d) CO_2 is carried by haemoglobin as carbamino-haemoglobin (about 20–25 per cent)

104. Receptors associated with aortic and carotid artery can recognize changes in ______ and ______ conc. and send necessary signal to _____ for remedial action.
(a) O_2, CO_2, pneumotaxic (b) CO_2, H+, rhythm centre
(c) CO_2,H^+, apneustic centre (d) O_2, H^+, pneumotaxic

105. Carbonic anhydrase is found in high concentration in
(a) leucocytes (b) blood plasma (c) erythrocytes (d) lymphocytes

106. Controlling centre of normal breathing in mammals lies in
(a) Cerebrum (b) Cerebellum
(c) Midbrain (d) Medulla oblongata

107. Number of RBCs per unit volume of blood is likely to be higher in a person living at high altitudes, because
(a) air is clean and unpolluted (b) more sunshine is available
(c) air is less dense (d) vegetation gives out more O_2

108. Wheezing sound is produced in
(a) Asthma (b) Emphysema (c) Silicosis (d) Pneumonia

109. Major cause of emphysema is
(a) cigarette smoking (b) allergy
(c) wine consumption (d) viral infection

110. Match the column:

Column A		**Column B**
1. Asthma	–	A. Inflammation of bronchi and bronchioles
2. Emphysema	–	B. Chronic disorder in which alveolar walls are damaged due to which respiratory surface is decreased
3. Occupational Respiratory Disorders	–	C. Long exposure of chemicals can give rise to inflammation leading to fibrosis (proliferation of fibrous tissues)

(a) 1–A, 2–B, 3–C (b) 1–B, 2–A, 3–C (c) 1–C, 2–A, 3–B (d) 1–C, 2–B, 3–A

111. Emphysema is a
(a) Cardiovascular disease (b) Pulmonary disease
(c) Renal disease (d) Pain in lungs

112. Which of the following is incorrect about occupational respiratory disorder?
(a) It occur in some industries, especially those involving grinding or stone-breaking
(b) Long exposure in such industries leading to fibrosis (proliferation of fibrous tissues)
(c) Workers in such industries can be protected from these disorders by wearing protective masks
(d) It is an allergic disease always

113. Respiratory control centre lies in
(a) pons (b) medulla oblongata
(c) both (d) cerebellum

114. Two friends are eating together in a dining table. One of them suddenly starts coughing while swallowing some food. This coughing would have been due to the improper movement of
(a) tongue (b) epiglottis (c) diaphragm (d) neck

115. Which one of the following is a possibility for most of us in regard to breathing, by making a conscious effort?
(a) One can breathe out air totally without oxygen
(b) One can breathe out air through Eustachian tubes by closing both the nose and the mouth
(c) One can consciously breathe out by moving the diaphragm alone without moving the ribs at all
(d) The lungs can be made fully empty by forcefully breathing out all air from them

116. Cartilaginous rings in respiratory passage are present in
(a) Trachea only (b) Trachea and initial bronchioles only
(c) Trachea, bronchi and initial bronchioles (d) None

117. Which of the following represents a larger volume of air than that is normally found in the resting tidal volume or a human lung?
(a) Residual volume
(b) Inspiratory reserve volume
(c) Expiratory reserve volume
(d) All

118. Mark the correct statement from the following:
(a) Tracheal rings are of hyaline cartilage
(b) Dorsal side of thoracic chamber is formed by sternum
(c) Expiration occurs when there is negative pressure in lungs
(d) All

119. 6000–8000 ml of air is the
(a) vital capacity of lungs
(b) volume of normal expiration per minute
(c) sum of IRV + ERV
(d) inspiratory capacity of lungs

120. The volume of air that remains in the lungs after normal expiration is
(a) residual volume
(b) vital capacity
(c) expiratory capacity
(d) functional residual capacity

121. A large proportion of oxygen is left unused in the human blood even after its uptake by the body tissues. This O_2
(a) helps in releasing more O_2 to the epithelium tissues
(b) acts as a reserve during muscular exercise
(c) raises the pCO_2 of blood to 75 mm of Hg
(d) is enough to keep oxyhaemoglobin saturation at 96%

122. Bulk of carbon dioxide (CO_2) released from body tissues into blood is present as
(a) bicarbonate in blood plasma and RBCs
(b) free CO_2 in blood plasma
(c) 70% Carbaminohaemoglobin and 30% as bicarbonate
(d) Carbaminohaemoglobin in RBCs

123. Name the blood vessel A to D.

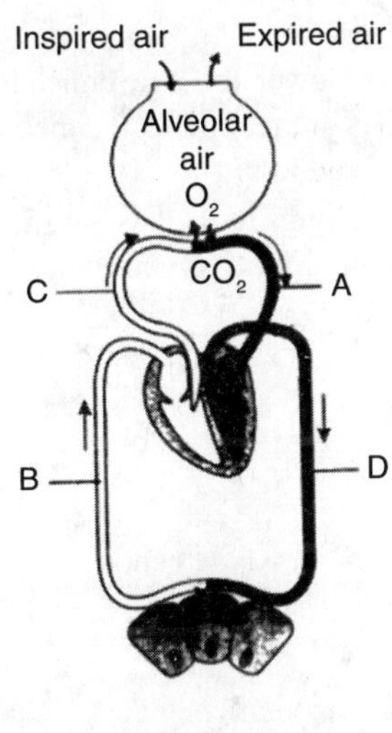

(a) A–Pulmonary vein, B–Systemic vein, C–Pulmonary artery, D–Systemic artery
(b) A–Systemic vein, B–Systemic artery, C–Pulmonary vein, D–Pulmonary artery
(c) A–Systemic artery, B–Pulmonary artery, C–Systemic vein, D–Systemic artery
(d) A–Pulmonary artery, B–Systemic vein, C–Systemic artery, D–Pulmonary vein

124. Study the accompanying figure.

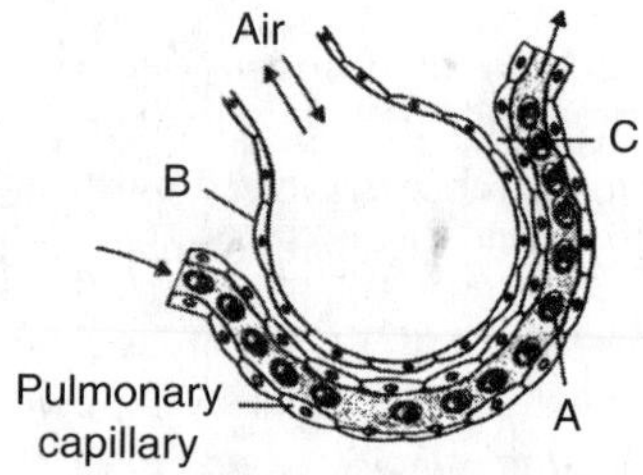

Identify A to C
(a) A–Basement substance, B–RBC, C–Alveolar wall
(b) A–Alveolar wall, B–Basement substance, C–RBC
(c) A–RBC, B–Basement substance, C–Alveolar wall
(d) A–RBC, B–Alveolar wall, C–Basement substance

125. How O_2 and CO_2 gets transported through blood?
(a) with the help of RBCs and blood plasma
(b) with the help of RBCs and WBCs
(c) with the help of WBCs and blood serum
(d) with the help of platelets and corpuscles

126. During oxygen transport the oxyhaemoglobin at the tissue level liberates oxygen to the cells because in tissue
(a) O_2 concentration is high and CO_2 is low
(b) O_2 concentration is low and CO_2 is also low
(c) O_2 tension is high and CO_2 tension is low
(d) O_2 tension is low and CO_2 tension is high

127. The blood leaving the lungs has all its hemoglobin oxygenated and gives up oxygen to the tissues because
(a) the tissue can absorb O_2 from oxyhaemoglobin
(b) O_2 concentration in tissues is lower and CO_2 concentration is higher as compared to lungs
(c) O_2 concentration in tissues is higher and CO_2 concentration is lower as compared to lungs
(d) oxyhaemoglobin undergoes reduction

128. During one circuit of blood from lungs to the tissues and back through circulatory system, the percentage of haemoglobin giving up its oxygen to tissues is
(a) 25%
(b) 50%
(c) 75%
(d) 100%

Read the ***assertion*** *and* ***reason*** *carefully to mark the correct option out of the options given below:*

(a) If both the assertion and the reason are true and the reason is a correct explanation of the assertion

(b) If both the assertion and reason are true but the reason is not a correct explanation of the assertion

(c) If the assertion is true but the reason is false

(d) If both the assertion and reason are false

129. **Assertion:** Fishes use tracheal tubes for respiration.
Reason: Fishes are amphibian.

130. **Assertion:** Humans can directly alter the pulmonary volume without change in the volume of thoracic cavity.
Reason: Our lungs are inelastic.

131. **Assertion:** We have the ability to increase the strength of inspiration and expiration.
Reason: We have some vestigeal abdominal muscles.

132. **Assertion:** During inspiration, pressure of air falls in the thorax.
Reason: There is a rise in volume of thorax during inspiration.

133. **Assertion:** During inspiration, the volume of thorax increases.
Reason: This happens due to the relaxation of diaphragm and inspiratory muscles.

134. **Assertion:** Forceful expiration occurs through expiratory muscles.
Reason: Expiratory muscles expires quickly.

135. **Assertion:** Vital capacity is higher in athletes than non-athletes.
Reason: Vital capacity is about 3.5–4.5 litres in a normal adult person.

136. **Assertion:** 70 % of CO_2 is carried as bicarbonate ion in plasma.
Reason: If it transported directly th pH of blood become acidic.

137. **Assertion:** In mammals, complex respiratory system has developed.
Reason: Mammalian skin is impermeable to gases.

138. **Assertion:** Emphysema is chronic disorder.
Reason: One of the major cause of emphysema is cigarette smoking.

139. **Assertion:** Respiratory rhythm is maintained by the respiratory centre in medulla region of brain.
Reason: A chemosensitive area in the medulla can alter respiratory mechanism.

140. **Assertion:** The maximum amount of CO_2 is converted in bicarbonate ion in RBCs
Reason: RBCs contain a very high concentration of the enzyme, carbonic anhydrase.

141. **Assertion:** Blood of insects is colourless
Reason: The blood of insect does not play any role in transport of oxygen.

142. **Assertion:** In mollusca, circulatory system is of closed type.
Reason: The blood of mollusca contains haemoglobin

143. **Assertion:** The amount of CO_2 that can diffuse through the diffusion membrane per unit difference in partial pressure is much higher compared to that of O_2.
Reason: The solubility of CO_2 is 20 – 25 times higher than that of O_2.

AIPMT PREVIOUS YEAR QUESTIONS

1. Listed below are four respiratory capacities (1 - 4) and four jumbled respiratory volumes of a normal human adult

Respiratory capacities	**Respiratory volumes**
(a) Residual volume	2500 mL
(b) Vital capacity	3500 mL
(c) Inspiratory reserve volume	1200 mL
(d) Inspiratory capacity	4500 mL

Which one of the following is the correct matching of two capacities and volumes?

[AIPMT PRE 2010]

(a) (b) 2500 mL   (c) 4500 mL
(b) (c) 1200 mL   (d) 2500 mL
(c) (d) 3500 mL   (a) 1200 mL
(d) (a) 4500 mL   (b) 3500 mL

2. What is true about RBCs in humans?

[AIPMT PRE 2010]

(a) They carry about 20-25 per cent of CO_2
(b) They transport 99.5 per cent of O_2
(c) They transport about 80 per cent oxygen only and the rest 20 per cent of it is transported in dissolved state in blood plasma
(d) They do not carry O_2 at all

3. Two friends are eating together on a dining table. One of them suddenly starts coughing while swallowing some food. This coughing would have been due to improper movement of:

[AIPMT PRE 2011]

(a) Diaphragm   (b) Neck
(c) Tongue   (d) Epiglottis

4. The figure given below shows a small part of human lung where exchange of gas takes place. In which one of the options given below, the one part A, B C or D is correctly identified along with its function.

[AIPMT PRE 2011]

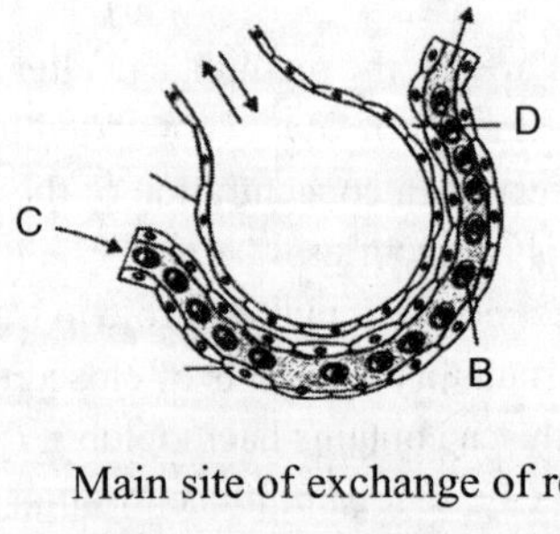

(a) A: Alveolar cavity   Main site of exchange of respiratory gases
(b) D: Capillary wall   Exchange of and takes place here
(c) B: Red blood cell   Transport of mainly
(d) C: Arterial capillary   Passes oxygen to tissues

5. Which one of the following is a possibility for most of us in regard the breathing by making a conscious effort?

[AIPMT MAINS 2011]

(a) One can breathe out air totally without oxygen
(b) One can breathe out air through Eustachian tube by closing both nose and mouth
(c) One can consciously breathe in and breathe out by moving the diaphragm alone, without moving the ribs at all
(d) The lungs can be made fully empty by forcefully breathing out all air from them

6. Bulk of carbon dioxide CO_2 released from body tissues into the blood is present as

[AIPMT MAINS 2011]

(a) Bicarbonate in blood plasma and RBCs
(b) Free CO_2 in blood plasma
(c) 70% carbamino-haemogloin and 30% as bicarbonate
(d) Carbamino-haemoglobin in RBCs

7. A large proportion of oxygen is left unused in the human blood even after its uptake by the body tissues. This O_2

[AIPMT PRE 2011]

(a) Raises the p_{CO_2} of blood to 75 mm of Hg
(b) Is enough to keep oxyhaemoglobin
(c) Helps in relasing more O_2 the epithelial tissue's
(d) Acts as a reserve during muscular exercise

8. Which one of the following is the correct statement for respiration in humans?

[AIPMT PRE 2012]

(a) Cigarette smoking may lead to inflammation of bronchi
(b) Neural signals form pneumotoxic centre in pons region of brain can increase the duration of inspiration
(c) Workers in grinding and stone-breaking industries may suffer, from lung fibrosis
(d) About 90% of carbon dioxide CO_2 is carried by haemoglobin as carbamino haemoglobin

9. The figure shows a diagrammatic view of human respiratory system with labels A, B, C and D. Select the option which gives correct identification and main function and / or characteristics.

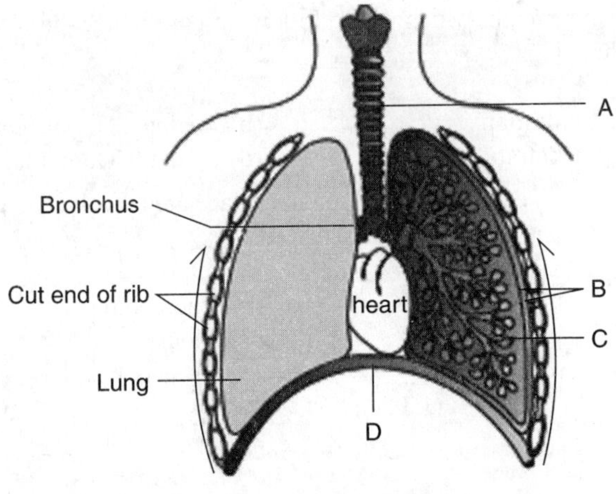

[AIPMT 2013]

(a) A – trachea – long tube supported by complete cartilaginous rings for conducting inspired air
(b) B – pleural membrane – surround ribs on both sides to provide cushion against robbing
(c) C – Alveoli – thin walled vascular bag like structures for exchange of gases
(d) D – Lower end of lungs – diaphragm pulls it down during inspiration

10. Figure shows schematic plant of blood circulation in humans wit labels A to D. Identify the label a give its function / s.

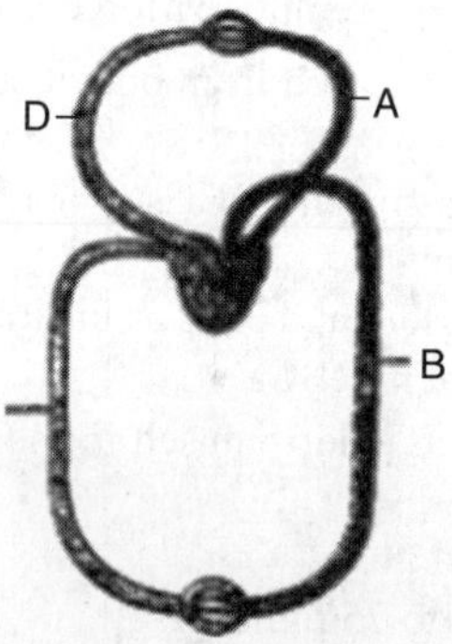

[AIPMT 2013]

(a) A – Pulmonary vein – takes impure blood from body parts, pO_2 = 60 mm Hg
(b) B – Pulmonary artery – takes blood from heart to lungs pO_2 = 90 mm Hg
(c) C – Vena Cava – takes blood from body parts to right auricle, pCO_2 = 45 mm Hg
(d) D – Dorsal aorta – takes blood from heart body parts, pO_2= 95 mm Hg

11. Approximately seventy percent of carbon –dioxide absorbed by the blood will be transported to the lungs:

[AIPMT 2014]

(a) As bicarbonate ions
(b) In the form of dissolved gas molecules
(c) By binding to R.B.C.
(d) As carbamino – haemoglobin

12. When you hold your breath, which of the following gas changes in blood would first lead to the urge in breathe?

[AIPMT 2015]

(a) Falling O_2 concentration
(b) Rising CO_2 concentration
(c) Falling CO_2 concentration
(d) Rising CO_2 and falling O_2 concentration

13. Name the pulmonary disease in which alveolar surface area involved in gas exchange is drastically reduced due to damage in the alveolar walls

[RE-AIPMT 2015]

(a) Emphysema
(b) Pneumonia
(c) Asthma
(d) Pleurisy

Answer Keys

1. (b)	2. (b)	3. (b)	4. (c)	5. (d)	6. (c)	7. (b)	8. (b)	9. (d)	10. (b)
11. (b)	12. (c)	13. (b)	14. (b)	15. (b)	16. (b)	17. (c)	18. (d)	19. (d)	20. (c)
21. (a)	22. (c)	23. (b)	24. (d)	25. (d)	26. (d)	27. (a)	28. (c)	29. (d)	30. (d)
31. (d)	32. (d)	33. (c)	34. (c)	35. (b)	36. (a)	37. (d)	38. (a)	39. (a)	40. (c)
41. (a)	42. (b)	43. (d)	44. (a)	45. (d)	46. (b)	47. (c)	48. (d)	49. (a)	50. (b)
51. (c)	52. (c)	53. (d)	54. (b)	55. (c)	56. (b)	57. (b)	58. (a)	59. (d)	60. (b)
61. (d)	62. (b)	63. (b)	64. (b)	65. (d)	66. (c)	67. (d)	68. (a)	69. (c)	70. (b)
71. (a)	72. (d)	73. (b)	74. (b)	75. (d)	76. (a)	77. (d)	78. (a)	79. (b)	80. (a)
81. (d)	82. (c)	83. (b)	84. (d)	85. (c)	86. (c)	87. (d)	88. (c)	89. (c)	90. (c)
91. (d)	92. (b)	93. (c)	94. (c)	95. (c)	96. (b)	97. (c)	98. (b)	99. (a)	100. (b)
101. (d)	102. (c)	103. (b)	104. (b)	105. (c)	106. (d)	107. (c)	108. (a)	109. (a)	110. (a)
111. (b)	112. (d)	113. (c)	114. (b)	115. (c)	116. (c)	117. (d)	118. (a)	119. (b)	120. (d)
121. (b)	122. (a)	123. (a)	124. (d)	125. (a)	126. (d)	127. (b)	128. (a)	129. (d)	130. (d)
131. (b)	132. (a)	133. (c)	134. (c)	135. (c)	136. (a)	137. (b)	138. (b)	139. (b)	140. (a)
141. (c)	142. (d)	143. (a)							

AIPMT Previous Year Questions

1. (c)	2. (a)	3. (d)	4. (a)	5. (c)	6. (a)	7. (d)	8. (c)	9. (c)	10. (c)
11. (a)	12. (b)	13. (a)							

CHAPTER 18

Body Fluids and Circulation

1. Select the incorrect statement from the following:
   (a) Simple organisms like sponges and coelenterates circulate water from their surroundings through their body cavities to facilitate the cells to exchange substances
   (b) Different groups of animals have evolved the same method for transport
   (c) Blood is the most commonly used body fluid by most of higher organisms for transport
   (d) Lymph also help in transport of certain substances in human
2. Blood is a special connective tissue consist of
   (a) fluid matrix (b) plasma (c) formed elements (d) all
3. Color of Plasma is
   (a) straw color (b) red color (c) colorless (d) blue color
4. How much % of plasma is water
   (a) 90–92% (b) 80–90% (c) 60–65% (d) 10–15%
5. How much protein is present in plasma (in %)
   (a) 2–4% (b) 6–8% (c) 10% (d) 15–20%
6. Which protein is required for coagulation?
   (a) fibrinogen (b) globulin (c) albumin (d) All
7. Formed element constitutes how much percent of blood
   (a) 55% (b) 45% (c) 35% (d) 65%
8. Find out incorrect statement
   (a) Globulins are primarly involved in defence mechanism of body
   (b) Albumin is main osmotic protein of blood
   (c) Plasma without clotting factor is called serum
   (d) factors for coagulation of blood are also present in the plasma in an active form
9. Most abundant cell in human blood are
   (a) Neutrophils (b) Monocytes (c) Lymphocytes (d) None
10. Number of erythrocyte in mm^3 of blood are
    (a) 4.5 to 5 million (b) 5 to 5.5 million
    (c) 5.5 to 6.5 million (d) 3 million
11. Shape of RBC in mammal is
    (a) oval (b) biconvex (c) biconcave (d) flattened
12. True statement about RBC is
    (a) RBCs have an average life span of 120 days
    (b) RBCs are destroyed in the spleen (graveyard of RBCs)
    (c) RBCs are devoid of nucleus in most of the mammals
    (d) All

13. Leucocytes are known as WBC as they are colorless due to
(a) Presence of nucleus (b) White pigment present in them
(c) Lack of haemoglobin (d) All

14. Basophil secrete
(a) histamine (b) serotonin (c) heparin (d) All

15. Which of the following is associated with allergic reactions?
(a) Neutrophils (b) Monocyte (c) Eosinophils (d) Lymphocyte

16. Which of the following is an incorrect statement about leucocytes?
(a) They are nucleated
(b) They are approx average 6000–8000 mm^{-3} of blood cells in numbers
(c) Two main types are found granulocyte and agranulocyte
(d) Monocytes are most abundant WBCs

17. Lymphocyte forms how much percent of WBCs?
(a) 20–25% (b) 2–3% (c) 6–8% (d) 60–65%

18. Which of the following cells are responsible for immune responses of the body
(a) T–lymphocyte (b) B–lymphocyte (c) both (d) Astrocyte

19. Platelets are
(a) cell fragments of megakaryocyte (b) 1.5 to 3.5 lac/mm^3 in blood
(c) also called thrombocytes (d) All

20. ABO grouping is based on how many antigens present or absent on WBCs
(a) 1 (b) 2 (c) 3 (d) None

21. Select the correct statement from the following:
(a) Surface antigen on RBC always induce autoimmune response
(b) Blood grouping (ABO) is example of multiple allelism
(c) AB blood group is universal recipient as well as donor
(d) 4 phenotype of blood group (ABO) are possible and 5 genotype of blood group (ABO) are possible

22. A patient with blood group ‘A’ was injured in an accident and has lost a lot of blood during injury. Which blood group the doctor should effectively use in this case?
(a) AB (b) A/O (c) B/O (d) AB/A/B

23. How many people are Rh+ve in human population?
(a) 80% (b) 20% (c) 60% (d) 40%

24. Rh incompatibility in first pregnancy occurs when
(a) Foetus develop its heart completely (b) During the delivery of first child
(c) When foetal organs completely develop (d) Never occur in the first pregnancy

25. Erythroblastosis foetalis is
(a) HDN (b) Rh incompatibility (c) Both (d) None

26. There is a vertical transmission of Rh antibody from mother to foetus because they are _________ type of antibody
(a) Ig M (b) IgG (c) Ig A (d) Ig D

27. Select incorrect statement from the following:
(a) Clot or coagulum formed mainly by network of fibrin in which died and damaged formed element of blood are trapped
(b) Inactive fibrinogen is converted to fibrin by hormone thrombin
(c) Prothrombin is converted into thrombin by enzyme complex, thrombokinase
(d) Platelet or injured tissue released certain factors which initiate coagulation

28. Select the incorrect statement from the following:
(a) When platelet releases certain factor which initiate clotting it is known as intrinsic pathway
(b) When injured tissue releases certain factor which initiate clotting it is known as extrinsic pathway
(c) Calcium plays a minor role in clotting
(d) Coagulation prevent excessive loss of blood from the body from injured part

29. Which enzyme causes conversion of prothrombin into thrombin?
(a) Thrombinase (b) Prothrombinase
(c) Thrombokinase (d) Rennin

30. Blood is a special type of connective tissue which
(a) consists of a fluid matric (Plasma)
(b) forms elements
(c) is the most commonly used body fluid in most of the higher organism
(d) all

31. How many mechanism are there for clotting in our body?
(a) 1 (b) 2 (c) 3 (d) 4

32. Lymph is known as
(a) tissue fluid (b) interstitial fluid (c) both of above (d) plasma

33. Lymph
(a) transports oxygen to brain (b) transport CO_2 to lungs
(c) returns interstitial fluid to blood (d) returns RBCs and WBCs to lymph nodes

34. Fill up the gaps given below in the table:

Blood group	Antigens on RBCs	Antibody in Plasma	Donor groups
A	A	Anti-B	A, O
B	B	__II__	B, O
AB	AB	nil	A,B,ABO,O
O	__I__	__III__	__IV__

	I	II	III	IV
(1)	Nil	Nil	Nil	O
(2)	Nil	Nil	Anti-A, B	AB
(3)	Nil	Anti-A, B	Nil	O
(4)	Nil	Anti-A	Anti-A, B	O

35. Find the correct descending order to percentage proportion of leucocytes in human blood.
(a) Neutrophils → Basophils → Lymphocytes → Acidophils (Eosinophils) → Monoytes
(b) Neutrophils → Monoytes → Lymphocytes → Acidophils → Basophils
(c) Neutrophils → Lymphocytes → Monoytes → Acidophils → Basophils
(d) Neutrophils → Acidophils → Basophils → Lymphocytes → Monocytes

36. In case of emergency, which blood group could be safely transfused?
(a) AB R– (b) AB Rh+ (c) O Rh– (d) O Rh+

37. Which of the following is expected if husband is Rh^+ and wife is Rh^-?
(a) No problem in the first pregnancy
(b) Problems in future pregnancies
(c) Both (a) and (b)
(d) No problem in any pregnancy

38. What is the correct order of these events?
1. Conversion of fibrinogen to fibrin
2. Clot retraction and leakage of serum
3. Thromoboplastin formation
4. Conversion of prothrombin to thrombin

(a) 3, 2, 1, 4 (b) 3, 4, 1, 2 (c) 3, 4, 2, 1 (d) 4, 1, 3, 2

39. Open circulatory system is found in
(a) Arthopods and molluscs (b) Annelids and Chordates
(c) Annelids and arthopods (d) Fishes and molluscs

40. Close circulatory system is found in
(a) Arthropod and chordates (b) Molluscs and chordates
(c) Amphibians and molluscs (d) Annelids and chordates

41. In an open circulatory system,
(a) there is no heart
(b) there is no need of blood vessels
(c) there are open spaces or sinuses in the body
(d) all

42. Which of the following has a closed type of circulatory system?
(a) Cockroach (b) Fish (c) Scorpion (d) Mollusc

43. Which of the following has a closed blood vascular system?
(a) Cockroach (b) Hydra (c) Sponge (d) Earthworm

44. Single heart circuit occurs in
(a) fishes (b) frogs (c) reptiles (d) man

45. Four chambered heart is found in
(a) cobra (b) tortoise (c) salamander (d) crocodile

46. Select correct matching:

Column I	Column II
(A) Fishes	(i) 3 chambered
(B) Amphibian	(ii) 4 chambered
(C) Reptiles	(iii) 1 chambered
(D) Birds	(iv) 2 chambered
(E) Mammals	
(F) Crocodile	

(a) (A), (B)–(iii) (b) (B), (C)–(i)
(c) (D), (E), (F)–(iv) (d) (A), (B), (C)–(ii)

47. Incomplete double circulation is found in
(a) Amphibia (b) Reptiles (c) Fishes (d) Both (a) and (b)

48.

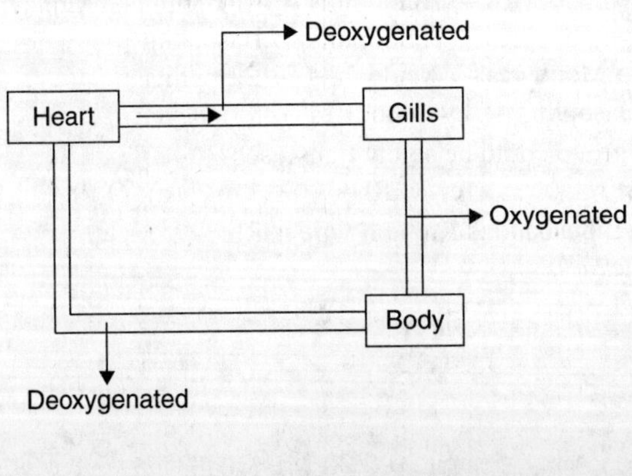

The given diagram represent circulation in

(a) Fishes (b) Amphibians (c) Birds (d) Reptiles

49.

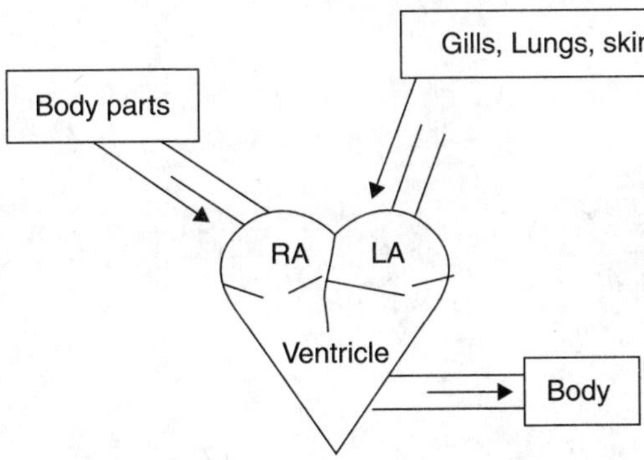

The given diagram shows circulation found in

(a) amphibian (b) reptiles (c) both (a) and (b) (d) birds

50. Double circulation is found in

(a) birds (b) crocodile (c) mammals (d) all

51. Heart is derived from

(a) ectoderm (b) endoderm (c) mesoderm (d) all

52. In fishes, the blood circulation is represented as

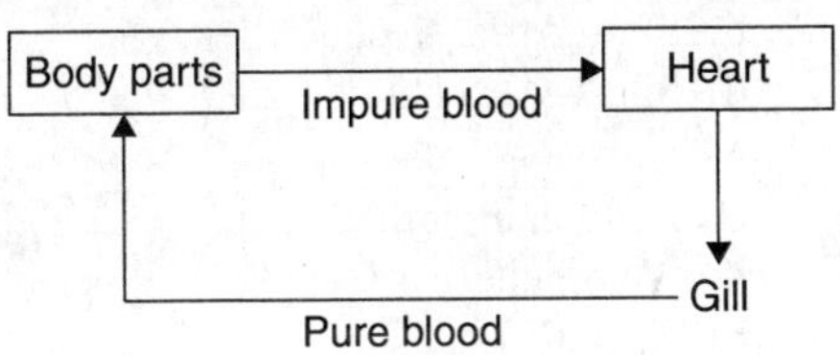

The given flow of blood indicates that it is a

(a) double circulation (b) single circulation
(c) incomplete single circulation (d) incomplete double circulation

53. Which of the following statements is not true?

(a) Heart is ectodermal in origin
(b) In human beings heart is situated in the thoracic cavity, in between the two lungs slightly tilted to the left
(c) Human heart has the size of a clenched fist
(d) Heart protected by double wall membranous bag (pericardium) with pericardial fluid

54. Select the total number of thick structure out of following:

(A) Interatrial septum (muscular wall) (B) Interventricular septum
(C) Atrioventricular septum (fibrous) (D) Walls of ventricles

(a) 1 (b) 2 (c) 3 (d) 4

55. How many papillary muscles are present in right ventricle?

(a) 1 (b) 2 (c) 3 (d) 4

56. Apex of heart is

(a) upper and tilted toward left (b) lower and tilted towards left
(c) upper and tilted towards right (d) lower and tilted towards right

57. Which of the following organs has papillary muscles?
(a) Ciliary body
(b) Legs
(c) Wall of heart
(d) Mammary glands

58. Full form of 'A' in diagram

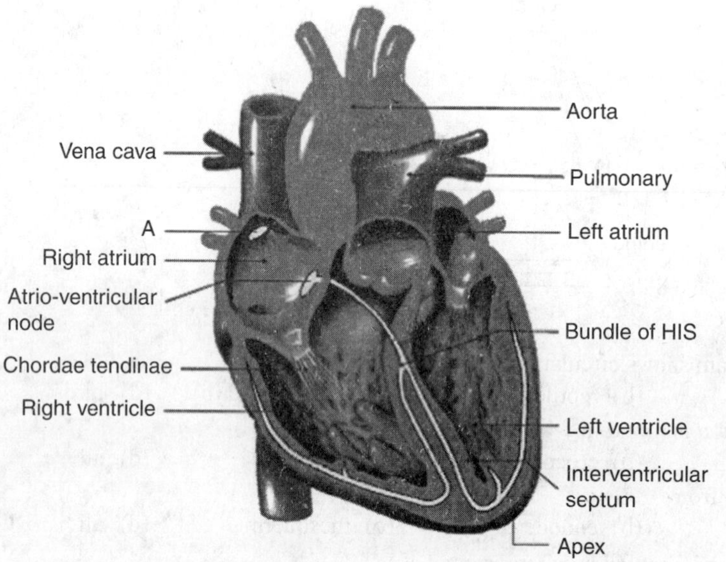

(a) Sin–Atrial–Node
(b) Sinu–Atrial–Node
(c) Sino–Atrial–Node
(d) Sinus–Atrial–Node

59. Bundle of HIS is consist of
(A) Right bundle branch
(B) Left bundle branch
(C) Purkinje fibres
(D) AV bundle
(a) A, B, C only
(b) A, B, C, D
(c) B, C, D only
(d) C, D only

60. Bicuspid valve/mitral valve is found between
(a) Left atrium and left ventricle
(b) Right atrium and right ventricle
(c) Right atrium and left ventricle
(d) Left atrium and right ventricle

61. Tricuspid valve is present between the
(a) two atria
(b) two ventricles
(c) left atrium and left ventricle
(d) right atrium and right ventricle

62. Chordae tendinae are found in
(a) joints
(b) atria of heart
(c) ventricles of heart
(d) ventricles of brain

63. Ventricles are thick-walled as compared to atrium because
(a) it is to receive blood from atria
(b) it is present on the posterior side
(c) it has to pump blood
(d) none

64. Papillary muscles are located in
(a) heart ventricles of human
(b) dermis of mammalian skin
(c) orbits of vertebrate eyes
(d) pylorus of vertebrate stomach

65. Purkinje fibres are found in
(a) brain
(b) kidneys
(c) skin
(d) heart

66. Which of the following has the thickest wall?
(a) Left auricle (b) Left ventricle
(c) Right auricle (d) Right ventricle

67. 'Heart of heart' is
(a) SA-node (b) AV-node
(c) Bundle of HIS (d) Purkinje fibres

68. SA node is located in
(a) upper left corner of right atrium (b) lower left corner of left atrium
(c) lower right corner of left atrium (d) upper right corner of right atrium

69. Human heart is
(a) neurogenic (b) myogenic
(c) cardiogenic (d) digenic

70. Which of the following term does not apply to human heart?
(a) Pacemaker (b) Four chambered
(c) Mitral valve (d) Neurogenic

71. Rate of heartbeat is determined by
(a) SA node (b) AV node
(c) Purkinje fibres (d) Papillary muscles

72. In amphibia, the heart has
(a) two auricles and two ventricles
(b) two auricles and one ventricle
(c) one auricle and two ventricles
(d) one auricle, one ventricle and one sinus venosus

73. SA node is called pace maker of the heart. Why?
(a) It can change contractile activity generated by AV node
(b) It delays the transmission of impulse between the atria and ventricles
(c) It gets stimulated when it receives neural signal
(d) It initiates and maintains the rhythmic contractile activity of heart

74. Sino-Atrial node (SAN) can generate impulses
(a) 70–75 min^{-1} (b) 50–55 min^{-1} (c) 35–40min^{-1} (d) 90–100 min^{-1}

75. The impulse of heartbeat originates from
(a) SAN (b) AVN (c) Vagus nerve (d) Cardiac nerve

76. Rate of heart is determined by
(a) SAN (b) AVN
(c) Purkinje fibres (d) Bundle of His

77. Bundle of HIS is a group of
(a) ganglia (b) nerve fibres
(c) muscular fibres (d) connective tissue

78. Bundle of HIS found in
(a) right atrium (b) left atrium
(c) both (d) interventricular septum

79. An atrioventricular valve prevents the back flow or leakage of blood from the
(a) right ventricle into the right atrium (b) left atrium into the left ventricle
(c) aorta into the left ventricle (d) pulmonary vein into the right atrium

80. How many double circulation are normally completed by the human heart in one minute?
(a) 8 (b) 16 (c) 36 (d) 72

81. The duration of cardiac cycle in a normal man is
(a) 0.8 seconds (b) 80 seconds (c) 60 seconds (d) 72 seconds

82. During systole of heart
(a) only atria contract
(b) only ventricles contract
(c) atria and ventricles contract separately
(d) atria and ventricles contract simultaneously

83. During diastole, blood
(a) enters the heart (b) leaves the heart
(c) leaves the ventricle (d) enters into lungs

84. During ventricular systole oxygenated blood is pumped into the
(a) aorta and deoxygenated blood is pumped into the pulmonary artery
(b) pulmonary artery and deoxygenated blood is pumped into the artery
(c) aorta and deoxygenated blood is pumped into pulmonary vein
(d) pulmonary vein and deoxygenated blood is pumped into pulmonary artery

85. To reach the left side of heart, the blood must pass through
(a) lungs (b) liver (c) kidneys (d) sinus venosus

86. Mammals are said to have double circulation. It means
(a) blood vessels are paired
(b) there are two types of blood vessels attached to every organ
(c) there are two systems, one from the heart to the lungs and back to the rest of the body
(d) blood circulates twice through the heart

87. In mammals, veins differs from arteries in having
(a) thicker walls (b) deeply present
(c) carry blood away from heart (d) internal valves

88. An artery is
(a) thick-walled in which blood flows under low pressure
(b) thin-walled in which blood flows under high pressure
(c) thick-walled in which blood flows under high pressure
(d) thin-walled in which blood flows under low pressure

89. Cells constituting the wall of capillaries are
(a) parietal (b) endothelial (c) oxyntic (d) haemocytes

90. A muscular wall is absent in
(a) Venule (b) Vein (c) Capillary (d) Arteriole

91. Contraction of right ventricle pumps blood into
(a) dorsal aorta (b) pulmonary vein
(c) coronary artery (d) pulmonary artery

92. Arteries carry oxygenated blood except in
(a) pulmonary (b) cardiac (c) hepatic (d) systemic

93. When ventricular systole occurs
(a) atrial diastole coincides
(b) tricuspid and bicuspid valves close
(c) semilunar valves guarding pulmonary artery and aorta are forced to open
(d) all

94. During cardiac cycle, about ________ % of ventricular filling occurs prior to atrial contraction. ________ % ventricular filling occurs due to atrial contraction
(a) 50, 50 (b) 70, 30 (c) 30, 70 (d) 10, 90

95. Which of the following events do not occur during joint diastole?
A. All four chambers of heart are in relaxed state
B. Tricuspid and bicuspid valves open
C. Action potential is conducted from SAN to AVN
D. Blood from the pulmonary veins and vena cava flows into the left and right ventricles respectively through the left and right atria
E. The Semilunar valves are closed
(a) Only E (b) Only C
(c) Only D (d) Only A and B

96. The amount of blood to be pumped out by each ventricle/minute is
(a) Stroke volume (b) Cardiac output
(c) ERV (d) ZRV

97. During cardiac cycle each ventricle pumps out about 70 ml of blood which is called
(a) Stroke volume (b) Cardiac output
(c) Tidal volume (d) Residual volume

98. Cardiac output is
(a) Stroke volume (SV) × Heart rate (HR) = 5L/m
(b) SV × HR = 500 ml
(c) SV × HR = 72 ml/m
(d) SV × HR = 70 ml/m

99. Which of the following statement is incorrect?
(a) Cardiac output of an athlet is much higher than that of an ordinary man
(b) In each minute a single cardiac cycle is performed
(c) During each cardic cycle two prominent sounds are produced
(d) Cardiac cycle includes atrial systole, ventricular systole and joint diastole

100. Identify the correct sequence of events in a cardiac cycle:
(a) Diastole, atrial systole, ventricular diastole
(B) Atrial systole, ventricular diastole, ventricular systole
(c) Atrial systole, ventricular systole, joint diastole
(d) Ventricular diastole, diastole, ventricular systole, atrial systole

101. First cardiac sound (lub) is associated with
(a) closure of tricuspid and bicuspid valves (b) opening of tricuspid valves
(c) closure of semilunar valves (d) opening of semi lunar valves

102. Which of the following statement is wrong for second cardiac sound?
(a) It is heard as dup
(b) It is produced due to the closure of semilunar valves
(c) It is clinically significant
(d) It is clinically nonsignificant

103. Which of the following is correct about human heart?
(a) The volume of both atria > the volume of both ventricles
(b) The volume of both ventricle > the volume of both atria
(c) The volume of both atria = the volume of both ventricles
(d) Ventricles are upper chambers and atria are lower chambers in our heart

104. Which of the following blood vessels possess semilunar valves?
(a) Vena cava and aorta (b) Aorta and pulmonary artery
(c) Pulmonary artery and pulmonary vein (d) Pulmonary vein and vena cava

105. The heartbeat of a person increases at the time of an interview due to the secretion of
(a) Renin (b) Adrenaline (c) ADH (d) ACTH

106. Which of the following set is correct?
(a) Sebum – Analgesic
(b) Vitamin – Nicotine
(c) Corpus callosum – Graafian follicle
(d) Bundle of His – Purkinje fibres

107. Cardiac centre lies in
(a) Medulla oblongata (b) Pons
(c) Cerebrum (d) Epithalamus

108. Cardiac centre can moderate the cardiac functions through
(a) somatic neural system
(b) parasympathetic nervous system only
(c) autonomic nervous system (ANS)
(d) sympathetic nervous system only

109. Neural signal through the sympathetic nervous (part of ANS) increase cardiac output because of
(a) increasing the rate of heat beat
(b) increasing the strength of ventricular contraction
(c) both (a) and (b)
(d) increasing the stimulation of vagus nerve

110. Parasympathetic neural signal decreases cardiac output by
(a) decreasing the rate of heartbeat
(b) decreasing the speed conduction of action potential
(c) both
(d) increasing adrenal medulla hormones secretion

111. Heartbeat increases
(a) on stimulation of sympathetic nerves
(b) on stimulation of vagus nerve (para sympathetic nerve)
(c) by adrenalin secreted by adrenal medulla
(d) both (a) and (c)

112. Select the total number of incorrect matching from the following:
(A) ECG–Electro Cardio Gram (B) AVN–Atrio Ventricular Node
(C) SAN–Sino Atrial Node (D) WBC–White Blue Cells
(E) RBC–Red Blood Cells
(a) 1 (b) 2 (c) 3 (d) 4

113. Heartbeat is accelerated by
(a) Sympathetic nerves and acetylcholine (b) Cranial nerves and adrenaline
(c) Cranial nerves and acetylcholine (d) Sympathetic nerves and epinephrine

114. Body has the capacity to alter
(a) stroke volume (b) heart rate
(c) cardiac output (d) all

115. To obtain standard ECG a patient is connect to the machine with three electrical leads attached to the following parts except

(a) right wrist (b) left wrist
(c) right ankle (d) left ankle

116. Find out the incorrect statement from the following:
(a) ECG is a graphical representation of the electrical activity of the heart during cardiac cycle
(b) For a detailed evaluation of heart's function, multiple leads are attached to the chest region (chest leads)
(c) P, R, T are +ve wave whereas Q and S are –ve wave in standard ECG
(d) Starting of T-wave marks the end of systole of ventricles

117. Select the correct statement from the following:
(a) ECG is of great clinical insignificance
(b) By counting the number of QRS complexes (in given time period), we can find pulse rate
(c) The contraction of atria starts with starting of Q wave
(d) T-wave represent repolarization of atria

118. Electrocardiogram is a measure of
(a) heart rate
(b) ventricular contraction
(c) volume of blood pumped
(d) electrical activity of heart

119. P-wave represents
(a) depolarization of ventricles (b) repolarization of ventricle
(c) repolarization of atria (d) depolarization of atria

120. QRS complex represents the
(a) depolarization of ventricles (b) repolarization of ventricles
(c) repolarization of atria (d) depolarization of atria

121. T-wave on an ECG represents
(a) depolarization of ventricles (b) repolarization of ventricles
(c) repolarization of atria (d) depolrization of atria

122. In an adult, normal blood pressure is
(a) 80/120 mmHg (b) 100/80 mm Hg
(c) 120/80 mmHg (d) 100/120 mmHg

123. Normal BP = 120/80 mmHg in an adult. In this measurement 120 mmHg is the ________ pressure and 80 mmHg is ________ pressure
(a) Diastolic, systolic (b) Systolic, diastolic
(c) Pulse, diastolic (d) Pulse, systolic

124. The difference of blood pressure between systolic and diastolic phase is
(a) 10 mm Hg (b) 40 mm Hg (c) 120 mm Hg (d) 180 mm Hg

125. Which one indicates hypertension?
(a) 120/80 mmHg (b) 80/120 mmHg
(c) 140/90 mmHg (d) 40/60 mmHg

126. Pulmonary circulation includes
(a) pulmonary artery (b) pulmonary vein
(c) lungs (d) all

127. The instrument by which BP of human beings are determined is called
(a) ultrasound (b) BP meter
(c) stethoscope (d) sphygmomanometer

128. The instrument used to hear heartbeats is called
(a) electrocardiograph (b) sphygmomanometer
(c) stethoscope (d) haemo meter

129. A system which supplies blood to heart is
(a) portal system (b) pulmonary system
(c) coronary system (d) all

130. Hepatic portal system starts from
(a) digestive system to liver (b) kidney to liver
(c) liver to heart (d) liver to kidney

131. A unique vascular connection exist between the digestive tract and liver is called
(a) Renal portal system
(b) Hypothalamus—Hypophyscal portal system
(c) Hepatic portal system
(d) All

132. Pulmonary circulation is required for
(a) nutrient supply to lungs
(b) elimination of waste products from the lungs
(c) oxygenation of deoxygenated blood
(d) nutrient supply to heart

133. Which of the following is true about hypertension?
(a) It leads to cardiac diseases
(b) It affect vital organs like brain and kidney
(c) It repeated checks of blood pressure of an individual is 140/90 or higher, it shows hypertensions
(d) All

134. Find the incorrect matching:
(a) CAD–Atherosclerosis (b) Angina–Angina pectoris
(c) Stroke volume–Beat volume (d) Heart failure–Heart attack

135. Match the Column I with Column II:

Column I		**Column II**
A. Heart failure	–	1. Heart muscle is suddenly damaged by an inadequate blood supply
B. Cardiac arrest	–	2. Chest pain due to inadequate O_2 reaching the heart muscles
C. Heart Attack	–	3. Atherosclosis
D. Coronary Artery disease	–	4. Heart not pumping blood effectively enough to meet the needs of the body (CAD)
E. Angina pectoris	–	5. Heart stops beating

	A	B	C	D	E
(a)	4	5	1	3	2
(b)	4	5	3	1	2
(c)	4	3	5	2	1
(d)	5	4	2	3	1

136. It is often referred to as atherosclerosis, affects the blood vessels that supply blood to the heart muscles. It is caused by deposition of Ca, fat, cholesterol and fibrous tissues making the lumen of arteries narrow

(a) CAD (b) SCID (c) Blue baby (d) myocarditis

137. The given figure describes the diagrammatic representation of standard ECG.

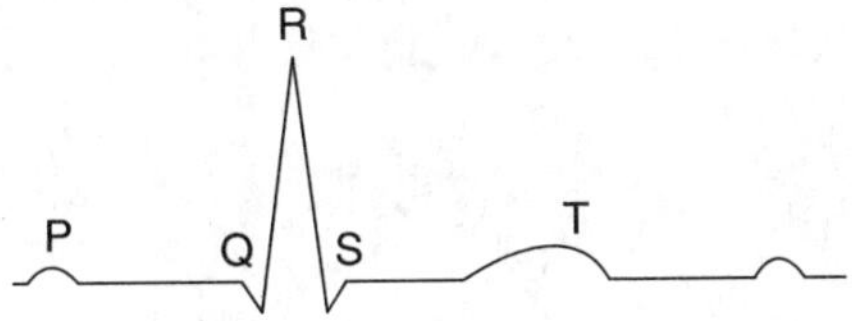

Column I		Column II
A. P-wave	–	I. Ventricular depolarization followed by ventricular contraction
B. QRS complex	–	II. Atrial depolarization followed by systole of both atria
C. T-wave	–	III. Ventricular repolarization followed by ventricular relaxation

(a) A–I, B–II, C–III (b) A–III, B–II, C–I
(c) A–II, B–I, C–III (d) A–II, B–III, C–I

138.

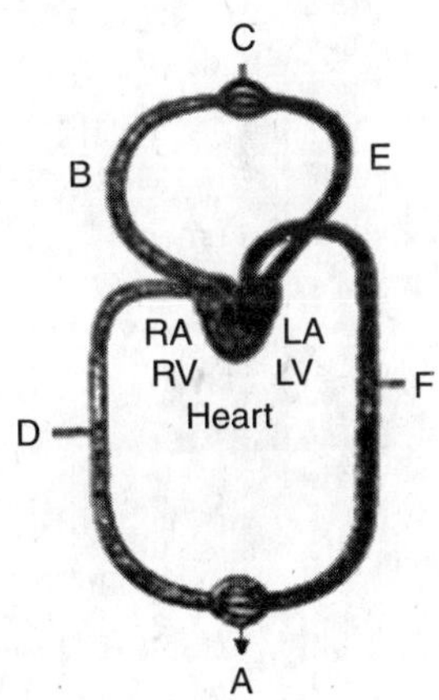

The given figure is the systematic plant of blood circulation in human. Identify from A to F.

	A	B	C	D	E	F
(a)	Body parts	Pulmonary vein	Lungs	Vena cava	Pulmonary artery	Dorsal aorta
(b)	Body parts	Pulmonary artery	Lungs	Vena cava	Pulmonary vein	Dorsal aorta
(c)	Body parts	Pulmonary artery	Lungs	Dorsal aorta	Pulmonary vein	Vena cava
(d)	Lungs	Pulmonary artery	Body parts	Dorsal aorta	Pulmonary vein	Vena cava

139. Which is the nature of blood passing through blood vessels (A, B, C and D)?

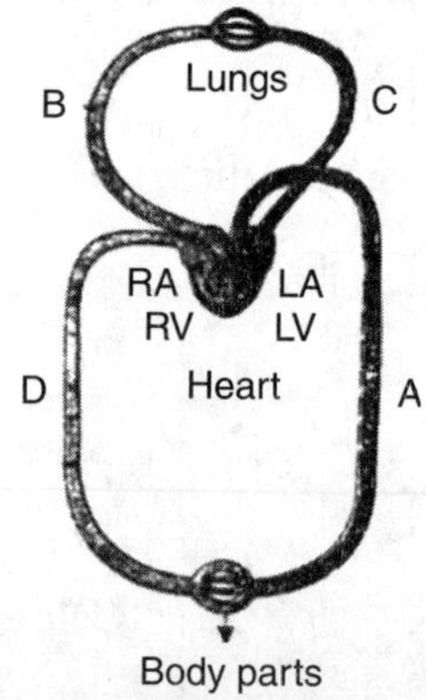

What is the nature of blood passing through blood vessels (A, B, C and D)?

	A	B	C	D
(1)	Oxygenated	Deoxygenated	Oxygenated	Deoxygenated
(2)	Oxygenated	Oxygenated	Deoxygenated	Deoxygenated
(3)	Deoxygenated	Deoxygenated	Oxygenated	Oxygenated
(4)	Deoxygenated	Oxygenated	Deoxygenated	Oxygenated

140. Identify the following blood vessels

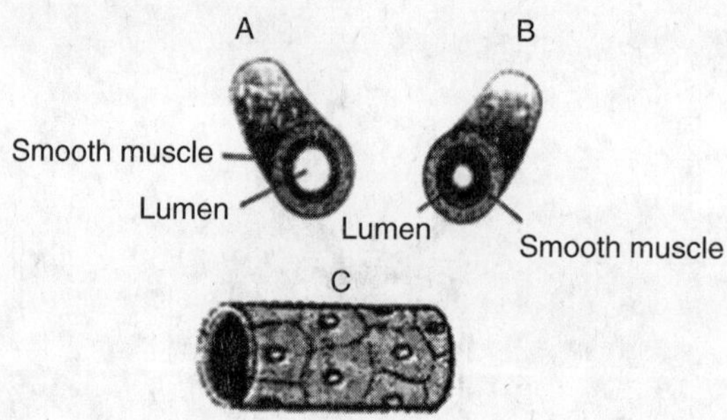

	A	B	C
(1)	Capillary	Artery	Vein
(2)	Vein	Capillary	Artery
(3)	Vein	Artery	Capillary
(4)	Artery	Vein	Capillary

141. The given diagram shows which cell of blood?

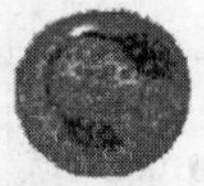

(a) Neturophil (b) Basophil (c) Eosinophil (d) Monocyte

142. Which of the following is a true statement about this diagram?

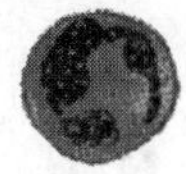

(a) This is the most abundant cell of blood
(b) This cell is phagocytic in nature
(c) Abundance in blood is 60–65%
(d) This cell secrete histamine, serotonin and heparin

143. The function of the cell fragments in blood (given in the diagram) is

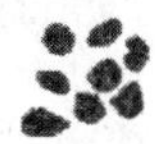

(a) to resist infection
(b) to be responsible for immune response
(c) to help in clotting of blood
(d) to resist allergy

144. Which cell represent surface antigen for ABO blood group?

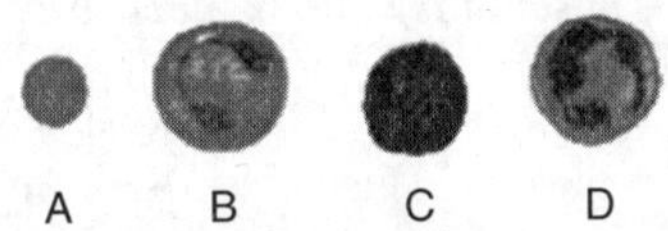

(a) A (b) B (c) C (d) D

145. Identify A, B, C, D, E, F, G and H in given diagram

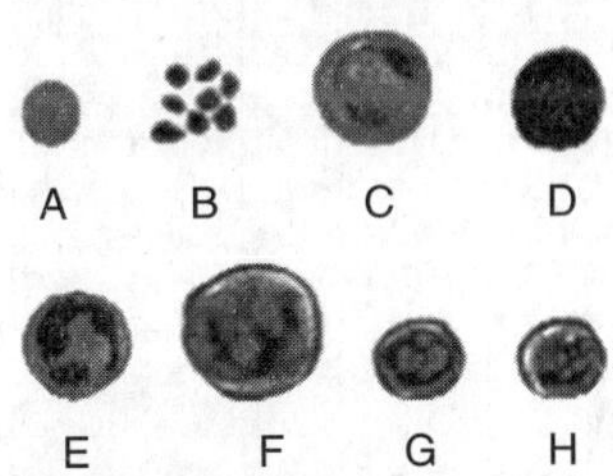

	A	B	C	D	E	F	G	H
(a)	Neturo-phil	Eosino-phil	Platelets	Basophil	Neutrophil	Monocyte	T lym-phocyte	B lym-phocyte
(b)	RBC	Platelets	Basophil	Eosinophil	Monocyte	Neutrophil	T lym-phocyte	B lym-phocyte
(c)	RBC	Platelets	Eosinophil	Basophil	Neutrophil	Monocyte	T lym-phocyte	B lym-phocyte
(d)	T lym-phocyte	B lym-phocyte	Platelets	Eosinophil	Basophil	Neutrophil	Monocyte	RBC

146. Rate of heartbeat is highest in
(a) Whale (b) Elephant (c) Mouse (d) Man

147. Which of the following pair of terms represent both one and the same thing?
(a) Plasma–Serum (b) Atrioventricular node–Pacemaker
(c) Leucocytes–Lymphocytes (d) Mitral valve–Bicuspid valve

148. How many times a red blood corpuscle will have to pass through the heart in its journey from hepatic artery to the aorta?
(a) Two times (b) Only once
(c) Several times (d) Four times

149. Maximum pressure of blood is experienced
(a) when blood enters from left atrium to aorta
(b) when blood enters from right atrium to aorta
(c) when blood enters from left ventricle to aorta
(d) when blood enters from right ventricle to aorta

150. The blood circulation, which starts and ends into capillaries, is
(a) portal circulation (b) renal circulation
(c) hepatic circulation (d) lymphatic circulation

151. Which one of the following is absent in the human beings?
(a) Hypophyseal-hypothalamotract (b) Hepatic portal vein
(c) Renal portal vein (d) None of these

*Read the **assertion** and **reason** carefully to mark the correct option out of the options given below:*

(a) If both the assertion and the reason are true and the reason is a correct explanation of the assertion
(b) If both the assertion and reason are true but the reason is not a correct explanation of the assertion
(c) If the assertion is true but the reason is false
(d) If both the assertion and reason are false

152. Assertion: Simple organism use special fluids within their bodies to transport materials.
Reason: Boold is the only fluid used by higher organism including human for transport of certain substances.

153. Assertion: Closed circulatory system is more effective than open type.
Reason: The closed circulatory system considerably enhances the speed, precision and efficiency of circulation.

154. Assertion: Cardiac output rises during exercise.
Reason: Cardiac output helps in less oxygen consumption.

155. Assertion: Plasma retains water.
Reason: Plasma contains an osmotic protein called albumin.

156. Assertion: An artificial pacemaker can replace the sinoatrial node of heart.
Reason: This is because, an artificial pacemaker is capable of stimulating the heart electrically to maintain its beats.

157. **Assertion:** When heart stops beating it is known as cardiac arrest.
Reason: Heart attack occur due to cardic arrest.

158. **Assertion:** Plasma without the clotting factors is called serum.
Reason: Serum contain immunoglobulins.

159. **Assertion:** Heart of fish contains only deoxygenated blood.
Reason: Oxygenated blood do not return back to the heart in fishes.

160. **Assertion:** Basophiles involved in inflammatory reaction.
Reason: Basophiles use to secrete histamine,serotonin,heparin etc.

161. **Assertion:** A reduction in number of platelets can leads to clotting disorders.
Reason: Platelets release a variety of sustances most of which are involved in the clotting of blood.

162. **Assertion:** Blood pressure is arterial blood pressure.
Reason: It is measured by sphygmomanometer

163. **Assertion:** Body has ability to alter cardiac output.
Reason: Body has ability to alter the stroke volume as well as the heart rate.

164. **Assertion:** QRS complex represent the depolarisation of atria
Reason: Biggining of the T-wave marks the end of systole

165. **Assertion:** WBCs accumulate at the site of wounds by diapedesis.
Reason: It is the sqeezing of leucocytes from the endothelium.

AIPMT PREVIOUS YEAR QUESTIONS

1. Given below are four statements (1-4) regarding human blood circulatory system [AIPMT MAINS 2010]
(A) Arteries are thick-walled and have narrow lumen as compared to veins
(B) Angina is acute chest pain when the blood circulation to the brain is reduced
(C) Persons with blood group AB can donate blood to any person with any blood group ABO system
(D) Calcium ions play a very important role in blood clotting
Which two of the above statements are correct?
(a) (a) & (d) (b) (a) & (b)
(c) (b) & (c) (d) (c) & (d)

2. The haemoglobin content per 100 ml of blood of a normal healthy human adult is: [AIPMT MAINS 2010]
(a) 5 – 11 mg (b) 25 – 30 mg
(c) 17 – 20 mg (d) 12 – 16 mg

3. If due to some injury the chordate tendinae of the tricuspid valve of the human heart is partially non-functional, what will be the immediate effect? [AIPMT PRE 2010]
(a) The flow of blood into the aorta will be slowed down
(b) The 'pacemaker' will stop working
(c) The blood will tend to flow back into the left atrium
(d) The flow of blood into the pulmonary artery will be reduced

4. Given below is the ECG of a normal human. Which one of its components is correctly interpreted below?

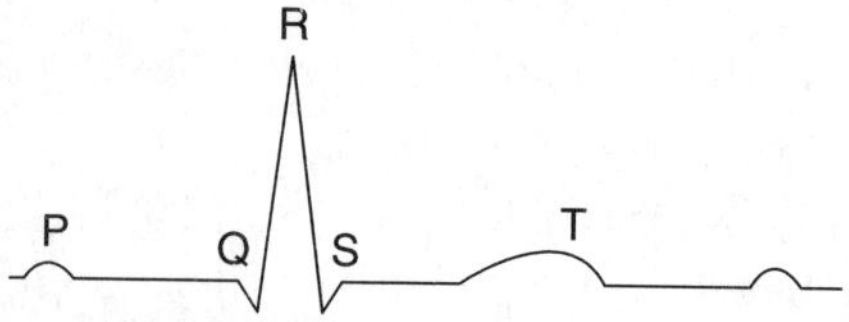

[AIPMT MAINS 2011]

(a) Complex QRS-one complete pulse
(b) Peak T-initiation of total cardiac contraction
(c) Peak P and peak R together – systolic and diastolic blood pressure
(d) Peak P – initiation of left atrial contraction only

5. Arteries are best defined as the vessels which:

[AIPMT PRE 2011]

(a) Carry blood away from the heart to different organs
(b) Break up into capillaries which reunite to form a vein
(c) Carry blood from one visceral organ to another visceral organ
(d) Supply oxygenated blood to the different organs

6. Which one of the following statements is correct regarding blood pressure?

[AIPMT PRE 2011]

(a) 100/55 mmHg is considered an ideal blood pressure
(b) 105/50 mmHg makes one very active
(c) 190/110 mmHg may harm vital organs like brain and kidney
(d) 130/90 mmHg is considered high and require treatment

7. A person with unknown blood group under ABO system has suffered much blood loss in an accident and needs immediate blood transfusion. His one friend, who has a valid certificate of his own blood type, offers for blood donation without delay. What would have been the type of blood group of the donor friend?

[AIPMT PRE 2011]

(a) Type AB
(b) Type O
(c) Type A
(d) Type B

8. 'Bundle of His' is a part of which one of the following organs in humans?

[AIPMT PRE 2011]

(a) Heart
(b) Kidney
(c) Pancreas
(d) Brain

9. Which one of the following plasma proteins is involved in the coagulation of blood?

[AIPMT PRE 2011]

(a) Serum amylase
(b) A globulin
(c) Fibrinogen
(d) An albumin

10. A certain road accident with unknown blood group needs immediate blood transfusion. His one doctor friend at once offers his blood. What was the blood group of the donor?

[AIPMT PRE 2012]

(a) Blood group B
(b) Blood group AB
(c) Blood group O
(d) Blood group A

11. The diagram given here is the standard ECG of normal person. The P – wave represents the:

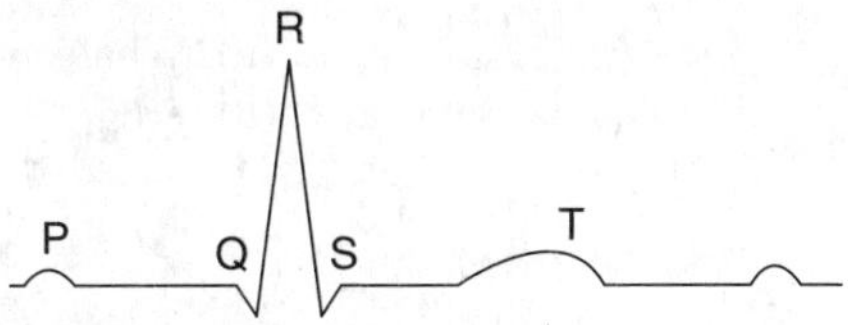

[AIPMT 2013]

(a) Constriction of both the atria
(b) Initiation of the ventricular contraction
(c) Beginning of the systole
(d) End of systole

12. Person with blood group AB is considered as universal recipient because he has:

[AIPMT 2014]

(a) Both A and B antigens on RBC but no antibodies in the plasma
(b) Both A and B antibodies in the plasma
(c) No antigen on RBC and no antibody in the plasma
(d) Both A and B antigens in the plasma but no antibodies

13. How do parasympathetic neural signals affect the working of the heart?

[AIPMT 2014]

(a) Reduce both heart rate and cardiac output
(b) Heart rate is increased without affecting the cardiac output
(c) Both heart rate and cardiac output increase
(d) Heart rate decreases but cardiac output increases

14. Erythropoiesis starts in:

[AIPMT 2015]

(a) Kidney (b) Liver
(c) Spleen (d) Red bone marrow

15. Blood pressure in the mammalian aorta is maximum during:

[AIPMT 2015]

(a) Systole of the left atrium (b) Diastole of the right ventricle
(c) Systole of the left ventricle (d) Diastole of the right atrium

16. Which one of the following is correct?

[AIPMT 2015]

(a) Plasma = Blood – Lymphocytes
(b) Serum = Blood + Fibrinogen
(c) Lymph = Plasma + RBC + WBC
(d) Blood = Plasma + RBC + WBC + Platelets

17. Doctors use stethoscope to hear the sounds produced during each cardiac cycle. The second sound is heard when:

[RE-AIPMT 2015]

(a) Ventricular walls vibrate due to gushing in of blood from atria
(b) Semilunar valves close down after the blood flows into vessels from ventricles
(c) AV node receives signal from SA node
(d) AV valves open up

18. Which one of the following animals has two separate circulatory pathways? [RE-AIPMT 2015]

(a) Lizard
(b) Whale
(c) Shark
(d) Frog

Answer Keys

1. (b) 2. (d) 3. (a) 4. (a) 5. (b) 6. (a) 7. (b) 8. (d) 9. (d) 10. (b)
11. (c) 12. (d) 13. (c) 14. (d) 15. (c) 16. (d) 17. (a) 18. (c) 19. (d) 20. (d)
21. (b) 22. (b) 23. (a) 24. (b) 25. (c) 26. (b) 27. (b) 28. (c) 29. (c) 30. (d)
31. (b) 32. (c) 33. (c) 34. (d) 35. (c) 36. (c) 37. (c) 38. (b) 39. (a) 40. (d)
41. (c) 42. (b) 43. (d) 44. (a) 45. (d) 46. (b) 47. (d) 48. (a) 49. (c) 50. (d)
51. (c) 52. (b) 53. (a) 54. (c) 55. (c) 56. (b) 57. (c) 58. (c) 59. (a) 60. (a)
61. (d) 62. (c) 63. (c) 64. (a) 65. (d) 66. (b) 67. (a) 68. (d) 69. (b) 70. (d)
71. (a) 72. (b) 73. (d) 74. (a) 75. (a) 76. (a) 77. (c) 78. (d) 79. (a) 80. (d)
81. (a) 82. (c) 83. (a) 84. (a) 85. (a) 86. (d) 87. (d) 88. (c) 89. (b) 90. (c)
91. (d) 92. (a) 93. (d) 94. (b) 95. (b) 96. (b) 97. (a) 98. (a) 99. (b) 100. (c)
101. (a) 102. (d) 103. (b) 104. (b) 105. (b) 106. (d) 107. (a) 108. (c) 109. (c) 110. (c)
111. (d) 112. (d) 113. (d) 114. (d) 115. (c) 116. (d) 117. (b) 118. (d) 119. (d) 120. (a)
121. (b) 122. (c) 123. (b) 124. (b) 125. (c) 126. (d) 127. (d) 128. (c) 129. (c) 130. (a)
131. (c) 132. (c) 133. (d) 134. (d) 135. (a) 136. (a) 137. (c) 138. (b) 139. (a) 140. (c)
141. (c) 142. (b) 143. (c) 144. (a) 145. (c) 146. (c) 147. (d) 148. (a) 149. (c) 150. (a)
151. (c) 152. (d) 153. (a) 154. (c) 155. (a) 156. (a) 157. (c) 158. (b) 159. (a) 160. (a)
161. (a) 162. (b) 163. (a) 164. (d) 165. (b)

AIPMT Previous Year Questions

1. (a) 2. (d) 3. (d) 4. (a) 5. (a) 6. (c) 7. (b) 8. (a) 9. (c) 10. (c)
11. (a) 12. (a) 13. (a) 14. (b) 15. (c) 16. (d) 17. (b) 18. (b)

CHAPTER

19

Excretory Products and Their Elimination

1. Select the incorrect statement from the following:
   (a) Animals accumulate ammonia, urea, uric acid, CO_2 and water by metabolic activities
   (b) Animal accumulate substance like ions (Na^+, K^+, Cl^-) and urea, ammonia, uric acid, CO_2 and water are removed totally or partially
   (c) Ammonia produced by metabolism is converted into urea in the liver of mammals
   (d) Kidneys play significant rote in removal of ammonia directly
2. Select ammonotelic from the following
   (a) Many bony fishes (b) aquatic amphibians
   (c) aquatic insects (d) All
3. Select order of toxicity of
   A. Ammonia B. Urea C. Uric acid
   (a) A > B > C (b) B > A > C (c) C > A > B (d) C > B > A
4. Which of the following excretory product require maximum water for its elimination?
   (a) Ammonia (b) Urea (c) Uric acid (d) Creatinine
5. Select incorrect statement from the following:
   (a) Ammonia is readily soluble in water
   (b) Ammonia is generally excreted by the process of diffusion
   (c) Ammonia is excreted as ammonium ion through gill surface in fishes
   (d) Ammonia is major and urea and uric acid are minor form of nitrogenous waste excreted by animals
6. Metabolic wastes containing nitrogen in our body are due to
   (a) Carbohydrates (b) Proteins (c) Fats (d) Vitamins
7. Excretion involves process in which
   (a) harmful substances in the body are chemically changed
   (b) substances of no further use or those present in excessive quantities are thrown out of the body
   (c) harmful substances are stored in cells before being eliminated
   (d) expulsion of urine from the urinary bladder and sweat from the skin
8. Which of the following is Ureotelic?
   (a) Mammals (b) Most of the terrestrial amphibians
   (c) Marine fishes (d) All

9. Ammonia which is produced by metabolism is converted into ___**A**___ in the liver of mammals and released into ___**B**___ which is filtered and ___**C**___ out by kidney
(a) A–Uric acid, B–Blood, C–excreted
(b) A–Urea, B–Blood, C–excreted
(c) A–Amino acid, B–Blood, C–excreted
(d) A–Sugar, B–Blood, C–excreted

10. Which of the following is uricotelic?
(A) Reptiles (B) Birds (C) Insects (D) Land snails
(a) A, B, C only (b) B and C only (c) A, D only (d) A, B, C, D all

11. With respect to the mode of excretion, bony fish falls into what category of organism?
(a) Ureotelic (b) Uricotelic
(c) Ammonotelic (d) Osmoconformers

12. Aquatic animals are mostly ammonotelic because
(a) ammonia helps in checking inflow of water into body
(b) excretion of ammonia requires large amount of water which is available to these animals
(c) water contains less nitrogen
(d) these get less light

13. What gets increased in blood if liver becomes functionless?
(a) Urea (b) Ammonia (c) Uric acid (d) Proteins

14. Nitrogenous excretory product of frog tadpole is
(a) Ammonia (b) Urea (c) Guanine (d) Uric acid

15. In aquatic organisms, the waste end product of nitrogen metabolism is
(a) Urea (b) Nitrogen (c) Ammonia (d) Allantois

16. Chief nitrogenous waste product present in urine of frog is
(a) Ammonia (b) Urea (c) Uric acid (d) Allantoin

17. Nitrogenous waste is excreted mainly as
(a) urea in both frog and tadpole (b) urea in frog and ammonia in tadpole
(c) uric acid in frog and urea in tadpole (d) urea in tadpole and ammonia in frog

18. Urea is derived from
(a) Fats (b) Amino acids
(c) Carbohydrates (d) Uric acid

19. Which of the following sets of animals produce the same substances as their chief excretory product?
(a) Fish, pigeon and frog (b) Camel, housefly and snake
(c) Frog, monkey and dog (d) Amoeba, ant and antelope

20. Which of the following sets of animals are uricotelic?
(a) Fish, snake, fowl and man (b) Fish, frog, lizard and fowl
(c) Crow, snake, cockroach and lizard (d) Camel, dog, monkey and man

21. Excretion of nitrogenous waste product mainly as uric acid by birds is helpful in
(a) conserving body heat (b) conserving water
(c) eliminating excess water (d) eliminating excess body heat

22. Uric acid is formed in human being from
(a) proteins (b) glucose (c) purines (d) pyrimidines

23. Uric acid is excreted by
(a) Pigeon (b) Frog (c) Rabbit (d) Man

24. The least toxic nitrogenous waste is
(a) Ammonia (b) Ammonia + Urea
(c) Urea (d) Uric acid

25. Marine teleost fishes excrete
(a) Uric acid (b) TMO (c) Ammonia (d) All

26. Select the correct statement from the following:
(A) In most of invertebrates, excretory structures are in complex tubular forms.
(B) Vertebrates have simple tubular organ as excretory structure like kidney
(C) Protonephridia is primarily concern with excretion
(D) Protonephridia are excretory structure in rotifers, some annelids and cephalochordates (Amphioxus)
(a) A (b) B (c) C (d) D

27. Excretory and osmoregulatory structure in cockroach is
(a) flame cells (b) green glands
(c) nephridia (d) malpighian tubules

28. The animal which retains urea for hypertonicity is (most appropriate):
(a) elasmobranch (b) man (c) bird (d) amphibian

29. Malpighian tubules are the excretory organs in
(a) platyhelminths (b) cockroach (c) pila (d) ascaris

30. In annelids, excretory organs are
(a) Nephridia (b) Malpighian tubules
(c) Green glands (d) Kidneys

31. The excretory organs in prawn are
(a) malpighian tubules (b) nephridia
(c) kidneys (d) green glands or antennal gland

32. Green glands are excretory organs of
(a) moths (b) crayfishes (c) scorpions (d) spiders

33. Coxal glands are excretory organs in
(a) spiders and scorpions (b) insects
(c) annelids (d) molluscs

34. Which of these parts in vertebrates functionally corresponds to the contractile vacuole of protozoans?
(a) Heart (b) Cloaca (c) Sweat glands (d) Kidneys

35. In human excretory system coexist of
(a) Pair of kidneys (b) Pair of Ureters
(c) A urinary bladder and A urethra (d) All

36. Kidneys in human situated between __________.
(a) T12–L3 (b) T11–L2 (c) T12–L1 (d) T12–L5

37. Correct dimensions of human kidney are

	Length	Width	Thickness	Weight
(a)	10–12 cm	5–7 cm	2–3 cm	120–170 gm
(b)	10–12 cm	2–3 cm	5–7 cm	120–140 gm
(c)	12–14 cm	5–7 cm	2–3 cm	120–140 gm
(d)	12–14 cm	2–3 cm	2–3 cm	120–170 gm

38. Which of the following is correct about hilum of kidney?
(a) It is present on convex outer surface
(b) It is present at inner convex surface
(c) It is notch through which ureter, nerve and blood vessel inter
(d) It is place where calyces open

39. Which of the following is incorrect about human kidney?
(a) Kidney is covered by tough capsule
(b) Kidney is divided into cortex and medulla on outer side
(c) The cortex extended in between the medullary pyramid are renal column of Bertini
(d) Kidney is situated close to the dorsal inner wall of abdominal cavity

40. Each kidney has (nearly) how many Nephrons?
(a) 1 million (b) 2 million (c) ½ million (d) 3 million

41. Extension of cortex in medulla is known as
(a) columnae carneae (b) columns of bertini
(c) renal columns (d) both (b) and (c)

42. Each nephron consists of
(a) glomerulus (b) renal tubules (c) both (d) calyces

43. Glomerules along with Bowman's capsule is called
(a) Renal Corpuscle (b) Malpighian tubule
(c) Malpighian body (d) Both (a) and (c)

44. Part of Nephron is situated in cortex completely
A. Malpighian Corpuscle B. PCT
C. DCT D. Loop of Henle
E. Collecting duct
(a) A, B, C only (b) B, C only (c) A, B, C, D only (d) D, E only

45. Select the incorrect statement from the following:
(a) The DCTs of many nephrons opens into a straight tube called collecting duct
(b) In cortical nephrons (majority), the loop of Henle is too short and extended only very little in medulla
(c) In juxta medullary nephrons (minority), the loop of Henle is very long and runs deeply into medulla
(d) Vasa recta is not a part of peritubular network

46. Two kidneys of human beings lie
(a) at the level of ovaries
(b) at the same level
(c) left kidney at a higher level than the right one
(d) right kidney at a higher level than the left one

47. Which term is used both for a part of kidney and a part of skeleton in the mammals?
(a) Centrum (b) Pelvis (c) Cortex (d) Medulla

48. Mammalian kidney serve to excrete
(a) excess water, urea and amino acids
(b) excess salts, urea and excess water
(c) excess salts, excess water and excess amino acids
(d) excess salts, urea and water

49. Part through which arteries and veins enter or leave the kidney is called
(a) major calyces (b) minor calyces
(c) hilus (d) renal pore

50. Cells named podocytes occur in the wall of
(a) neck region of nephrons
(b) glomerular capillaries
(c) outer wall of Bowman's capsules
(d) inner wall of Bowman's capsules

51. A malpighian corpuscle is
(a) another name for nephron
(b) an excretory structure of insects
(c) combined name for glomerulus and Bowman's capsule
(d) none

52. Blood vessel leading to glomerulus is called
(a) renal artery
(b) renal vein
(c) efferent arteriole
(d) afferent arteriole

53. Blood vessel draining the glomerulus in a mammalian nephron is called
(a) afferent arteriole and is narrower than the vessel entering it
(b) efferent venule and is narrower than the vessel entering it
(c) efferent arteriole and is narrower than the vessel entering it
(d) renal artery and is wider than the vessel entering it

54. In mammalian kidneys, Bowman's capsules or Malpighian corpuscles occur in
(a) Cortex
(b) Medulla
(c) Pelvis
(d) All

55. In a glomerulus
(a) afferent arteriole is thicker than efferent arteriole
(b) afferent capillaries are thicker than efferent capillaries
(c) afferent capillaries are thinner than efferent capillaries
(d) afferent arteriole is thinner than efferent arteriole

56. Which one of these is not a part of uriniferous tubule?
(a) Loop of Henle
(b) Collecting duct
(c) Bowman's capsule
(d) Distal convoluted tubule

57. Bowman's capsule is lined by
(a) Ciliated epithelium
(b) Squamous epithelium
(c) Cuboidal epithelium
(d) Cuboidal and columnar epithelium

58. Brush border is characteristic of
(a) Neck of nephron
(b) Collecting tube
(c) Proximal convoluted tubule
(d) All

59. Filtration of blood occurs in
(a) loop of Henle
(b) Bowman's capsule
(c) lungs
(d) renal papillae

60. The glomerular filtrate, i.e. the liquid collected in the cavity of Bowman's capsule, is
(a) blood minus proteins
(b) blood minus proteins and corpuscles
(c) water
(d) urine

61. Glomerular filtrate will not contain, normally,
(a) Albumin
(b) Glucose
(c) NaCI
(d) Creatinine

62. Glomerular filtration rate would be decreased by
(a) constriction of the efferent arteriole
(b) an increase in afferent arteriolar pressure
(c) compression of the renal capsule
(d) an increase in renal blood flow

63. A minute vessel runs parallel to the Henle's loop forming 'U' shape vasa recta is a part of
(a) Peritubular network
(b) Afferent arteriole
(c) Efferent arteriole
(d) Bowman's capsule

64. Urine formation mainly involve the process of
(a) ultrafiltration
(b) selective reabsorption
(c) secretion
(d) all

65. How much amount of blood is filtered out by kidney's/min?
(a) 500 ml (b) 1100–1200 ml (c) 1500 ml (d) 125 ml

66. How many layers do filtration membrane consist of?
(a) 1 (b) 2 (c) 3 (d) 4

67. Filtration membrane consist of
(a) endothelium of glomerular blood vessels
(b) epithelium of Bowman's capsule
(c) basement membrane between above two layers
(d) all

68. Which of the following is incorrect about ultrafiltration?
(a) Podocytes are arranged in intricate manner so as to leave minute space called filtration slits and slit pore, filtration occur finely through these pores
(b) Filtration is so fine that almost all constituent of blood except protein pass onto the lumen of Bowman's capsule
(c) Filtrated fluid is isotonic to blood plasma
(d) JGA control filtration rate of Ultrafiltration

69. The values of GFR in healthy individual is
(a) 125 ml/min (b) 150 ml/min (c) 100 ml/min (d) 200 ml/min

70. The amount of the filtrate formed by the kidneys are
(a) 125 ml/min (b) 7.5 litre/hr (c) 180 litre/day (d) All

71. Select the total number of correct matching
(1) JGA → Juxtaglomerular Apparatus
(2) GFR → Glomerular Filtration Rate
(3) PCT → Proximal Conducting Tube
(4) DCT → Distal Convoluted Tubule
(5) CD → Conducting Duct
(6) ADH → Antidiuretic Hormone
(a) 6 (b) 5 (c) 4 (d) 2

72. JGA is formed by
(a) part of DCT
(b) part of afferent arteriole
(c) both
(d) none

73. Following are the points of mechanism of JGA. Arrange them accordingly.
(A) Activation of JG cells
(B) Activated JG cells release renin
(C) Fall in GFR
(D) Increase of glomerular blood flow
(E) GFR back to normal
(a) E, A, D, C, B (b) C, A, B, D, E (c) A, B, C, D, E (d) C, A, D, B, E

74. Nearly how much percent of the filtrate reabsorbed by the renal tubules
(a) 70–80% (b) 85% (c) 99% (d) 90%

75. Choose the correct statement about absorption in renal tubules from the following:
(a) Glucose, amino acids and Na^+ reabsorbed actively
(b) Nitrogenous waste an absorbed by passive transport
(c) 70–80% of electrolyte and water are absorbed in PCT
(d) All

76. Tubular secretion helps in
(a) ionic balance of body fluid
(b) acid base balance of body fluid
(c) both
(d) none

77. Which of the following is an incorrect statement about filtration?
(a) Selective process
(b) Non-selective process
(c) Performed by glomerulus
(d) It occurs through the usage of capillary (glomerulus) blood pressure

78. Which of the following is incorrect about PCT?
(a) Lined with simple cuboidal brush border epithelium
(b) All essential nutrient and 70–80% electrolyte and water are reabsorbed here
(c) It helps in PH maintenance of body fluid by selective of secration H^+ ion and by absorption of HCO_3^-
(d) It does not help in maintenance of ionic balance of body fluid

79. Which of the following part has minimum reabsorption?
(a) PCT (b) HL (c) DCT (d) Collecting duct

80. Select total number of correct statement about loop of Henle.
(1) Descending limb is permeable to water
(2) Descending limb almost impermeable to electrolyte
(3) Ascending limb impermeable to water
(4) It allows transport of electrolyte only actively
(5) At the tip of loop of Henle concentration of filtrate is 1200 m osmol/l
(6) It helps in maintenance of high osmolarity in medullary interstitium.
(a) 6 (b) 3 (c) 4 (d) 5

81. Which segment help in pH maintenance of body fluid?
(a) PCT (b) DCT (c) Collecting duct (d) All

82. DCT helps in
(A) conditional reabsorption of Na^+ and water
(B) HCO_3^- absorption
(C) pH maintenance
(D) selective secretion of H^+ and K^+
(a) A, C, D only (b) B, C, D only (c) all (d) C, D only

83. Which of the following segment allows passage of small amount of urea into modularly interstitium to keep up the osmolarity?
(a) PCT (b) DCT (c) HL (d) Collecting duct

84. At which place we first time use the term 'urine' for filtrate
(a) PCT
(b) DCT
(c) HL
(d) Collecting duct (end)

85. Counter-current mechanism is present in
(a) HL (b) Vasa recta (c) Both (a) and (b) (d) DCT

86. Which of the following is incorrect about counter-current mechanism?
(a) Flow of filtrate in two limbs of vasa recta is in opposite direction

(b) Flow of blood in two limbs of vasa recta is also in opposite direction
(c) NaCI is transported by ascending limb of HL which is exchanged with the descending limb of vasa recta
(d) NaCI is returned to in interstitium by the ascending portion of vasa recta.

87. Counter current mechanism maintains concentration gradient in the medullary interstitium. It helps in
(a) easy passage of water from PCT
(b) easy passage of water from DCT
(c) easy passage of water from HL
(d) easy passage of water from collecting duct

88. Total filtrate formed in 24 hours in human kidney is
(a) 1.8 litre (b) 8.0 litre (c) 18 1itre (d) 180 litre

89. Which of the following is most likely to cause an increase in the glomerular filtration rates?
(a) Blockage of ureter
(b) Dilation of the afferent arterioles
(c) Release of renin from the juxtaglomerular apparatus
(d) Volume depletion

90. Which of these will be completely reabsorbed from glomerular filtrate under normal conditions in the nephrons?
(a) Urea (b) Salts (c) Uric acid (d) Glucose

91. What are mainly reabsorbed from Henle's loops?
(a) Potassium (b) Glucose
(c) Water and NaCl (d) Urea and NaCl

92. The part of the nephron that helps in active reabsorption of sodium is
(a) Bowman's capsule (b) Distal convoluted tubule
(c) Ascending limb of Henle's loop (d) Proximal convoluted tubules

93. Which of the following substance is actively secreted into glomerular filtrate of the kidney tubule?
(a) Amino acids (b) Chloride ions
(c) Na^+ (d) K^+

94. The effect of antidiuretic hormone (ADH) on the kidney is to increases the
(a) excretion of water
(b) excretion of Na'
(c) permeability of the distal nephron to water
(d) glomerular filtration rate

95. In deficiency of ADH, rate of micturition
(a) decreases (b) increases
(c) remains the same (d) none

96. Volume of urine is regulated by
(a) aldosterone (b) aldosterone and ADH
(c) aldosterone, ADH and testosterone (d) ADH alone

97. When a person is suffering from poor renal reabsorption, which one of the following will not help in maintenance of blood volume?
(a) Increased ADH secretion (b) Decreased glomerular filtration
(c) Increased arterial pressure in kidneys (d) Decreased arterial pressure in kidneys

98. The number of nephrons in a kidney is equal to the
(a) number of Bowman's capsules
(b) sum of Bowman's capsules and glomeruli
(c) double the number of Bowman's capsules
(d) sum of Bowman's capsules and Malpighian corpuscles

99. If Henle's loop were absent from mammalian nephron, which of the following is to be expected?
(a) The urine will be more dilute
(b) There will be no urine formation
(c) The urine will have more concentration
(d) There will be hardly any change in the quality and quantity of urine formed

100. Which of the following statements is/are true?
1. urine is hypertonic in distal convoluted tubule
2 when the urine passes into the collecting tubule it becomes hypotonic
3. urine is isotonic in proximal convoluted tubule
4. urine becomes more and more hypotonic as it passes through the Henle's loop
(a) 1 and 4 only (b) 1, 2 and 3 only
(c) 2 and 3 only (d) 3 only

101. Which one of the following groups of structures/organs have similar function?
(a) Typhlosole in earthworm, intestinal villi in rat and contractile vacuole in Amoeba
(b) Nephridia in earthworm, Malpighian tubules in cockroach and urinary tubules in rat
(c) Antennae of cockroach, tympanum of frog and clitellum of earthworm
(d) Incisors of rat, gizzard (proventriculus) of cockroach and tube feet of starfish

102. Ducts of Bellini are present in
(a) liver (b) kidney
(c) intestine (d) medulla oblongata

103. Human kidney produce how much concentrated urine than initial filtrate formed
(a) 2 times (b) 4 times (c) 6 times (d) 3 times

104. What is the ratio of concentration of outer medulla to outer portion of inner medulla?
(a) $\frac{1}{3}$ (b) $\frac{2}{3}$ (c) $\frac{4}{3}$ (d) $\frac{1}{4}$

105. The functioning of kidney is regulated by
(a) Hypothalamus (b) JGA (c) Heart (d) All

106. ADH causes
(a) increase water absorption from DCT and CT
(b) increase GFR by increasing blood pressure
(c) increase reabsorption of electrolyte from distal tubules
(d) all

107. Arrange the following steps in order
(1) excessive loss of fluid
(2) stimulation of osmoreceptor
(3) stimulation of Hypothalamus
(4) release of ADH or Vasopressin
(5) ADH facilitate water reabsorption from distal tubules
(6) Increase in body fluid switch off osmoreceptor and suppress release of ADH
(a) 1, 2, 3, 4, 5, 6 (b) 1, 3, 2, 4, 5, 6 (c) 6, 1, 2, 3, 4, 5 (d) 2, 3, 4, 1, 5, 6

108. Stimulus for activation of JG cells to release rennin is/are
(a) ↓ glomerular blood flow (b) ↓ glomerular blood pressure
(c) ↓ GFR (d) All

109. RAAS involve
(a) JGA apparatus (b) Angiotensinogen (c) Adrenal cortex (d) All

110. Select the incorrect from the following:

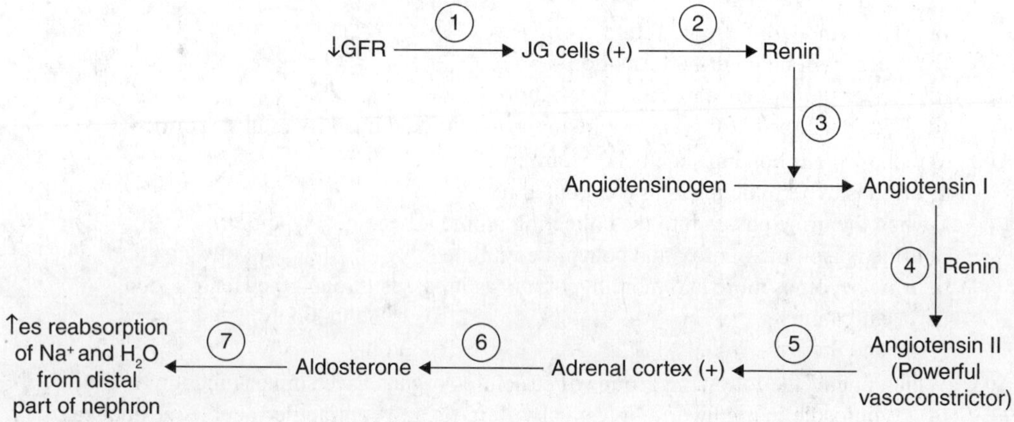

(a) 2, 3 (b) 1, 3 (c) 4 (d) 5, 6

111. Increase in blood pressure is caused by
(a) ↑es ADH secretion (b) ↑es Aldosterone secretion
(c) ↑es Angiotensinogen II (d) All

112. Which of the following is true about ANF?
(a) Full form is Autonomic Nervous Factor
(b) Antagonistic to Renin–Angiotensin mechanism
(c) It causes Vasoconstriction
(d) All are true

113. Find the correct steps for micturition (arrange in order)
(A) Urine filled in urinary bladder
(B) Stretch–receptor activation
(C) Wall of bladder send signal to CNS
(D) Motor message from CNS to urinary bladder and urethral sphincter
(E) Bladder contracts and sphincter dilates leads to micturition
(a) A → B → C → D → E (b) C → B → A → D → E
(c) B → A → C → D → E (d) A → B → C → E → D

114. Neural mechanism of micturition is called
(a) micturition reflex (b) simple reflex
(c) conditioned reflex (d) All

115. An adult human excrete how much urine per day?
(a) 1–1.5 litre (b) 1.5–2 litre (c) 5–1 litre (d) 3 litre

116. On an average _________ gm of urea is excreted out per day
(a) 20–25 gm (b) 25–30 gm (c) 25–30 mg (d) 40–45 gm

117. Analysis of urine help in the clinical diagnosis of
(a) Metabolic disorders (b) Malfunctioning of kidney
(c) Diabetes mellitus (d) All

118. Select the correct matching:

Colour	pH	Odour
(a) Light yellow	7.0	Characteristic
(b) Light yellow	6.0	Characteristic
(c) Light yellow	6.5	Pungent
(d) Light yellow	6.0	Almond

119. Presence of glucose and ketone bodies in urine is called
(a) Glycosuria and ketonuria (b) glycogenic and ketonuria
(c) Glycosuria and ketonemia (d) Gluconeogenesis and ketonemia

120. Glycosuria and ketonuria is indicative of
(a) starvation (b) diabetes mellitus
(c) diabetes insipidus (d) all

121. Sweat contains
(a) watery fluid with NaCl (b) urea
(c) lactic acid (d) all

122. Primary function of sweat is
(a) removal of excess of water (b) removal of urea
(c) cooling of body surface (d) all

123. Nitrogenous waste is eliminated through
(a) kidney (b) saliva
(c) sweat gland (d) all

124. Sterols, hydrocarbons and waxes are eliminated through
(a) liver (b) lungs
(c) sebaceous gland (d) sweat gland

125. Select the incorrect statement from the following
(a) Liver is the second largest gland in our body
(b) Sebum provide protective oily covering for skin
(c) Bile contain substance like bilirubin, biliverdin, cholesterol, degraded steroid hormones, vitamins and drugs are passed with digestive waste
(d) Other than kidney lungs, liver and skin also help in elimination of excretory waste

126. Which is not a part of renal tubule?
(a) PCT (b) Bowman's capsule
(c) DCT (d) Collecting duct

127. Select the total number of excretory organ from the following found in various animals: **Protonephridia, SA node, Nephridia, Hepatic Cecae, Atrium, Malpighian tubules, green glands, kidney, pons, ommatidia, parapodia**
(a) 4 (b) 5 (c) 6 (d) 7

128. Excretory organs help in
(a) excretion only (b) maintenance of acid–base balance
(c) maintenance of ionic balance (d) all

129. Our lung remove how much of CO_2 per hour from the body
(a) 10L (b) 20L (c) 18L (d) 2L

130. Inflammation of glomeruli of kidney is
(a) renal failure (b) renal calculi
(c) glomerulonephritis (d) cystitis

131. Stone and insoluble mass of crystallized salts, formed within the kidney, is generally made up of
(a) calcium carbonate (b) calcium oxalate
(c) silica (d) any of the above

132. Which is the ultimate method for the correction of acute renal failure?
(a) Haemodialysis
(b) Renal transplantation
(c) Blood transfusion
(c) Angioplasty

133. Following are the steps of dialysis:
A. Blood is passed into a vein
B. Blood is mixed with heparin
C. Blood is mixed with anti-heparin
D. Blood is drained from convenient artery.
E. Blood is passed through a coiled and porous cellophane tube bathing in dialysis fluid.
F. Removal of nitrogenous wastes from blood.
The correct sequence of steps is
(a) $A \rightarrow B \rightarrow C \rightarrow D \rightarrow E \rightarrow F$
(b) $D \rightarrow B \rightarrow E \rightarrow F \rightarrow C \rightarrow A$
(c) $F \rightarrow C \rightarrow E \rightarrow B \rightarrow A \rightarrow D$
(d) $D \rightarrow C \rightarrow E \rightarrow F \rightarrow B \rightarrow A$

134. Malfunctioning of kidney may lead to the accumulation of ________ in blood.
(a) glucose (b) amino acid
(c) urea (d) all

135. Which of the following is true about renal transplantation?
(a) Kidney transplantation is the ultimate method at the stage where drug or dialysis do not help
(b) Immunosuppressive agent are used in kidney transplant patient
(c) Close relatives are often used as kidney donors to minimise risk of rejection
(d) All

136. In the diagram of excretory system of human beings given below, different parts have been indicated by alphabets; choose the answer in which these alphabets have been correctly matched with the parts which they represent.

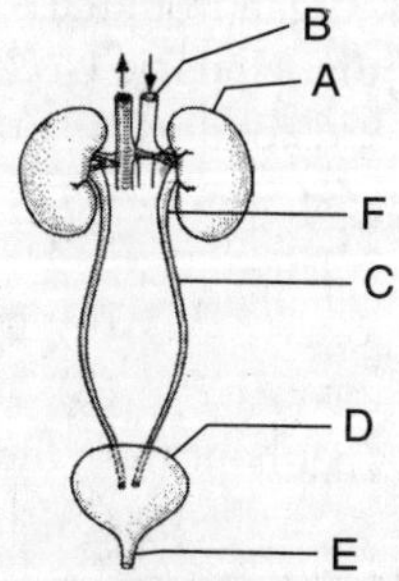

(a) A–Kidney, B–Abdominal aorta, C–Ureters, D–Urinary bladder, E–Urethra, F–Renal pelvis

(b) A–Kidney, B–Abdominal aorta, C–Urethra, D–Urinary bladder, E–Ureters, F–Renal pelvis
(c) A–Kidney, B–Renal pelvis, C–Urethra, D–Urinary bladder, E–Ureters, F–Abdominal aorta
(d) A–Kidney, B–Abdominal aorta, C–Urethra, D–Urinary bladder, E–Renal pelvis, F–Ureters

137. Match the excretory functions of section I with the parts of the excretory system in section II. Choose the correct combinations from among the answers given.

Section I			**Section II**
(i)	Ultrafiltration	–	(a) Henle's loop
(ii)	Concentration of urine	–	(b) Ureter
(iii)	Transport of urine	–	(c) Urinary bladder
(iv)	Storage of urine	–	(d) Malpighian corpuscles
			(e) Proximal convoluted tubules

(a) (i)–(d), (ii)–(a), (iii)–(b), (iv)–(c)
(b) (i)–(d), (ii)–(c), (iii)–(b), (iv)–(a)
(c) (i)–(e), (ii)–(d), (iii)–(a), (iv)–(c)
(d) (i)–(e), (ii)–(d), (iii)–(a), (iv)–(b)

138. Observe the following figure.

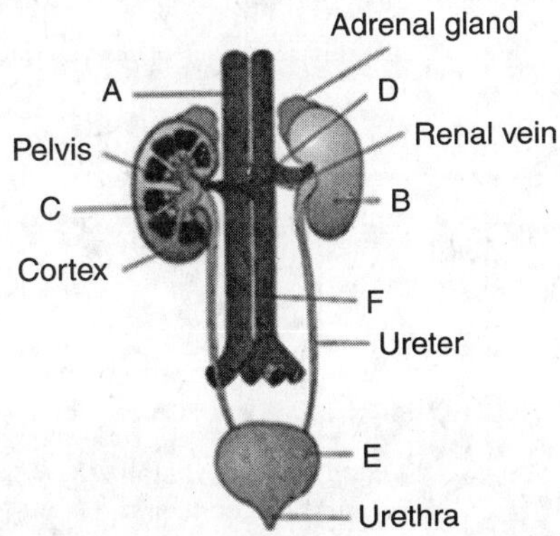

Identify A to E structure:

	A	**B**	**C**	**D**	**E**
(a)	Renal artery	Urinary bladder	Inferior vena cava	Kidney	Medulla
(b)	Inferior vena cava	Kidney	Medulla	Renal artery	Urinary bladder
(c)	Urinary bladder	Medulla	Kidney	Inferior vena cava	Renal artery
(d)	Kidney	Renal artery	Inferior vena cava	Urinary bladder	Medulla

139. Go through the following figure:

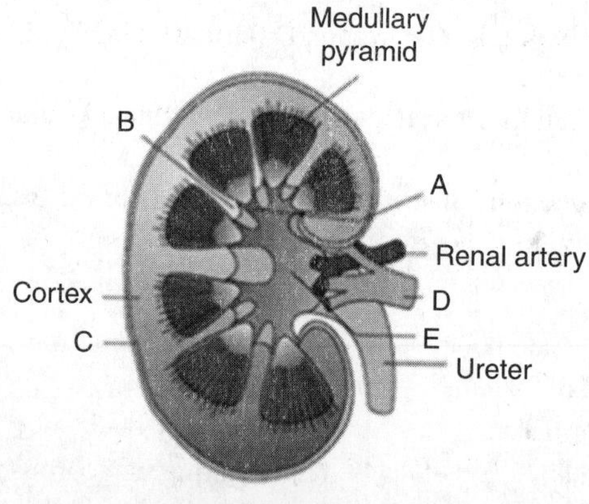

Identify A to D.

	A	B	C	D
(a)	Renal column	Renal capsule	Calyx	Renal pelvis
(b)	Renal capsule	Renal pelvis	Renal vein	Calyx
(c)	Calyx	Renal column	Renal capsule	Renal vein
(d)	Renal vein	Calyx	Renal column	Renal capsule

140. Match the following:

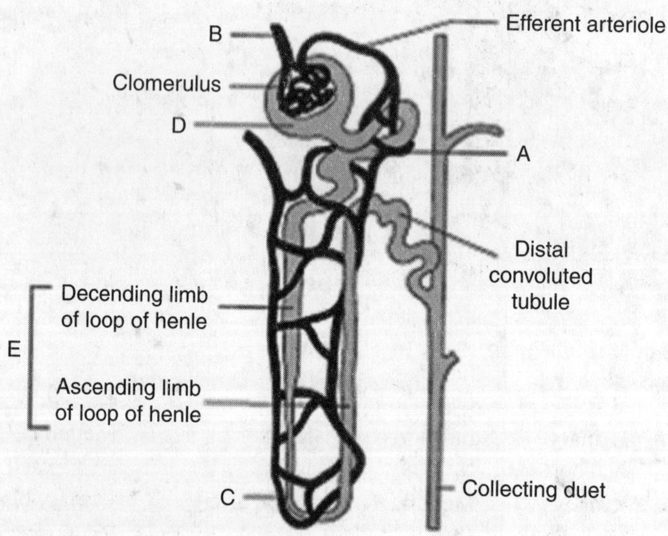

(a) A–Proximal convoluted tubule, B–Afferent arteriole, C–Vasa recta, D–Bowman's capsule, E–Henle's loop

(b) A–Henle's loop, B–Vasa recta, C–Proximal convoluted tubule, D–Bowman's capsule, E–Afferent arteriole

(c) A–Bowman's capsule, B–Henle's loop, C–Proximal convoluted tubule, D–Vasa recta, E–Afferent arteriole

(d) A–Vasa recta, B–Proximal convoluted tubule, C–Bowman's capsule, D–Afferent arteriole, E–Henle's loop

141. The following diagram represent the Malpighian body. Identify A to D.

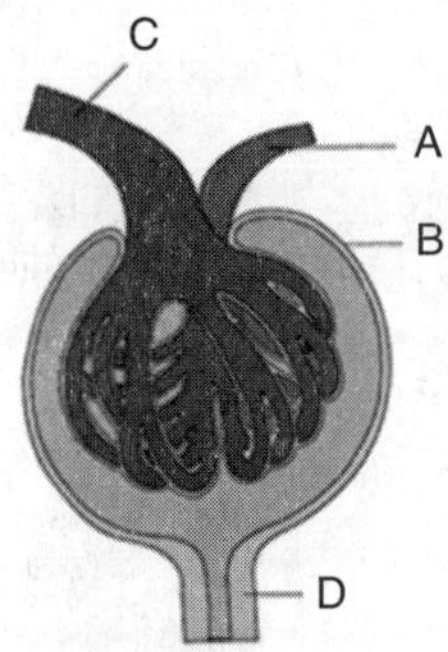

(a) A–Efferent arteriole, B–Afferent arteriole, C–Bowman's capsule, D–DCT

(b) A–Afferent arteriole, A–Efferent arteriole, C–renal corpuscle, D–Proximal convoluted tubule

(c) A–Efferent arteriole, B–Bowman's capsule, C– Afferent arteriole, D–PCT

(d) A–Afferent arteriole, B–Efferent arteriole, C–Bowman's capsule, D–DCT

142. The diagram following the different parts absorb:

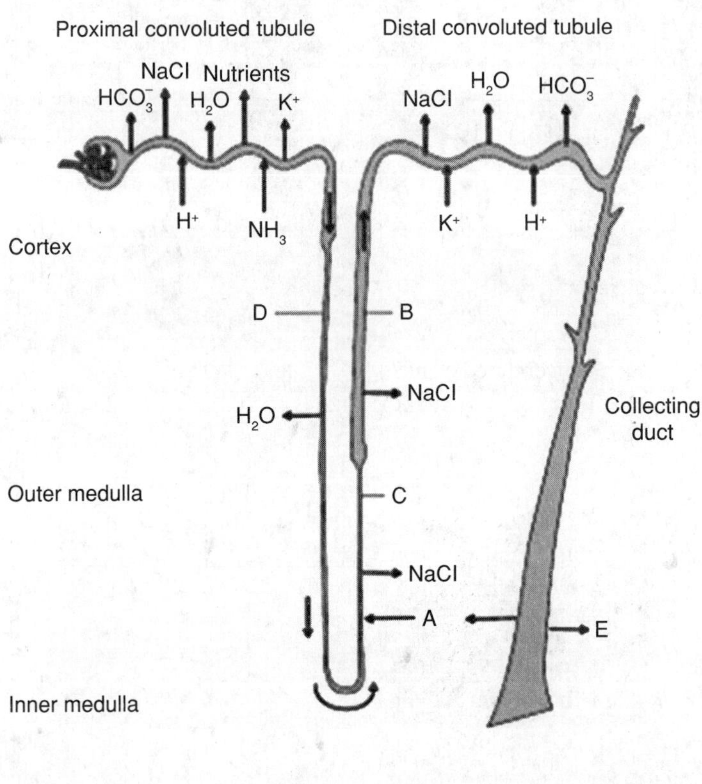

Identify A, B and D

(a) A–Urea, B–Thick segment of ascending limb, D–Descending limb of loop of Henle
(b) A–Descending limb of loop of Henle, B–Thick segment of ascending limb, D–Urea
(c) A–Thick segment of ascending limb, B–Descending limb of loop of Henle, D–Urea
(d) A–Thick segment of ascending limb, B–Thick segment of ascending limb, D–Urea

143.

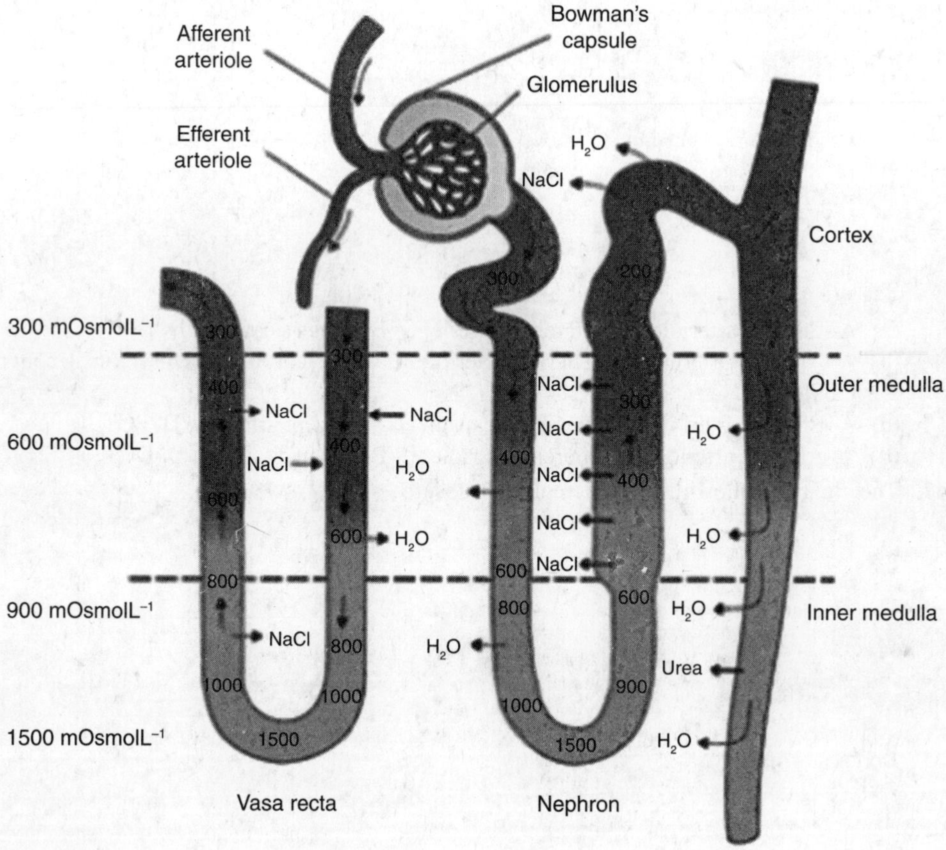

Nephron produces how much concentrated urine?

(a) 4 times (b) 5 times (c) 3 times (d) 2 times

144.

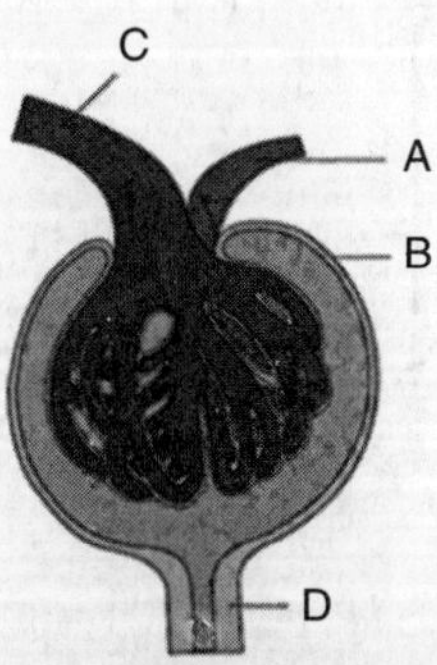

Glomerulus is formed by branching of

(a) A (b) B (c) C (d) D

145.

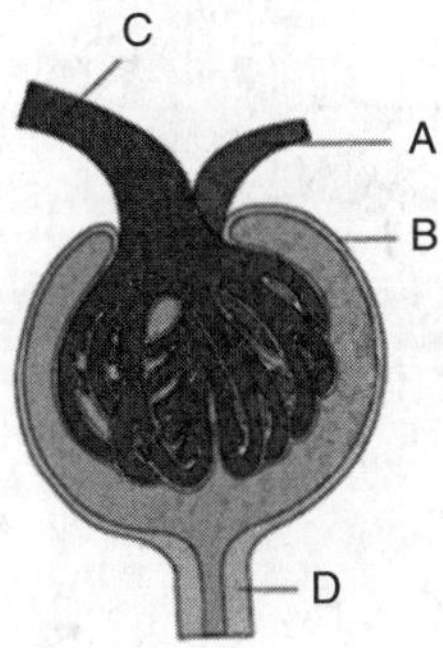

'B' in above diagram is lined with

(a) cuboidal epithelium (b) columnar epithelium

(c) squamous epithelium (d) brush border epithelium

146.

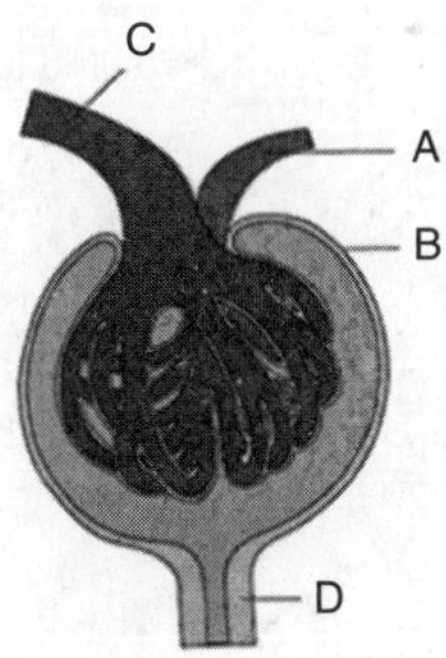

Which part of above diagram is lined with podocytes

(a) A (b) B (c) C (d) D

147.

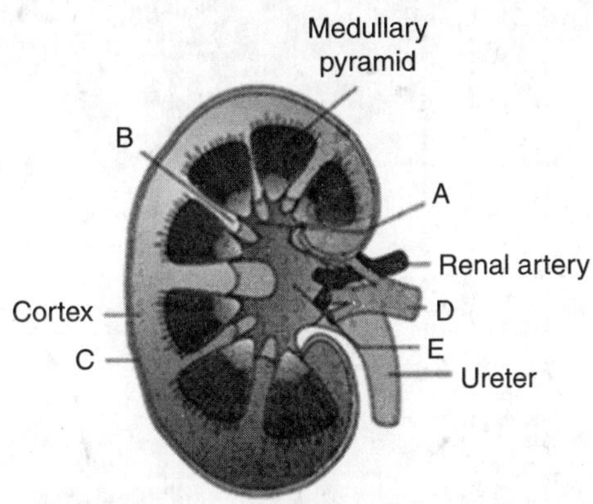

B part of above diagram contains

(a) PCT (b) DCT (c) HL (d) Blood Vessels

148.

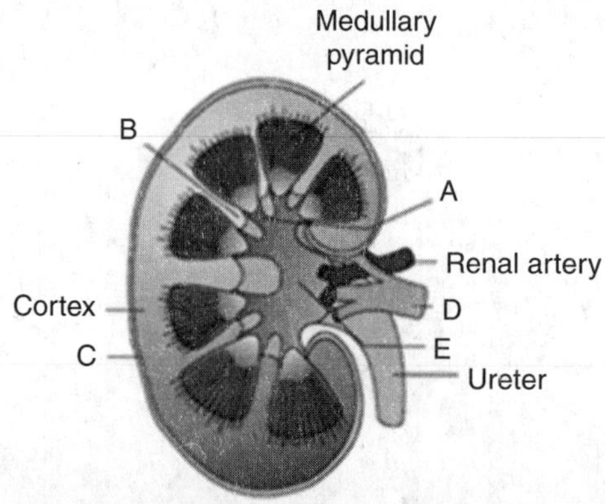

In which part of the diagram calyces opens

(a) A (b) B (c) C (d) E

149. In the below diagram, identify the end excretory product which remains in body to maintain concentration of medullary interstitium?

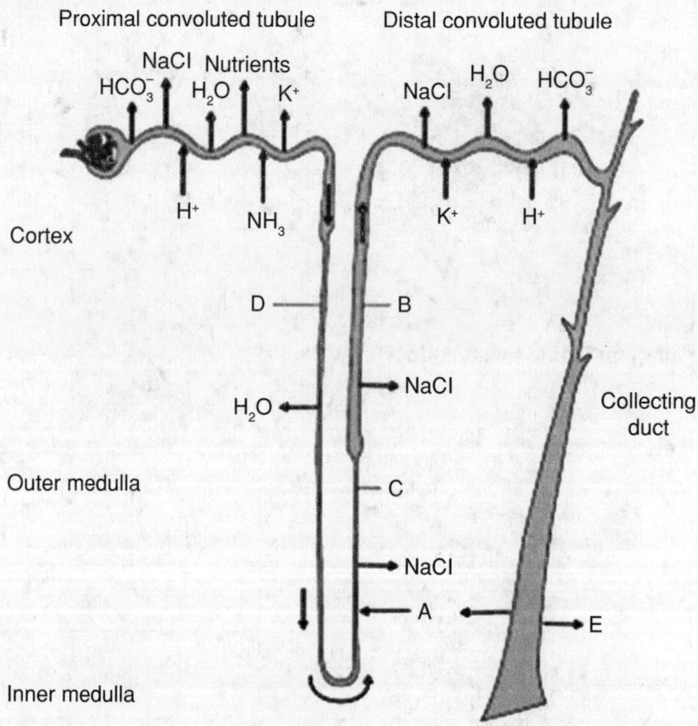

(a) F (b) G (c) A (d) E

Read the **assertion** *and* **reason** *carefully to mark the correct option out of the options given below:*

(a) If both the assertion and the reason are true and the reason is a correct explanation of the assertion
(b) If both the assertion and reason are true but the reason is not a correct explanation of the assertion
(c) If the assertion is true but the reason is false
(d) If both the assertion and reason are false

150. **Assertion:** Diabetes insipidus is marked by excessive urination and too much thirst for water.
Reason: Anti-diuretic hormone (ADH) is secreted by the posterior lobe of pituitary gland.

151. **Assertion:** Filteration is a selective process performed by the glomerulus using the glomerular capillary blood pressure.
Reason: Blood is filtered through fine pores present in PCT.

152. **Assertion:** The antidiuretic hormone increases the water permeability of distal convoluted tubule.
Reason: In absence of ADH, water re-absorption is considerably reduced.

153. **Assertion:** Presence of glucose and ketone bodies in urine are indicative of diabetes mellitus.
Reason: Malfunctioning of kidney can lead to accumulation of urea in blood a condition called uremia.

154. **Assertion:** In the descending limb of loop of Henle, the urine is hypertonic, while in ascending limb of loop of Henle, the urine is Hypotonic.
Reason: Descending limb is impermeable to Na^+, while ascending limb is impermeable to H_2O.

155. **Assertion:** Vasa recta is absent or highely reduced in cortical nephrons.
Reason: PCT and DCT are situated in cortical region of kidney.

156. **Assertion:** Ammonia is excretory product of aquatic amphibian.
Reason: Ammonia is readily soluble in water and require large amount of water for excretion.

157. **Assertion:** Urinary bladder and ureters are lined by transitional epithelium.
Reason: Ureters carry the urine to urinary bladder where it is stored temporarily.

158. **Assertion:** Kidneys maintain the osmotic concentration of the blood.
Reason: Kidneys eliminate either hypotonic or hypertonic urine according to the need of the body.

159. **Assertion:** In vertebrates, the liver is also referred as an accessory excretory organ.
Reason: Liver helps kidneys in the secretion of urine.

160. **Assertion:** Sharks are said to be ammonotelic animals.
Reason: Sharks can retain considerable amounts of ammonia in their blood.

161. **Assertion:** The glomerular filtrate resembles the protein free plasma in composition and osmotic pressure.
Reason: The glomerular capillary wall and inner membrance of Bowman's capsule are impermeable to large molecules.

162. **Assertion:** PCT reabsorb nearly all essential nutrients and 70–80% of electrolyte and water from filterate.
Reason: PCT is lined with lined with brush border epitelium.

163. **Assertion:** Conter current mechanism responsible for concentration of urine..
Reason: Counter current mechanism help to maintain concentration gradient in the medullary interstitium.

164. **Assertion:** Aldosterone leads to increase in blood pressure.
Reason: Aldosterone causes reabsorbtion of sodium ion and water from distal part of tubules.

AIPMT PREVIOUS YEAR QUESTIONS

1. In which one of the following organisms its excretory organs are correctly stated? [AIPMT MAINS 2010]

   (a) Humans – Kidneys, sebaceous glands
   (b) Earthworm – Pharyngeal, integumentary and septal nephridia
   (c) Cockroach – Malpighian tubules and enteric caeca
   (d) Frog – Kidneys, skin and buccal epithelium

2. Which one of the following statements in regard to the excretion by the human kidneys is correct? [AIPMT PRE 2010]

   (a) Descending limb of Loop of Henle is impermeable to water
   (b) Distal convoluted tubule is incapable of reabsorbing HCO_3^-
   (c) Nearly 99 per cent of the glomerular filtrate is reabsorbed by the renal tubules
   (d) Ascending limb of loop of Henle is impermeable to electrolytes

3. The principal nitrogenous excretory compound in humans is synthesised [AIPMT PRE 2010]

   (a) In kidneys but eliminated mostly through liver
   (b) In kidneys as well as eliminated by kidneys
   (c) In liver and also eliminated by the same through bile
   (d) In the liver, but eliminated mostly through kidneys

4. Which one of the following correctly explains the function of a specific part of a human nephron? [AIPMT PRE 2011]

   (a) Henle's loop – Most reabsorption of the major substance from the glomerular filtrate
   (b) Distal convoluted tubule – Reabsorption of ions into the surrounding blood capillaries
   (c) Afferent arteriole – Carries the blood away from the glomerulus towards the renal vein
   (d) Podocytes – Create minute space (slit pores) for the filtration of blood into the Bowman's capsule

5. Which one of the following is not a part of a renal pyramid? [AIPMT PRE 2011]

   (a) Convoluted tubules (b) Collecting ducts
   (c) Loops Henle (d) Peritubular capillaries

6. Uricotelic mode of passing out nitrogenous wastes is found in:

[AIPMT PRE 2011]

(a) Birds and annelids
(b) Amphibians and reptiles
(c) Insects and amphibians
(d) Reptiles and birds

7. Which one of the following statements is correct with respect to kidney function regulation?

[AIPMT PRE 2011]

(a) Exposure to cold temperature stimulates ADH release
(b) An increase in glomerular blood flow stimulates formation of angiotensin II
(c) During summer when body loses lot of water by evaporation, the release of ADH is suppressed
(d) When someone drinks lot of water ADH release is suppressed

8. A fall in glomerular filtration rate (GFR) activates:

[AIPMT MAINS 2012]

(a) Adrenal cortex to release aldosterone
(b) Adrenal medulla to release adrenaline
(c) Posterior pituitary to release vasopressin
(d) Juxta glomerular cells to release rennin

9. Which one of the following option gives the correct categorization of six animals according to the type of nitrogenous wastes {A (Ammonotelic), B (Ureotelic), C (Uricotelic)} they give out?

[AIPMT MAINS 2012]

(a) A: Frog, Lizards, B: Aquatic Amphibia, Humans, C: Cockroach, Pigeon
(b) A: Aquatic Amphibia, B: Frog, Humans, C: Pigeon, Lizards, Cockroack
(c) A: Aquatic Amphibia, B: Cockroach, Humans, C: Frog, Pigeon, Lizards
(d) A: Pigeon, Humans, B: Aquatic Amphibia, Lizards, C: Cockroach, Frog

10. The maximum amount of electrolytes and water (70–80 percent) from the glomerular filtrate is reabsorbed in which part of the nephron?

[AIPMT PRE 2012]

(a) Ascending limb of loop of Henle
(b) Distal convoluted tubule
(c) Proximal convoluted tubule
(d) Descending limb of loop of Henle

11. Figure shows humans urinary system with structures labelled A to D. Select option which correctly identifies them and gives their characteristics and / or functions.

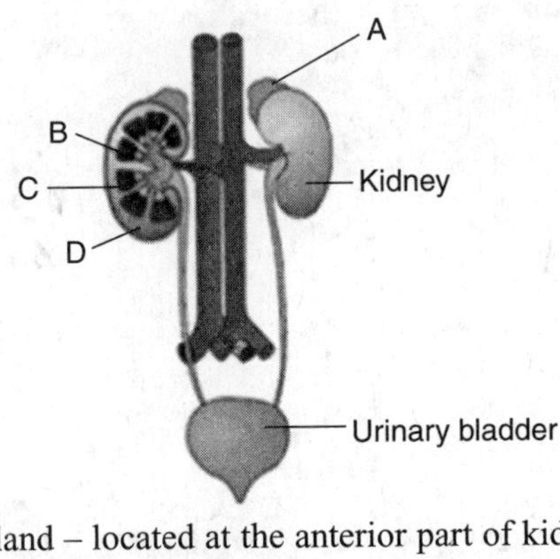

[AIPMT 2013]

(a) A: Adrenal gland – located at the anterior part of kidney, secrete catecholamine's, which stimulate glycogen breakdown
(b) B: Pelvis – broad funnel shaped space inner to hilum, directly connected to loop of Henle
(c) C: Medulla – inner zone of kidney and contains complete nephrons
(d) D: Cortex – outer part of kidney and do not contain any part of nephrons

12. Which of the following causes an increase in sodium reabsorption in the distal convoluted tubule? [AIPMT 2014]
(a) Increase in aldosterone levels
(b) Increase in antidiuretic hormone levels
(c) Decrease in aldosterone levels
(d) Decrease in antidiuretic hormone levels

13. Removal of proximal convoluted tubule from the nephron will result in : [AIPMT 2015]
(a) More diluted urine
(b) More concentrated urine
(c) No change in quality and quantity of urine
(d) No urine formation

14. Which of the following does not favour the formation of large quantities of dilute urine? [AIPMT 2015]
(a) Alcohol
(b) Caffeine
(c) Renin
(d) Atrial-natriuretic factor

15. Human urine in usually acidic because: [RE-AIPMT 2015]
(a) Excreted plasma proteins are acidic
(b) Potassium and sodium exchange generates acidity
(c) Hydrogen ions are actively secreted into the filtrate
(d) The sodium transporter exchange one hydrogen ion for each sodium ion, in peritubular capillaries.

Answer Keys

1. (d)	2. (d)	3. (a)	4. (a)	5. (d)	6. (b)	7. (b)	8. (d)	9. (b)	10. (d)
11. (c)	12. (b)	13. (b)	14. (a)	15. (c)	16. (b)	17. (b)	18. (b)	19. (c)	20. (c)
21. (b)	22. (c)	23. (a)	24. (d)	25. (b)	26. (d)	27. (d)	28. (a)	29. (b)	30. (a)
31. (d)	32. (b)	33. (a)	34. (d)	35. (d)	36. (a)	37. (a)	38. (c)	39. (b)	40. (a)
41. (d)	42. (c)	43. (d)	44. (a)	45. (d)	46. (c)	47. (b)	48. (b)	49. (c)	50. (d)
51. (c)	52. (d)	53. (c)	54. (a)	55. (a)	56. (b)	57. (b)	58. (c)	59. (b)	60. (b)
61. (a)	62. (c)	63. (a)	64. (d)	65. (b)	66. (c)	67. (d)	68. (b)	69. (a)	70. (d)
71. (c)	72. (c)	73. (b)	74. (c)	75. (d)	76. (c)	77. (a)	78. (d)	79. (b)	80. (d)
81. (d)	82. (c)	83. (d)	84. (d)	85. (c)	86. (a)	87. (d)	88. (d)	89. (b)	90. (d)
91. (c)	92. (b)	93. (d)	94. (c)	95. (b)	96. (b)	97. (c)	98. (a)	99. (a)	100. (d)
101. (b)	102. (b)	103. (b)	104. (b)	105. (d)	106. (d)	107. (a)	108. (d)	109. (d)	110. (c)
111. (d)	112. (b)	113. (a)	114. (a)	115. (a)	116. (b)	117. (d)	118. (b)	119. (a)	120. (b)
121. (d)	122. (c)	123. (d)	124. (c)	125. (a)	126. (d)	127. (b)	128. (d)	129. (c)	130. (c)
131. (b)	132. (b)	133. (b)	134. (c)	135. (d)	136. (a)	137. (a)	138. (b)	139. (c)	140. (a)
141. (c)	142. (a)	143. (b)	144. (c)	145. (c)	146. (b)	147. (d)	148. (d)	149. (c)	150. (b)
151. (d)	152. (b)	153. (b)	154. (a)	155. (b)	156. (a)	157. (b)	158. (a)	159. (c)	160. (d)
161. (a)	162. (a)	163. (a)	164. (a)						

AIPMT Previous Year Questions

1. (b)	2. (c)	3. (d)	4. (d)	5. (a)	6. (d)	7. (d)	8. (d)	9. (b)	10. (c)
11. (a)	12. (a)	13. (a)	14. (c)	15. (c)					

CHAPTER

20

Locomotion and Movement

1. Which of the following is a simple form of movement?
   (a) Streaming of protoplasm in amoeba
   (b) Ciliary movement in paramecium
   (c) Flagellar movement in Euglena
   (d) All
2. The movement results in a change of place or location is known as
   (a) Contraction
   (b) Adduction
   (c) Abduction
   (d) Locomotion
3. Select the correct matching:

Column I		Column II		Column III
A. Paramecium	–	1. Cilia	–	X. Movement of food through cytopharynx and locomotion.
B. Hydra	–	2. Tentacles	–	Y. Capturing of prey and for locomotion
C. Human	–	3. Limbs	–	Z. Changes in body posture and for locomotion

   (a) A–1–X, B–2–Y, C–3–Z
   (b) A–1–Z, B–3–X, C–2–Y
   (c) A–3–Z, B–1–X, C–2–Y
   (d) A–2–Y, B–3–X, C–1–Z
4. Select the incorrect statement?
   (a) Plant and animal both exhibit movement
   (b) All locomotion are movement but all movement are not locomotion
   (c) Methods of locomotion performed by animal very with their habitats and the demand of the situation
   (d) None
5. Locomotion is used for
   (A) Search of food and Shelter
   (B) Search for mate
   (C) Search for suitable breeding ground
   (D) Escaping from enemies/Predators
   (a) All except B (b) All except C (c) All except D (d) All
6. Which is the movement exhibited by cell of a human body?
   (a) Amoeboid (b) Ciliary (c) Fagellar (d) All
7. Which of the following cells exhibit amoeboid movement?
   (a) Macrophages (b) Leucocytes (c) RBC (d) Both (a) and (b)
8. Which of the following is correct about pseudopodia?
   (a) Formed by streaming of protoplasm
   (b) Formed in amoeba and neutrophile
   (c) Both
   (d) None

9. Which of the following is involved in amoeboid movement?
(a) Centriole (b) Cilia
(c) Flagella (d) Microfilament

10. Which of the following organs is lined with cilia?
(a) Fallopian tube (b) Trachea (c) Intestine (d) Both (a) and (b)

11. Locomotion requires a perfect coordinated activity of
(a) muscular system (b) skeletal system (c) neural system (d) all

12. Muscle is derived from
(a) Mesoderm (b) Ectoderm (c) Endoderm (d) All

13. Muscle forms __________ % of adult human body
(a) 30–40% (b) 40–50% (c) 50–60% (d) 60–70%

14. Muscles are characterized by
(a) Excitability and Contractility (b) Extensibility
(c) Elasticity (d) All

15. Muscles can be classified on which of the following criterion?
(a) Location (b) Appearance
(c) Nature of regulation of their activities (d) All

16. How many types of muscles can be identified depending upon the location?
(a) 1 (b) 2 (c) 3 (d) 4

17. Which of the following is incorrect about skeletal muscles?
(a) Striped appearance under microscope hence called striated muscle
(b) They are Voluntary muscle
(c) Primarily involved in locomotory actions and changes of body postures
(d) They are Involuntary muscles

18. Which of the following is incorrect about visceral muscles?
(a) Non-striated muscle (Smooth muscle)
(b) Involuntary muscle
(c) Located in inner walls of hollow visceral organs of the body
(d) They are under in voluntary control

19. Smooth muscles help in
(a) transportation of food through the digestive tract
(b) transfer of gametes through genital tract
(c) micturition by urinary bladder
(d) all

20. Cardiac muscle is characterized by
(a) striated appearance (b) involuntary control
(c) branching pattern (d) all

21. Which muscle is not under direct control of nervous system?
(a) Skeletal (Striated muscles) (b) Smooth (Non-striated muscles)
(c) Cardiac muscles (d) All

22. Muscle fibre is a
(a) anatomical unit of muscle (b) physiological unit of muscle
(c) biochemical unit of muscle (d) none

23. Identify A, B, C and D in the given figure.

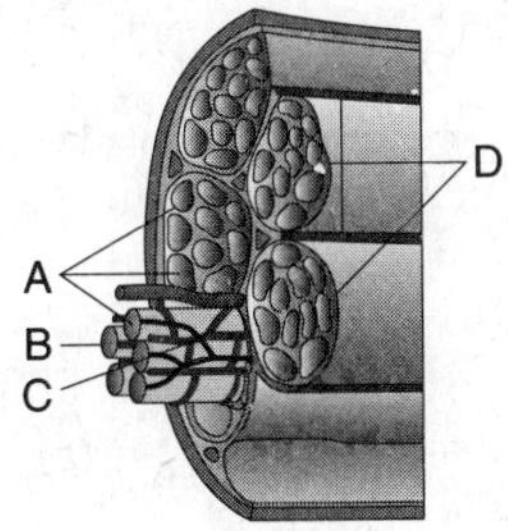

(a) A–Sarcolemma, B–Blood capillary, C–Fascicle (muscle bundle), D–Muscle fibre (muscle cell)
(b) A–Blood capillary, B–Muscle fibre (muscle cell), C–Fascicle (muscle bundle), D–Sarcolemma
(c) A–Sacrolemma, B–Muscle fibre (muscle cell), C–Fesicle (muscle bundle), D–Blood capillary
(d) A–Muscle fibre (muscle cell), B–Sarcolemma, C–Blood capillary, D–Fascicle (muscle bundles)

24. Each organized skeletal muscle in our body is made up of a number of muscle bundles or fascicles held together by a common collagenous connective tissue layer called
(a) Tunicine (b) Fascia (c) Pellicle (d) Capsule

25. Select the correct matching from the following:
(a) Plasma membrane of muscle fibre – Sarcolemma
(b) Cytoplasm of muscle fiber – Sarcoplasm
(c) Endoplasmic reticulum of muscle fiber – Sarcoplasmic reticulum
(d) All

26. Sarcoplasmic reticulum is a storehouse of which ion
(a) Ca^{2+} (b) Na^+ (c) K^+ (d) Fe^{2+}

27. Sarcolemma is a membrane found over
(a) nerve fibre (b) cardiac muscle
(c) skeletal muscle fibre (d) heart

28. The functional unit of the contractile system in the striped muscle is
(a) Z-band (b) A-band (c) Myofibril (d) Sarcomere

29. Contraction of a muscle is caused by
(a) Myosin (b) Actin (c) ATP (d) Actomyosin

30. The dark bands (A-bands) of a skeletal muscle are known as
(a) Isotropic bands (b) Anisotropic bands
(c) Intercalated disc (d) Cross bridges

31. The light bands (I-bands) of a skeletal muscles are known as
(a) Isotropic bands (b) Anisotropic bands
(c) Intercalated disc (d) Cross bridges

32. Ciliary muscles are found in
(a) Diaphragm of a mammal
(b) Eyes of vertebrates
(c) Heart of vertebrates
(d) Stomach of frog

33. Intercostal muscles are found in
(a) Fingers (b) Thoracic ribs (c) Femur (d) Radius-ulna

34. The special contractile protein actin is found in
(a) thick filaments of A-bands
(b) thin filaments of I-bands
(c) both thick and thin bands
(d) whole of myofibril

35. Striped muscles have
(a) one nucleus (b) many nuclei (c) two nuclei (d) no nuclei

36. Contractile fibrils of muscles are called
(a) neurofibrils (b) collagen fibres (c) myofibrils (d) elastin

37. Myofibrils show alternate dark and light bands in
(a) Cardiac muscles
(b) Smooth muscles
(c) Skeletal muscles
(d) both (a) and (c)

38. Select the correct statement:
(a) A-band is made up of thick myosin filament
(b) H-zone is present in the middle of A-band
(c) Actin and myosin are polymerised protein with contractility
(d) All

39. Match the columns:

Column I		**Column II**
(A) Inflammation of joints	–	(1) H-zone
(B) Protein of thick filament	–	(2) Myosin
(C) Protein of thin filament	–	(3) Actin
(D) The central part of thick filament not overlapped by thin filament	–	(4) Arthritis

(a) A–1, B–2, C–3, D–4
(b) A–1, B–3, C–2, D–4
(c) A–4, B–1, C–2, D–3
(d) A–4, B–2, C–3, D–1

40. Which of the following statements about the striated muscles is false?
1. Thick filaments in the 'A' band are also held together in the middle of this band by a thin fibrous membrane called 'M' line.
2. In the centre of each 'I' band is an elastic fibre called 'Z' line which bisects it.
3. The thin filaments are firmly attached to the 'Z' line.
4. This central part of thick filament, not overlapped by thin filaments is called the 'H' zone.

(a) All (b) only 2 (c) 1 and 4 only (d) None

41. Which of the following statements about the molecular arrangement of actin in myofibrils is incorrect?
1. Each actin (thin) filament is made of two 'F' (filamentous) actins helically wound to each other.
2. Each 'F' actin is a polymer of monomeric 'G' (Globular) actins.
3. Two filaments of another protein, tropomyosin also run close to the 'F' actins throughout its length.
4. A complex protein Troponin is distributed at regular intervals on the tropomyosin.

(a) 1, 2 only (b) 3 only (c) only 4 (d) None

42. Select the total number of true statement from the following.

1. Each myosin (thick) filament is also a polymerised protein.
2. Many monomeric proteins called Meromyosins constitute one thick filament.
3. Each meromyosin has two important parts, a globular head with a short arm and a tail, the former being called the heavy meromyosin (HMM) and thelatter, the light meromyosin (LMM).
4. The HMM component, i.e., the head and short arm projects outwards at regular distance and angle from each other from the surface of a polymerised myosin filament and is known as cross arm.
5. The globular head is an active ATPase enzyme and has binding sites for ATP and active sites for actin.

(a) 1 (b) 2 (c) 4 (d) 5

43. Binding of Ca^{2+} with _____ in the skeletal muscles and leads to the exposure of the binding site for _____ on the filament _____.

(a) Troponin, myosin, actin (b) Troponin, actin, relaxin
(c) Actin, myosin, troponin (d) Tropomysin, myosis, actin

44. Following is the figure of actin (thin) filaments. Identify A, B and C.

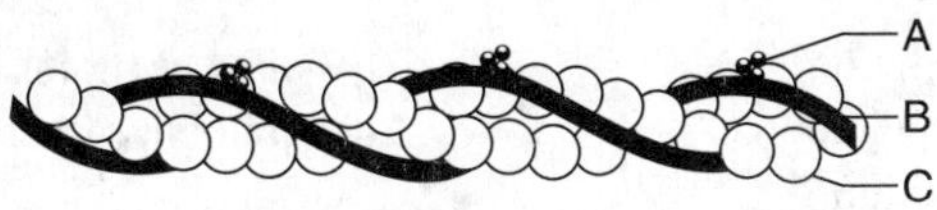

(a) A–Tropomyosin, B–Troponin, C–F actin
(b) A–Tropomyosin, B–Myosin, C–F Tropomyosin
(c) A–Troponin, B–Tropomyosin, C–Myosin
(d) A–Troponin, B–Tropomyosin, C–F actin

45.

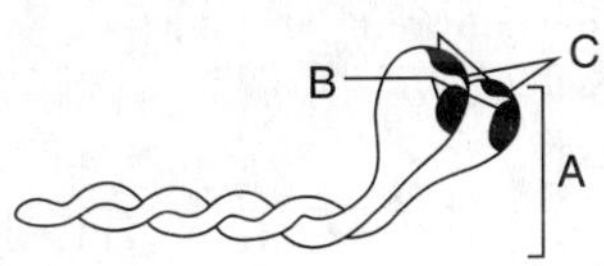

The above figure is related to the myosin monomer (meromyosin). Identify A to C.

(a) A–head, B–cross arm, C–GTP binding sites
(b) A–Cross arm, B–ATP Binding sites, C–Head
(c) A–head, B–cross arm, C–ATP binding sites
(d) A–cross arm, B–head C–ATP binding sites

46. Identify A–D in the below figure.

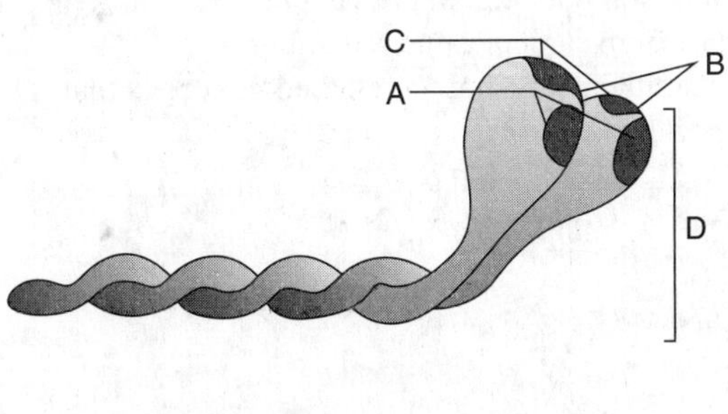

(a) A–Actin binding sites, B–Head, C–Cross arm, D–ATP binding sites
(b) A–Cross arm, B–Actin binding sites, C–ATP binding sites, D–Head
(c) A–ATP binding sites, B–Head, C–Actin binding sites, D–Cross arm
(d) A–Head, B–Cross arm, C–ATP binding sites, D–Actin binding sites

47. Mechanism of muscle contraction is best explained by
(a) all or no law
(b) sliding filament theory
(c) Balckmann's law
(d) all

48. ATP provides energy for muscle contraction by allowing for
(a) an action potential formation in his muscle cell
(b) cross-bridge detachment of myosin from actin
(c) cross-bridge attachment of myosin to actin
(d) release of Ca^{2+} from sarcoplasmic reticulum

49. A motor unit is best described as
(a) all the nerve fibres and muscle fibres in a single muscle bundle
(b) one muscle fibres and its single nerve fibre
(c) a single motor neuron and all the muscle fibres that it innervates
(d) as the neuron which carries the message from muscle to CNS

50. Motor end plate is a
(a) neuromuscular junction
(b) plate of motor neuron
(c) dendron of motor neuron
(d) gradient of protein motive force

51. During muscle contraction,
(a) chemical energy is changed into electrical energy
(b) chemical energy is changed into mechanical energy
(c) chemical energy is changed into physical energy
(d) mechanical energy is changed into chemical energy

52. Electron microscopic studies of the sarcomeres have revealed that during muscle contraction
(a) the width of A-band remains constant
(b) the width of the H-zone increases
(c) the width of I-band increases
(d) the diameter of the fibre increases

53. According to the sliding filament theory
(a) actin (thin filament) moves over myosin (thick filament)
(b) myosin moves over actin
(c) both myosin and actin move on each other
(d) none

54. Put the following statement in proper order to describe muscle contraction.
1. Signal sent by CNS via motor neuron.
2. Generation of action potential in the sarcolemma.
3. Release of Ca^{+2} from sarcoplasmic reticulum
4. The neurotransmitter acetycholine released motorend plate.
5. Sarcomere shortern

(a) 1→2→4→3→5
(b) 1→4→2→3→5
(c) 1→4→3→2→5
(d) 5→4→3→2→1

55. Go through the following diagram describing muscle contraction. Identify A to E.

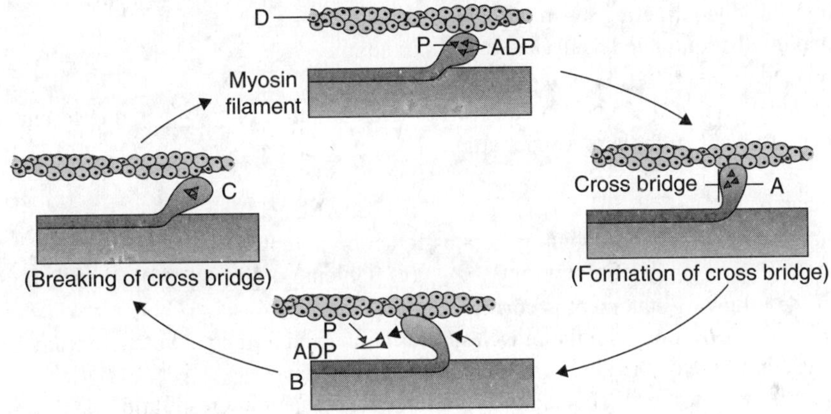

(a) A–Sliding/Rotation, B–Actin Filament, C–Myosin Head, D–ATP
(b) A–Myosin head, B–Sliding/Rotation, C–ATP, D–Actin filament
(c) A–Sliding/Rotation, B–Myosin head, C–Actin Filament, D–ATP
(d) A–Actin Filament, B–Sliding/Rotation, C–ATP, D–Myosin head

56. Which of the following muscle gets into fatigue very early?
(a) Skeletal muscle (b) Smooth muscle
(c) Cardiac muscle (d) All

57. Relaxation of muscle is due to the
(a) pumping of Ca^{+2} into sarcoplasmic cisternae
(b) presence of ATP
(c) conformational change in troponin and masking of actin filaments
(d) both (a) and (c)

58.

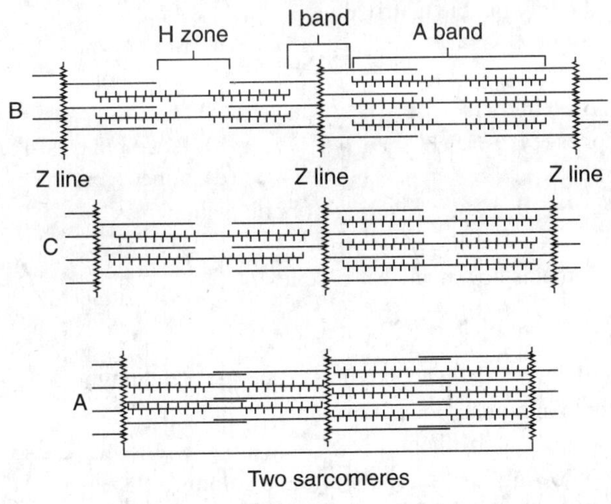

The diagrams given above 3 different condition of sarcomeres. Identify these conditions:

(a) A–contracting, B–relaxed, C–maximally contracted
(b) A–relaxed, B–contracting, C–maximally contracted
(c) A–maximally contracted, B–Relaxed, C–contracting
(d) A–relaxed, B–maximally contracted, C–contracting

59. Repeated activation of the muscles can lead to accumulation of _______ due to anaerobic breakdown of glycogen in there, cause fatigue
(a) Ethanol (b) Lactic acid
(c) Citric acid (d) Butyric acid

60. A neurotransmitter ________ which generates an action potential in the sarcolemma.
(a) GABA (b) Epinephrine (c) Glycine (d) Acetyt choline

61. Which of the following statement is correct?
(a) A motor neuron along with the muscles fibres connected to it constitute a motor unit
(b) The reaction time of the fibres can vary in different muscles
(c) Muscle fatigue is due to lactic acid formation due to anaerobic respiration
(d) All

62. The protein which maintains the muscular storage of oxygen is
(a) Myoglobin (b) Actomyosin (c) Myosin (d) Haemoglobin

63. Which is not a correct difference between white and red muscles fibre?

White Muscle fibre		**Red muscle fibre**
1. Less Myoglobin	–	1. More myglobin
2. Number of mitochondria less	–	2. Number of mitochondria more
3. Amount of Sarcoplasmic reticulum low	–	3. Amount of Sarcoplasmic reticulum high
4. Aerobic muscle	–	4. Anaerobic muscle

(a) 1 (b) 2 (c) 3 (d) 4

64. Skeletal system consists of
(a) framework of bone (b) few Cartilages
(c) both (d) none

65. Cartilage has slightly pliable matrix due to
(a) Ca^{2+} (b) Mg^{2+}
(c) chondroitin salts (d) phosphorus

66. Skull is composed of
(a) cranial bones (8) (b) facial bones (14)
(c) both (d) none

67. The hard and protective outer covering of brain is known as
(a) Cranium (b) Condyle (c) Meninges (d) All

68. Human body contains how many ear osscíles?
(a) 3 (b) 4 (c) 5 (d) 6

69. Human skull is
(a) Monocondylic (b) Dicondylic (c) Tricondylic (d) Acondylic

70. Vertebral column in human body is present
(a) Dorsally (b) Ventrally (c) Laterally (d) All

71. Which of the following is true about vertebral column?
(a) Each vertebra in vertebral column has a central hollow protein (Neural canal) through which spinal cord pass
(b) The first vertebra in vertebral column is atlas and it articulates with the occipital condyle

(c) Vertebral column protects spinal cord, supports the head and serves as the point of attachment for the ribs and musculature of the back
(d) All

72. Bone present on ventral midline of thorax
(a) Vertebral column (b) Ribs
(c) Scapula (d) Sternum

73. Which of the following is incorrect about ribs?
(a) Each rib is a thin and cat bone connected dorsally to the vertebral column and ventrally to the sternum
(b) Ribs has two articulation surfaces on its dorsal end which are called bicephalic
(c) Ventrally ribs are connected to sternum by elastic cartilage
(d) First 7 pairs are called true ribs. 8, 9 and 10th pair is known as false (vertebracondral) ribs, and 2 pair (11th and 12th) known as floating ribs

74. Scapula is an example of
(a) Long bone (b) short bone (c) flat bone (d) irregular bone

75. Number of bones in the adult human body is
(a) 206 (b) 406 (c) 106 (d) 306

76. Number of bones in human axial skeleton is
(a) 120 (b) 142 (c) 80 (d) 206

77. The number of bones in the skull of man is
(a) 14 (b) 28 (c) 8 (d) 22

78. Cranium of man is made up of
(a) 8 bones (b) 12 bones (c) 16 bones (d) 14 bones

79. Vertebral column of human body is made up of
(a) 33 vertebrae (b) 52 vertebrae (c) 45 vertebrae (d) 23 vertebrae

80. The number of bones in the vertebral column of man is
(a) 32 (b) 26 (c) 35 (d) 20

81. Human vertebral formula is
(a) C7T12L5S5Cd4 (b) C7T9L5S4Cd1 (c) C7T12L5S1Cd1 (d) C7T12L4S4Cd1

82. The vertebra which bears the whole weight of the skull is
(a) Atlas (b) Axis (c) Cervical (d) Sacral

83. In man, ribs are attached to
(a) Clavicle (b) Ileum (c) Sternum (d) Scapula

84. In the case of most of the mammals including man and Giraffe, the numbers of cervical vertebrae are
(a) 8 (b) 7 (c) 9 (d) 10

85. The eighth and ninth ribs are known as false ribs because their external portions are attached to
(a) xiphisternum (b) costa of 7th rib
(c) they have no costa (d) they are not true ribs

86. Number of bones of face is
(a) 12 (b) 30 (c) 40 (d) 14

87. Axial skeleton is made up of
(a) Skull only (b) Sternum only
(c) Complete vertebral column (d) All

88. What is the right sequence of bones in the ear ossicles of a mammal starting from the tympanum inwards?
(a) Malleus, Incus, Stapes (b) Malleus, Stapes, Incus
(c) Incus, Malleus, Stapes (d) Stapes, Incus, Malleus

89. Malleus is a part of
(a) fore limbs of vertebrates (b) reproductive organs of cockroach
(c) auditory ossicles of middle ear of human (d) skull of frog

90. In human beings, the thoracic basket is composed of
(a) Ribs and thoracic vertebrae (b) Ribs and sternum
(c) Ribs, sternum and vertebrae (d) Ribs, sternum and thoracic vertebrae

91. The bone which is U-shaped is
(a) Frontal (b) Vomer (c) Hyoid (d) Molar

92. Match the following:

Bone		Number
1. Skull	–	1. 24
2. Vertebrae	–	2. 60
3. Ribs	–	3. 22
4. Sternum	–	4. 1
5. Pectoral girdles	–	5. 2
6. Arms	–	6. 4
7. Ear ossicles	–	7. 6
8. Pelvic girdles	–	8. 33

The correct pairing sequence is
(a) 8–3, 1–4, 6–2, 5–7 (b) 3–8, 1–4, 6–2, 7–5
(c) 3–8, 1–4, 2–6, 7–5 (d) None

93. The number of floating ribs in human body is
(a) 6 pairs (b) 3 pairs (c) 5 pairs (d) 2 pairs

94. Foramen magnum, occipital condyles are found in
(a) Parietal bone (b) Ethmoid bone (c) Sphenoid bone (d) Occipital bone

95. The acromion process articulates with the
(a) Scapula (b) Clavicle
(c) Ribs (d) Vertebral column

96. The number of lumbar vertebrae in human vertebral column is
(a) 12 (b) 7 (c) 5 (d) 2

97. How many ribs are present in human beings?
(a) 6 pairs (b) 9 pairs (c) 12 pairs (d) 15 pairs

98. The cup-shaped cavity for the articulation of the head of the femur is called
(a) Glenoid cavity (b) Acetabulum (c) Obturator (d) Sigmoid notch

99. Ribs attached to sternum are
(a) First seven pairs (b) All ten ribs
(c) First ten rib pairs (d) First five rib pairs

100. Which part is indicated as A, B, C, D, and E in the given figure?

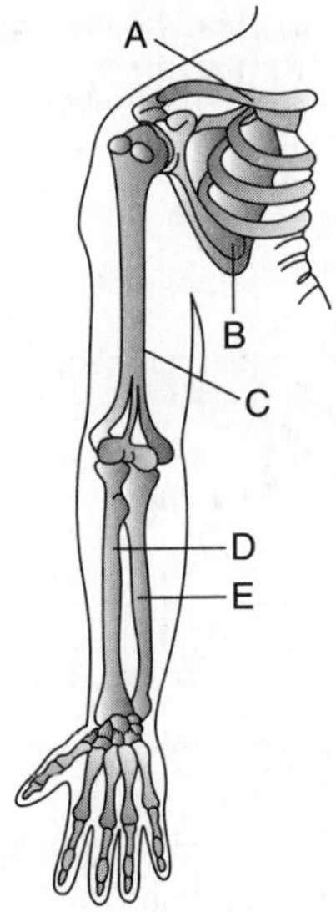

(a) A–Clavicle, B–Scapula, C–Humerus, D–Radius, E–Ulna
(b) A–Humerus, B–Clavicle, C–Ulna, D–Scapula, E–Radius
(c) A–Ulna, B–Humerus, C–Clavicle, D–Radius, E–Scapula
(d) A–Radius, B–Ulna, C–Scapula, D–Clavicle, D–Humerus

101. In human radius and ulna are (shown in diagram of question number 100.)
(a) completely fused together
(b) completely separated
(c) fused in middle and separated at both the ends
(d) separated but united at both the ends

102. A shallow depression in the scapula which receives the head of the upper arm bone is known as the
(a) acetabulum (b) neural arch
(c) glenoid cavity (d) none

103. Patella, the sesamoid bone is also known as
(a) pisiform (b) replacing bone
(c) knee cap (d) none

104. Humerus bone is situated in
(a) thigh (b) lower arm (c) upper arm (d) shank

105. The cup-shaped structure of pelvic girdle, the acetabulum in man is formed by
(a) ilium, ischium and pubis (b) ilium, ischium and cotyloid
(c) ilium and ischium (d) ilium and cotyloid

106. The pectoral and pelvic girdles and the bones of limb form
(a) axial skeleton (b) appendicular skeleton
(c) visceral skeleton (d) outer skeleton

107. The total number of bones in your right arm is
(a) 30 (b) 32 (c) 35 (d) 40

108. An acromian process is characteristically found in mammals in
(a) Pelvic girdle (b) Pectoral girdle (c) Skull (d) Sternum

109. Which one of the following component is the part of pectoral girdle?
(a) Acetabulum (b) Hilum (c) Sternum (d) Glenoid cavity

110. Pelvic girdle of human consist of
(a) ilium, ischium and pubis (b) ilium, ischium and coracoid
(c) coracoid, scapula and clavicle (d) ilium, coracoid and scapula

111. Innominate or hip bone is formed by the fusion of how many bones
(a) 2 (b) 3 (c) 4 (d) 5

112. Phallangeal formula of hand of man is
(a) 1, 2, 2, 2, 2 (b) 2, 1, 1, 1, 1 (c) 2, 3, 3, 3, 3 (d) 2, 3, 3, 2, 2

113. Appendicular skeleton includes all except
(a) hind limb (b) fore limb
(c) amphicoelous vertebra (d) pectoral and pelvic girdle

114. Patella is associated with
(a) elbow (b) knee (c) neck (d) wrist

115. Which one of the cartilage helps in early birth of a child, without damage to the pelvic girdle?
(a) Hyaline cartilage (b) Elastic cartilage
(c) Calcified cartilage (d) Fibrous cartilage

116. Total number of bones in the hind limb of a man is
(a) 14 (b) 21 (c) 24 (d) 30

117. Which of the following is an example of appendicular skeleton?
(a) Bones of skull (b) Bones of vertebral column
(c) Ribs (d) Bones of fore and hind limbs

118. Longest bone of human body is
(a) femur (thigh bones) (b) tibia
(c) patella (knee cap) (d) humerus

119. All are bones of forelimb except
(a) radius (b) ulna (c) humerus (d) tibia

120. Carpals, metacarpals, tarsals, Metatarsals are ____ and ____ in numbers respectively
(a) 8, 5, 7, 5 (b) 8, 7, 5, 5 (c) 8, 5, 8, 5 (d) 8, 5, 5, 7

121. How many ankle bones are present in the human body?
(a) 7 (b) 5 (c) 8 (d) 14

122. Each girdle of appendicular skeleton is made up of
(a) two halves (b) three halves (c) four halves (d) five halves

123. Each of Pectoral girdle is consist of
(a) Clavicle (b) Scapula (c) Humerus (d) Both (a) and (b)

124. Scapula is a large triangular and flat bone situated in the dorsal part of the thorax between ____ to ____ ribs.
(a) 2, 5 (b) 2, 7 (c) 2, 6 (d) 2, 8

125. Which of the folowing is correct about clavicle?
(a) Known as collar bone (b) Long bone
(c) It has two curvatures (d) All

126. Scapula has slightly elevated ridge called the spine, which projects as a flat, expanded process known as
(a) coracoid
(b) greater tubercle
(c) acromian
(d) lesser tubercle

127. Joints are lubricated by
(a) epidermis
(b) dermis
(c) tympanic membrane
(d) synovial fluid

128. Ball and socket joints can be seen in
(a) wrist (b) fingers (c) neck (d) shoulders

129. The knee joint in between the thigh and lower leg is a
(a) Hinge joint (b) Gliding joint (c) Pivot joint (d) Fixed joint

130. When the head of humerus fits into glenoid cavity, joint is
(a) Ball and socket joint
(b) Hinge joint
(c) Pivot joint
(d) Saddle joint

131. The joint between the carpal bones and tarsal bones is
(a) Gliding joint
(b) Ball and socket joint
(c) Hinge joint
(d) Saddle joint

132. Joint between femur and tibio–fibula is
(a) Hinge joint (b) Saddle joint (c) Pivot joint (d) Imperfect joint

133. Articulation of the atlas with the axis is an example of
(a) Hinge joint
(b) Ball and socket joint
(c) Gliding joint
(d) Pivot joint

134. Sutural joints are found between
(a) Parietals of skull
(b) Humerus and radio-ulna
(c) Glenoid cavity and pectoral girdle
(d) Thumb and metatarsal

135. Synovial joints is
(a) Pivot joint
(b) Hinge joint
(c) Ball and socket joint
(d) All

136. Which of the following pairs is correctly matched?
(a) Hinge joint – Between vertebrae
(b) Gliding joint – Between carpal and metacarpal of thumb
(c) Cartilaginous joint – between carpels
(d) Fibrous joint – Flat skull bones

137. What is the joint between sternum and the ribs in humans?
(a) Fibrous joint
(b) Gliding joint
(c) Cartilaginous joint
(d) Angular joint

138. The shoulder and hip are
(a) Pivot joint
(b) Hinge joint
(c) ellipsoid joint
(d) ball and socket joint

139. Symphysis is made up of
(a) fibro cartilage (b) synovial fluid (c) elastic cartilage (d) hyaline cartilage

140. Inflammation of joints due to accumulation of uric acid crystals occurs in
(a) Osteoporosis (b) Gout (c) Tetany (d) Rickets

141. Myasthenia gravis is
   (a) auto immune disorder affecting neuromuscular junction leading to fatigue, weakening and paralysis of skeletal muscle
   (b) progressive degeneration of skeletal muscle mostly due to genetic disorder
   (c) rapid spasms (wild contractions) in muscle due to low Ca^{++} in body fluid
   (d) inflammation of joints
142. Progressive degeneration of skeletal muscle, mostly due to genetic disorder, is
   (a) Osteoporosis (b) Gout
   (c) Tetany (d) Muscular dystrophy
143. Tetany is due to
   (a) low Ca^{2+}in body fluid
   (b) high Ca^{2+}in body fluid
   (c) high concentration of uric acid in boy fluid
   (d) all
144. Which is age-related disorder characterized by decreased bone mass and increased chances of fractures. Decreased levels of estrogen are a common cause.
   (a) Osteoporosis (b) Gout
   (c) Tetany (d) Muscular dystrophy
145. Smooth muscle fibres are
   (a) cylindrical, unbranched, striated, multinucleate and voluntary
   (b) spindle-shaped, unbranched, non-striated, uninucleate and involuntary
   (c) cylindrical, unbranched, non-striated, multinucleate and involuntary
   (d) spindle-shaped, unbranched, striated, uninucleate and voluntary

*Read the **assertion** and **reason** carefully to mark the correct option out of the options given below:*

(a) If both the assertion and the reason are true and the reason is a correct explanation of the assertion
(b) If both the assertion and reason are true but the reason is not a correct explanation of the assertion
(c) If the assertion is true but the reason is false
(d) If both the assertion and reason are false

146. **Assertion:** Ciliary movement occurs in most of our internal tubular organs which are lined by ciliated epithelium.
   Reason: Passage of ova through the female reproductive tract is also facilitated by the ciliary movement.
147. **Assertion:** All locomotions are movements but all movements are not locomotion.
   Reason: Movement is one of the significant features of living beings.
148. **Assertion:** Ball and socket joints are the most mobile joints.
   Reason: Synovial fluid is present here in synovial cavity such arrangement allows considerable movement.
149. **Assertion:** Arthritis or inflammation of a joint makes the joint painful.
   Reason: Some toxic substances are deposited at the joint.

150. **Assertion:** Movement of body parts serves to change the body posture.
Reason: Body parts move in relation to body axis.

151. **Assertion:** There are similarities between the locomotion of unicellular organisms and multi-cellular animal.
Reason: Ciliary, flagellar and amoeboid movement occur in unicellular organisms.

152. **Assertion:** White muscle fibres have very less quantity of myoglobin.
Reason: White muscle fibres have high number of sarcoplasmic reticulum.

153. **Assertion:** Each myosin filament is a polemerised carbohydrate.
Reason: Actin filament is made up of meromysin.

154. **Assertion:** Skeleton helps in blood cell formation.
Reason: Blood flows through skeleton.

155. **Assertion:** Biceps and triceps are called antagonistic muscles.
Reason: This is due to the fact that they contract and relax together.

156. **Assertion:** Muscle contraction force increases with rise in strength of stimulus.
Reason: This is due to increased contraction of individual muscle fibres with increase in stimulus strength.

157. **Assertion:** Muscle as a whole doesn't obey All or None law.
Reason: Each muscle fibre contracts maximally whenever it contracts.

AIPMT PREVIOUS YEAR QUESTIONS

1. Which one of the following pairs of structures is correctly matched with their corrected description?

[AIPMT MAINS 2010]

Structures		**Description**
(a) Tibia and fibula	→	Both form parts of knee joint
(b) Cartilage and cornea	→	No blood supply but do require oxygen for respiratory need
(c) Shoulder joint and elbow joint	→	Ball and socket type of joint
(d) Premolars and molars	→	20 in all and 3 rooted

2. Which one of the following is the correct description of a certain part of a normal human skeleton?

[AIPMT MAINS 2010]

(a) Parietal bone and the temporal bone of the skull are joined by fibrous joint
(b) First vertebra is axis which articulates with the occipital condyles
(c) The 9th and 10th pairs of ribs are called the floating ribs
(d) Glenoid cavity is a depression to which the thigh bone articulates

3. There of the following pairs of the human skeletal parts are correctly matched with their respective inclusive skeletal category and one pair is not matched. Identify the non-matching pair

[AIPMT MAINS 2011]

Pair of skeletal parts	**Category**
(a) Sternum and ribs	Axial skeleton
(b) Clavicle and glenoid cavity	Pelvic girdle
(c) Humerus and ulna	Appendicular skeleton
(d) Malleus and stapes	Ear ossicles

4. Which one of the following pairs of chemical substances is correctly categorized? [AIPMT MAINS 2012]
   (a) Pepsin and prolactin - Two digestive enzymes secreted in stomach
   (b) Troponin and myosin - Complex proteins in striated muscles
   (c) Secretin and rhodopsin - Polypeptide hormones
   (d) Calcitonin and thymosin - Thyroid hormones
5. Select the correct statement regarding the specific disorder of muscular or skeletal system: [AIPMT PRE 2012]
   (a) Muscular dystrophy: age related shortening of muscles
   (b) Osteporosis: decrease in bone mass and higher chances of fractures with advancing age
   (c) Myasthenia gravis: Auto immune disorder which inhibits sliding of myosin filaments
   (d) Gout: inflammation of joints due to extra deposition of calcium
6. The H – zone in the skeletal muscles fibre is due to: [AIPMT 2013]
   (a) The absence of myofibrils in the central portion of A – band
   (b) The central gap between myosin filaments in the A – band
   (c) The central gap between actin filaments extending through myosin filaments in the A – band
   (d) Extension of myosin filaments in the central portion of the A – band
7. Select the correct statement with respect to locomotion in humans: [AIPMT 2013]
   (a) A decreased level of progesterone causes osteoporosis in old people
   (b) Accumulation of uric acid crystals in joints causes their inflammation
   (c) The vertebral column has 10 thoracic vertebrae
   (d) The joint between adjacent vertebrae is a fibrous joint
8. The characteristics and an example of a synovial joint in humans is: [AIPMT 2013]

	Characteristics		Examples
(a)	Fluid cartilage between two bones, limited movements	→	Knee joint
(b)	Fluid filled between two joints, provides cushion	→	Skull bones
(c)	Fluid filled synovial cavity between two bones	→	Joint between atlas and axis
(d)	Lymph filled between two bones, limited movement	→	Gliding joint between carpals

9. Select the correct matching of the type of the joint with the example in human skeletal system: [AIPMT 2014]

	Type of joint	Example
(a)	Cartilaginous joint	Between frontal and pariental
(b)	Pivot joint	Between third and fourth cervical vertebrae
(c)	Hinge joint	Between humerus and pectoral girdle
(d)	Gliding joint	Between carpals

10. Stimulation of a muscle fiber by a motor neuron occurs at: [AIPMT 2014]
    (a) The neuromuscular junction
    (b) The transverse tubules
    (c) The myofibril
    (d) The sacroplasmic reticulum

11. Sliding filament theory can be best explained as:

[AIPMT 2015]

(a) When myofilaments slide pass each other Actin filaments shorten while Myosin filament do not shorten
(b) Actin and Myosin filaments shorten and slide pass each other
(c) Actin and Myosin filaments do not shorten but rather slide pass each other
(d) When myofilaments slide pass each other, Myosin filaments shorten while Actin filaments do not shorten

12. Glenoid cavity articulates :

[AIPMT 2015]

(a) Clavicle with acromion (b) Scapula with acromion
(c) Clavicle with scapula (d) Humerus with scapula

13. Which of the following joints would hallow no movement?

[RE-AIPMT 2015]

(a) Cartilaginous joint (b) Synovial joint
(c) Ball and Socket joint (d) Fibrous joint

14. Which of the following is not a function of the skeletal system?

[RE-AIPMT 2015]

(a) Storage of minerals (b) Production of body heat
(c) Locomotion (d) Production of erythrocytes

Answer Keys

1. (a)	2. (d)	3. (a)	4. (d)	5. (d)	6. (d)	7. (d)	8. (c)	9. (d)	10. (d)
11. (d)	12. (a)	13. (b)	14. (d)	15. (d)	16. (c)	17. (d)	18. (d)	19. (d)	20. (d)
21. (c)	22. (a)	23. (d)	24. (b)	25. (d)	26. (a)	27. (c)	28. (d)	29. (d)	30. (b)
31. (a)	32. (b)	33. (b)	34. (b)	35. (b)	36. (c)	37. (d)	38. (d)	39. (d)	40. (d)
41. (d)	42. (d)	43. (a)	44. (d)	45. (b)	46. (c)	47. (b)	48. (c)	49. (c)	50. (a)
51. (b)	52. (a)	53. (a)	54. (b)	55. (b)	56. (a)	57. (d)	58. (c)	59. (b)	60. (d)
61. (d)	62. (a)	63. (d)	64. (c)	65. (c)	66. (c)	67. (a)	68. (d)	69. (b)	70. (a)
71. (d)	72. (d)	73. (c)	74. (c)	75. (a)	76. (c)	77. (d)	78. (a)	79. (a)	80. (b)
81. (a)	82. (a)	83. (c)	84. (b)	85. (b)	86. (d)	87. (d)	88. (a)	89. (c)	90. (d)
91. (c)	92. (d)	93. (d)	94. (d)	95. (b)	96. (c)	97. (c)	98. (b)	99. (a)	100. (a)
101. (d)	102. (c)	103. (c)	104. (c)	105. (a)	106. (b)	107. (a)	108. (b)	109. (d)	110. (a)
111. (b)	112. (c)	113. (c)	114. (b)	115. (d)	116. (d)	117. (d)	118. (a)	119. (d)	120. (a)
121. (d)	122. (a)	123. (d)	124. (b)	125. (d)	126. (c)	127. (d)	128. (d)	129. (a)	130. (a)
131. (a)	132. (a)	133. (d)	134. (a)	135. (d)	136. (d)	137. (c)	138. (d)	139. (a)	140. (b)
141. (a)	142. (d)	143. (a)	144. (a)	145. (b)	146. (b)	147. (a)	148. (a)	149. (c)	150. (b)
151. (b)	152. (b)	153. (d)	154. (c)	155. (c)	156. (c)	157. (b)			

AIPMT Previous Year Questions

1. (b)	2. (a)	3. (b)	4. (b)	5. (b)	6. (c)	7. (b)	8. (c)	9. (d)	10. (a)
11. (c)	12. (d)	13. (d)	14. (b)						

CHAPTER 21

Neural Control and Co-ordination

1. Select the incorrect statement:
   (a) Co-ordination is the process through which two or more organ interact and complement the function of one another
   (b) Neural system provides on organised network of point to point connection for quick coordination
   (c) Neural organisation is complex in lower invertebrates
   (d) Vertebrates have more developed neural system
2.

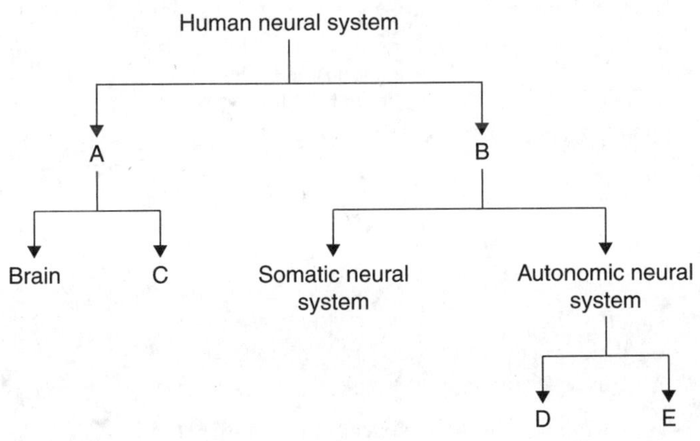

   Identify A, B, C, D and E:
   (a) A–Central Nervous System (CNS), B–Peripheral Nervous System (PNS), C–Spinal Cord, D–Sympathetic Neural System, E–Parasympathetic Neural System
   (b) A–Peripheral Nervous System (PNS), B–Parasympathetic Neural System, C–Central Nervous System (CNS), D–Sympathetic Neural System, E–Spinal Cord
   (c) A–Parasympathetic Neural System, B–Spinal Cord, C–Central Nervous System (CNS), D–Sympathetic Neural System, E–Peripheral Nervous System (PNS)
   (d) A–Central Nervous System (CNS), B–Spinal Cord, C–Peripheral Nervous System (PNS), D–Sympathetic Neural System, E–Parasympathetic Neural System

3. Somatic Neural System transmits impulse to
   (a) Skeletal muscle (b) Involuntary organs
   (c) Smooth muscles (d) All
4. Which of the following lacks a neural system?
   (a) Hydra (b) Silver fish
   (c) Spongia (Sponges) (d) Ophiura
5. Nervous system of Hydra is composed of
   (a) Ganglia chain
   (b) Vertical glanglion chain interconnected by commissure
   (c) Network of nerves
   (d) Brain
6. Nissl's granules are found in all except
   (a) Cyton (b) Dendrites
   (c) Axon (d) Cell body
7. Which of the following system relays impulse from CNS to skeletal muscles?
   (a) Somatic neural system
   (b) Sympathetic neural system
   (c) Parasympathetic neural system
   (d) Autonomic neural system
8. Dendrites transmit impulse ____ cell body and axon transmits impulse ____ cell body.
   (a) Towards, away from (b) away, towards
   (c) towards, towards (d) away, away
9. Bipolar axons are found in
   (a) Retina of eye (b) Cerebral cortex
   (c) Mesencephalon (d) Embryonic stage
10. Unipolar axons are found in
    (a) Respiratory Epithelium (b) Retina
    (c) Embryo (d) Cerebral cortex
11. Schwann cell is absent in
    (a) Myelinated neuron (b) Non myelinated
    (c) Astrocytes (d) Both (b) and (c)
12. Neuron can
    (a) Detect stimuli (b) Receive stimuli
    (c) Transmit stimuli (d) All
13. Neuron is a _____ structure composed of three major parts cell body, _____ and axon.
    (a) Macroscopic, dendrites (b) Microscopic, dendrites
    (c) Microscopic, cyton (d) Microscopic, soma

14.

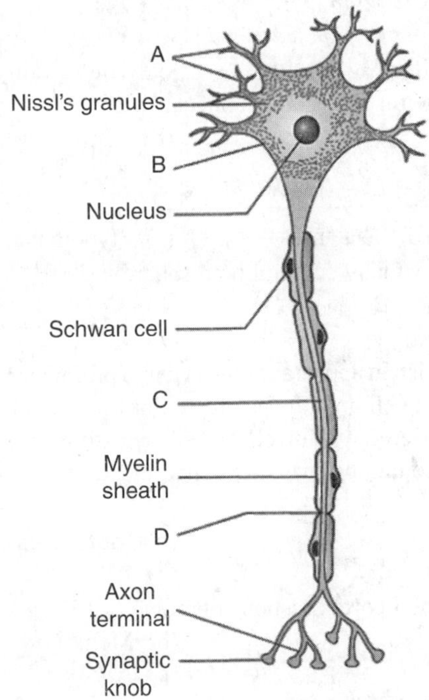

Structure of a neuron

A) Which part do not contain Nissl's granule?

(a) A (b) B (c) C (d) All

B) Which path of transmission is correct?

(a) $A \rightarrow B \rightarrow C$ (b) $B \rightarrow A \rightarrow C$
(c) $C \rightarrow B \rightarrow A$ (d) $B \rightarrow A \rightarrow B \rightarrow C$

15. Match the Column:

Column I		**Column II**
A. Unipolar	–	1. Cell body with one axon only, found usually in the embryonic stage
B. Bipolar	–	2. Cell body with one axon and two or more dendrites, found in cerebral cortex
C. Multipolar	–	3. Cell body with one axon and one dendrite, found in retina of eye

(a) A–1, B–3, C–2 (b) A–2, B–1, C–3
(c) A–3, B–2, C–1 (d) A–1, B–2, C–3

16. Myelinated nerve fibre found in

(a) Spinal Nerve (b) Cranial Nerve
(c) Both (d) None

17. Unmyelinated Nerve fibres commonly found in

(a) ANS (b) Somatic Neural System
(c) Both (d) None

18. The outermost of the 3 cranial meninges is
(a) Arachnoid (b) Dura (c) Pia (d) Sclera
19. Brain stem is formed by
(a) Fore Brain (b) Mid Brain (c) Hind Brain (d) Both (b) and (c)
20. Right and left cerebral hemispheres are connected via
(a) Corpus striatum (b) Corpus callosum
(c) Thalamus (d) Hippocampus
21. Forebrain consist of
(a) Cerebrum (b) Thalamus (c) Hypothalamus (d) All
22. Cerebrum is made of how many cerebral hemisphere
(a) 1 (b) 2 (c) 3 (d) 4
23. Select incorrect statement:
(a) Cerebral cortex, greyish in appearance thrown into prominent folds known as Sulci and Gyri
(b) Concentrated Neuron cell body gives grey color to cerebral cortex
(c) Fibres of the tract, covered with myelin sheath, constitute inner part of cerebral hemisphere
(d) Cerebrum is wrap around the structure called medulla
24. Cerebral cortex contain
(a) Sensory area (b) Motor area
(c) Large association area (d) All
25. Association area in cerebral cortex responsible for
(a) Inter sensory association (b) Memory
(c) Communication (d) All
26. Major coordinating centre for sensory and motor signaling is
(a) Thalamus (b) Hypothalamus (c) Medulla (d) Pons
27. Hypothalamus contain centre which control
(a) Body temperature (b) Urge for eating
(c) Urge for drinking (d) All
28. True about hypothalamus
(a) Situated at the base of thalamus (b) Contain neurosecretory cell which
(c) It contain centre for thermoregulation (d) All
29. Limbic system consist of
(a) Amygdala (b) Hippocampus (c) Both (d) None
30. Part of brain located between thalamus hypothalamus of fere brain and pons is known as
(a) Mid brain (b) Hind brain (c) Limbic system (d) All
31. True about midbrain:
(a) A canal called cerebral aqueduct passes through the mid brain
(b) Dorsal portion of mid-brain consist of four round swelling called corpora quadrigemina
(c) It forms part of brain stem
(d) All
32. Hind brain consist of
(a) Pons (b) Medulla oblongata
(c) Cerebellum (d) All
33. Hypothalamus controls
(a) Body's thermostat (b) Respiration
(c) Gastric secretions (d) All

34. Limbic system controls
(a) Sexual behaviour (b) Motivation
(c) Affection (d) All
35. Corpora quadrigemina are present on _____ portion of Mesencephalon (midbrain)
(a) Anterior (b) Dorsal (c) Ventral (d) Lateral
36. False about hind brain
(a) Pons a part of it consist of fibre tracts that interconnect different region of brain
(b) Cerebellum part of it has very convoluted surface to accommodate many neurons
(c) Medulla of this part connected to spiral cord
(d) Hind brain regular excitement, pleasure, rag and fear
37. Medulla contain centre for
(a) Respiration (b) Cardiovascular Reflex
(c) Gastric Secretion (d) All
38. Which of the following consists of fibre tracts interconnecting different regions of brain?
(a) Cerebellum (b) Pons varoli (c) Medulla (d) All
39. Which of the following help in regulation of respiration?
(a) Medulla (b) Cerebral cortex (c) Pons (d) Both (a) and (c)
40. Reflex action is under
(a) CNS (b) Spiral cord
(c) Peripheral Nervous Stimulation (d) Voluntary response
41. Dorsal nerve root ganglion is
(a) Bipolar (b) Unipolar (c) Pseudo unipolar (d) Multipolar
42. In spiral cord of humans grey matter is _____ shaped.
(a) Circular (b) Irregular (c) Butterfly (d) None
43. White matter is _____ in brain and _____ in spiral cord (in case of humans)
(a) Outside, inside (b) In, out (c) In, in (d) Out, out
44. Resting axonal membrane is
(a) Unpolarised (b) Unpolarised and more permeable to K^+
(c) Polarised and more permeable to Na^+ (d) Polarised and more permeable to K^+
45. Na/K pumps transports
(a) $3Na^+$ out for $2K^+$ in (b) $3Na^+$ in for $2K^+$ out
(c) $2Na^+$ out for $3K^+$ in (d) $2Na^+$ in for $3K^+$ out
46. True about Neural membrane
(a) Different type of ion channels present
(b) Ion channels are selectively permeable
(c) Impermeable to negatively charged protein present in axoplasm
(d) All
47. Axoplasm have (polarised)
(a) High K^+ ion (b) Low Na^+ ion
(c) Negatively charge proteins (d) All
48. The electrical potential difference across the resting plasma membrane is called as
(a) Spike potential (b) Action potential
(c) Resting potential (d) All
49. Depolarisation occur due to
(a) Influx of Na^+ (b) Eflux of Na^+ (c) Influx of K^+ (d) Eflux of K^+

50. Correct sequence for depolarisation and repolarisation
(A) Stimulus applied at a site on polarised membrane
(B) increase permeability for Na^+
(C) Generation of A.P.
(D) increase permeability for K^+
(E) Restoration of membrane potential
(a) $A \rightarrow B \rightarrow C \rightarrow D \rightarrow E$
(b) $B \rightarrow A \rightarrow C \rightarrow D \rightarrow E$
(c) $A \rightarrow D \rightarrow C \rightarrow B \rightarrow E$
(d) $A \rightarrow B \rightarrow D \rightarrow C \rightarrow E$

51. Unidirectional transmission of the nerve impulse is maintained by
(a) Interneurons
(b) Myelin sheath
(c) Synapse
(d) Membrane polarity

52. Select total number of true statement from the followinG—
1) There are two types of synapses, namely electrical synapses and chemical synapses
2) Electrical synapses are rare in our system
3) At chemical synapse, the membranes of pre- and post-synaptic neuron are in very close proximity
4) Transmission of an impulse across electrical synapses is very similar to impulse conduction along a single axon
5) At a chemical synapse, the membrane of the pre- and post-synaptic neurons are separated by a fluid-filled space called synaptic cleft

(a) 2 (b) 3 (c) 4 (d) 5

53. Chemicals called _____ are involved in the transmission of impulses at chemical synapse
(a) Neurohormones
(b) Neurotransmitters
(c) Receptors
(d) Interferon

54. Which ion helps in releasing Ach at synaptic left?
(a) Na^+ (b) K^+ (c) Ca^{+2} (d) PO_4^{3-}

55. The new potential developed on post-synaptic membrane is
(a) excitatory always
(b) inhibitory always
(c) May be excitatory or inhibitory
(d) Neither excitatory nor inhibitory

56. Identify A–H in the given figure.

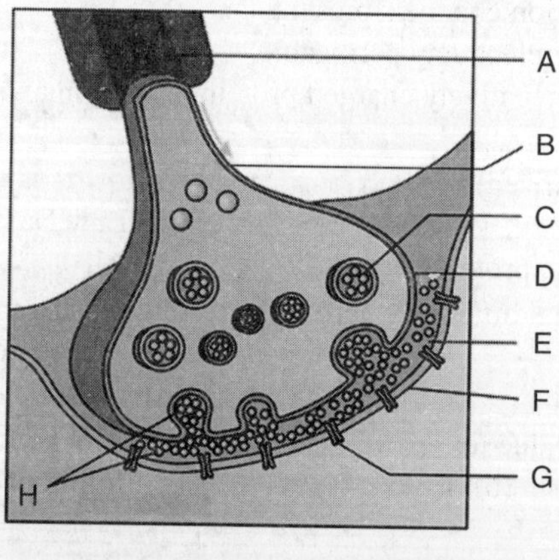

(a) A—Neurotransmitters, B—Pre-synaptic membrane, C—Receptors, D—Axon, E—Synaptic vesicles, F—Axon terminal, G—Synaptic cleft, H—Post-synaptic membrane
(b) A—Axon, B—Axon terminal, C—Synaptic vesicles, D—Pre-synaptic membrane, E—Synaptic cleft, F—Post-synaptic membrane, G—receptors, H—Neurotransmitters
(c) A—Receptors, B—Post-synaptic membrane, C—Pre-synaptic membrane, D—Axon terminal, E—Neurotransmitters, F—Synaptic clef, G—Synaptic vesicles, H—Axon
(d) A—Axon termina, B—Neurotransmitters, C—Synaptic vesicles, D—Axon, E—Pre-synaptic membrane, F—Post-synaptic membrane, G—Synaptic vesicles, H—Synaptic cleft

57. Reflex action
(a) Occur involutary
(b) Require involvement of CNS
(c) Protective
(d) All

58. Smallest reflex are consist of
(a) Afferent neuron (Receptor)
(b) Efferent neuron (effector or excitor)
(c) Both
(d) None

59. In reflex action, the reflex arc is formed by
(a) Muscle, receptor, brain
(b) Brain, spinal cord, muscle
(c) Receptor, spinal cord, muscle
(d) receptor, muscle, spinal cord

60. Following are due to reflex action
(a) Vomiting
(b) Sneezing
(c) Coughing
(d) All

61. Following are example of reflexes
(a) Knee-jerk reflex
(b) Corneal reflex
(c) Papillary reflex
(d) All

62. In the diagram of the lateral view of the human brain, parts are indicated by alphabets. Choose the answer in which these alphabets have been correctly matched with the parts which they indicate?

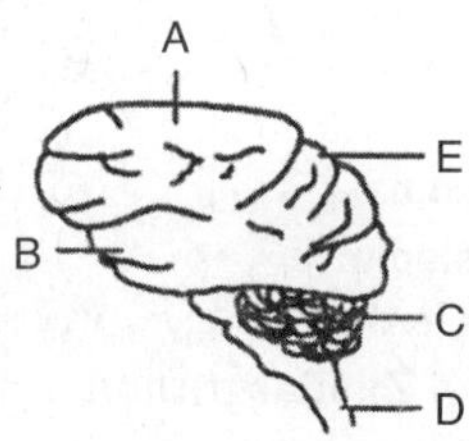

(a) A–Temporal lobe, B–Parietal lobe, C–Cerebellum, D–Medulla oblongata, E–Frontal lobe
(b) A–Frontal lobe, B–Temporal lobe, C–Cerebrum, D–Medulla oblongata, E–Occipital lobe
(c) A–Temporal lobe, B–Parietal lobe, C–Cerebrum, D–Medulla oblongata, E–Frontal lobe
(d) A–Frontal lobe, B–Temporal lobe, C–Cerebellum, D–Medulla oblongata, E–Occipital lobe

63. Site for processing of vision, hearing, speech, memory, intelligence, emotions and thoughts is
(a) Brain
(b) Hear
(c) Lungs
(d) Kidney

64. Eyes are located in
(a) Eye orbits (b) Depression in sphenoid bone
(c) Both (d) None

65. Choroid is blue due to _________
(a) Lack of O_2 in tissue (b) Due to pigment
(c) Excess of blood vessels (d) None

66. Choroid thickens anteriorly to form
(a) Iris (b) Ciliary body
(c) Suspensory ligaments (d) None

67. Diameter of pupil is regulated by
(a) Lens (b) Ciliary muscles
(c) Muscles of iris (d) All

68. Cells located in retina are
(a) Photo receptor cells (b) Bipolar cell
(c) Ganglion cells (d) All

69. Layers in wall of eyeballs from inside outwards are
(a) Retina, choroid, sclerotic (b) Sclerotic, choroid, retina
(c) Choroid, retina, sclerotic (d) Choroid, sclerotic, retina

70. Which layer of the wall of an eyeball contains abundant blood vessels?
(a) Lens (b) Retina (c) Choroid (d) Sclerotic

71. Iris is a part of
(a) Choroid only (b) Retina only
(c) Sclera and choroid (d) Choroid and retina

72. The size of aperture of the pupil of one eye is controlled by
(a) iris (b) retina (c) cornea (d) conjunctiva

73. Eye lens of man is
(a) Biconcave (b) Biconvex (c) Concave (d) Convex

74. Cornea is a transparent part of
(a) Choroid (b) Sclera (c) Conjunctiva (d) Retina

75. The second layer of the eyeball is called
(a) Choroid (b) Retina (c) Cornea (d) Sclera

76. The iris of the eye is an extension of
(a) Cornea (b) Sclerotic (c) Retina (d) Choroid

77. Suspensory ligament (zonule of Zinn) is part of:
(a) Tongue (b) Brain (c) Heart (d) Eye

78. The choroid layer is thin over the _________ of the eye ball
(a) Anterior two-third (b) Posterior two-third
(c) Lateral two-third (d) Posterior one-third

79. Find out the incorrect statement:
(a) Lens is transparent and crystalline structure
(b) Iris is pigmented and opaque layer
(c) Aperture surrounded by iris is called pupil
(d) Twilight vision is the function of cones

80. Aqueous humor is present
(a) In front of the retina (b) in front of cornea
(c) Behind the conjunctiva (d) in front of lens

81. Retinal cells involved in colour vision are
(a) Cones (b) Rods (c) Neurons (d) Neuroglial cells

82. Which of the following is not a basic colour in trichromatic vision?
(a) Red (b) Yellow (c) Green (d) Blue

83. Anterior chamber of the eye is the space between
(a) Cornea and lens (b) Cornea and iris (c) Lens and retina (d) Lens and iris

84. Which of the following passes from lens to blindspot?
(a) Eustachian canal (b) Canal of Schlemm
(c) Hyaloid canal (d) Semicircular canal

85. Colour vision in man is
(a) Trichromatic (b) Bichromatic (c) Monochromatic (d) Achromatic

86. Quantum of light entering the eye through the pupil is dependent on
(a) Ciliary body (b) Lens (c) Retina (d) Iris

87. Rhodopsin is a constituent of
(a) Choroid (b) Sclera (c) Cornea (d) None

88. In nocturnal birds, the retina contains mostly
(a) Cones (b) Rods
(c) Both in equal numbers (d) None

89. Macula lutea is located
(a) in the middle of retina (b) below lens
(c) below pupil (d) at posterior polelateral to blind spot

90. Photopic vision is associated with
(a) Rods (b) Cones (c) Both (d) None

91. Retina is most sensitive at
(a) Optic disc (b) Periphery (c) Macula lutea (d) Fovea centralis

92. Aperture controlling light passage in eye is
(a) Pupil (b) Sclerotic (c) Blindspot (d) Iris

93. Space between cornea and lens is
(a) Aqueous chamber (b) Vitreous chamber
(c) Canal of Schlemm (d) Fovea centralis

94. Cones are sensitive to
(a) Dim light only (b) Bright light only
(c) Both dim and bright light (d) None

95. Colour is perceived by
(a) Rods in retina (b) Cones in retina
(c) Corneal-lens complex (d) Lens

96. Rhodopsin (visual purple) of the eye will require
(a) Guava (b) Carrot (c) Mango (d) Wheat

97. Area of most acute vision in the eye where sharp and bright image formed is
(a) Yellow spot (b) Blindspot (c) Pupil (d) Lens

98. An area of the retina which does not have rods or cones are
(a) red spot (b) blue spot (c) blind spot (d) black spot

99. Vitamin A combines with a protein in the retina to produce
(a) Glaucoma (b) Night blindness (c) Rhodopsin (d) Colour blindness

100. The fovea is a ________ portion of the ________

(a) Thick-out, sclera (b) Thin-out, choroid
(c) Thin-out, retina (d) Thick-out, retina

101. When all three types of cones are stimulated equally, a sensation of ________ light is produced?

(a) Black (b) White
(c) Blue (d) Green

102 Select the incorrect matching:

	Part		Function
(a)	Optic nerve	–	Carry impulse to visual cortex
(b)	Cones	–	Colour vision
(c)	Cornea and lens	–	Focusing of light on retina
(d)	Pupil	–	Generate action potential

103. Vitreous chamber is filled with

(a) Transparent sol called vitreous humor
(b) Transparent gel called vitreous humor
(c) Opaque sol called vitreous humor
(d) Opaque gel called vitreous humor

104. Select the incorrect statement:

(a) Rhodopsin is also known as visual purple
(b) Rods contain a purplish-red protein, which in turn contain derivative of VitaminA
(c) In human eye three type of cones are present
(d) At fovea of retina resolution (visual acuity) is minimum

105. Optic nerve leaves the eye balls at which location

(a) Slightly below the posterior pole of eye ball
(b) Slightly above the posterior pole of eye ball
(c) Anterior pole of eye ball
(d) Macula lutea

106. Orderly arrange following steps of mechanism of vision:

(1) Light induce dissociation of the retinal from opsin
(2) Change in structure of opsin
(3) Change in membrane permeability
(4) Potential differences are generated in photoreceptor cells
(5) Generation of AP is ganglion cell through bipolar cells
(6) AP transmitted via optic nerve to visual cortex
(7) At visual cortex, nerve impulses are analysed and image formed on retina is recognised based on earlier memory and experience
(8) Focusing of visible light on retina

(a) 8,1,2,3,4,5,6,7 (b) 8,1,7,2,6,3,5,4 (c) 1,2,3,4,5,6,7,8 (d) 8,7,6,5,4,3,2,1

107. Ear performs which of the following sensory function

(A) Vision (B) Olfaction
(C) Hearing (D) Maintenance of body balance

(a) A, B, C (b) B, C Only (c) C, D Only (d) C Only

108. Identify A–F in the given figure.

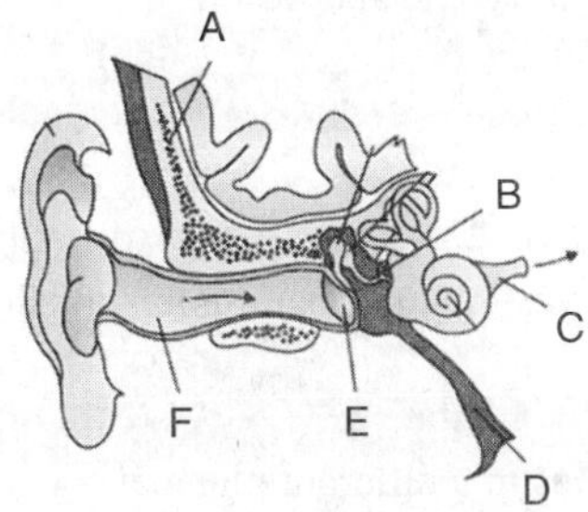

(a) A–Cochlear nerve, B–Incus, C–Eustachian tube, D–Cochlea, E–Exernal auditory canal, F–Tympanic membrane
(b) A–External auditory canal, B–Eustachian tube, C–Temporal bone, D–Steps in oval window, E–Tympanic membrane, F–Cochlear nerve
(c) A–Cochlea, B–Tympanic membrane, C–Incus, D–Cochlear nerve, E–Eustachian tube, F–External auditory canal
(d) A–Temporal bone, B–Steps in oval window, C–Cochlear nerve, D–Eustachian tubem E–Tympanic membrane, F–External auditory canal

109. Anatomically the ear can be divided into how many major sections
(a) 1 (b) 2 (c) 3 (d) 4

110. Ear is divided into
(a) Outer ear (b) Middle ear (c) Inner ear (d) All

111. Tympanic membrane consist of
(a) Skin on outside (b) Connective tissue middle part
(c) Mucus membrane on inside (d) All

112. The _________ is attached to the tympanic membrane and the _________ is attached to the oval window of the cochlea.
(a) Malleus, Incus (b) Incus, Stapes (c) Malleus, Steps (d) Steps, Malleus

113. Select the incorrect statement:
(a) Eustachian tube connects middle ear cavity with the pharynx
(b) The Eustachian tube helps in equalizing the pressure on either sides of ear drum
(c) Oval window is part of cochlea
(d) The ear ossicle decreases the efficiency of transmission of sound waves to the inner ear

114. Select the correct matching:
(a) Inner ear ossicle → Malleus, incus and steps
(b) Scala media → Filled with perilymph
(c) Fluid filled inner ear → Labyrinth
(d) Bony labyrinth → Surrounded by tympanic membrane

115. Inner ear contain all except
(a) Reissner's membrane (b) Basilar membrane
(c) Cochlea (d) Stapes

116. Select the total number of true statement from the following:
(1) Scala vestibuli end at the oval window
(2) Scala tympani terminates at round window

(3) Vestibular apparatus located above cochlea
(4) Otolith organ consist of sccule and utricle
(a) 1 (b) 2 (c) 3 (d) 4

117. Vestibular apparatus consists of
(a) Three semicircular canal (b) Saccule
(c) Utricle (d) All

118. Specific receptors of the vestibular apparatus responsible for maintenance of balance of the body and posture
(a) Macula (b) Crista (c) Organ of corti (d) Both (a) and (b)

119. Each semicircular canal lies in a different plane at ________ angle to each other
(a) 45° (b) 60° (c) 90° (d) 120°

120. In man the receptors stimulated by sound waves are
(a) Organ of corti (b) Semicircular canal
(c) Utriculus (d) Sacculus

121. Scala vestibuli is connected with
(a) scala media (b) fenestra ovalis
(c) scala tympani (d) fenestra rotundus

122. Cochlea of mammalian internal ear is concerned with
(a) hearing (b) balance of body posture
(c) both (a) and (b) (d) perception changes of atmospheric pressure

123. Identify the correct sequence of organs/regions in the organization of human ear as an auditory mechanoreceptor organ
(a) Pinna–Cochlea–Tympanic membrane–Auditory canal–Malleus–Stapes–Incus–Auditory nerve
(b) Pinna–Auditory canal–Tympanic membrane–Malleus–Incus–Stapes–Cochlea–Auditory nerve
(c) Pinna–Tympanic membrane–Auditory canal–Incus–Malleus–Stapes–Cochlea–Auditory nerve
(d) Pinna–Malleus–Incus–Stapes–Auditory canal–Tympanic membrane–Cochlea–Auditory nerve

124. Internal ear is filled with
(a) perilymph (b) endolymph (c) lymph (d) both (a) and (b)

125. Reissner's membrane is found in
(a) Cochlea of mammal (b) Eye of mammal
(c) Heart of mammal (d) Nasal duct of mammal

126. In the internal ear, the organ of Corti' which bears hair cells is located in
(a) sacculus (b) scala media (c) scala tympani (d) scala vestibuli

127. Equilibrium of the body is maintained by
(a) Sacculus and cochlea (b) Semicircular canals and utriculus
(c) Eustachian tube (d) Ear ossicles

128. Which of the following senses is affected if the tectorial membrane is removed from human?
(a) Balance (b) Hearing (c) Vision (d) Smell

129. Malleus (hammer shape), incus (anvil shape) and stapes (stirrup shape) are present in
(a) Internal ear of frog (b) Middle ear of human
(c) Eye of rabbit (d) Eye of frog

130. The waxy substance which coats the surface of auditory canal is produced by
(a) Harderian glands (b) Meibomian glands
(c) Zeis glands (d) Ceruminous glands (sebaceous gland)

131. Macula in man are present in
(a) Semicircular canals (b) Utriculus
(c) Sacculus (d) Both utriculus and sacculus

132. Which of the following parts in your body is concerned with the sense of balance?
(a) Eustachian tube (b) Cochlea
(c) Eardrum (d) Semicircular canals

133. The fluid present in the semicircular canals of the internal ear of human is
(a) Endolymph (b) Perilymph (c) Lymph (d) Coelomic fluid

134. Identify A, B, C, D, E, F and G in the given figure.

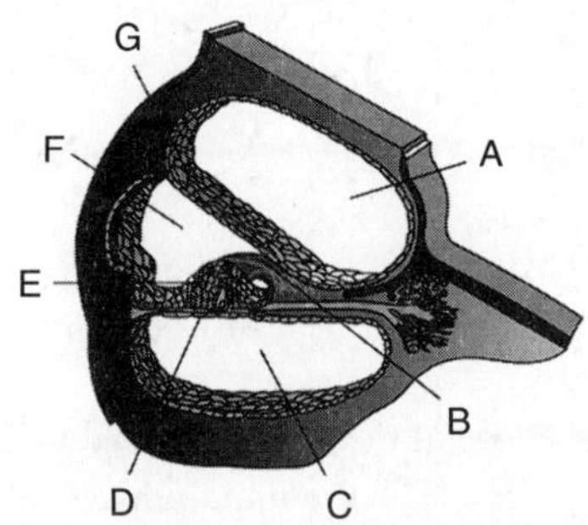

(a) A–Scala vestibuli, B–Tectorial membrane, C–Scala tympani, D–Basilar membrane, E–Organ of corti, F–Scala media, G–Reissner's membrane
(b) A–Scala tympani, B–Reissner's membrane, C–Scala vestibuli, D–Basilar membrane, E–Scala media, F–Organ of corti, G–Tectorial membrane
(c) A–Reissner's membrane, B–Tectorial membrane, C–Scala media, D–Organ of corti, E–Scala vestibuli, F–Scala tympani, G–Basilar membrane
(d) A–Tectorial membrane, B–Scala tympani, C–Reissner's membrane, D–Basilar membrane, E–Scala vestibuli, F–Scala vestibuli, G–Organ of corti

135. Which one of the following is not a part of ear?
(a) Eustachian tube (b) Cone cell
(c) Utriculus (d) Sacculus

136. The base of semicircular canals is swollen and is called _________ which contain a projecting ridges called _________ which ahs hair cells.
(a) Papilla, macula ampullaris (b) Ampulla, crista ampullaris
(c) Ampulla, macula ampullaris (d) Macula, crista ampullaris

137. Otolith organ consisting of
(a) Saccule (b) Utricle
(c) Semicircular canal (d) Both (a) and (c)

138. Select the correct statement:
(a) Neural system co-ordinates and integrates functions as well as metabolic and homeostatic activities of all organs
(b) Chemical involved in the transmission of impulse at chemical synapses are always proteins

(c) The electrical potential difference across the resting neural membrane is called the action potential

(d) Organ of Corti influenced by gravity and movement and helps in maintaining balance of the body and posture

*Read the **assertion** and **reason** carefully to mark the correct option out of the options given below:*

(a) If both the assertion and the reason are true and the reason is a correct explanation of the assertion

(b) If both the assertion and reason are true but the reason is not a correct explanation of the assertion

(c) If the assertion is true but the reason is false

(d) If both the assertion and reason are false

139. Assertion: The sensation of different colors are produced by various combinations of five types of cones found in our eyes.
Reason: Cones are responsible for vision in dim light.

140. Assertion: Nerve impulse can never be transmitted from dendrite or cell body of one neuron to the axon of the next neuron, across a synapse.
Reason: This happens because of the synaptic delay at each synapse.

141. Assertion: After hearing a sound, nerve impulse passes from neurons to the brain.
Reason: The neurons which pass nerve impulses from the body organ to the brain is called afferent neuron.

142. Assertion: Cerebrospinal fluid is present throughout the central nervous system.
Reason: CSF has no function.

143. Assertion: Cerebellum has very convoluted surface.
Reason: It provide additional space for many more neurons.

144. Assertion: Some areas of the brain and spinal cord look white.
Reason: This is because cell bodies of neurons are situated in those areas.

145. Assertion: Motor neuron terminates on a motor end plate at the neuromuscular junction.
Reason: Motor end plate acts as receptor for detecting changes in the muscle fibres.

146. Assertion: Crista and macula are the specific receptors of vestibular apparatus responsible for the maintenance of balance of the body and postur.
Reason: Cochlea helps in hearing.

147. Assertion: Spinal cord has a column of both grey and white matter.
Reason: Grey matter forms the central spinal canal.

148. Assertion: All motor neurons are efferent neurons.
Reason: Motor neurons conduct nerve impulses from the spinal cord to the brain.

149. Assertion: The chemical stored in the synaptic vesicles are termed as neurotransmitters.
Reason: Synaptic vesicles release these chemicals in the synaptic cleft.

150. Assertion: Medulla oblongata causes reflex actions like vomiting, coughing and sneezing.
Reason: It has many nerve cells which control autonomic reflexes.

151. Assertion: Transmission of the nerve impulse across a synapse is accomplished by neurotransmitters.

Reason: Transmission across a synapse usually requires neurotransmitters because there is small space i.e. synaptic cleft, that separates one neuron from another.

152. Assertion: Place in retina from where optic nerve leave is known as blind spot.

Reason: Because this place is devoid of photoreceptor cells.

AIPMT PREVIOUS YEAR QUESTIONS

1. Select the answer with correct matching of the structure, its location and function.
[A: Structure, B: Location, C: Function]

[AIPMT MAINS 2010]

Structure	Location	Function
(a) Eustachian tube	Anterior part of internal ear	Equalizes air pressure on either sides of tympanic membrane
(b) Cerebellum	Midbrain	Controls respiration and gastric secretions
(c) Hypothalamus	Fore brain	Controls body temperature, urge for eating and drinking
(d) Blind spot	Near the place where optic nerve leaves the eye	Rods and cones are present but inactive here

2. The nerve centres which control the body temperature and the urge for eating are contained in [AIPMT PRE 2010]

(a) Hypothalamus (b) Pons
(c) Cerebellum (d) Thalamus

3. The purplish red pigment rhodopsin contained in the rods type of photoreceptor cells of the human eyes is a derivative of:

[AIPMT PRE 2011]

(a) Vitamin – C (b) Vitamin – D
(c) Vitamin – A (d) Vitamin - B

4. When a neuron is an resting state, ie, not conducting any impulse, the axonal membrane is: [AIPMT PRE 2011]

(a) Equally permeable to both Na^+ and K^+ ions
(b) Impermeable to both Na^+ and K^+ ions
(c) Comparatively more permeable to K^+ ions and nearly impermeable to Na^+ ions
(d) Comparatively more permeable to Na^+ ions and nearly impermeable to K^+ ions

5. The human hind brain comprises three parts, one of which is:

[AIPMT PRE 2012]

(a) Spinal cord (b) Corpus callosum
(c) Cerebellum (d) Hypothalamus

6. Which part of the human ear plays no role in hearing as such but is otherwise very much required?

[AIPMT PRE 2012]

(a) Eustachian tube (b) Organ of Corti
(c) Vestibular apparatus (d) Ear ossicles

7. A person entering an empty room suddenly finds a snake right in front on opening the door. Which one of the following is likely to happen in his neuro-hormonal control system? [AIPMT PRE 2012]

(a) Sympathetic nervous system is activated releasing epinephrine and norepinephrin from adrenal medulla.
(b) Neurotransmitters diffuse rapidly across the cleft and transmit a nerve impulse.
(c) Hypothalamus activates the parasympathetic division of brain.
(d) Sympathetic nervous system is activated releasing epinephrine and system is activated releasing epinephrine and norepinephrin from adrenal cortex.

8. A diagram showing axon terminal and synapse is given. Identify correctly at least two of A – D.

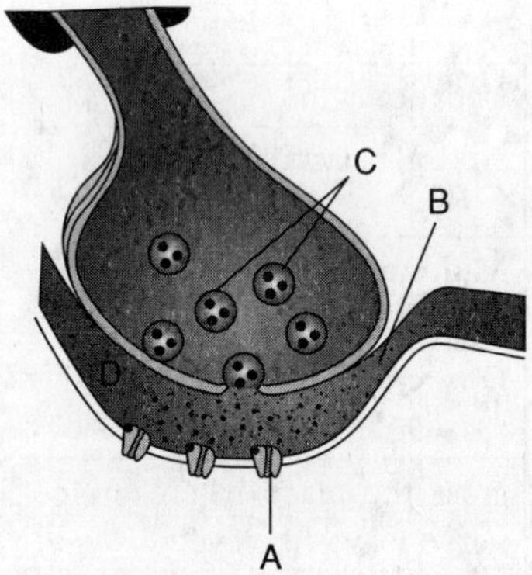

[AIPMT 2013]

(a) A – Receptor C – Synaptic vesicles
(b) B – Synaptic connections D – K^+
(c) A – Neurotransmitter B – Synaptic cleft
(d) C – Neurotransmitter D – Ca^{++}

9. Parts A, B, C and D of the human eye are shown in the diagram. Select the option which gives correct identification along with its function / characteristics.

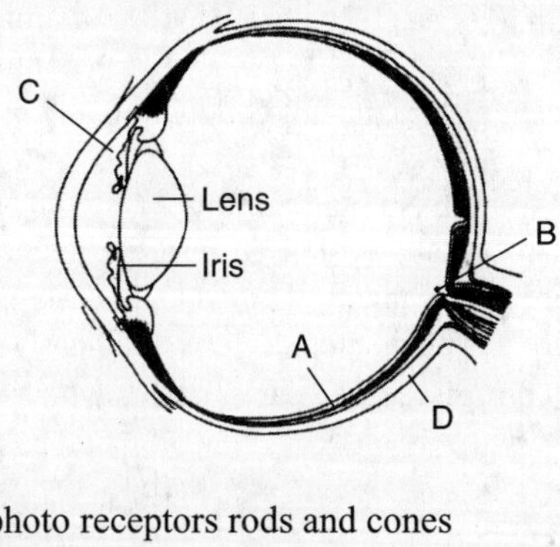

[AIPMT 2013]

(a) A – Retina – contains photo receptors rods and cones
(b) B – Blind spot –has only a few rods and cones
(c) C – Aqueous chamber – reflects the light which does not pass through the lens
(d) D – Choroid – its anterior part forms ciliary body

10. Injury localized to the hypothalamus would most likely disrupt:

[AIPMT 2014]

(a) Short-term memory
(b) Co-ordination during locomotion
(c) Executive functions, such as decision making
(d) Regulation of body temperature

11. Which one of the following statements is not correct?

[AIPMT 2014]

(a) Retinal is the light absorbing portion of visual photo pigments
(b) In retina the rods have the photopigment rhodopsin while cones have three different photopigments
(c) Retinal is a derivative of Vitamin C
(d) Rhodopsin is the purplish red protein present in rods only

12. Which of the following regions of the brain is incorrectly paired with its function?

[AIPMT 2015]

(a) Medulla oblongata – homeostatic control
(b) Cerebellum – language comprehension
(c) Corpus callosum – communication between the left and right cerebral cortices
(d) Cerebrum – calculation and contemplation

13. A gymnast is able to balance his body upside down even in the total darkness because of:

[AIPMT 2015]

(a) Cochlea (b) Vestibular apparatus
(c) Tectorial membrane (d) Organ of corti

14. In mammalian eye, the 'fovea' is the center of the visual field, where:

[RE-AIPMT 2015]

(a) The optic nerve leaves the eye
(b) Only rods are present
(c) More rods than cones are found
(d) High density of cones occur, but has no rods

15. Destruction of the anterior horn cells of the spinal cord would result in loss of:

[RE-AIPMT 2015]

(a) Voluntary motor impulse
(b) Commissural impulses
(c) Integrating impulses
(d) Sensory impulses

Answer Keys

1. (c)	2. (a)	3. (a)	4. (c)	5. (c)	6. (c)	7. (a)	8. (a)	9. (a)	10. (c)
11. (c)	12. (d)	13. (b)	14. (i) (c)(ii) (a)	15. (a)	16. (c)	17. (c)	18. (b)	19. (d)	
20. (b)	21. (d)	22. (b)	23. (d)	24. (d)	25. (d)	26. (a)	27. (d)	28. (d)	29. (c)
30. (a)	31. (d)	32. (d)	33. (a)	34. (d)	35. (b)	36. (d)	37. (d)	38. (b)	39. (d)
40. (c)	41. (c)	42. (c)	43. (b)	44. (d)	45. (a)	46. (d)	47. (d)	48. (c)	49. (a)
50. (a)	51. (c)	52. (c)	53. (b)	54. (c)	55. (c)	56. (b)	57. (d)	58. (c)	59. (c)
60. (d)	61. (d)	62. (d)	63. (a)	64. (c)	65. (c)	66. (b)	67. (d)	68. (d)	69. (a)
70. (c)	71. (a)	72. (a)	73. (b)	74. (b)	75. (a)	76. (d)	77. (d)	78. (b)	79. (d)

80. (d)	81. (a)	82. (b)	83. (b)	84. (c)	85. (a)	86. (d)	87. (d)	88. (b)	89. (d)
90. (b)	91. (d)	92. (a)	93. (a)	94. (b)	95. (b)	96. (b)	97. (a)	98. (c)	99. (c)
100. (c)	101. (b)	102. (d)	103. (b)	104. (d)	105. (b)	106. (a)	107. (c)	108. (d)	109. (c)
110. (d)	111. (d)	112. (c)	113. (d)	114. (c)	115. (d)	116. (d)	117. (d)	118. (d)	119. (c)
120. (a)	121. (c)	122. (a)	123. (b)	124. (d)	125. (a)	126. (b)	127. (b)	128. (b)	129. (b)
130. (d)	131. (d)	132. (d)	133. (a)	134. (a)	135. (b)	136. (b)	137. (d)	138. (a)	139. (a)
140. (c)	141. (c)	142. (c)	143. (a)	144. (c)	145. (c)	146. (b)	147. (b)	148. (c)	149. (b)
150. (a)	151. (a)	152. (a)							

AIPMT Previous Year Questions

1. (c)	2. (a)	3. (c)	4. (c)	5. (c)	6. (c)	7. (a)	8. (a)	9. (a)	10. (d)
11. (c)	12. (c)	13. (b)	14. (d)	15. (a)					

CHAPTER

22

Chemical Co-ordination and Integration

1. Select the incorrect statement from the following:
   (a) Neural System provide point to point rapid co-ordination among organs
   (b) Neural co-ordination is fast
   (c) Neural co-ordination is short-lived
   (d) Nerve fibres innervates all the cells of body so cellular function be continuously regulated
2. Which system jointly coordinate and regulate the physiological functions in the body
   (a) Nervous System (b) Endocrine System
   (c) Both (d) None
3. Hormonal System is very important because
   (a) neural co-ordination is fast
   (b) nerve fibre do not innervate all the cells of body
   (c) neural system provide point to point coordination among organ
   (d) neural co-ordination is short-lived
4. Endocrine glands
   (a) are ductless (b) secrete hormones
   (c) pour their secretion in blood (d) all of the above
5. Identify A–F in the given figure.

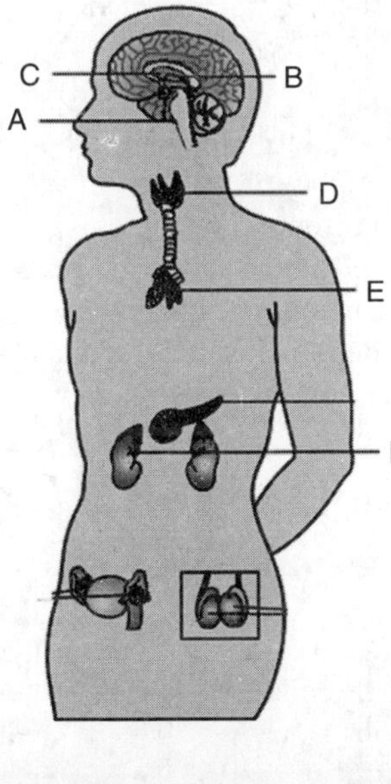

(a) A–Hypothalamus, B–Pineal, C–Thymus, D–Adrenal, E–Pituitary, F–Thyroid and parathyroid
(b) A–Pituitary, B–Pineal, C–Hypothalamus, D–Thyroid and parathyroid, E–Thymus, F–Adrenal
(c) A–Thymus, B–Pituitary, C–Thyroid and parathyroid, D–Pineal, E–Hypothalamus, F–Adrenal
(d) A–Pineal, B–Thyroid and parathyroid, C–Pituitary, D–Hypothalamus, E–Adrenal, F–Pineal

6. Hormones are
(a) non-nutrient chemical (b) intercellular messengers
(c) produced in traces (d) all

7. Select from the following the total number of endocrine glands:
Pituitary, pineal, thyroid, parathyroid, adrenal, pancreas, thymus, gonads
(a) 7 (b) 8 (c) 6 (d) 5

8. Following organs produce hormones except
(a) GIT (b) liver and kidney
(c) Heart (d) Urinary bladder

9. Hypothalamus contains several groups of neurosecretory cells called ________ which produce hormones.
(a) ganglion (b) plexus
(c) nuclei (d) astrocytes

10. Hypothalamus is a part of
(a) forebrain (b) mid brain
(c) hind brain (d) none

11. Hypothalamus is
(a) Roof of diencephalon (b) Basal part of diencephalon
(c) Lateral wall of diencephalon (d) All

12. Hypothalamus regulates directly ________ endocrine gland
(a) Pituitary (b) Thyroid (c) Thymus (d) Pancreas

13. Releasing hormones and inhibiting hormones are produced by
(a) Pituitary (b) Thyroid (c) Thymus (d) Hypothalamus

14. Pars distalis produces how many trophic hormones
(a) 4 (b) 5
(c) 6 (d) 8

15. Following hormones are released by hypothalamus except
(a) GnRH (b) Somatostatin (c) TSH–RH (d) PRL

16. Select the incorrect statement from following:
(a) Invertebrates possess very simple endocrine system
(b) Anterior pituitary is under control of hypothalamus by portal system
(c) Posterior pituitary is under direct neural regulation of hypothalamus
(d) Hypothalamus secretes tropic hormones

17. Which of the following is incorrect about pituitary
(a) Located in bony cavity called sella turcica
(b) Attached to hypothalamus by stalk
(c) Divided anatomically into adenohypophyis and neurohypophysis
(d) Secrete released and inhibitory hormones

18. Identify A–E in the given figure.

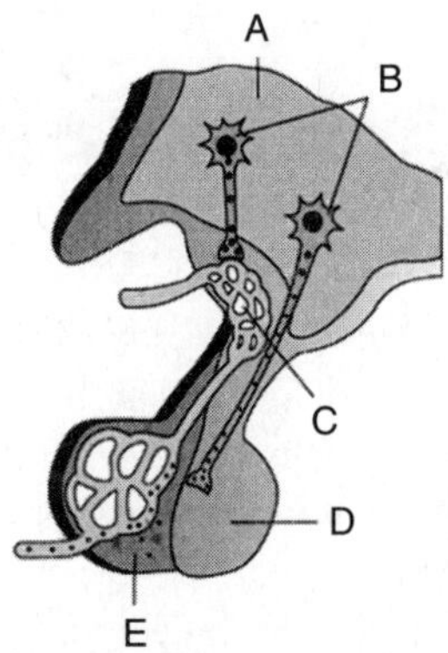

(a) A–Hypothalamus, B–Hypothalamic neurons, C–Portal circulation, D–Posterior pituitary, E–Anterior pituitary
(b) Posterior pituitary, B–Hypothalamic neurons, C–Hypothalamus, D–Anterior pituitary, E–Posterior pituitary
(c) A–Anterior pituitary, B–Portal circulation, C–Hypothalamus, D–Posterior pituitary, E–Hypothalamic neurons
(d) A–Hypothalamic neurons, B–Posterior pituitary, C–Anterior pituitary, D–Portal circulation, E–Hypothalamus

19. Adenohypophyis consists of
(a) pars distalis (b) pars intermedia
(c) pars nervosa (d) both (a) and (b)

20. Neurohypophysis consist of
(a) Pars distalis (b) Pars intermedia (c) Pars Nervosa (d) All

21. Which is commonly called anterior pituitary?
(a) Pars distalis (b) Pars intermedia (c) Pars Nervosa (d) All

22. Which is commonly called posterior pituitary?
(a) Pars distalis (b) Pars intermedia (c) Pars Nervosa (d) All

23. Which of the following hormones are secreted by pars distalis (find out total numbers)
GH, PRL, MSH, FSH, LH, TSH, ACTH, ADH
(a) 4 (b) 5 (c) 6 (d) 8

24. Pars intermedia secretes
(a) follicle stimulating hormone (b) melanocyte stimulating hormone
(c) melatonin (d) prolactin

25. Posterior pituitary stores and release two hormones
(a) oxytocin (b) vasopressin (ADH)
(c) growth hormone (d) both (a) and (b)

26. Where oxytocin and ADH is synthesized?
(a) Ant pituitary (b) Post pituitary (c) Hypothalamus (d) Thalamus
27. Following hormones regulate the growth of the mammary glands and formation of milk:
(a) GH (b) TSH
(c) Prolactin (PRL) (d) ACTH
28. Which of the hormone stimulates the synthesis and secretion of thyroid hormone is
(a) GH (growth hormone) (b) TSH (thyroid stimulating hormone)
(c) PRL (Prolactin) (d) ACTH (Adrenocorticotropic hormone)
29. Which of the following hormone stimulates the synthesis and secretion of steroid hormones called glcorticorticoids from the adrenal cortex?
(a) TSH (b) ACTH
(c) LH (d) FSH
30. ________ stimulates the synthesis and secretion of hormone called androgens from testis
(a) FSH (b) ACTH (c) LH = ICSH (d) GH
31. ________ induces ovulation of fully mature follicle (Graffian follicles) and maintains the corpus leuteum, formed from the remnants of the Graffian follicles after ovulation.
(a) FSH (b) ACTH (c) LH (d) GH
32. ________ stimulate growth and development of ovarian follicles in females
(a) FSH (b) LH (c) PRL (d) TSH
33. Which of the following hormones of anterior pituitary together called gonadotrohins?
(a) LH and ACTH (b) FSH and LH (c) TSH and PRL (d) MSH and LH
34. Over-secretion of GH (growth hormone) in child leads to
(a) Dwarfism (b) Cretinism
(c) Gigantism (d) Tetany
35. Low secretion of GH in child leads to
(a) Pituitary dwarfism (b) Gigantism
(c) Cretinism (d) Tetany
36. ________ acts on the smooth muscles of our body and stimulate their contraction
(a) LH (b) FSH (c) Oxytocin (d) GH
37. In females ________ stimulates a vigorous contraction of uterus at the time of child birth
(a) LH (b) FSH (c) Oxytocin (d) Relaxin
38. From which part of nephron ADH stimulates reabsorption of water and electrolyte
(a) PCT (b) HL
(c) Distal tubules (d) Bowman capsule
39. Following hormone is known as Antidiuretic hormone
(a) Oxytocin (b) Prolactin
(c) Luteinizing Hormone (d) Vasopressin
40. Diuresis is reduced by
(a) oxytocin (b) prolactin
(c) luteinizing hormone (d) vasopressin
41. ________ acts on melanocyte (melanin contains cells) and regulates pigmentation of skin.
(a) LH (b) Melatonin (c) MSH (d) TSH
42. Pineal gland is located on
(a) dorsal side of mid brain (b) dorsal side of hind brain
(c) dorsal side of forebrain (d) Vertical side of forebrain

43. Pineal gland secretes ________ hormone
(a) MSH (b) Melatonin
(c) FSJ (d) Insulin

44. Melatonin influences
(a) metabolism, pigmentation (b) menstrual cycle
(c) defence capability (d) all

45. 24 hr diurnal rhythms of our body is maintained by
(a) Melatonin (b) Glucagon (c) Thymosin (d) Oxytocin

46. Menstruation cycle is affect by the following hormones except
(a) Thyroid (b) Melatonin (c) Oestrogen (d) Oxytocin

47. Thin flap of connective tissue connect two lobes of thyroid is known as
(a) lobes (b) ileum (c) isthmus (d) ampulla

48. Which of the following is incorrect about thyroid gland?
(a) It is composed of follicles and stromal tissues
(b) It secretes tetraiodothyronine or thyroxine (T_4) and triiodothyronine (T_3), TCT
(c) It consists of 4 lobes
(d) It is stimulated by hormone TSH

49. Enlargement of thyroid gland is called
(a) Hypothyroidism (b) Hyperthyroidism
(c) Goitre (d) Isthmus

50. The features of cretinism includes
(a) stunted growth (b) mental retardation and low IQ
(c) abnormal skin and deaf mutism (d) all

51. Hypothyroidism in during pregnancy cause defective development and maturation of growing baby leading to
(a) addison's disease (b) cretinism
(c) creatinin (d) tetany

52. Hypothyroidism caused by
(a) cancer of thyroid gland (b) development of nodule of thyroid gland
(c) iodine deficiency (d) both (a) and (b)

53. Hypothyroidism causes
(a) irregular menstrual cycle (b) reduced BMR
(c) reduced production of RBC (d) all

54. Thyroid gland secrete
(a) T_3 (b) T_4 (c) TCT (d) All

55. Thyroid controls the metabolism of
(a) Carbohydrates (b) Proteins (c) Lipids (fat) (d) All

56. A. Melatonin influences menstrual cycle and our defence capability
B. In adult women, hypothyroidism may cause menstrual cycle to become irregular.
C. Protein hormone secreted by thyroid, TCT (Thyrocalcitonin) regulates the blood Calcium level.
D. Maintenance of water and electrolytes balance is also influence by thyroid hormone.
E. Oxytocin causes milk ejection from mammary gland.

Select the correct statement:
(a) A, B, C only (b) A, B, C, E only
(c) All except D (d) All statement are correct

57. Which of the following hormones affect Ca^{2+} ion metabolism?
(a) TCT (Thyrocalcitonin) (b) Parathyroid hormone (PTH)
(c) Both (d) Cortisol

58. Correct full form of PTM is
(a) Parathyroid hormone (b) Prethyroid hormone
(c) Prothyroid hormone (d) Pretectile hormone

59. PTH is
(a) Protein hormone (b) peptide hormone
(c) biogenic amines (d) steroid

60. Process by which PTH increase blood Ca^{2+} level except
(a) acts on bones and stimulates the process of bone reabsorption/dissolution/demineralisation
(b) reabsorption of Ca^{2+} by the renal tubules
(c) increases Ca^{2+} absorption from the digested food
(d) increases osteoblastic activity

61. Which of the following is correct about thymus?
(a) Globular structure located on the dorsal side of the heart and aorta
(b) It plays minor role in the development of the immune system
(c) Thymus size increase with age
(d) Thymus doesn't affect production of Antibodies

62. Thymosin is
(a) Peptide hormone (b) Secreted by pituitary
(c) Helps in RBC production (d) Decreases WBC production

63. Which gland play major role in the differentiation of T-lymphocyte?
(a) Thyroid (b) Thymus (c) Adrenal (d) gonads

64. Immune response of old persons are weak because
(a) thymus is degenerated in old individual (b) thymus production decreases
(c) both (d) none

65. Position of Adrenal gland is
(a) anterior part of each kidney (b) posterior part of each kidney
(c) ventral part of each kidney (d) dorsal part of each kidney

66. 'Cortex' terms used in
(a) Brain (b) kidney (c) Adrenal gland (d) All

67. The adrenal medulla secretes two hormone called adrenaline or epinephrine and nor-adrenaline or nor-epinephrine. These are commonly called as
(a) Steroids (b) Terpens
(c) catecholamine (d) Cytokinin

68. Emergency hormone and hormones of fight or fight are
(a) adrenalin (b) nor adrenaline
(c) cortisol (d) both (a) and (b)

69. A. Increase alertness
B. pupilary constriction
C. piloerection
D. increase heart rate
E. increase respiratory rate
F. sweating

Which of the above are effect of Adrebaline/Nor-Adrenalin
(a) All Except C
(b) All except B, F
(c) All except B
(d) All except B,E,F

70. Catecholamine causes
(a) Glycogenolysis (b) Proteolysis (c) Lipolysis (d) All

71. Glucocorticoid causes all except
(a) Proteolysis
(b) Lipolysis
(c) Glycogenolysis
(d) Gluconeogenesis

72. Histological adrenal cortex is divided into how many layers
(a) 1 (b) 2 (c) 3 (d) 4

73. Following layers are present in the adrenal cortex inner to outer
(a) Zona reticularis, zona fasciculate, zona glomerulosa
(b) Zona fasciculata, zona glomerulosis, zona reticularis
(c) Zona glomerulosa, zona reticularis, zona fasciculata
(d) Zona glomerulosa, zona fasciculate, zona reticularis

74. The adrenal cortex secret many hormones commonly called
(a) Catecholamine
(b) Peptide
(c) Corticoids
(d) All

75. In our body main Glucocorticoid is
(a) Adrenaline (b) Aldosterone (c) ADH (d) Cortisol

76. In our body main mineral corticoid is
(a) Adrenaline (b) Aldosterone (c) ADH (d) Cortisol

77. Which of the following is incorrect about Glucocorticoid?
(a) Inhibit cellular uptake and utilization of amino-acids
(b) Maintain cardio vascular system as well as kidney function
(c) Anti-inflammatory and suppresses the immune response
(d) Glucocorticoid stimulates gluconeogenesis, lipogenesis and proteolysis

78. Following are effects of Cortisol
(a) Anti-inflammatory
(b) Immune suppressant
(c) Increase RBC production
(d) All

79. Aldosterone causes all except
(a) Reabsorption of electrolyte and water from renal tubule
(b) Excretion of K^+
(c) Excretion of PO^{3-}_4 ion
(d) Absorption of K^+

80. Aldosterone helps in the maintenance of
(a) Electrolyte and body fluid volume
(b) Osmotic pressure
(c) Blood pressure
(d) All

81. Androgenic steroids are also secreted by adrenal cortex which causes
(a) growth of axial hair
(b) growth of pubic hair
(c) growth of facial hair
(d) all

82. Adrenal cortex secretes all except
(a) cortisol
(b) aldosterone
(c) androgenic steroid
(d) relaxin

83. 1 to 2 million Islets of Langerhans in a human pancreas represents ________ percent of the pancreatic tissue.
(a) 2–3 (b) 4–6 (c) 10 (d) 1–2

84. Islet of langerhans consists of
(a) ∝–cells (b) β cells (c) δ–cells (d) All

85. Following are the petide hormone except
(a) Insulin (b) PTH (c) Thymosin (d) T_4

86. A. Act mainly on liver cells
B. Stimulate Glycogenolysis
C. Stimulate gluconeogenesis
D. Reduces glucose uptake and utilization
Which of the following is correct about action of glucagon from above statements?
(a) A, B only (b) B, C only (c) A, B, C only (d) A,B,C,D All

87. Select the incorrect statement:
(a) Insulin and glucagon are peptide hormones
(b) Insulin acts mainly on hepatocyte and adipoaytes and enhance glucose uptake and utilization
(c) Insulin stimulate glycogeneis
(d) Glucagon inhibits process of gluconeogenesis

88. Following are the function of insulin except
(a) glycogenesis (b) ↑glucose utilization by hepatocyte
(c) ↑ glucose utilization by adipocyte (d) gluconeogenesis

89. Diabetes mellitus is characterised by
(a) Ketonuria (b) Glycosuria
(c) Prolonged hyperglyemia (d) All

90. Select the correct matching
(a) Insulin — ↓es uptake of glucose utilization by hepatoyte and adipocytes
(b) Cortisol — ↓es RBC production, causes inflammation
(c) Thymosin — Promotes production of antibodies to provide humoral immunity also
(d) Thyroxine — No role in water and electrolyte balance

91. Select the incorrect matching.
(a) Zona fasciculata — Glucocorticoids (b) ∝–cell — Glucagon
(c) β–cell — Insulin (d) Follicular cells of thyroid — TCT

92. Testis act as the
(a) primary sex organ (b) endocrine gland
(c) both (d) none

93. Leydig cells or interstitial cells secret
(a) Estrogens (b) Progesterone (c) Testosterone (d) Relaxin

94. Androgens, from the following are
(a) Estrogens (b) Progesterone
(c) Testosterone (d) Relaxin

95. A. Anabolic effect on protein and carbohydrate metabolism
B. Influences male sexual behaviour (libido)
C. Stimulates spermatogenesis
D. Muscular growth, aggressiveness, low pitch voice
Above are the functions of which of the following hormones?
(a) Estrogens (b) Progesterone (c) Testosterone (d) Relaxin

96. Select the total number of male accessory sex organs from the following:
Epididymis, Vas, Deferens, Seminal Vesicle, Prostate, Urethra.
(a) 2 (b) 3 (c) 4 (d) 5

97. Androgen regulates ________ of male accessory sex organ
(a) development (b) maturation (c) function (d) all

98. Testis is composed of
(a) Uriniferous tubules (b) Seminiferous tubules
(c) Nephron (d) Neuron

99. Select the correct matching:
(a) Interstitial cells–Testosterone (b) β-cells–Glucagon
(c) ∝-cells–Insulin (d) Follicular cells–TCT

100. Which one is correct about testis in human?
(a) Situated in scrotal sacs (outside the abdomen)
(b) Consist of seminiferous tubule and Leydig cells
(c) Secretion effect male sexual behaviour (libido)
(d) All

101. ANF leads to
(a) Dilation of blood vessels (b) ↓es blood pressure
(c) Both 1 and 2 (d) ↑es blood pressure

102. Match the column:

Column I (Production Site)		Column II (Hormones)
A. Atrial wall	–	1. ANF
B. Thyroid gland	–	2. PTH
C. Parathyroid	–	3. T_3, T_4, TCT
D. GIT	–	4. CCK, GIP, gastrin and secretin

(a) A–2, B–4, C–1, D–3 (b) A–1, B–3, C–2, D–4
(c) A–4, B–2, C–3, D–1 (d) A–4, B–3, C–2, D–1

103. Match the Column:

Hormone		Function
A. Gastrin	–	1. Act on exocrine pancrease and stimulate secretion of water and bicarbonate ion
B. Secretin	–	2. Action both pancrease and gall bladder and stimulate secretion of pancreatic enzyme and bile juice respectively
C. CCK (Cholesystokinin)	–	3. Act on gastric gland and stimulate secretion of HCl and pepsinogen
D. GIP (Gastric Inhibitory Peptide)	–	4. Inhibit gastric secretion and motility

(a) A–3, B–1, C–2, D–4 (b) A–1, B–3, C–4, D–2
(c) A–1, B–2, C–3, D–4 (d) A–4, B–3, C–1, D–2

104. The ________ of kidney produce peptide hormone called ________ which stimulate erythropoiesis.
(a) Podocyte, Erythropoietin (b) JG cells, Erythropoietin
(c) JG cells, Rennin (d) JG cells, Renin

105. Select the incorrect statement:
(a) GIT secrete four major peptide hormone
(b) Several other non–endocrine tissues secrete hormones called growth factors
(c) Hormone receptors are located in target tissues only
(d) Hormone receptors are non-specific in nature

106. Hormones are secreted by following organs which are non endocrine gland:
(a) Heart (b) Kidney (c) GIT (d) All

107. Select the incorrect matching:
Hormone Target organ
(a) Secretin Pancrease (b) CCK Pancrease and Gall bladder
(c) ANF Atrial wall (d) Gastrin Gastric glands

108. Match the source gland with its respective hormone as well as the function.

Source gland	Hormone	Function
(a) Posterior pituitary	Vasopressin	Stimulates reabsorption of water in the distal tubules in the nephron
(b) Corpus luteum	Oestrogen	Supports pregnancy
(c) Thyroid	Thyroxine	Regulated blood calcium level
(d) Anterior	Oxytocin	Contraction of uterus muscles during child birth

109. Select the total number of peptide hormones from the following:
Erythropoietin, Gastrin, Secretin, GIP, CCK, Insulin, Glucagon, Thymosin, PTH, ANF
(a) 8 (b) 7 (c) 9 (d) 10

110. Match the Column I with Column II:

Column I		Column II
A. Peptide, polypeptide protein hormones	–	1. Epinephrine.
B. Steroid	–	2. T_3 and T_4 (thyroid hormones)
C. Iodothyronines	–	3. Cortisol, testosterone, estradiol, progesterone, Aldosterone
D. Amino acid derivatives	–	4. Pituitary hormones, pancreatic hormones, hypothalamic hormone

(a) A–1, B–2, C–3, D–4 (b) A–4, B–3, C–2, D–1
(c) A–4, B–3, C–1, D–2 (d) A–1, B–4, C–3, D–2

111. A steroid hormone typically alters the activity of its target cells by
(a) changing membrane permeability of cells
(b) entering the cell and altering gene expression
(c) Activation of IP_3
(d) conversion ATP to cAMP

112. Hormone receptors are located in target tissue only. There position is
(a) In plasma membrane
(b) In cytoplasm
(c) In nucleus
(d) Any of the above depending on type of hormone

113. Find out the correct statement from the following:
1) Hormones interact with membrane bound receptors normally do not enter the target cells
2) Iodothyronines have membrane bound receptors
3) Hormones which interact with intracellular receptors mostly regulate gene expression
4) Steroid hormones generate second messengers
(a) 1 and 2 only (b) 2 and 3 only (c) 1 and 3 only (d) 2 and 4 only

114. Identify A, B, C and D in the given figure.

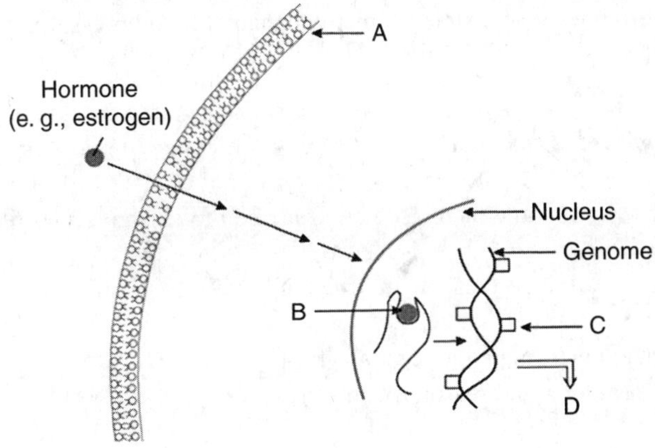

(a) A–Physiological response, B–Proteins, C–Receptor-hormone complex, D–Uterine cell membrane
(b) A–Receptor-hormone complex, B–Proteins, C–Uterine cell membrane, D–Physiological response
(c) A–Uterine cell membrane, B–Receptor-hormone complex, C–Proteins, D–Physiological response
(d) A–Proteins, B–Uterine cell membrane, C–Physiological response, D–Receptor-hormone complex

115. Find the total no. of hormones from the following which binds to intracellular receptors.
Cortisol, Testosterone, T3, Glucagon, Oxytocin, FSH, Progesterone, ICSH, Estrogen, GH
(a) 4 (b) 5 (c) 6 (d) 7

116. Which of the following act as secondary messenger?
(a) Ca^{2+} (b) IP_3 (c) cAMP (d) All 2Ca 3IP

117. Following hormones are iodothyronines
(a) T3 (b) T4 (c) TCT (d) Both (a) and (b)

118. Which in steroid hormone?
(a) GH (b) Insulin (c) Aldosterone (d) Epinephrine

119. Which of the following hormones do not act by a second messenger system?
(a) GH (b) Epinephrine (c) ICSH (d) Estrogen

120. Chemically epinephrine is
(a) Amino acid derivative (b) Peptide hormone
(c) Steroid hormone (d) Iodothyronines

121. Which hormone receptors are present in cytoplasm of target cell?
(a) Thyroxin (b) Estrogen (c) Insulin (d) All

122. Arrange in sequence, working of 'FSH'?
(1) Binding to membrane receptor
(2) Biochemical response
(3) Generation of second messenger
(4) Physiological response (ev. Ovarian growth)
(a) $1 \rightarrow 2 \rightarrow 3 \rightarrow 4$ (b) $1 \rightarrow 3 \rightarrow 2 \rightarrow 4$ (c) $4 \rightarrow 3 \rightarrow 2 \rightarrow 1$ (d) $3 \rightarrow 1 \rightarrow 4 \rightarrow 2$

123. Which hormone directly affect transcription by acting on gene?
(a) FSH (b) GH (c) Estrogen (d) CCK

124. Following hormones responsible for maintenance of blood pressure.
(a) Aldosterone (b) Renin (c) ANF (d) All

*Read the **assertion** and **reason** carefully to mark the correct option out of the options given below:*

(a) If both the assertion and the reason are true and the reason is a correct explanation of the assertion
(b) If both the assertion and reason are true but the reason is not a correct explanation of the assertion
(c) If the assertion is true but the reason is false
(d) If both the assertion and reason are false

125. Assertion: Aldosterone increases the volume of blood and other extracellular fluids.
Reason: The secretion of aldosterone is stimulated by a fall in the circulating volume of blood.

126. Assertion: FSH is also known as interstitial cell stimulating hormone.
Reason: It is because of the fact that FSH stimulates the interstitial cells of testis.

127. Assertion: Oxytocin is also known as Anti Diuretic hormone (ADH).
Reason: Oxytocin can cause an increase in the renal reabsorption of water.

128. Assertion: Failure of secretion of thyroid gland hormones from childhood causes cretinism disease.
Reason: Thyrotropin hormone maintains BMR and promote growth of body tissues.

129. Assertion: Hormones are similar to enzymes in their action and chemical nature.
Reason: Hormones and enzymes are proteinaceous in nature and act as informational molecules.

130. Assertion: Glucagon is said to lower down the blood sugar level.
Reason: Glucagon increase the utilisation of glucose in the tissue and the synthesis of liver glycogen.

131. Assertion: Prolactin is also called the 'Milk ejection hormone'.
Reason: Prolactin stimulates the smooth muscle contractions of the mammary glands.

132. Assertion: A tumor of adrenal cortex may cause addison's disease.
Reason: This happens due to over secretion of cortisol by the tumor.

133. Assertion: Neurohypophysis(Pars nervosa) also known as posterior pitutary.
Reason: Posterior pitutary stores and releases two hormones called oxytocin and vasopressin.

134. Assertion: Vasopressin is also known as anti- diueretic hormone.
Reason: vasopressin stimulate reabsorbtion of water and electrolyte by distal tubules and there by reduce diuresis.

135. Assertion: Enlargement of throid gland is known as goitre.
Reason: Goitre occur due to deficiency of iodine only.

136. Assertion: Immune response of old person become weak.
Reason: Thymus is degenerate in old individuals.

137. **Assertion:** Adrenal cortex can be removed without causing death.
Reason: Adrenal cortex is not vital for survival.

138. **Assertion:** Failure of secretion of somatotropin from an early age causes dwarfism in the patient.
Reason: Somatotropin hormone stimulates the body growth and elongation of long bones.

AIPMT PREVIOUS YEAR QUESTIONS

1. Select the correct matching of a hormone, its source and function.
[AIPMT MAINS 2010]

Hormone	Source	Source
(a) Vasopressin	Posterior pituitary	Increases loss of water through urine
(b) Norepinephrine	Adrenal medulla	Increases heart beat, rate of respiration and alterness
(c) Glucagon	Beta-cells of islets of lengerhans	Stimulates glycogenolysis
(d) Prolactin	Posterior pituitary	Regulates growth of mammary glands and milk formation in females

2. Injury to adrenal cortex is not likely to affect the secretion of which one of the following?
[AIPMT PRE 2010]
(a) Aldosterone
(b) Both androstenedione and dehydroepiandrosterone
(c) Adrenalin
(d) Cortisol

3. Low Ca^{2+} in the body fluid may be the cause of
[AIPMT PRE 2010]
(a) Tetany (b) anaemia
(c) Angina pectoris (d) Gout

4. Which one of the following pairs is incorrectly matched?
[AIPMT PRE 2010]
(a) Glucagon – Beta cells (source)
(a) Somatostatin – Delta cells (source)
(b) Corpus luteum – Relaxin (secretion)
(c) Insulin – Diabetes mellitus (disease)

5. Toxic agents present in food which interfere with thyroxin synthesis lead to the development of:
[AIPMT PRE 2010]
(a) Toxic goitre (b) Cretinism
(c) Simple goitre (d) Thyrotoxicosis

6. Match the source gland with its respective hormone as well as the function. [AIPMT PRE 2011]

Source gland	Hormone	Function
(a) Posterior pituitary	Vasopressin	Stimulates reabsorption of water in the distal tubules in the nephron
(b) Corpus luteum	Oestrogen	Supports pregnancy
(c) Thyroid	Thyroxine	Regulated blood calcium level
(d) Anterior	Oxytocin	Contraction of uterus muscles during child birth

7. Given ahead is an incomplete table about certain hormones, their source glands and one major effect of each on the body in humans. Identify the correct option for the three blanks A, B and C.

Gland	Secretion	Effect on body
A	Oestrogen	Maintenance of secondary sexual characters
Alpha cells of islets of Langerhans	B	Raises blood sugar level
Anterior pituitary	C	Over secretion leads to gigantism

[AIPMT PRE 2011]

Options:
(a) A: Placenta, B: Insulin, C: Vasopressin
(b) A: Ovary, B: Insulin, C: Calcitonin
(c) A: Placenta, B: Glucagon, C: Calcitonin
(d) A: Ovary, B: Glucagon, C: Growth hormone

8. The 24 hours (diurnal) rhythm of our body such as the sleep-wake cycle is regulated by the hormone [AIPMT MAINS 2011]
(a) Calcitonin (b) Prolactin
(c) Adrenaline (d) Melatonin

9. The Leydig cells as found in the human body are the secretory source of: [AIPMT PRE 2012]
(a) Progesterone (b) Intestinal mucus
(c) Glucagon (d) Androgens

10. Which one of the following pairs of hormones are the examples of those that can easily pass through cell membrane the target cell and bind to a receptor inside it (mostly in the nucleus). [AIPMT PRE 2012]
(a) Insulin, glucagon (b) Thyroxin, insulin
(c) Somatostatin, oxytocin (d) Cortisol, testosterone

11. What is correct to say about the hormone action in humans? [AIPMT PRE 2012]
(a) Glucagon is secreted by β-cells of Islets of Langerhans and stimulates glycogenolysis
(b) Secretion of thymosins is stimulated with aging
(c) In females, FSH first binds with specific receptors on ovarian cell membrane
(d) FHS stimulates the secretion of estrogen and progesterone

12. Which of the following statements is correct in relation to the endocrine system? [AIPMT 2013]

(a) Adenopophysis is under direct neural regulation of the hypothalamus.
(b) Organs in the body like gastrointestinal tract, heart, kidney and liver do not produce any hormones
(c) Non – nutrient chemicals produced by the body in trace amount that act as intercellular messenger are known as hormones.
(d) Releasing and inhibitory hormones are produced by the pituitary gland

13. A pregnant female delivers a baby who suffers from stunted growth, mental retardation, low intelligence quotient and abnormal skin. [AIPMT 2013]

(a) Deficiency of iodine in diet
(b) Low secretion of growth hormone
(c) Cancer of the thyroid gland
(d) Over secretion of pars distalis

14. Select the answer which correctly matches the endocrine gland with the hormone it secretes and its function / deficiency symptom. (A: Endocrine gland, B: Hormone, C: Function/deficiency symptoms) [AIPMT 2013]

A	B	C
(a) Anterior pituitary	Oxytocin	Stimulates uterus contraction during child birth
(b) Posterior pituitary	Growth hormone (GH)	Over secretion stimulates abnormal growth
(c) Thyroid	Thyroxin	Lack of iodine in diet results in goitre
(d) Corpus luteum	Testosterone	Stimulates spermatogenesis

15. Identify the hormone with its correct matching of source and function: [AIPMT 2014]

(a) Oxytocin – posterior pituitary, growth and maintenance of mammary glands
(b) Melatonin – pineal gland, regulates the normal rhythm of sleepwake cycle
(c) Progesterone – corpus-luteum, stimulation of growth and activities of female secondary sex organs
(d) Atrial natriuretic factor – ventricular wall increases the blood pressure.

16. Fight-or-flight reactions cause activation of: [AIPMT 2014, RE-AIPMT 2015]

(a) The parathyroid glands, leading to increased metabolic rate
(b) The kidney, leading to suppression of rennin-angiotensin-aldosterone pathway
(c) The adrenal medulla, leading to increased secretion of epinephrine and norepinephrene
(d) The pancreas leading to a reduction in the blood sugar levels

17. Which one of the following hormones is not involved in sugar metabolism? [AIPMT 2015, RE-AIPMT 2015]

(a) Aldosterone (b) Insulin
(c) Glucagon (d) Cortisone

18. A chemical signal that has both endocrine and neural roles is: [AIPMT 2015]

(a) Melatonin (b) Calcitonin
(c) Epinephrine (d) Cortisol

19. Which one of the following hormones though synthesized elsewhere, is stored and released by the master gland? [RE-AIPMT 2015]

(a) Luteinizing hormone (b) Prolactin
(c) Melanocyte stimulating hormone (d) Antidiuretic hormone

Answer Keys

1. (d)	2. (c)	3. (b)	4. (d)	5. (b)	6. (d)	7. (b)	8. (d)	9. (c)	10. (a)
11. (b)	12. (a)	13. (d)	14. (c)	15. (d)	16. (d)	17. (d)	18. (a)	19. (d)	20. (c)
21. (a)	22. (c)	23. (c)	24. (b)	25. (d)	26. (c)	27. (c)	28. (b)	29. (b)	30. (c)
31. (c)	32. (a)	33. (b)	34. (c)	35. (a)	36. (c)	37. (c)	38. (c)	39. (d)	40. (d)
41. (c)	42. (c)	43. (b)	44. (d)	45. (a)	46. (d)	47. (c)	48. (c)	49. (c)	50. (d)
51. (b)	52. (d)	53. (d)	54. (d)	55. (d)	56. (d)	57. (c)	58. (a)	59. (b)	60. (d)
61. (a)	62. (a)	63. (b)	64. (c)	65. (a)	66. (d)	67. (c)	68. (d)	69. (c)	70. (d)
71. (c)	72. (c)	73. (a)	74. (c)	75. (d)	76. (b)	77. (d)	78. (d)	79. (d)	80. (d)
81. (d)	82. (d)	83. (d)	84. (d)	85. (d)	86. (d)	87. (d)	88. (d)	89. (d)	90. (c)
91. (d)	92. (c)	93. (c)	94. (c)	95. (c)	96. (d)	97. (d)	98. (b)	99. (a)	100. (d)
101. (c)	102. (b)	103. (a)	104. (b)	105. (d)	106. (d)	107. (c)	108. (a)	109. (d)	110. (b)
111. (b)	112. (d)	113. (c)	114. (c)	115. (b)	116. (d)	117. (d)	118. (c)	119. (d)	120. (a)
121. (a)	122. (b)	123. (c)	124. (d)	125. (b)	126. (d)	127. (d)	128. (c)	129. (d)	130. (d)
131. (d)	132. (d)	133. (b)	134. (a)	135. (c)	136. (a)	137. (d)	138. (a)		

AIPMT Previous Year Questions

1. (b)	2. (c)	3. (a)	4. (a)	5. (c)	6. (a)	7. (d)	8. (d)	9. (d)	10. (d)
11. (c)	12. (c)	13. (a)	14. (c)	15. (b)	16. (c)	17. (d)	18. (c)	19. (d)	

Unit

VI

Reproduction

This unit is divided into four chapters—Reproduction in Organisms, Sexual Reproduction in Flowering Plants, Human Reproduction and Reproductive Health. The unit is very important in understanding the process of reproduction, both in plants and animals. The chapter titled 'Human Reproduction' should be dealt with particular care as 3–5 questions are asked from this chapter. Figure-based questions are very important and should be dealt with careful and special attention.

CHAPTER 23 Reproduction in Organisms

1. Clones are
   (a) Morphologically similar
   (b) Genetically similar
   (c) Both (a) and (b)
   (d) None of the above
2. The approximate life span of a parrot is
   (a) 60 yrs
   (b) 1–2 weeks
   (c) 15 yrs
   (d) 140 yrs
3. The approximate life span of a crocodile is
   (a) 60 yrs
   (b) 15 yrs
   (c) 150 yrs
   (d) 140 yrs
4. Arrange the following in decreasing order of their life span
   (1) Crocodile
   (2) Dog
   (3) Crow
   (4) Parrot
   (a) 1 > 2 > 3 > 4
   (b) 2 > 3 > 4 > 1
   (c) 4 > 1 > 2 > 3
   (d) 4 > 1 > 3 > 2
5. Life span of a tortoise is approx
   (a) 50–100 yrs
   (b) 100–150 yrs
   (c) 150–200 yrs
   (d) 200–250 yrs
6. The given diagram shows:

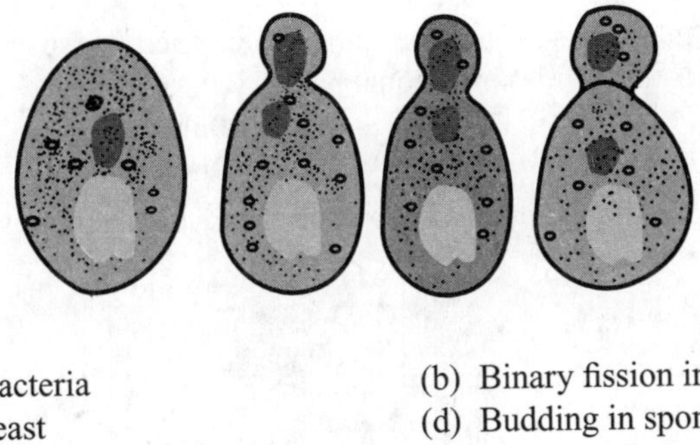

   (a) Budding in Bacteria
   (b) Binary fission in amoeba
   (c) Budding in yeast
   (d) Budding in sponge
7. Sexual reproduction is characterized by:
   (a) Two parent participation
   (b) Formation of gametes
   (c) Fusion of gametes
   (d) All of the above
8. Asexual reproduction is common among all except:
   (a) Unicellular organisms
   (b) Plants with simple organization
   (c) Animals with simple organization
   (d) Animals with complex organization

9. In which of these organisms is cell division in itself a mode of reproduction?
(a) Amoeba
(b) E. coli
(c) Euglena
(d) All

10. The given diagram shows:
(a) Budding in Bacteria
(b) Binary fission in amoeba
(c) Budding in yeast
(d) Budding in sponge

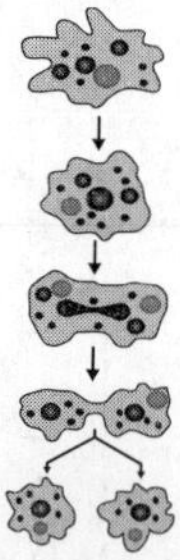

11. Cell division is synonymous with reproduction in:
(a) Plants and Fungi
(b) Animal and Plant
(c) Protista and Monera
(d) Monera and Algae

12. Binary fission is seen in:
(a) Amoeba
(b) Paramecium
(c) Vorticella
(d) All of these

13. Which of these organisms show budding?
(a) Yeast
(b) Hydra
(c) Sponge
(d) All

14. Find the false statement.
(A) In yeast unequal division leads to bud formation.
(B) When offspring is produced by a single parent with or without the involvement of gamete formation, the reproduction is asexual.
(C) Size of crows and parrots are not very different yet their life span shows a wide difference.
(D) In binary fission cell divides in unequal parts.
(a) Only B and D
(b) Only C
(c) Only D
(d) Only A and B

15. Approximate life span of the organism shown in the given diagram is:

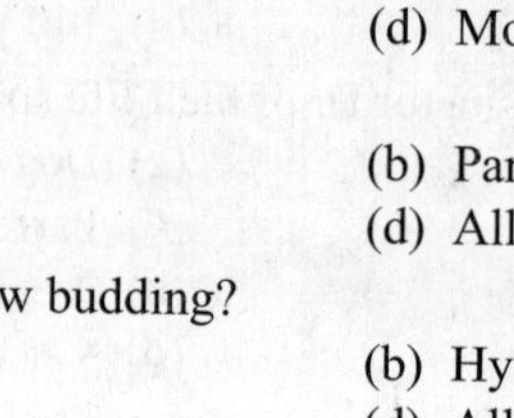

(a) 5 yrs
(b) 15 yrs
(c) 25 yrs
(d) 50 yrs

16. Match column-I (Organism) with column-II (reproductive structure).

Column-I	Column-II
(A) Penicillium	(1) Conidia
(B) Hydra	(2) Exogenous bud
(C) Sponge	(3) Gemmules (Endogenous buds)
(D) Paramecium	(4) Binary fission

(a) A:1, B:2, C:3, D:4
(b) A:4, B:1, C:3, D:2
(c) A:1, B:3, C:4, D:2
(d) A:2, B:1, C:4, D:3

17. Select the incorrect statement.
(a) Members of the Kingdom Fungi and simple plants such as algae reproduce through special asexual reproductive structures.
(b) Zoospores are generally microscopic motile structures.
(c) Zoospores are usually macroscopic motile structures.
(d) Clones are morphologically and genetically similar individuals.

18. Which are the units of vegetative propagation in plants?
(a) Runners and rhizomes
(b) Suckers and bulbs
(c) Tuber and offset
(d) All of these

19. In plants, the units of vegetative propagation are capable of giving rise to new offspring. These structures are called:
(a) Zoospores
(b) Asexual spores
(c) Vegetative propagules
(d) Rhizomes

20. Match Column-I (Structure) with Column-II (Name of structure and its parent plant).

Column-I	Column-II
A. 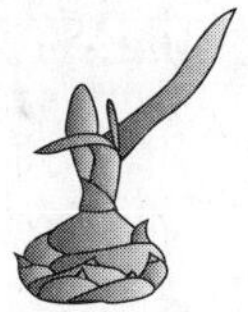	1. Bulbil of Agave
B. 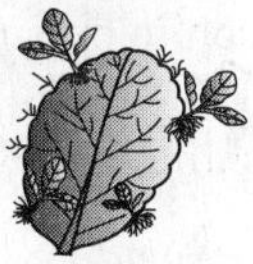	2. Leaf buds of Bryophyllum
C. 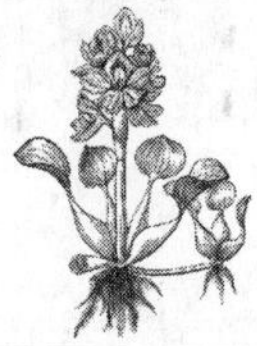	3. Offset of water hyacinth (Terror of Bengal)

(a) A:2, B:1, C:3
(b) A:1. B:2, C:3
(c) A:3, B:2, C:1
(d) A:2, B:3, C:1

21. Which is the incorrect statement about water hyacinth?
    (a) Introduced in India for their lovely flowers and shape of leaves.
    (b) It is world's most problematic terrestrial weed.
    (c) It reproduce asexually through offsets
    (d) Its botanical name is *Eicchornia crassipes*
22. Vegetative propagules of Agave i
    (a) Tuber (b) Rhizome
    (c) Bulbil (d) Runner
23. Vegetative propagules of *Solanum tuberosum* is:
    (a) Tuber (b) Rhizome
    (c) Bulbil (d) Offset
24. Select the odd one out.
    (a) Tuber (b) Rhizome
    (c) Bulbil (d) Zoospores
25. Rhizomes are vegetative propagules of:
    (a) Apple (b) Banana
    (c) Mango (d) Grapes
26. Which of these points is false about the diagram?

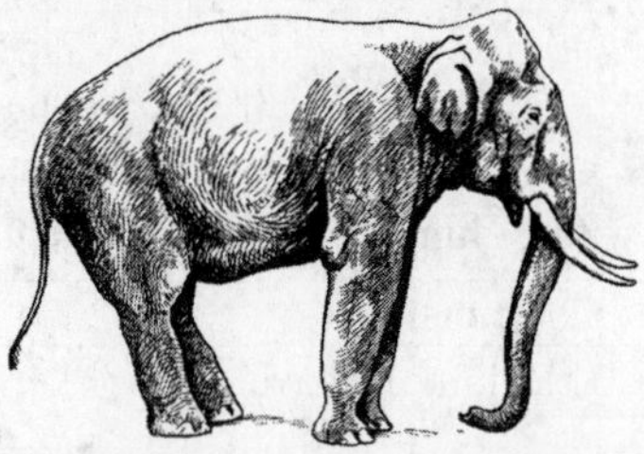

    (a) Belongs to class mammalia (b) Life span is approx 40 yrs
    (c) Belongs to genus Elephas (d) Crepuscular animal.
27. Choose the correct statement.
    (A) Asexual reproduction method is the common method of reproduction in organisms with relatively simple organization like algae and fungi.
    (B) Organism with relatively simple organization like algae and fungi shifted to sexual mode of reproduction just before onset of adverse conditions.
    (C) Vegetative as well as sexual mode of reproduction is exhibited by the higher plants
    (D) Only sexual mode of reproduction is present in most of the animals.
    (a) A and B only (b) B and C only
    (c) C and D only (d) All A, B, C and D
28. Sexual reproduction as compared to asexual reproduction is a:
    (A) Slow process (B) Fast process
    (C) Simple process (D) Complex process
    (a) A and D only (b) A and C only
    (c) B and D only (d) B and C only

29. Plants, animals or fungi differ in all of these aspects except:
(a) External morphology (b) Internal structure
(c) Physiology (d) Pattern of sexual mode of reproduction

30. Which of these plants which do not show clear cut vegetative, reproductive and senescent phase?
(a) Annual plant (b) Biennial plant
(c) Perennial plant (d) All of these

31. Which information is false about the organism shown in the diagram?

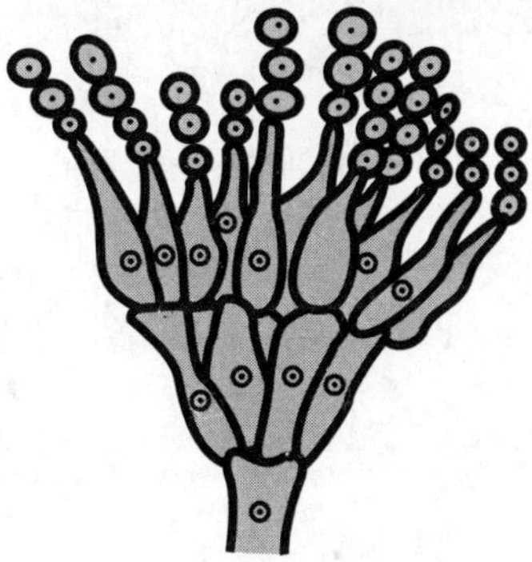

(a) Reproduce by basidiospores (b) It is a multicellular fungus.
(c) It is conidia of penicillium. (d) Belongs to ascomycetes.

32. Which of the following flowers only once in their lifetime?
(a) Mango (b) Neem
(c) Bamboo (d) All of these

33. Which of the following plant flowers once in 12 years?
(a) *Mangifera indica* (b) *Strobilanthus kunthiana* (Neelakuranji)
(c) *Helianthus annus* (d) *Papver somniferum*

34. Which of these statement is true about *Strobilanthus kunthiana*?
(a) This plant flowered during September–October 2006.
(b) Its mass flowering transformed large tracks of hilly areas in Kerala, Karnataka and Tamil Nadu into blue stretches.
(c) It flowers once in 12 years.
(d) All of the above

35. In animals, the juvenile phase is followed by – changes prior to active reproductive behaviour.
(a) Morphological changes (b) Physiological changes
(c) Genetical changes (d) Both (a) and (b)

36. Which of the following mammals show menstrual cycle?
(a) Monkeys (b) Apes
(c) Humans (d) All of these

37. The diagram shows:

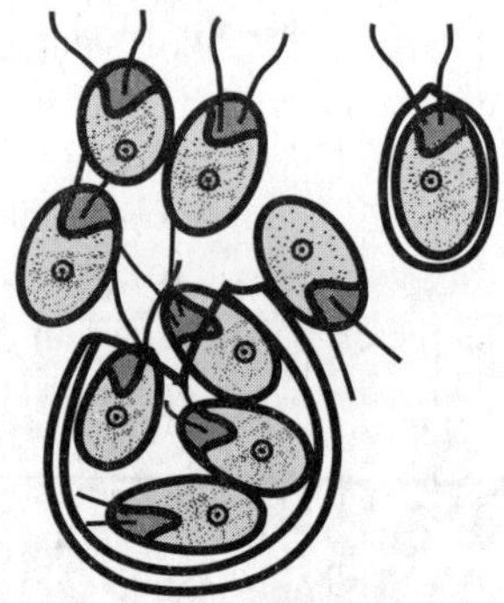

(a) Zoospores of hydra
(b) Conidia of Penicillium
(c) Gemmules in sponge
(d) Zoospores of chlamydomonas

38. Oestrous cycle occurs in:
(a) Cows
(b) Rats
(c) Deer
(d) All of these

39. Find the correct statement.
(a) 'Reproductive phase' is of same duration in all organisms.
(b) Birds in captivity can be made to lay eggs throughout the year.
(c) Female of non-primates shows cyclical changes during reproductive phase which is known as menstrual cycle.
(d) Perennial plants show clear cut vegetative, reproductive and senescent phase.

40. Most wild mammals are:
(a) Continuous breeder
(b) Seasonal breeder
(c) Continuous for half year, seasonal for next half year.
(d) None of the above

41. Which of these statements is false about the diagram?

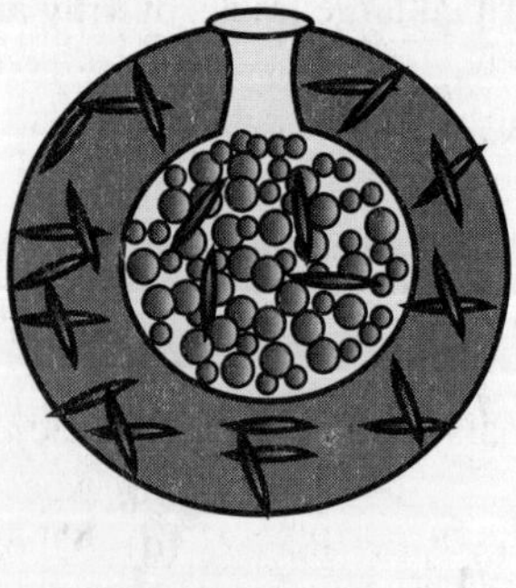

(a) It represents asexual reproductive structure of hydra.
(b) It contains archeocyte cells.
(c) It represents asexual reproductive structure of sponges.
(d) It shows gemmules in sponges.

42. 'Humans' are:
(a) Seasonal breeder
(b) Continuous breeder
(c) Both
(d) None of these

43. Which of the following can be considered as one of the parameter of senescence or old age?
(a) End of Juvenile or vegetative phase
(b) End of Reproductive phase
(c) Hormonal imbalance
(d) Slowing of metabolism due to disease

44. Pre-fertilization events among these are:
(a) Syngamy
(b) Gametogenesis and Gamete transfer
(c) Formation of zygote
(d) Embryogenesis

45. Gametes are generally:
(a) Haploid
(b) Triploid
(c) Diploid
(d) Hexaploid

46. The diagram shows:

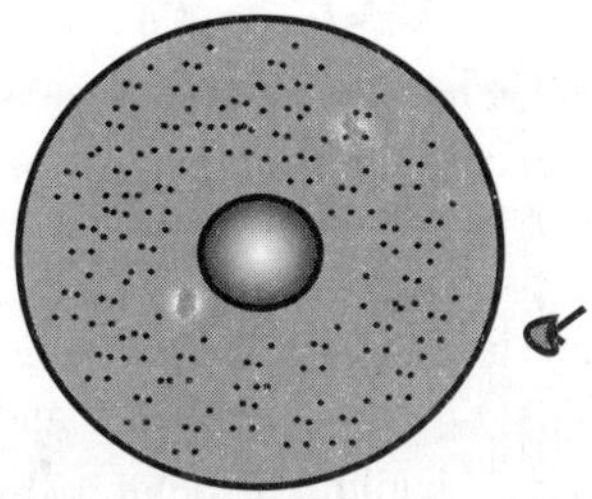

(a) Homogametes of cladophora
(b) Heterogametes of Fucus
(c) Hetrogametes of cladophora
(d) Heterogametes of Fungus

47. Which of the following is/are male gametes?
(a) Egg
(b) Ovum
(c) Antherozoids
(d) Zygote

48. Count the total number of organisms which are monoecious.
Cucurbits, Coconut, Papaya, Date palm, Chara, Marchantia
(a) 1
(b) 2
(c) 3
(d) 4

49. Archegoniophore is present in:
(a) Chara
(b) Papaya
(c) Marchantia
(d) Fucus

50. Select the incorrect statement.
(a) Unisexual male flower is staminate.
(b) Unisexual female flower is pistillate.
(c) Heterothallic and dioecious are terms used to describe unisexual condition.
(d) Cockroach is a hermaphrodite.

51. Select the example/s of hermaphrodite organism/s among these.
(a) Earthworm
(b) Tapeworm
(c) Leech
(d) All of these

52. Identify A, B, C in the diagram.

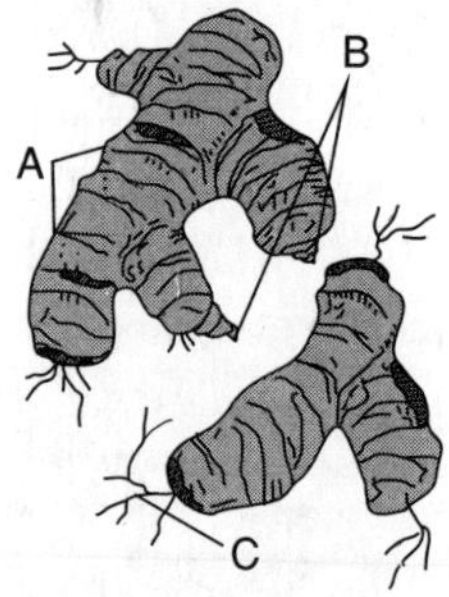

(a) A: Nodes, B: Buds, C: Adventitious root
(b) A: Buds, B: Nodes, C: Top root
(c) A: Adventitious root, B: Nodes, C: Buds
(d) A: Tape root, B: Nodes, C: Buds

53. Monoecious plants means:
(A) Only male flowers are present in the plant
(B) Only female flowers are present in the plant
(C) Bisexual flowers are present in the plants
(D) Separate male and female flowers are present in the same plant.
(a) Only A
(b) Only D
(c) Only C
(d) C and D both

54. Which of these organisms has/have haploid parental body?
(a) Monera and fungi
(b) Algae
(c) Bryophytes
(d) All of these

55. Which of these organisms has/have diploid parental body?
(a) Pteridophyte and gymnosperm
(b) Angiosperm
(c) Most of animals
(d) All of the above

56. Anthridiophore is present in:
(a) Chara
(b) Fucus
(c) Marchantia
(d) Sweet potato

57. The diagram shows:

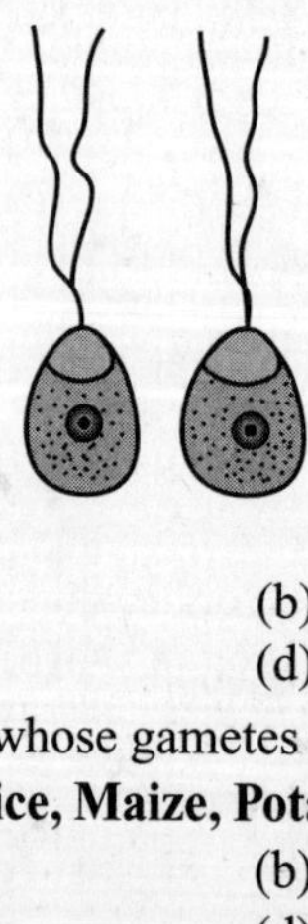

(a) Homogametes of cladophora
(b) Homogametes of Fucus
(c) Hetrogametes of cladophora
(d) Heterogametes of Fungus

58. Find out total number of organism whose gametes contain odd number of chromosomes.
Rat, Housefly, Dog, Cat, Apple, Rice, Maize, Potato, Onion
(a) 3
(b) 4
(c) 5
(d) 6

59. Meiocyte of which organism contain maximum number of chromosomes?
(a) Fruit fly (b) Butterfly
(c) Ophiglossum (a fern) (d) Human

60. Meiocyte of cat contains how many chromosomes?
(a) 8 (b) 12
(c) 42 (d) 38

61. Identify the plant part given in below diagram belongs to which plant given in option.

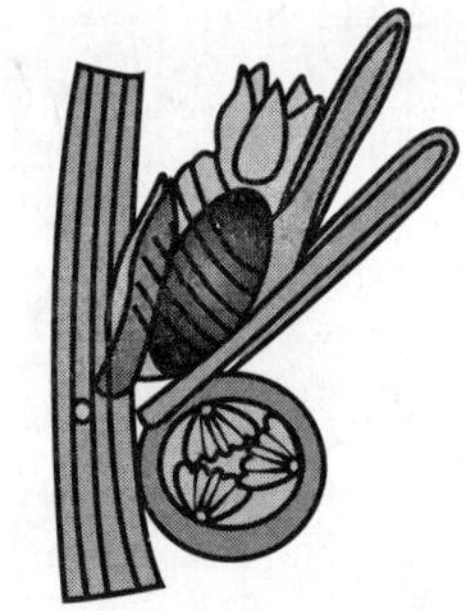

(a) 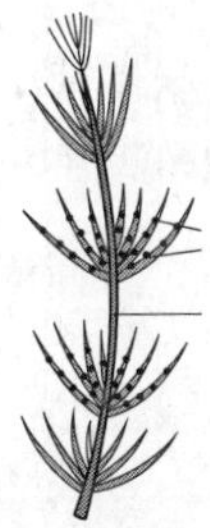

(b) 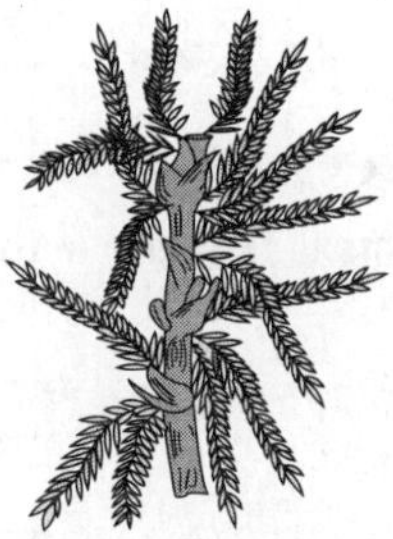

(c) 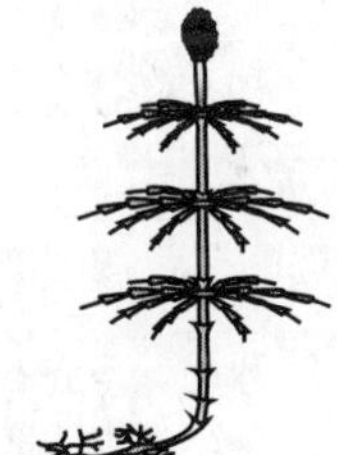

(d) 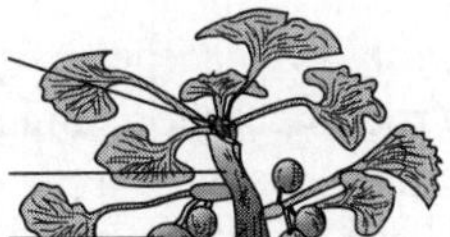

62. Water is a medium for gamete transfer in:
(a) Bryophytes (b) Pteridophyte
(c) Algae (d) All of these

63. Which of these are carriers of male gamete in seed plants?
(a) Microspore mother cell (b) Megasporemother cell
(c) Anther (d) Pollen grains

64. Transfer of pollen grains from anther to stigma is known as:
(a) Emasculation (b) Pollination
(c) Bagging (d) Fertilization

65. Most critical event in sexual reproduction is:
(a) Gametogenesis
(b) Gamete transfer
(c) Fertilization (Syngamy)
(d) Embryogenesis

66. Match column-I (Organism) with column-II (Chromosome number in meiocyte).

Column-I	Column-II
(A) Housefly	(1) 12
(B) Apple	(2) 34
(C) Rice	(3) 24
(D) Rat	(4) 42
(E) Onion	(5) 32

(a) A:1, B:2, C:3, D:4, E:5
(b) A:2, B:3, C:1, D:4, E:5
(c) A:5, B:4, C:3, D:2, E:1
(d) A:3, B:2, C:1, D:4, E:5

67. Select the incorrect statement from the following.
(a) Few fungi and algae have motile male and motile female gametes.
(b) Most vital event of sexual reproductive is the fusion of gametes.
(c) Pea is a bisexual self fertilizing plant.
(d) In majority of organisms male gamete is non-motile and female gamete is motile.

68. Parthenogenesis is shown by:
(a) Rotifers
(b) Honeybees
(c) Some lizards and birds (turkey)
(d) All of above

69. Which of these statements is false about the diagram?

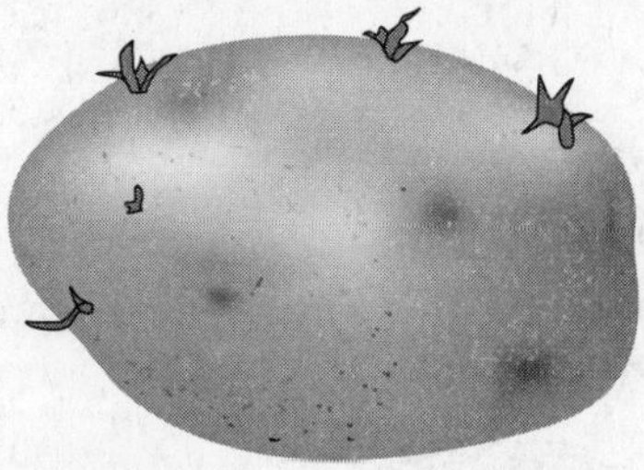

(a) It belongs to family solanaceae.
(b) It is a modified root meant for storage.
(c) It is a modified stem meant for reproduction.
(d) Eyes of the above structure are axillary buds.

70. External fertilization is seen in all of these except:
(a) Algae
(b) Amphibians
(c) Fishes
(d) Mammals

71. Find the incorrect statement.
(a) Large number of gametes are released in surrounding water in external fertilization
(b) Offspring produced by external fertilization are extremely vulnerable to predators.
(c) External fertilization is shown by bony fishes and frogs.
(d) In seed plant motile male gametes are carried to female gamete by pollen tubes.

72. Internal fertilization is seen in:
(a) Reptiles
(b) Birds
(c) Mammals
(d) All of these

73. Internal fertilization is seen in:
(a) Bryophytes
(b) Pteridophytes
(c) Gymnosperm and Angiosperm
(d) All of the above

74. Which of these characteristics belong to organisms showing internal fertilization?
(a) Eggs are formed inside the female body where they fuse with male gamete.
(b) Male gametes are motile
(c) Number of eggs produced less in number
(d) All of the above

75. Development of embryo from zygote is:
(a) Parthenogenesis
(b) Embryogenesis
(c) Blastulation
(d) Gastrulation

76. Life in all organism starts from:
(a) Single cell zygote
(b) Two celled zygote
(c) Single cell embryo
(d) Multicellular embryo

77. Select the total number of true statements.
(A) In organisms belonging to fungi and algae, the zygote develops a thick wall that is resistant to dessication and damage.
(B) Formation of diploid zygote is universal in all sexually reproducing organisms.
(C) Syngamy occurs inside the body of the organism in internal fertilization.
(D) In organism with haplontic life cycle zygote divides by meiosis to form haploid spores that grow into haploid individuals.
(a) 1
(b) 2
(c) 2
(d) 4

78. Following are oviparous except:
(a) Crocodile
(b) Crow
(c) Parrot
(d) Horse

79. In oviparous animals like birds and reptiles the fertilized egg in covered by shell made up of ________.
(a) SiO_2
(b) Na_2CO_3
(c) $CaCO_3$
(d) $MgCO_3$

80. Chances of survival of the young one is greater in:
(a) Internal fertilization
(b) External fertilization
(c) Oviparous animals
(d) Viviparous animals

81. After fertilization which part of flower generally withers and falls off?
(a) Sepals
(b) Petals
(c) Stamens
(d) All of these

82. Select the false statement.
(a) Ovule develops into seed.
(b) Ovary develops into fruit.
(c) Zygote develops into embryo.
(d) Placenta develops into pericarp.

83. A, B, C and D shows which type of placentation respectively?

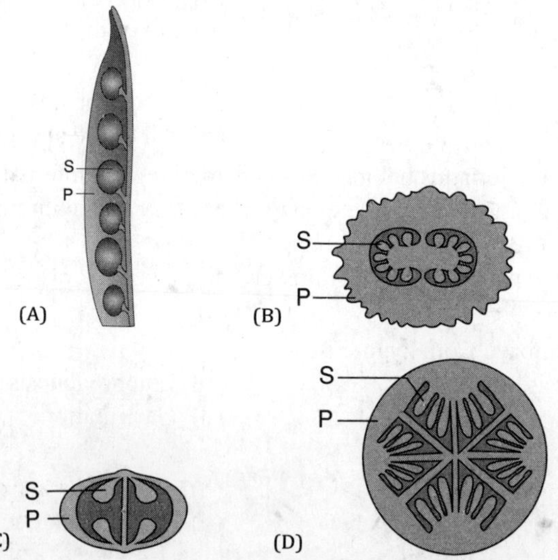

(a) A: Marginal, B: Free central, C: Perietal, D: Axile
(b) A: Perietal, B: Marginal, C: Axile, D: Free central
(c) A: Axile, B: Free central, C: Marginal, D: Perietal
(d) A: Axile, B: Perietal, C: Free central, D: Marginal

84. Gametes in haploid organisms are produced by:
(a) Amitosis (b) Mitosis
(c) Meiosis (d) Cleavage

85. Embryonal protection and care are better in:
(a) Oviparity (b) Parthenogenesis
(c) Viviparity (d) Polyembryony

86. After fertilization in angiosperms, ovules develop into:
(a) Pericarp (b) Fruit
(c) Seed (d) Embryo

87. 'A' in the diagram shows:

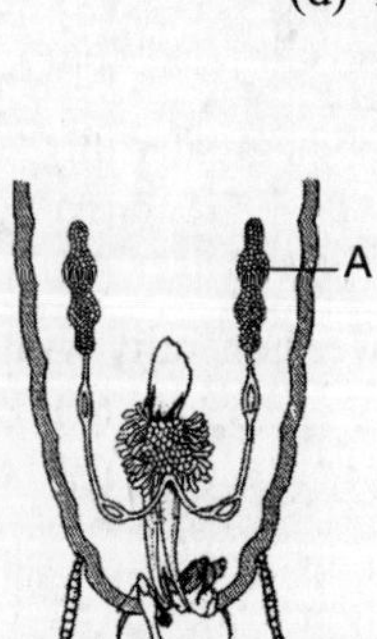

(a) Testis of a male cockroach (b) Ovary of a female cockroach
(c) Testis of an earthworm (d) Ovary of an earthworm

88. The progenitor of the next generation inside the mature seed is known as:
(a) Micropyle (b) Pericarp
(c) Embryo (d) Zygote

89. Identify the ploidy of the following parts of flowering plants.
Ovary, Anther, Egg, Pollen, Male gamete and Zygote
(a) 2n, 2n, n, n, n, 2n (b) 2n, 3n, n, n, 2n, 2n
(c) 2n, n, n, n, n, 2n (d) 2n, 2n, n, 2n, n, 2n

90. Select the correct statement from the following.
(A) In flowering plants, the zygote is formed inside the ovule.
(B) In reptiles and birds, the fertilized eggs covered by hard calcareous shell (Cleidoic) are laid in a safe place in environment,
(C) In organisms belonging to fungi and algae, the zygote develops a thick wall that is vulnerable to dessication and damage.
(D) During embryogenesis, zygote undergoes cell division and cell differentiation
(a) A and C only (b) A, B and C only
(c) C and D only (d) A, B and D only

91. Which of these statements is true about chara?
(a) Oogonium and Anthredium are present on different plants.
(b) Oogonium is placed in the upper part andAnthredium in the lower part.
(c) Oogonium is placed in the lower part andAnthredium in upper part
(d) Chara belongs to angiosperm

92. Identify A and B in this diagram.

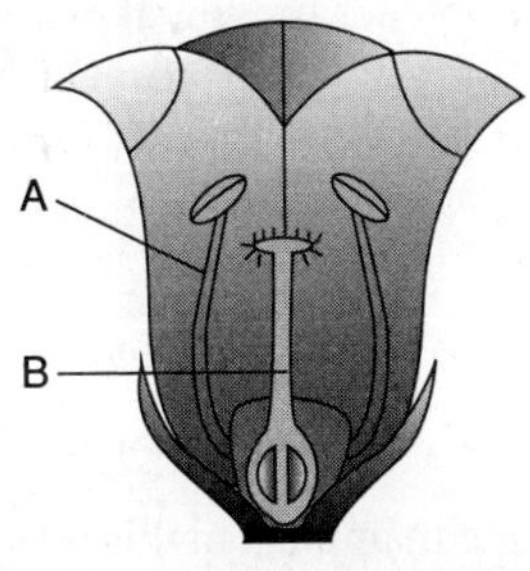

(a) A: Anther, B: Sepals (b) A: Petals, B: Anther
(c) A: Stamen, B: Carpel (d) A: Pistil, B: Stamen

93. Find the chromosome numbers in gamete (n) of the following organisms respectively.
Human, Housefly, Rat, Dog, Cat, Fruitfly, Apple, Rice, Maize, Potato, Butterfly, Onion
(a) 23, 12, 12, 39, 19, 6, 17, 12, 10, 24, 190, 16
(b) 23, 12, 21, 39, 19, 6, 17, 12, 20 24, 190, 16
(c) 23, 6, 21, 39, 19, 4, 17, 12, 10, 24, 190, 16
(d) 23, 6, 12, 39, 19, 4, 17, 21, 10, 24, 190, 16

94. Identify A, B, C in the diagram.

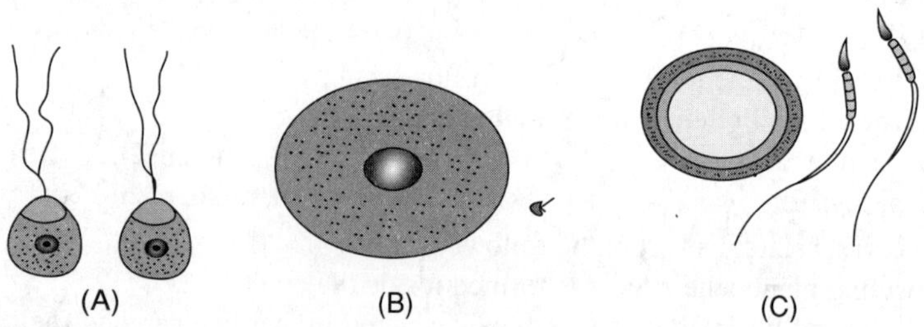

(a) A: Heterogametes of Chlamydomonas
B: Homogametes of fucus
C: Hetrogametes of Homo sapiens
(b) A: Homogametes of Chara
B: Heterogametes of Fucus
C: Heterogamete of Homo sapiens
(c) A: Homogamete of Claldophora (a bryophyte)
B: Heterogamete of Fucus (an alga)
C: Heterogamete of Homo sapiens
(d) A: Isogametes of Cladophora (an alga)
B: Heterogametes of Fucus (an alga)
C:Heterogametes of Homo sapiens

95. Adventitious buds arise from the notches present at margins of leaves in:
(a) Potato (b) Offset
(c) Bryophyllum (d) Turmeric

96. Most of the animals shows which type of reproduction?
(a) Asexual
(b) Vegetative
(c) Sexual
(d) Gemmules formation

97. What is the number of non-primate mammals in this series?
Cow, Sheep, Rat, Deer, Dog, Tiger, Monkey, Human and Ape
(a) 3 (b) 4
(c) 6 (d) 7

98. Rhizomes are present in:
(a) Banana (b) Ginger
(c) Potato (d) Both (a) and (b)

99. Identify A, B and C in the figure.

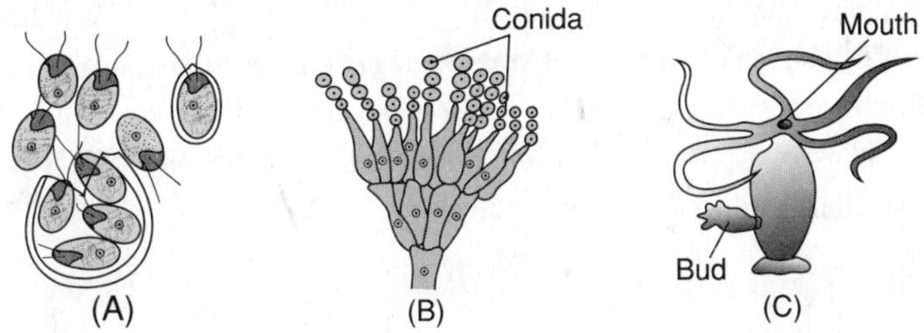

(a) A: Zoospores of chlamydomonas, B: Conidia of Penicillium, C: Buds in Hydra
(b) A: Zoospores of chlamydomonas, B: Conidia of yeast, C: Buds in Hydra
(c) A: Conidia of Penicillium, B: Zoospores of Chymydomonas, C: Buds in Hydra
(d) A: Zoospores of chlamydomonas, B: Ascospores of Penicillium, C: Buds in Hydra

100. Bulbils are vegetative propagules in:
(a) Water hyacinth
(b) Agave
(c) Potato
(d) Tomato

*Read the **assertion** and **reason** carefully to mark the correct option out of the options given below:*

(a) If both the assertion and the reason are true and the reason is a correct explanation of the assertion
(b) If both the assertion and reason are true but the reason is not a correct explanation of the assertion
(c) If the assertion is true but the reason is false
(d) If both the assertion and reason are false

101. Assertion: Asexual as well as sexual modes of reproduction are exhibited by the higher plants.
Reason: Only sexual mode of reproduction is present in most animals.

102. Assertion: In sexual reproduction offspring are not identical to parents or amongst themselves.
Reason: Sexual reproduction involves fusion of male & female gamete.

103. Assertion: Humans are called continuous breeder
Reason: Humans are reproductively active throughout.

104. Assertion: Zygote is the vital link that ensures continuity of species between organisms.
Reason: Most vital events of sexual reproduction is the fusion of gametes.

105. Assertion: In flowering plant after fertilization, ovary develops into seeds.
Reason: Ovules mature into fruits.

106. Assertion: In angiosperms the ovule develops into a seed after fertilization.
Reason: Fertilization is not essential for formation of fruit.

107. Assertion: Sexual reproduction is simple & fast process.
Reason: Asexual reproduction is complex & slow process

108. **Assertion:** Organisms exhibiting external fertilization releases large number of gametes in to surrounding medium.

Reason: It will enhance chance of syngamy.

109. **Assertion:** The chance of survival of young ones is greater in viviparous organism.

Reason: Proper embryonic care and protection is available inside the body of female organism.

110. **Assertion:** All members of bee are diploid except the queen.

Reason: Queen is produced parthenogentically.

AIPMT PREVIOUS YEAR QUESTIONS

1. Which one of the following is monoecious?

[AIPMT MAINS 2010]

(a) Marchantia (b) Cycas
(c) Pinus (d) Data palm

2. Examine the figures (A – D) given below and select the right option out (a – d), in which all the four structures A, B, C and D are identified correctly.

[AIPMT MAINS 2010]

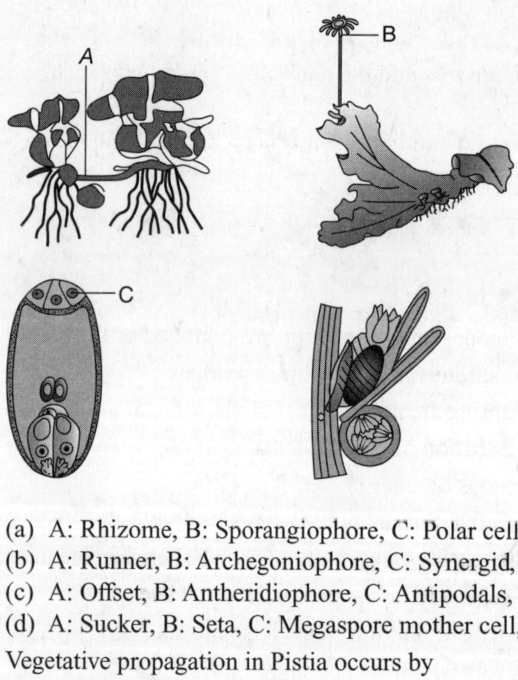

(a) A: Rhizome, B: Sporangiophore, C: Polar cell, D: Globule
(b) A: Runner, B: Archegoniophore, C: Synergid, D: antheridium
(c) A: Offset, B: Antheridiophore, C: Antipodals, D: Oogonium
(d) A: Sucker, B: Seta, C: Megaspore mother cell, D: Gemma cup

3. Vegetative propagation in Pistia occurs by

[AIPMT MAINS 2010]

(a) Stolon (b) Offset
(c) Runner (d) Sucker

4. Which one of the following pairs is wrongly matched while the remaining three are correct? [AIPMT MAINS 2011]

(a) Penicillium - conidia
(b) Water hyacinth - runner
(c) Bryophyllum - leaf buds
(d) Agave - bulbils

5. Which one of the following is correctly matched? [AIPMT PRE 2012]

(a) Onion – Bulb
(b) Ginger – Sucker
(c) Chlamydomonas – Conidia
(d) Yeast – Zoospores

6. Product of sexual reproduction generally generates: [AIPMT 2013]

(a) Longer viability of seeds
(b) Prolonged dormancy
(c) New genetic combination leading to variation
(d) Large biomass

7. Meiosis takes place in: [AIPMT 2013]

(a) Meiocyte
(b) Conidia
(c) Gemmule
(d) Megaspore

8. Monoecious plant of Chara shows occurrence of: [AIPMT 2013]

(a) Antheridiophore and archegoniophore on the same plant
(b) Stamen and carpel on the same plant
(c) Upper antheridium and lower oogonium on the same plant
(d) Upper oogonium and lower antheridium on the same plant

9. Which one of the following is wrong about chara? [AIPMT 2014]

(a) Upper oogonium and lower round antheridium
(b) Globule and nucule present on the sap plant
(c) Upper antheridium and lower oogonium
(d) Globule is male reproductive structure

10. In ginger vegetative propagation occurs through [AIPMT 2015]

(a) Rhizome
(b) Offsets
(c) Bulbils
(d) Runners

11. Which of the following pairs is not correctly matched? [RE-AIPMT 2015]

Mode of reproduction	**Example**
(a) Rhizome	Banana
(b) Binary fission	Sargassum
(c) Conidia	Penicillium
(d) Offset	Water hyacinth

12. Roots play insignificant role in absorption of water in: [RE-AIPMT 2015]

(a) Pistia
(b) Pea
(c) Wheat
(d) Sunflower

Answer Keys

1. (c)	2. (d)	3. (a)	4. (c)	5. (b)	6. (c)	7. (d)	8. (d)	9. (d)	10. (b)
11. (c)	12. (d)	13. (d)	14. (c)	15. (b)	16. (a)	17. (c)	18. (d)	19. (c)	20. (b)
21. (b)	22. (c)	23. (a)	24. (d)	25. (b)	26. (b)	27. (d)	28. (a)	29. (d)	30. (c)
31. (a)	32. (c)	33. (b)	34. (d)	35. (d)	36. (d)	37. (d)	38. (d)	39. (b)	40. (b)
41. (a)	42. (b)	43. (b)	44. (b)	45. (a)	46. (b)	47. (c)	48. (c)	49. (c)	50. (d)
51. (d)	52. (a)	53. (d)	54. (d)	55. (d)	56. (c)	57. (a)	58. (b)	59. (c)	60. (d)
61. (a)	62. (d)	63. (d)	64. (b)	65. (c)	66. (a)	67. (d)	68. (d)	69. (b)	70. (d)
71. (d)	72. (d)	73. (d)	74. (d)	75. (b)	76. (a)	77. (d)	78. (d)	79. (c)	80. (d)
81. (d)	82. (d)	83. (a)	84. (b)	85. (c)	86. (c)	87. (a)	88. (c)	89. (a)	90. (d)
91. (b)	92. (c)	93. (c)	94. (d)	95. (c)	96. (c)	97. (c)	98. (d)	99. (a)	100. (b)
101. (b)	102. (a)	103. (a)	104. (b)	105. (d)	106. (c)	107. (d)	108. (a)	109. (a)	110. (d)

AIPMT Previous Year Questions

1. (c)	2. (c)	3. (b)	4. (b)	5. (a)	6. (c)	7. (a)	8. (d)	9. (c)	10. (a)
11. (b)	12. (a)								

CHAPTER

24

Sexual Reproduction in Flowering Plant

1. Flowers convey important human feelings such as
   (a) Love and affection (b) Happiness and grief
   (c) Mourning (d) All of the above
2. Flowers are considered as object of
   (a) Aesthetic value (b) Ornamental value
   (c) Religious and cultural value (d) All of the above
3. Biologist consider flower to be objects of
   (a) Morphological marvels (b) Embryological marvels
   (c) Sites of sexual reproduction (d) All of the above
4. When does plant decides to flower?
   (a) In embryonic development
   (b) When flower bud appears
   (c) Before the actual flower appear on plant
   (d) All are correct
5. Identify A, B, C and D in this figure?

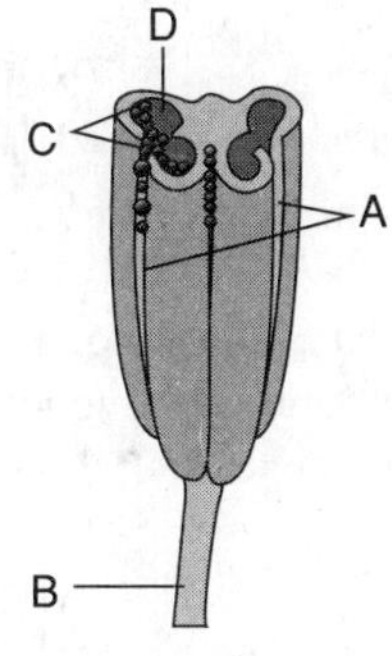

   (a) A: Pollen grains, B: Filament (Stalk), C: Line of dehiscence, D: Pollen sacs
   (b) A: Line of dehiscence, B: Filament (Stalk), C: Pollen sacs, D: Pollen grains
   (c) A: Filament (Stalk), B: Pollen grains, C: Line of dehiscence, D: Pollen sacs
   (d) A: Line of dehiscence, B: Pollen sacs, C: Pollen grains, D: Filament (Stalk)

6. The initiation and development of floral primordium takes place by
(a) Only by hormonal changes in plant
(b) Only structural changes in plant
(c) Changes in seasonal variation
(d) Both by hormonal and structural changes in plant

7. Whorl of stamens in flower represents
(a) Gynoecium (b) Androecium
(c) Calyx (d) Corolla

8. Whorl of carpel in flower represents
(a) Gynoecium (b) Androecium
(c) Calyx (d) Corolla

9. What indicates 'A' in below figure?

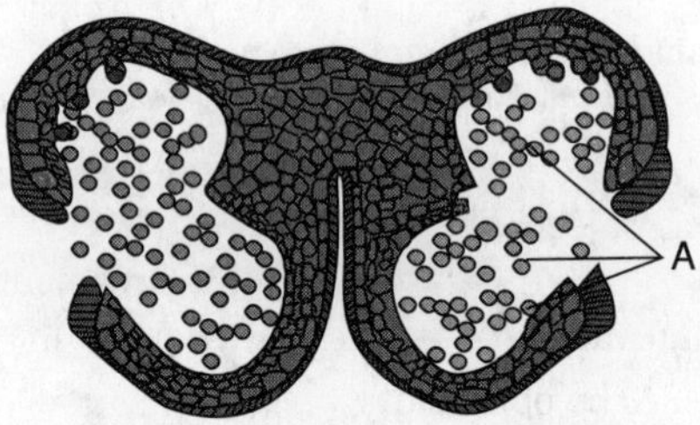

(a) Pollen grains (b) Pollen sacs
(c) Generative cell (d) Vacuoles

10. Whorl of petals in flower represents
(a) Gynoecium (b) Androecium
(c) Calyx (d) Corolla

11. Whorl of sepals in flower represents
(a) Androecium (b) Gynoecium
(c) Calyx (d) Corolla

12. Stamens consist of the following parts
(a) Filament (b) Style, stigma
(c) Anther (d) Both (a) and (c)

13. The number and length of stamens in flowers are
(a) Variable in different species
(b) Same in plants present in similar climatic condition
(c) Variable and depend on the amount of hormonal secretion
(d) Variable in different species and depend on the seasonal variation

14. Typical angiosperm anther is
(a) Unilobed and dithecous (b) Bilobed and dithecous
(c) May be both (a) and (b) (d) Bilobed and tetrathecous

15. The anther in transverse section appears to be
(a) Diagonal (b) Tetragonal
(c) Unilobed (d) Mosaic

16. What are A, B, C and D in this figure?

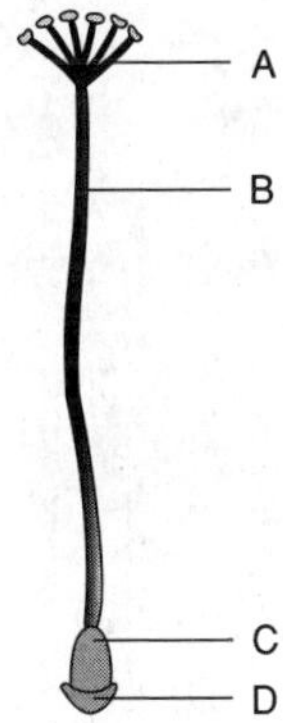

(a) A: Thalamus, B: Style, C: Ovary, D: Stigma
(b) A: Style, B: Ovary, C: Stigma, D: Thalamus
(c) A: Stigma, B: Style, C: Ovary, D: Thalamus
(d) A: Ovary, B: Stigma, C: Thalamus, D: Style

17. Tetragonal anther consist of
(a) One microsporangia (b) Two microsporangia
(c) Three microsporangia (d) Four microsporangia

18. How many microsporangia are there in each lobe of anther?
(a) One microsporangia (b) Two microsporangia
(c) Three microsporangia (d) Four microsporangia

19. Pollen sacs develop from
(a) Microspore (b) Microspore mother cell
(c) Microsporangium (d) Megaspore

20. Typical microsporangium appear ________ in transverse section.
(a) Wavy (b) Circular
(c) Oval (d) Irregular

21. Which one amongst the given perform the function of protection in typical microsporangium?
(A) Epidermis (B) Endothecium
(C) Tapetum (D) Middle layer
(a) A and B (b) A and C
(c) A and D (d) A, B and D

22. Which of the following layer of microsporangium provide nourishment to the developing anther?
(a) Middle layers (b) Tapetum
(c) Endothecium (d) Epidermis

23. Outer three layers of microsporangium, perform the function of
(a) Protection to developing pollen
(b) Provide nourishment to developing pollen
(c) Help in dehiscence of anther to release pollen
(d) Both (a) and (c)

24. Identify the parts A to I in this figure.

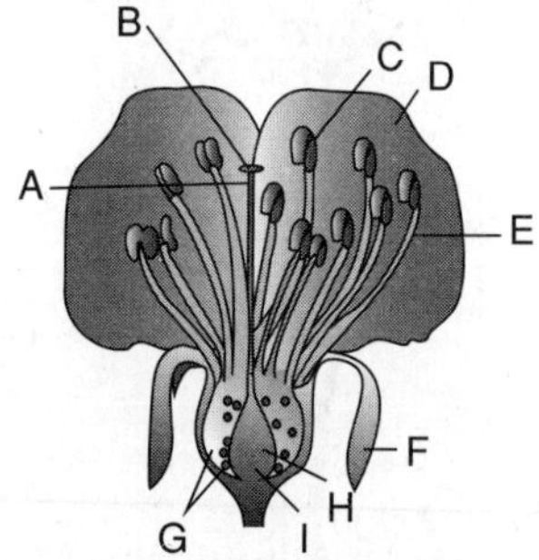

(a) A: Ovary, B: Anther, C: Filament, D: Nectariferous area, E: Sepal, F: Stigma, G: Style, H: Ovule, I: Petal
(b) A: Anther, B: Ovule, C: Stigma, D: Anther, E: Petal, F: Filament, G: Sepal, H: Nectariferous area, I: Ovary
(c) A: Ovary, B: Ovule, C: Nectariferous area, D: Sepal, E: Filament, F: Petal, G: Anther, H: Stigma, I: Style
(d) A: Style, B: Stigma, C: Anther, D: Petal, E: Filament, F: Sepal, G: Nectariferous area, H: Ovule, I: Ovary

25. The microsporangium cells which posses dense cytoplasm and have more than one nucleus is the characteristic of
(a) Middle layers (b) Tapetum
(c) Endothecium (d) Epidermis

26. In young anther the tissue occupying the centre of each microsporangium is called
(a) Megaspore mother cell (b) Sporogenous tissue
(c) Parietal tissue (d) None of the above

27. Identify A to E in this figure?

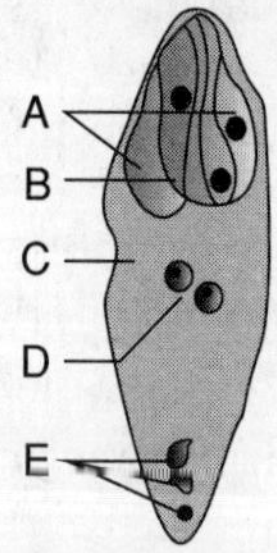

(a) A: Synergids, B: Egg, C: Central cell, D: 2 polar nuclei, E: Antipodals
(b) A: Antipodals, B: Synergids, C: Central cell, D: Egg, E: 2 polar nuclei
(c) A: Synergids, B: Central cell, C: 2 polar nuclei, D: Antipodals, E: Egg
(d) A: Egg, B: 2 polar nuclei, C: Antipodals, D: Antipodals, E: Synergids

28. Arrange the following layers of microsporangium from inside to outside
(A) Endothecium (B) Middle layer
(C) Tapetum (D) Epidermis
(a) A, B, C, D (b) B, A, C, D
(c) D, C, B, A (d) C, B, A, D

29. Sporogenous tissue of microsporangia is
(a) Groups of compactly arrange homogenous cells
(b) Occupies the centre of microsporangium
(c) Present inside young anther
(d) All are correct

30. Each cell of microspore tetrad is
(a) 2n (b) n
(c) Some n and some 2n (d) 3n

31. Which type of cell division occurs in the cell of sporogenous tissue to form microspore?
(a) Reduction division (b) Equational division
(c) Both (a) and (b) (d) Amitosis

32. Formation of pollen from pollen mother cell is referred to as
(a) Pollenogenesis (b) Megasporogenesis
(c) Microsporangesis (d) Ovulation

33. Pollen grains are
(a) Microspore tetrad (b) Dehydrated microspores
(c) Megaspore tetrad (d) Pollen mother cells

34. Male gametophyte in angiosperm is represented by
(a) Anther (b) Androecium
(c) Microsporangium (d) Pollen grain

35. Pollen grains are
(a) Spherical (b) Oval
(c) Generally spherical (d) Irregular

36. Diameter of pollen grain is
(a) 20–50 μm (b) 25–50 μm
(c) 30–50 μm (d) 10–50 μm

37. Exine of pollen is
(A) Hard outer layer of pollen grain
(B) Most resistant organic matter known
(C) Layer made up of sporopollenin
(D) Layer which can withstand high temperature, strong acids and alkali
(E) Layer which cannot be degraded by any known enzyme
Which one of the following is correct?
(a) A and B (b) A, B, C, D
(c) A, B, C, D, E (d) A, C, E

38. What are the parts A and B in this figure?

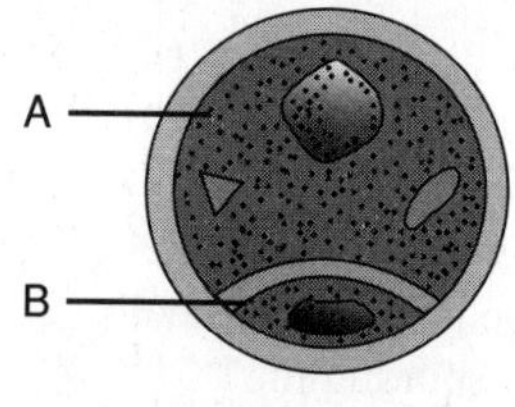

(a) A: Generative cell, B: Vegetative cell
(b) A: Tapetal cell, B: Generative cell
(c) A: Vegetative cell, B: Generative cell
(d) A: Homogenous cell, B: Tapetal cell

39. Sporopollenin is
(a) Most resistant organic matter known
(b) Present in exine of pollen grain
(c) Absent in the germ pole of pollen grain
(d) All of the above

40. Pollen grains can be preserved as fossil because
(a) They vary from species to species
(b) They have variety of architecture
(c) They are made up of sporopollenin
(d) They exhibit a fascinating array of pattern and design

41. Which part of pollen exhibit a fascination array of pattern and design?
(a) Intine
(b) Exine
(c) Germ pore
(d) None of them

42. Intine of pollen grain is
(a) Inner layer of pollen grain
(b) A thin and continuous layer
(c) Made up of cellulose and pectin
(d) All are correct

Figure based questions 43 to 47.

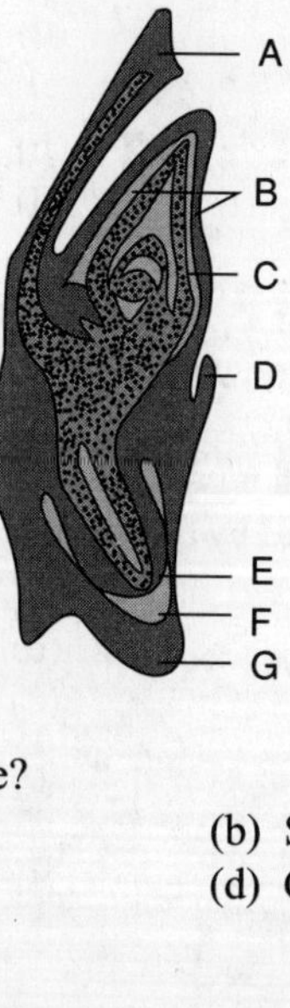

43. What does 'A' indicate in this figure?
(a) Scutellum
(b) Shoot apex
(c) Radicle
(d) Coleorhiza

44. What 'C' is showing in the given figure?
(a) Epiblast (b) Scutellum
(c) Shoot apex (d) Radicle

45. Identify the part 'D'.
(a) Radicle (b) Root cap
(c) Coleorhiza (d) Epiblast

46. What is 'G' in the given figure?
(a) Scutellum (b) Coleorhiza
(c) Coleoptile (d) Shoot apex

47. What is 'B' showing in the given figure?
(a) Scutellum (b) Coleorhiza
(c) Coleoptile (d) Shoot apex

48. Pollen grains are mature when:
(a) It contains vegetative and generative cell
(b) It contains only single haploid cell
(c) Contains two haploid cell
(d) Both (a) and (c)

49. Thin and continuous layer of pollen made up of cellulose and pectin
(a) Intine (b) Exine
(c) Germ pore (d) None of them

50. Pollen grains are shed in 2-celled stage in
(a) $>$ 90% Angiosperm plant (b) $<$ 50% Angiosperm plant
(c) $>$ 60% Angiosperm plant (d) $<$ 40% Angiosperm plant

51. Generate cell floats in the cytoplasm of
(a) Vegetative cell (b) Microspore mother cell
(c) Pollen mother cell (d) Mega sporangium

52. Below figure represents

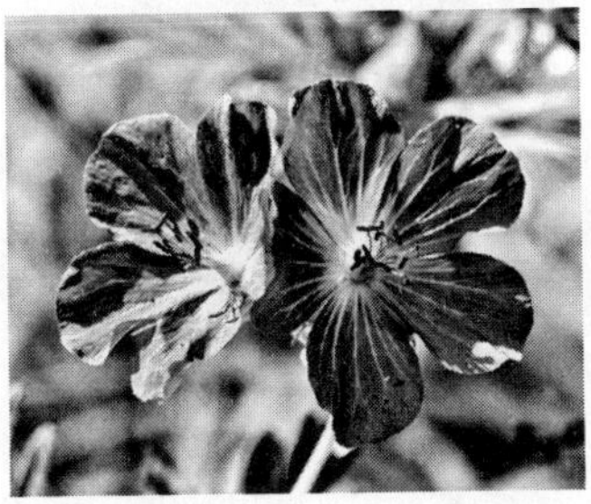

(a) Self-pollinated flowers (b) Cross-pollinated flowers
(c) Chasmogamous (d) None of these

53. The bigger cell that receives abundant food and has irregularly shaped nucleus is called
(a) Generative cell (b) Vegetative cell
(c) Germ cell (d) Sperm cell

54. Spindle-shaped cell with dense cytoplasm and nucleus in pollen grain is called
(a) Vegetative cell (b) Generative cell
(c) Sperm cell (d) Egg cell

55. Match the following

Column – I	Column – II
A. Vegetative cell	1. Sporopollenin
B. Generative cell	2. Spindle-shaped cell
C. Exine	3. Large sized and has abundant food reserve
D. Intine	4. Cellulose and pectin

(a) A:1, B:2, C:3, D:4
(b) A:4, B:3, C:2, D:1
(c) A:3, B:2, C:1, D:4
(d) A:2, B:1, C:4, D:3

56. Male gametes in angiosperms are formed by
(a) Mitotic division in vegetative cell
(b) Meiotic division in pollen mother cell
(c) Meiotic division in vegetative cell
(d) Mitotic division in generative cell

57. The pollen grains are shed in 3-celled stage in
(a) > 60% Angiospermic plant
(b) > 70% Angiospermic plant
(c) < 40% Angiospermic plant
(d) < 20% Angiospermic plant

58. Which of the following statement is correct?
(A) Pollen grains are shed in 2-celled stage in > 40% plants
(B) Pollen grains are shed in 3-celled stage in < 60% plant
(C) Generative cell divides meiotically to form male gametes
(D) Intine of pollen is made up of sporopollen in
(a) A, B, C
(b) All are correct
(c) All are wrong
(d) Only C

59. Plant came in India as a contaminant with imported wheat
(a) Vinca
(b) Parthenium
(c) Striga
(d) Orobanche

60. Below figure represents

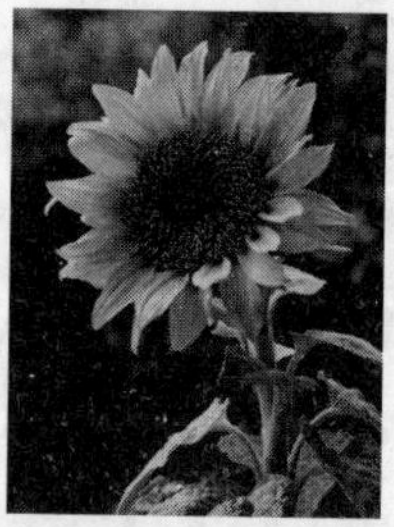

(a) Self-pollinated flowers
(b) Cross-pollinated flowers
(c) Cleistogamous flowers
(d) None of these

61. Which one of the following is incorrect?
(A) Parthenium or carrot gases causes pollen allergy
(B) Vegetative cell of pollen has abundant food reserve
(C) All pollen's cause severe allergies and bronchial afflictions
(D) Sporopollenin is the most resistant organic matter known
(a) All are correct
(b) A
(c) B
(d) C

62. What are A and B in this figure?

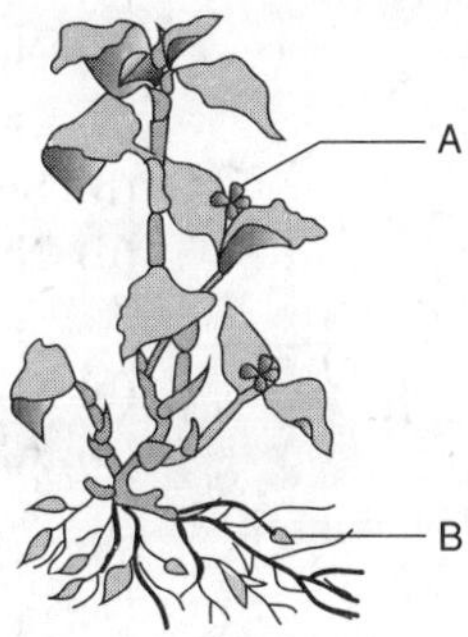

(a) A: Chasmogamous flower,
B: Cleistogamous flower
(b) A: Cleistogamous flower,
B: Chasmogamous flower
(c) A: Chasmogamous flower,
B: Chasmogamous flower
(d) A: Cleistogamous flower,
B: Self-pollinated flower

63. Pollen grains
(A) Represent gametophytic phase of plant
(B) Can cause severe allergies like asthma and bronchitis
(C) Are rich in nutrient
(D) Are used as food supplements
(E) Are available in form of tables and syrups in market of western countries
(a) Only A is correct
(b) All are correct
(c) All are wrong
(d) Only A, B and C are correct

64. Viability of pollen grains depend upon
(a) A particular species
(b) Prevailing temperature
(c) Humidity
(d) All of the above

65. Rice pollen grains are viable for
(a) 6.0 mins
(b) 30 mins (approx)
(c) 60 mins (approx)
(d) 40 mins

66. Pollens are stored in
(a) Oxygen (–196°C)
(b) Nitrogen (–196°C)
(c) Oxygen (196°C)
(d) Nitrogen (+196°C)

67. Syncarpous condition is referred to as
(a) Gynoecium containing single pistil
(b) More than one pistil fused together
(c) More than one pistil free from one another
(d) Gynoecium containing many pistils

68. Landing platform for pollen grains is
(a) Stigma
(b) Style
(c) Ovary
(d) None of them

69. Bulged basal part of pistil is
(a) Stigma (b) Style
(c) Ovary (d) None of them

70. Elongated slender part of pistil is
(a) Stigma (b) Style
(c) Ovary (d) None of them

71. Megasporangia is referred to as
(a) Ovule (b) Ovary
(c) Gynoecium (d) All of the above

72. What are parts A to E in this below figure?

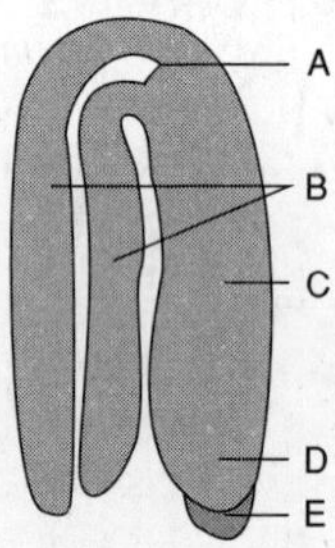

(a) A: Plumule, B: Cotyledons, C: Hypocotyl, D: Radicle, E: Root cap
(b) A: Root cap, B: Hypocotyl, C: Plumule, D: Radicle, E: Cotyledons
(c) A: Cotyledons, B: Root cap, C: Cotyledons, D: Plumule, E: Hypocotyl
(d) A: Plumule, B: Cotyledons, C: Root cap, D: Radicle, E: Hypocotyl

73. Plants having single ovule in ovary are
(a) Wheat (b) Paddy
(c) Mango (d) All of them

74. What represents 'A' in the following figure?

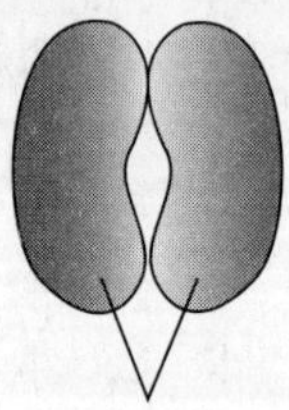

(a) Cotyledons (b) Scutellum
(c) Shoot apex (d) Radicle

75. More than one ovule is found in ovary of
(a) Wheat (b) Paddy
(c) Papaya (d) None of these

76. The stalk attaching ovule to placenta is
(a) Funiculus (b) Hilum
(c) Raphe (d) Chalaza

77. The junction between ovule and funiculus is
(a) Placenta (b) Hilum
(c) Raphe (d) Chalaza

78. The tips on the ovule where integument are absent are called
(a) Germ pore (b) Micropyle
(c) Both are correct (d) None of the above

79. The end opposite to micropyles end is called
(a) Funicle (b) Chalaza
(c) Germ pore (d) Hilum

80. Mass of cell present inside the integuments of megasporangium having abundant food reserve is
(a) Ovule (b) Nucellus
(c) Sporogenous cells (d) None of them

81. Female gametophyte of angiosperm is referred to as
(a) Megasporangium (b) Megaspore
(c) Embryo sac (d) Nucleus

82. Embryo sac is formed by
(a) Reduction division in megaspore
(b) Equational division in megaspore
(c) Reduction division followed by equational division in megaspore mother cell
(d) Both (b) and (c)

83. How many embryo sacs are present in an ovule?
(a) One embryo sac (b) More than one embryo sac
(c) One embryo sac (generally) (d) Two embryo sacs

84. What is functional megaspore referred to as?
(a) The megaspore that degenerates after formation
(b) The megaspore that only develops in female gametophyte
(c) The megaspore that undergoes reduction division
(d) The megaspore that is functionally inocuve

85. Identify the parts of A to F in the following figure?

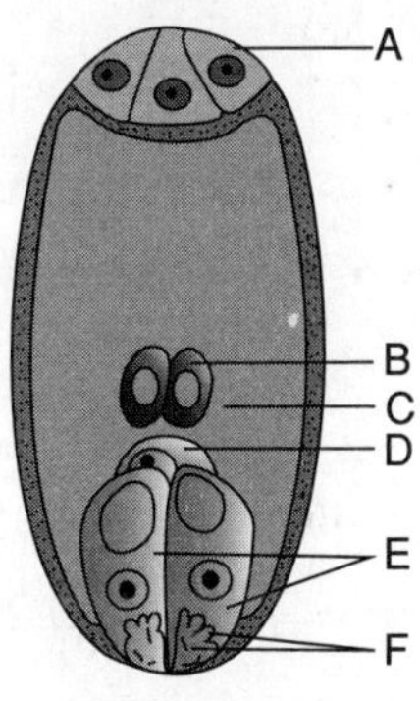

(a) A: Filiform apparatus, B: Polar nuclei, C: Antipodals, D: Synergids, E: Egg, F: Central cell
(b) A: Antipodals, B: Polar nuclei, C: Central cell, D: Egg, E: Synergids, F: Filiform apparatus
(c) A: Antipodals, B: Central cell, C: Polar nuclei, D: Egg, F: Synergids, G: Filiform apparatus
(d) A: Eggs, B: Central cell, C: Filiform apparatus, D: Polar nuclei, E: Antipodals, F: Synergids

86. Monosporic development referred to as
(a) Single megaspore developing in embryo sac
(b) Single megaspore mother cell undergoing meiosis
(c) Presence of single ovule in ovary
(d) None of them is correct

87. What is the ploidy level of nucleus, MMC, functional megaspore and female gametophyte?
(a) 2n, n, 2n, 2n (b) 2n, n, 2n, n
(c) 2n, 2n, n, n (d) n, 2n, n, n

88. How many mitotic division takes place for complete development of embryo sac?
(a) 4 (b) 3
(c) 2 (a) 1

89. The inside three mitotic division which occur the megaspore are
(a) Followed by cytoplasmic division immediately
(b) Strictly free nuclear not immediately followed by cell wall formation
(c) Wall formation occurs after completion of the second mitosis
(d) Wall formation will never occur

90. Typical female gametophyte is
(a) 7-celled 8 nucleate (b) 6-celled 8 nucleate
(c) 4-celled 6 nucleate (d) 5-celled 6 nucleate

91. What is 'A' in this figure?

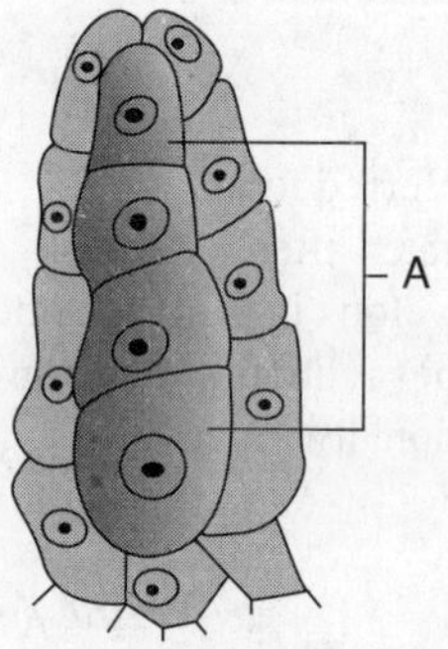

(a) Megaspore mother cell (b) Megaspore tetrad
(c) Embryo sac (d) Micropyle

92. Egg apparatus consist of
(a) Two synergids (b) Two antipodals
(c) Egg cell (d) (a) and (c) both

93. The cellular thickening at the tip of micropyle is
(a) Synergids (b) Egg apparatus
(c) Filiform apparatus (d) All are correct

94. The cells located at chalazal ends are called as
(a) Synergids (b) Antipodals
(c) Egg apparatus (d) None of them

95. Identify the parts A and B in this figure.

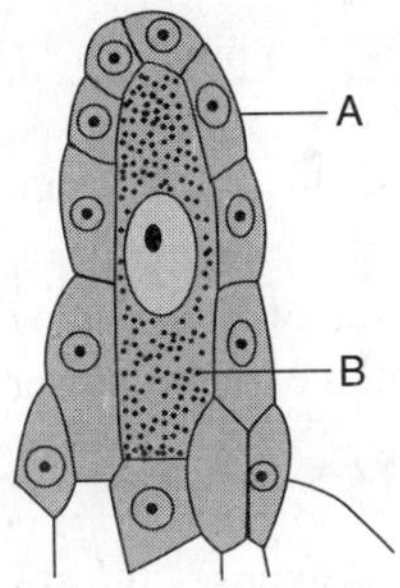

(a) A: Megaspore tetrad, B: Nucleus
(b) A: Central cell, B: Megaspore dyad
(c) A: Nucellus, B: Megaspore mother cell
(d) A: Nucellus, B: Central cell

96. The central cell
(a) Contains two haploid nuclei
(b) Has two polar nuclei
(c) Located in the centre of embryo sac
(d) All are correct

97. The cells in embryo sac located at the micropyles end are
(a) Egg apparatus
(b) Only synergid
(c) Antipodal cell
(d) Central cell

98. The male and female gametes of angiosperm are respectively
(a) Motile, non-motile
(b) Non-motile, motile
(c) Motile, motile
(d) Non-motile, non-motile

99. After three meiotic divisions in the functional megaspore, the gametophyte (embryosac) has how many cells.
(a) 7 cells
(b) 4 cells
(c) 5 cells
(d) 8 cells

100. Pollination is essential in angiosperm plants because
(a) It decreases the time required for fertilization
(b) Both of the male and female gametes are non-motile and they need to be brought together for fertilization
(c) It is a useless process
(d) Both (a) and (b)

101. Below figure represents

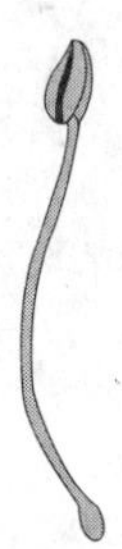

(a) Anther
(b) Typical stamen
(c) Pollen grain
(d) Microsporangium

102. Pollination in plants is referred to as
(a) Fusion of male and female gametes
(b) Transfer of pollen grain to stigma of pistil
(c) Germination of pollen of stigma
(d) Production of pollen grew inside the microsporangium

103. Autogamy refers to
(a) Transfer of pollen grain to stigma of another flower
(b) Transfer of pollen grain to stigma of same flower
(c) Both of the above
(d) None of the above

104. In a normal flower which opens and exposes the stigma and anther will have which type of pollination?
(a) Autogamy is absent
(b) Complete autogamy is rare
(c)
(d)

105. Plants which produce two types of flowers are
(a) Viola
(b) Oxalis
(c) Commelina
(d) All of them

106. Two types of flowers found in autogamous plant
(a) Flower similar to flowers of other species with exposed anthers and stigma
(b) Flowers which do not open at all
(c) Both (a) and (b)
(d) Flowers with only stigma and no anther

107. ________ flowers produce assured seed set even in the absence of pollinators
(a) Cleistogamous flower
(b) Chasmogamous flowers
(c) Both of them
(d) Flowers showing geitonogamy

108. A type of cross pollination involving a pollinating agent is genetically similar to autogamy since pollen grain come from same plant
(a) Xenogamy
(b) Geitonogamy
(c) Autogamy
(d) All are correct

109. What are the parts A, B, C, D and E in the below figure?

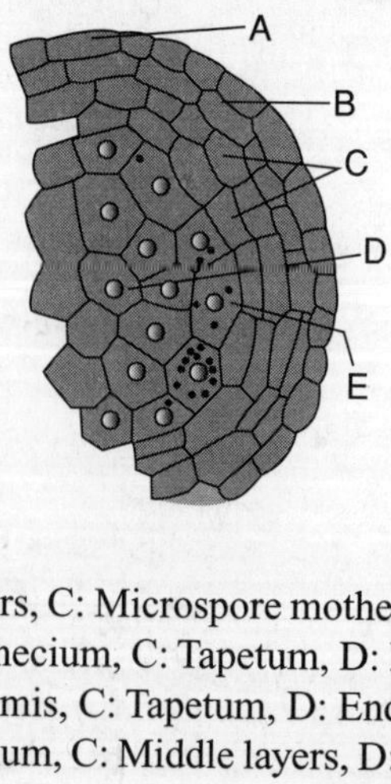

(a) A: Tapetum, B: Middle layers, C: Microspore mother cells, D: Endothecium, E: Epidermis
(b) A: Middle layers, B: Endothecium, C: Tapetum, D: Epidermis, E: Microspore mother cell
(c) A: Endothecium, B: Epidermis, C: Tapetum, D: Endothecium, E: Microspore mother cell
(d) A: Epidermis, B: Endothecium, C: Middle layers, D: Microspore mother cells, E: Tapetum

110. The only type of pollination during which pollination bring genetically different types of pollen grains to stigma
(a) Xenogamy (b) Geitonogamy
(c) Autogamy (d) All are correct

111. Majority of plants uses which types of pollinating agents
(a) Biotic (b) Abiotic
(c) Both (d) None

112. What are A and B in the following figure?

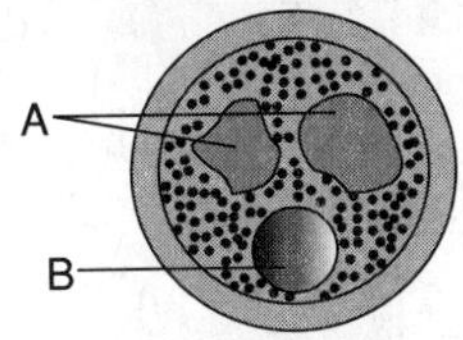

(a) A: Vacuoles, B: Intine (b) A: Vacuoles, B: Nucleus
(c) A: Nucleus, B: Intine (d) A: Exine, B: Intine

113. ________ proportion of plants uses abiotic agents for pollination.
(a) Major (b) Most
(c) Small (d) Can be small or major

114. ________ factor is responsible for contact of pollen with stigma in wind and water pollinated plants.
(a) Luck (b) Chance
(c) Time (d) Temperature

115. Enormous amount of pollens are produced in wind and water pollinated plants
(a) To compensate for uncertainties for contact of pollen with stigma.
(b) To compensate for loss of pollen grains
(c) To ensure pollination for large number of ovules present
(d) Both (a) and (b)

116. Most common abiotic pollinating agent for plant is
(a) Anemophily (b) Hydrophily
(c) Pollination by bees (d) Pollination by Ants

117. Light and non-sticky pollen grains are favourable for
(a) Water-pollinated plant (b) Wind-pollinated plant
(c) Plants with fatherly sigma (d) Both (a) and (c)

118. Which of the following are true for wind-pollinated plants?
(A) Well-exposed statements
(B) Large and often feathery stigma
(C) Single ovule in each ovary
(D) Large no. of flower packed into an inflorosence
(a) Only A (b) Only B and C
(c) Only C (d) All are correct

119. Flowers which are wind pollinated have
(a) Single ovule in one ovary (b) More than one ovule in ovary
(c) Been packed into an inflorosence (d) Both (a) and (c)

120. The tassels of corn cob are
(a) Stigma and style
(b) Meant to trap pollen grains in wind
(c) Both (a) and (b)
(d) All are incorrect

121. Wind pollination commonly found in
(a) Large trees
(b) Shrubs
(c) Grasses
(d) All of them

122. Identify A to G in this figure.

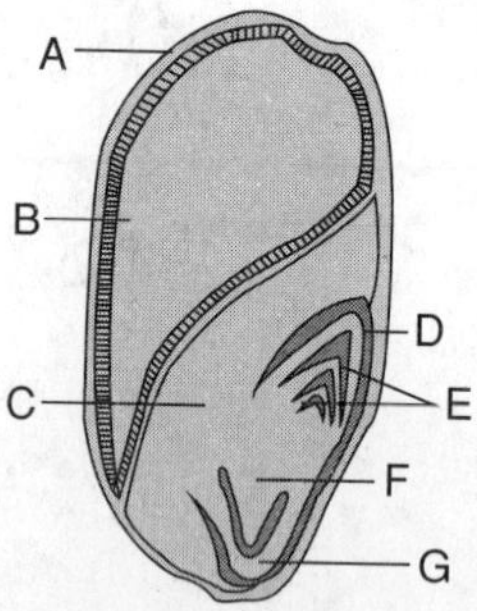

(a) A: Plumule, B: Endosperm, C: Pericarp, D: Radicle, E: Coleorhiza, F: Scutellum, G: Coleoptile
(b) A: Coleorhiza, B: Radicle, C: Endosperm, D: Pericarp, E: Plumule, F: Coleoptile, G: Scutellum
(c) A: Pericarp, B: Scutellum, C: Endosperm, D: Coleoptile, E: Plumule, F: Coleorhiza, G: Radicle
(d) A: Pericarp, B: Endosperm, C: Scutellum, D: Coleoptile, E: Plumule, F: Radicle, G: Coleorhiza

123. Pollination by water is
(a) Rare in flowering plants
(b) Limited to about 30 genera
(c) Most genera are monocotyledons
(d) All are correct

124. Water is the main medium of transport for male gametes of
(a) Algae
(b) Bryophytes
(c) Pteridophyte
(d) All of them

125. The distribution of pteridophytes and bryophytes is limited to some geographical zones only
(a) Because their spores can germinate in only specific kind of soil only
(b) Because they require water for fertilization
(c) Because they have only specific pollination which are available in narrow geographical range
(d) Only some weather conditions permit fruit formation in them

126. What indicates 'A' in below figure?

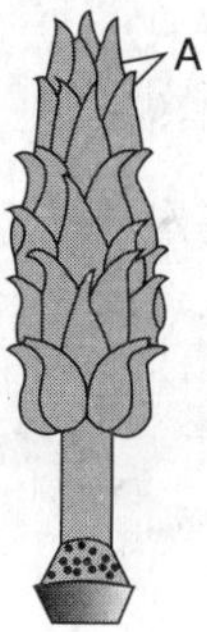

(a) Pericarp
(b) Scutellum
(c) Carpels
(d) Radicle

127. Which of the following is incorrect for equate plants?
(A) Vallisneria and Hydrilla are fresh water plants pollinated by wind
(B) Zostera a marine grass uses water as its pollinating agent
(C) Water hyacinth and water lily are pollinated by insects or wind.
(D) Most of the aquatic plant flowers emerges out of water and are pollinated by wind or insects.
(a) Only B
(b) Only A
(c) Only A, B, C
(d) All are incorrect

128. Which one of the following is correct for aquatic plants?
(a) All aquatic plants use water for pollination
(b) Not all aquatic plants use water for pollination
(c) Vallisneria flowers are pollinated by water under the water surface
(d) All are correct

129. Which one of the following is correct for Vallisneria?
(A) It grows in fresh water
(B) Female flowers or pollen grains reach the surface by long stalk
(C) Male flowers are released on to the surface of water
(D) Pollen grains are carried passively by water currents
(a) Only A
(b) Only A and B
(c) Only A, B and C
(d) A, B, C and D

130. In water pollinated species
(A) Pollen grains are long and ribbon like
(B) All pollen grains are protected from getting wet
(C) Flowers are not very colourful
(D) They do not produce nectar
(a) Only A and B are correct
(b) Only A and B are wrong
(c) All are correct
(d) All are wrong

131. Identify A and B in this figure.

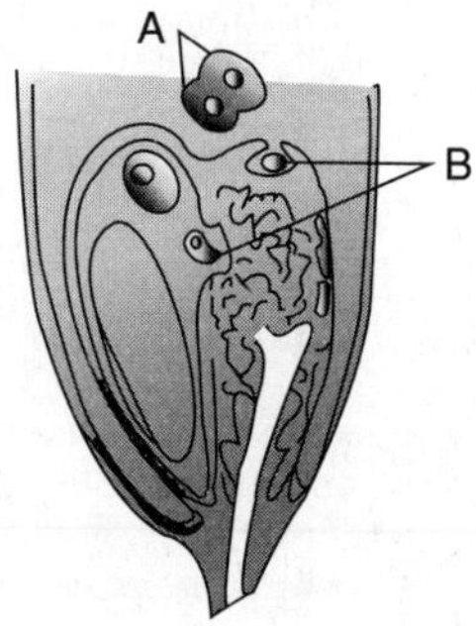

(a) A: Polar nuclei, B: Male gametes
(b) A: Female gametes, B: Polar nuclei
(c) A: Synergid, B: Egg cell
(d) A: Male gametes, B: Synergid

132. Amongst the pollinating agent which one is most dominant?
(a) Butterflies and flies
(b) Bees
(c) Beetles and wasps
(d) Moths and birds

133. Which of the following is correct in reference to animal pollinated plants?
(a) Butterflies, flies, beetles, wasps, ants, moths and bats are common pollinating agents
(b) Rodents, lizards, and primates are also pollinators in some species
(c) Animal pollinated plants are specifically adapted for particular species
(d) All are correct

134. What are the parts A, B, C, D and E in this figure?

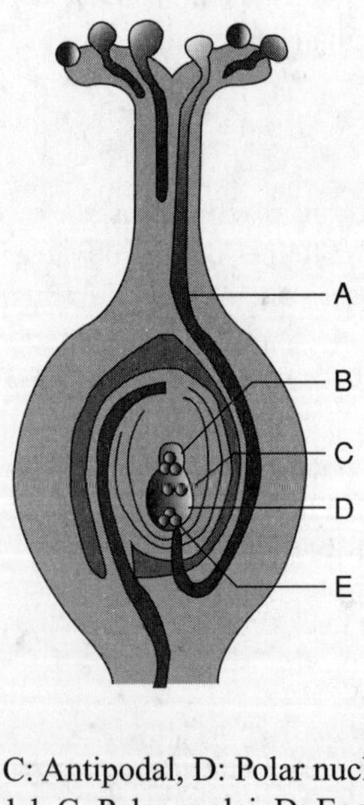

(a) A: Egg cell, B: Synergid, C: Antipodal, D: Polar nuclei, E: Pollen tube
(b) A: Pollen tube, B: Antipodal, C: Polar nuclei, D: Egg cell, E: Synergid
(c) A: Pollen tube, B: Egg cell, C: Polar nuclei, D: Antipodal, E: Synergid
(d) A: Synergid, B: Pollen tube, C: Egg cell, D: Antipodal, E: Polar nuclei

135. Insect pollinated plants are
(a) Large and colourful (b) Fragrant
(c) Rich in nectar (d) All are correct

136. Foul odour secreted by flowers which are pollinated by
(a) Flies and beetles (b) Wasps and ants
(c) Birds (d) None of them

137. The reward produced by plants to their animal visitors is in form of
(a) Nectar (b) Pollen grain
(c) Both (a) and (b) (d) None is correct

138. Which one of the following is correct for animal pollinated plants?
(a) Nectar and pollen grains are usual floral rewards
(b) To harvest the rewards from the flower, animal come in contact with anther and stigma
(c) Animal carrying pollen when come in contact with stigma, it brings about pollination
(d) All are correct

139. Amorphophallus provide floral rewards in the form of
(a) Providing safe place to lay eggs (b) Tallest flower
(c) Both are correct (d) None of them is correct

140. Which of the following is correct for relationship exists between moth and yucca plant?
(a) Moth and the plant cannot complete their life cycle without each other
(b) Moth deposit egg in the locule of the ovary and the flower and in turn flower gets pollinated by the moth
(c) Larva of the moth comes out of the eggs as the seeds start developing
(d) All are correct

141. What indicate A, B, C and D in the below figure?

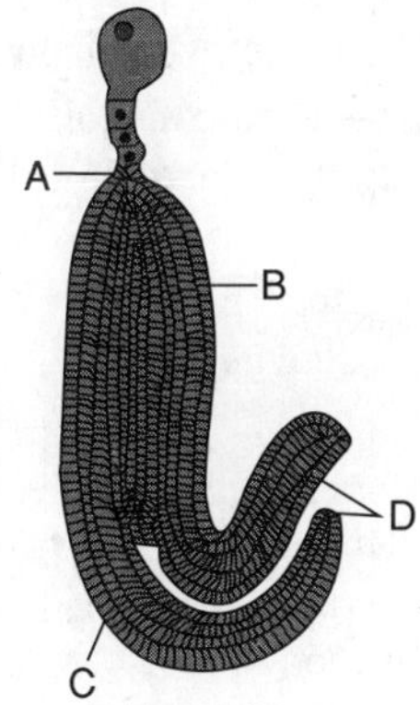

(a) A: Radicle, B: Plumule, C: Cotyledon, D: Suspensor
(b) A: Plumule, B: Suspensor, C: Radicle, D: Cotyledon
(c) A: Suspensor, B: Radicle, C: Plumule, D: Cotyledon
(d) A: Cotyledon, B: Suspensor, C: Cotyledon, D: Radicle

142. Seed is
(a) Fertilized ovule (b) Fertilized endosperm
(c) Modification of integument (d) Formed from pericarp

143. Typical seed is consist of
(a) Seed coat (b) Cotyledon
(c) Embryo axis (d) All of them

144. All are examples of albuminous seeds except
(a) Wheat (b) Sunflower
(c) Castor (d) Groundnut

145. Following figure represents

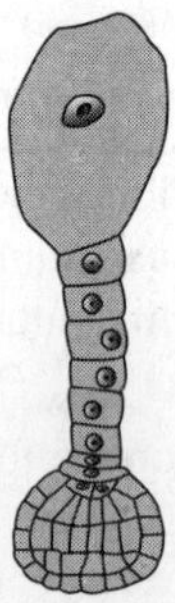

(a) Globular embryo (b) Heart-shaped embryo
(c) Zygote (d) Syngamy

146. Persistent nucleus perisperm is found in
(a) Wheat and maize (b) Pea + ground nut
(c) Barley and castor (d) Black paper + bect

147. Wheat is ploidy of perisperm
(a) n (b) 2n
(c) 3n (d) 4n

148. Select total number of albuminous seed from the following
Pea, Groundnut, Wheat, Maize, Barely, Castor, Sunflower
(a) 4 (b) 5
(c) 2 (d) 6

149. Mature seed contain how much moisture generally
(a) 10–15% by mass (b) 5–10% by mass
(c) 25–30% by mass (d) 40% by mass

150. Select false statement from the following
(a) Persistent Nucleus is the perisperm
(b) Integuments of ovule harden as though protective seed coat
(c) Micropyle remain as a small pore in seed coat and facilitates entry of oxygen and water into seed during germination
(d) General metabolic activity of embryo is high

151. Favourable conditions available for germination are
(a) Adequate moisture (b) Oxygen
(c) Suitable temperature (d) All of the above

152. Example of false fruit
(a) Apple (b) Strawberry
(c) Cashew (d) All of the above

153. Thalamus takes part in fruit formation in
(a) Guava (b) Orange
(c) Strawberry (d) Mango

154. Identify parts A, B, C and D in this figure.

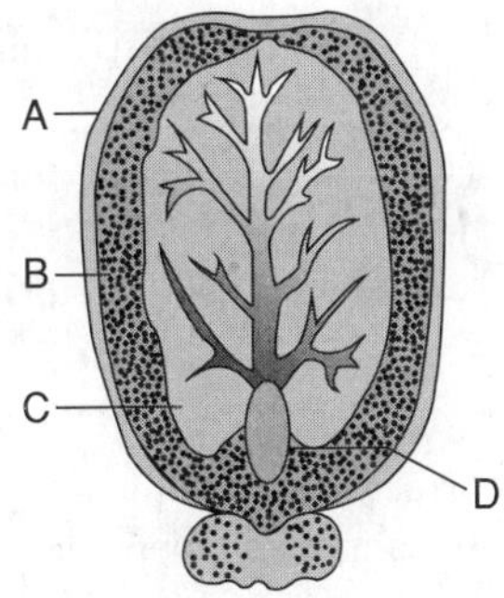

(a) A: Seed coat, B: Endosperm, C: Cotyledon, D: Hypocotyl root axis
(b) A: Cotyledon, B: Seed coat, C: Hypocotyl root axis, D: Endosperm
(c) A: Endosperm, B: Cotyledon, C: Seed coat, D: Hypocotyl root axis
(d) A: Hypocotyl root axis, B: Endosperm, C: Seed coat, D: Cotyledon

155. Which of the following is example of dry fruit?
(a) Groundnut (b) Mustard
(c) Both (a) and (b) (d) Mango

156. Fruit develops from
(a) Sepals (b) Petals (c) Thalamus (d) Ovary

157. Fruit developed without fertilization is known as
(a) Parthenocarpy (b) Anuphimixis
(c) Apomixes (d) Polyembryony

158. True about parthenocarpic fruit
(a) Seedless (b) Banana is an example
(c) Can be induced by growth hormones (d) All of the above

159. Select false statement
(a) Hard seed coat provide protection to young embryo
(b) Generally seed is the product of sexual reproduction, so they generate new genetic combination leading to variation
(c) Seeds have better adaptive strategies for dispersal to new habitat and help the species to colonize in other areas
(d) Pollination and fertilization in angiosperm depend on water

160. Which oldest seed is excavated form Arctic Tundra?
(a) Lupin arcticus (b) Phoenix dactylitera
(c) Solanum nigrum (d) Raphanus sativus

161. Phoenix dactylifera is
(a) 2000 year old viable seed
(b) a type of date palm
(c) excavated from king Herod's palace near the Dead sea
(d) All of the above

162. Apomixis is seen in
(a) Asteraceae
(b) Grasses
(c) Both (a) and (b)
(d) None of them

163. Apomixis means
(a) Fruit without seed
(b) Fruit with seed
(c) Seed without fertilization
(d) Fruit without fertilization

164. Polyembryony is
(a) One embryo in one seed
(b) More than one embryo in a seed
(c) More seed in one embryo
(d) Seed development without fertilization

165. Polyembryony seen in
(a) Citrus fruits
(b) Coconut
(c) Date palm
(d) Pineapple

166. Which one of the following is correct for yucca plant?
(a) Moth species and yucca plant cannot complete their life cycles without each other
(b) The moth deposits is egg in the locule of ovary of yucca plant
(c) The larva of the moth came out of the eggs as the seed starts developing of yucca
(d) All are correct

167. The devices developed by plants to discourage self-pollination include
(A) In some species pollen release and receptive stigma are not synchronised
(B) In some species, the anther and stigma are placed at different positions, so they do not come in contact
(C) Self-incompatibility
(a) All are correct
(b) A and B only
(c) A only
(d) B only

168. Dioecy is the mechanism for some plants to
(a) Promote autogamy
(b) Promote self-fertilization
(c) Promote cross pollination
(d) All are incorrect

169. P_n Castor and maize plant, flowers are
(a) Unisexual
(b) Both male and female flowers on same plants (monoecious)
(c) Both male and female flowers on different plants
(d) All are incorrect

170. Autogamy and geitonogamy absent in
(a) Papaya
(b) Maize
(c) Castor
(d) All are correct

171. Pollen pistil interaction refers to
(a) Pistil's ability to recognize the pollen
(b) Acceptance of pollen to promote post-pollination events
(c) Both are incorrect
(d) Both (a) and (b) are correct

172. The acceptance and rejection by continuous dialogue between pollen grain and pistil mediated by chemical components of pollen and pistil result in
(a) Autogamy (b) Pollen pistil interaction
(c) Geitonogamy (d) Pollination

173. During pollen pistil interaction chemical components are released from
(a) Only pollen (b) Only pistil
(c) Both pollen and pistil (d) The ovary

174. What happens when the pollen falls on the stigma?
(a) Pollination (b) Reject of pollen
(c) Only the compatible pollen germinates (d) Autogamy

175. The pore from which the pollen tube germinates
(a) Seed pore (b) Germ pore
(c) Intine (d) Exine

176. Which way of pollen to ovary is sequentially correct?
(a) Ovary → Style → Stigma
(b) Style → Stigma → Ovary
(c) Stigma → Ovary → Style
(d) Stigma → Style → Ovary

Figure based Questions 177 to 180.

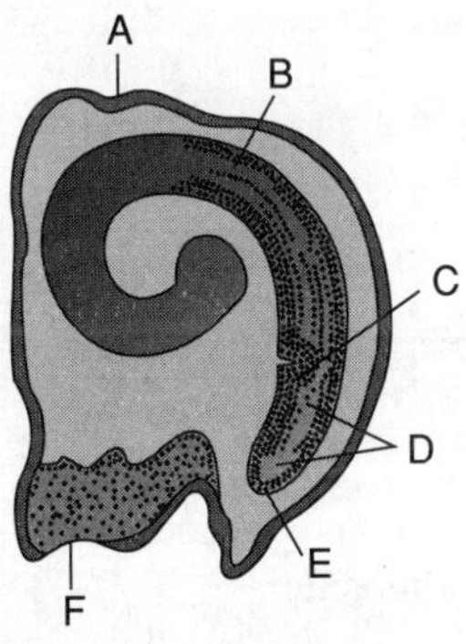

177. What indicates 'A' in above figure?
(a) Cotyledon (b) Hypocotyl root axis
(c) Seed coat (d) Endosperm

178. What indicates 'C' in above figure?
(a) Shoot apical meristem (b) Root tip
(c) Cotyledon (d) Seed coat

179. What indicates 'F' in above figure?
(a) Root tip (b) Shoot apical meristem
(c) Cotyledon (d) Endosperm

180. What indicates 'D' in above figure?
(a) Seed coat (b) Cotyledon
(c) Shoot apical meristem (d) Hypocotyl root axis

181. During pollination in plants which shed pollens in 2-celled stage, the cells are called as
(a) Two vegetative cell
(b) Two generative cell
(c) Both are correct
(d) One vegetative and one generative cell

182. Generative cell in pollen tube divides and forms
(a) One male gamete
(b) Two male gamete
(c) Three male gamete
(d) Four male gamete

183. The plants in which pollen are shed in 3-celled stage contain?
(a) Two male gametes only
(b) A large vegetative cell only
(c) Both (a) and (b)
(d) None of these

184. What indicates 'A' in the following figure?

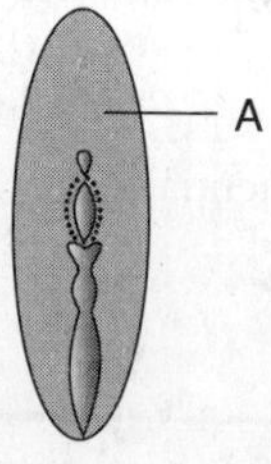

(a) Micropyle
(b) Cotyledon
(c) Endosperm
(d) Scutellum

185. The pollen tube after reaching the ovary enters inside the ovule generally through which part of ovule?
(a) Chalazal end
(b) Micropyle end
(c) Any of them
(d) Integument of ovule

186. The pollen enters one of the synergids through
(a) Micropyles end
(b) Filiform apparatus
(c) Integument
(d) Both (a) and (b)

187. The knowledge of pollen pistil interaction is helpful to plant breeders in which manner?
(a) Manipulating pollen-pistil interaction
(b) To get desired hybrids in incompatible pollination
(c) None of them
(d) Both (a) and (b) are correct

188. Which one of the following is correct for artificial hybridization?
(A) Combine desirable characters to produce superior varieties
(B) Approach towards crop improvement programme
(C) Desired pollen grains are used for pollination
(D) Stigma is exposed to receive pollen
(a) All are correct
(b) Only A
(c) Only A, B
(d) Only A, B and C

189. Artificial hybridization is achieved by
(a) Emasculation
(b) Bagging
(c) Both are required
(d) None of them

190. Emasculation is
(a) Removal of anther from unisexual flowering a pair of forecps.
(b) Removal of anther from flower bud after its dehisces using a pair of forceps
(c) Removal of anther from bisexual flower bud before it dehisces using a pair of forceps
(d) All of the above

191. Emasculated flowers are covered with bag of suitable size; the process is referred to as
(a) Emasculation
(b) Bagging
(c) Both
(d) None

192. Why bagging is done in an emasculated flower?
(a) To prevent contamination of its stigma with unwanted pollen
(b) To pollinate the stigma with required anthers only
(c) Both are correct
(d) None of them

193. Emasculation is not required in flowers with
(a) Only having pistil (unisexual)
(b) Having both pistil and anthers (bisexual)
(c) Having only anthers (unisexual)
(d) All are correct

194. The female parent plants produce unisexual flowers
(a) Do not require emasculation
(b) Require emasculation
(c) The flowers are bagged during bud stage
(d) Both (a) and (c)

195. During syngamy
(a) Male gamete fuses with two polar nuclear
(b) Male gamete fuses with egg cell
(c) Both of the above
(d) None of them

196. Primary endosperm nucleus is a result of
(a) Fusion of two polar nuclei with male gamete
(b) Fusion of egg cell with male gamete
(c) Both are correct
(d) None of them

197. Triple fusion is a result of
(a) Fusion of three haploid nuclei
(b) Fusion of two polar nuclei with male gamete
(c) Both are correct
(d) None of them

198. Double fertilization is
(A) Unique to flowering plant
(B) Results in formation of Zygote and Primary endosperm cell
(C) A process in which triple fusion and syngamy takes place
(D) A process in which triple fusion takes place only.
(a) Only A and B
(b) Only A, B and C
(c) All are correct
(d) Only A

199. Triple fusion results in ________ while syngamy results in ________.
(a) Zygote and endosperm
(b) Endosperm and Zygote
(c) Both form of Zygote
(d) Both fern endosperm

200. Identify A and B in this figure.

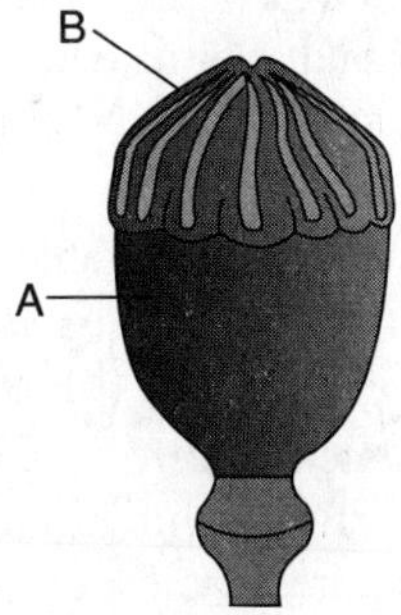

(a) A: Ovary, B: Syncarpous ovary
(b) A: Filament, B: Ovary
(c) A: Stigma, B: Filament
(d) A: Syncarpous ovary, B: Stigma

201. Endosperm is a product of ________ and embryo is a product of ________.
(a) Triple fusion, syngamy
(b) Syngamy, triple fusion
(c) Syngamy, Syngamy
(d) Triple fusion, Triple fusion

202. Post-fertilization events do not include
(A) Formation of primary endosperm cell
(B) Maturation of ovules in seed
(C) Formation of ovary into fruit
(D) Formation of embryo inside seed
(a) Only A
(b) Only B
(c) Only C
(d) None of them

203. Which of the following precedes the other?
(a) Development of embryo before endosperm
(b) Endosperm developing before embryo
(c) Both the development of embryo and endosperm occurs simultaneously
(d) All are correct

204. Which one of the following is correct for endosperm?
(a) The cells of this tissue are filled with reserve food material
(b) Used for nutrition of developing embryo
(c) PEN undergoes nuclear division followed by cytokinesis
(d) All are correct

205. Endosperm is earlier ________ and then develops into ________
(a) Cellular, Nuclear
(b) Nuclear, Cellular
(c) Cellular, Cellular
(d) Nuclear, Nuclear

206. The number of nuclei in free nuclear endosperm before cellularization is
(a) Fixed
(b) Varies greatly
(c) Fixed in species
(d) None of them

207. Coconut water is ________ part of endosperm
(a) Cellular
(b) Free nuclear
(c) Cellular as well as nuclear
(d) Neither cellular nor free nuclear

208. White kernel of coconut is which part of endosperm?
(a) Cellular (b) Free nuclear
(c) Cellular as well as nuclear (d) Neither cellular nor free nuclear

209. Endosperm is completely consumed during seed formation in
(a) Pea, caster and coconut (b) Castor and coconut
(c) Pea and beans (d) Groundnut and caster

210. Endosperm persist in mature seed of
(a) Pea, caster and coconut (b) Castor and coconut
(c) Pea and beans (d) Groundnut and caster

211. Development of embryo takes place at
(a) Chalazal end of embryo sac (b) Micropyle end of embryo sac
(c) Near only integument of embryo sac (d) All are correct

212. Zygote divides after formation of endosperm
(a) To provide assured nutrition to developing endosperm
(b) To provide assured nutrition to developing embryo
(c) None of them
(d) Both are correct

213. The development of embryo in both monocotyledons and dicotyledons
(a) Same (b) Differ greatly
(c) Biennials in early staples of development (d) Both (b) and (c)

214. Which of the following is correct?
(a) Proembryo → Mature embryo → Globular embryo
(b) Proembryo → Globular embryo → Mature embryo
(c) Globular embryo → Proembryo → Mature embryo
(d) Mature embryo → Globular embryo → Proembryo

215. The portion of embryo above the cotyledon is called ________ and below the cotyledon is called as ________
(a) Epicotyl, hypocotyl (b) Hypocotyl, epicotyl
(c) Plumule, radical (d) Radical and Plumule

216. Epicotyl terminates into
(a) Stem tip (b) Root tip
(c) Plumule (d) Both (a) and (c)

217. Hypocotyl terminates into
(a) Root tip (b) Stem tip
(c) Plumule (d) Both (a) and (c)

218. Embryo of monocotyledon posses only
(a) Two cotyledon (b) One cotyledon
(c) Scutellum (d) Both (b) and (c)

219. The root cap of monocot is covered in
(a) Coleoptile (b) Coleorrhiza
(c) Root tip (d) None of them

220. The leaf primordia enclosed in hollow foliar structure called as
(a) Coleoptile
(b) Coleorrhiza
(c) Root tip
(d) None of them

221. Identify A and B in this figure.

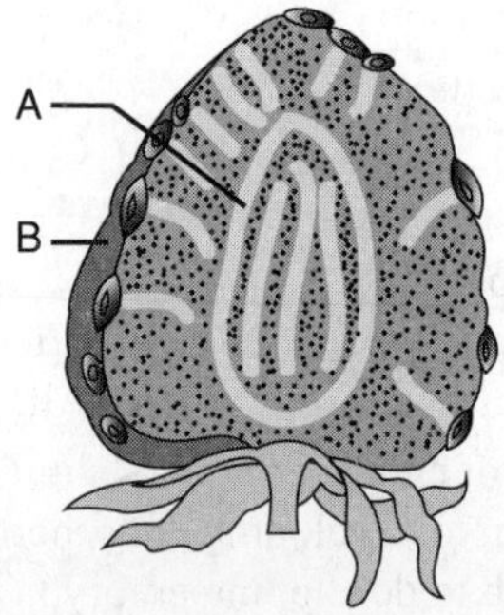

(a) A: Thalamus, B: Endocarp
(b) A: Thalamus, B: Achene
(c) A: Endocarp, B: Mesocarp
(d) A: Mesocarp, B: Endocarp

*Read the **assertion** and **reason** carefully to mark the correct option out of the options given below:*

(a) If both the assertion and the reason are true and the reason is a correct explanation of the assertion
(b) If both the assertion and reason are true but the reason is not a correct explanation of the assertion
(c) If the assertion is true but the reason is false
(d) If both the assertion and reason are false

222. **Assertion:** Pollen grains are well preserved as fossils.
Reason: Pollen posses sporopollenin.

223. **Assertion:** Pollen tables used as food supplement.
Reason: Pollen grains are rich in nutrient.

224. **Assertion:** Pollen tube enters the ovule through micropyle.
Reason: Pollen tube enters in one of synergids through filiform apparatus.

225. **Assertion:** Coconuts water is cellular endosperm.
Reason: White kernel of coconut is free nuclear endosperm.

226. **Assertion:** Most zygote divide only after certain amount of endosperm is formed.
Reason: This is an adaptation to provide assumed nutrition to the developing embryo.

227. **Assertion:** Embryos of monocotyledons posses only one cotyledon.
Reason: In the grass family the cotyledon is called scutellum.

228. **Assertion:** Parthenocarpic fruits are seedless
Reason: Parthenocarpic fruits develop without fertilization.

229. Assertion: Angiospermic can colonise is other areas easily.
Reason: Angiosperms have seeds, and seeds have better adoptive strategies for dispersal to new habitats.

230. Assertion: Seed is the basis to our agriculture.
Reason: Dehydration & dormancy of mature seed is not crucial for storage of seeds.

231. Assertion: Polyembryony is found in all angiosperm.
Reason: All angiosperm are produced by a apomixis.

AIPMT PREVIOUS YEAR QUESTIONS

1. Apomictic embryos in Citrus arise from [AIPMT PRE 2010]
(a) Synergids (b) Maternal sporophytic tissue in ovule
(c) Antipodal cells (d) Diploid egg

2. Transfer of pollen grains from the anther to the stigma of another flower of the same plant is called [AIPMT PRE 2010]
(a) Xenogamy (b) Geitonogamy
(c) Karyogamy (d) Autogamy

3. The scutellum observed in a grain of wheat or maize is comparable to which part of the seed in other monocotyledons? [AIPMT PRE 2010]
(a) Cotyledon (b) Endosperm
(c) Aleurone layer (d) Plumule

4. Wind pollinated flowers are [AIPMT PRE 2010]
(a) Small, brightly coloured, producing large number of pollen grains
(b) Small, producing large number of dry pollen grains
(c) Large, producing abundant nectar and pollen
(d) Small, producing nectar and dry pollen

5. Filliform apparatus is a characteristic feature of: [AIPMT PRE 2011]
(a) Egg (b) Synergid
(c) Zygote (d) Suspensor

6. What would be the number of chromosomes of the aleurone cells of a plant with 42 chromosomes in its root tip cells? [AIPMT PRE 2011]
(a) 63 (b) 84
(c) 21 (d) 42

7. Wind pollination is common in: [AIPMT PRE 2011]
(a) Lilies (b) Grasses
(c) Orchids (d) Legumes

8. Nucellar polyembryony is reported in species of: [AIPMT PRE 2011]

(a) Gossypium (b) triticum
(c) Brassica (d) Citrus

9. In which one of the following pollination is autogamous? [AIPMT PRE 2011]

(a) Xenogamy (b) Chasmogamy
(c) Cleistogamy (d) Geitonogamy

10. In angiosperms, functional megaspore develops into: [AIPMT MAINS 2011]

(a) Embryo sac (b) Ovule
(c) Endosperm (d) Pollen sac

11. What is common between vegetative reproduction and apomixes? [AIPMT MAINS 2011]

(a) Both are applicable to only dicot plants
(b) Both bypass the flowering phase
(c) Both occur round the year
(d) Both produce progeny identical to the parent

12. Plants with ovaries having only one or a few ovules are generally pollinated by: [AIPMT MAINS 2012]

(a) Butterflies (b) Birds
(c) Wind (d) Bees

13. What is the function of germ pore? [AIPMT MAINS 2012]

(a) Absorption of water for seed germination
(b) Initiation of pollen tube
(c) Release of male gametes
(d) Emergence of radical

14. Which one of the following statements is wrong? [AIPMT MAINS 2012]

(a) Vegetative cell is larger than generative cell
(b) Pollen grains in some plants remain viable for months
(c) Intine is made up of cellulose and pectin
(d) When pollen is shed at two-called stage, double fertilization does not take place

15. An organic substance that can withstand environmental extremes and cannot be degraded by any enzyme is: [AIPMT PRE 2012]

(a) Cuticle (b) Sporopollenin
(c) Lignin (d) Cellulose

16. Even in absence of pollinating agents seed - setting is assure in: [AIPMT PRE 2012]

(a) Commellina (b) Zostera
(c) Salvia (d) Fig

17. The coconut water and the edible part of coconut are equivalent to: [AIPMT PRE 2012]

(a) Endosperm (b) Endocarp
(c) Mesocarp (d) Embryo

18. Both, autogamy and geitonogamy are prevented in [AIPMT PRE 2012]

(a) Papaya (b) Cucumber
(c) Castor (d) Maize

19. The gynoecium consists of many free pistils in flowers of: [AIPMT PRE 2012]

(a) Aloe (b) Tomato
(c) Papaver (d) Michelia

20. Which one of the following statements is correct? [AIPMT 2013]

(a) Hard outer layer of pollen is called intine
(b) Sporogenous tissue is haploid
(c) Endothecium produces the microcspores
(d) Tapetum nourishes the developing pollen

21. Advantage of cleistogamy is: [AIPMT 2013]

(a) Higher genetic variability (b) More vigorous off spring
(c) No dependence on pollinators (d) Vivipary

22. Perisperm differs from endosperm in: [AIPMT 2013]

(a) Being a haploid tissue
(b) Having no reserve food
(c) Being a diploid tissue
(d) Its formation by fusion of secondary nucleus with several sperms

23. Geitonogamy involves: [AIPMT 2014]

(a) Fertilization of a flower by the pollen from another flower of the same plant
(b) Fertilization a flower by the pollen from the same flower
(c) Fertilization of a flower by the pollen from a flower of another plant in the same population
(d) Fertilization of a flower by the pollen from a flower of another plant belonging to a distant population

24. Male gametophyte with least number of cells is present in: [AIPMT 2014]

(a) Pteris (b) Funaria
(c) Lilium (d) Pinus

25. Pollen tablets are available in the market for: [AIPMT 2014]

(a) In vitro fertilization (b) Breeding programmes
(c) Supplementing food (d) Ex situ conservation

26. Function of filiform apparatus to: [AIPMT 2014]

(a) Recognize the suitable pollen at stigma
(b) Stimulate division of generative cell
(c) Produce nectar
(d) Guide the entry of pollen tube

27. Non – albuminous seed is produced in:

[AIPMT 2014]

(a) Maize (b) Castor
(c) Wheat (d) Pea

28. Which one of the following may required pollinators, but genetically similar to autogamy?

[AIPMT 2015]

(a) Geitonogamy (b) Xenogamy
(c) Apogamy (d) Cleistogamy

29. Which one of the following statements is not true?

[AIPMT 2015]

(a) Pollen grains are rich in nutrients, and they are used in the form on tablets and syrups
(b) Pollen grains of some plants cause severe allergies and bronchial afflications in some people.
(c) The flowers pollinated by flies and bats secrete foul odour to attract them
(d) Honey is made by bees by digesting pollen collected from flowers

30. Transmission tissue is characteristic feature of

[AIPMT 2015]

(a) Hollow style (b) Solid style
(c) Dry stigma (d) Wet stigma

31. Which of the following are the important floral rewards to the animal pollinators?

[AIPMT 2015]

(a) Colour and large size of flower
(b) Nectar and pollen grains
(c) Floral fragrance and calcium crystals
(d) Protein pellicle and stigmatic exudates

32. Male gametophyte in angiosperms producers:

[RE-AIPMT 2015]

(a) Single sperm and a vegetative cell (b) Single sperm and two vegetative cells
(c) Three sperms (d) Two sperms and a vegetative cell

33. Coconut water from a tender coconut is:

[RE-AIPMT 2015]

(a) Free nuclear endosperm (b) Innermost layers of the seed coat
(c) Degenerated nucellus (d) Immature embryo

34. Which one of the following fruits is parthenocarpic?

[RE-AIPMT 2015]

(a) Apple (b) Jackfruit
(c) Banana (d) Brinjal

35. Filiform apparatus is characteristic feature of:

[RE-AIPMT 2015]

(a) Nucellar embryo (b) Aleurone cell
(c) Synergids (d) Generative cell

36. In angiosperms, microsporogeneis and megasporogenesis:

[RE-AIPMT 2015]

(a) From gametes without further divisions (b) Involve meiosis
(c) Occur in ovule (d) Occur in anther

Answer Keys

1. (d)	2. (d)	3. (d)	4. (c)	5. (b)	6. (d)	7. (b)	8. (a)	9. (a)	10. (d)
11. (c)	12. (d)	13. (a)	14. (b)	15. (b)	16. (c)	17. (d)	18. (b)	19. (c)	20. (b)
21. (d)	22. (b)	23. (d)	24. (d)	25. (b)	26. (b)	27. (a)	28. (d)	29. (d)	30. (b)
31. (a)	32. (c)	33. (b)	34. (d)	35. (c)	36. (b)	37. (c)	38. (c)	39. (d)	40. (c)
41. (b)	42. (d)	43. (a)	44. (c)	45. (d)	46. (b)	47. (c)	48. (d)	49. (a)	50. (c)
51. (a)	52. (a)	53. (b)	54. (b)	55. (c)	56. (d)	57. (c)	58. (c)	59. (b)	60. (b)
61. (d)	62. (a)	63. (b)	64. (d)	65. (b)	66. (b)	67. (b)	68. (a)	69. (c)	70. (b)
71. (a)	72. (a)	73. (d)	74. (a)	75. (c)	76. (a)	77. (b)	78. (b)	79. (b)	80. (b)
81. (c)	82. (d)	83. (c)	84. (b)	85. (b)	86. (a)	87. (c)	88. (b)	89. (b)	90. (a)
91. (b)	92. (d)	93. (c)	94. (b)	95. (c)	96. (d)	97. (a)	98. (d)	99. (a)	100. (b)
101. (b)	102. (b)	103. (b)	104. (b)	105. (d)	106. (c)	107. (a)	108. (b)	109. (d)	110. (a)
111. (a)	112. (b)	113. (c)	114. (b)	115. (d)	116. (a)	117. (b)	118. (d)	119. (d)	120. (c)
121. (c)	122. (d)	123. (d)	124. (d)	125. (b)	126. (c)	127. (b)	128. (b)	129. (d)	130. (c)
131. (a)	132. (b)	133. (d)	134. (b)	135. (d)	136. (a)	137. (c)	138. (d)	139. (a)	140. (d)
141. (c)	142. (a)	143. (d)	144. (d)	145. (a)	146. (d)	147. (b)	148. (b)	149. (a)	150. (d)
151. (d)	152. (d)	153. (c)	154. (a)	155. (c)	156. (d)	157. (a)	158. (d)	159. (d)	160. (a)
161. (d)	162. (c)	163. (c)	164. (b)	165. (a)	166. (d)	167. (a)	168. (c)	169. (b)	170. (a)
171. (d)	172. (b)	173. (c)	174. (c)	175. (b)	176. (d)	177. (c)	178. (a)	179. (d)	180. (d)
181. (d)	182. (b)	183. (c)	184. (a)	185. (b)	186. (b)	187. (d)	188. (d)	189. (c)	190. (c)
191. (b)	192. (c)	193. (a)	194. (d)	195. (b)	196. (a)	197. (c)	198. (b)	199. (b)	200. (d)
201. (a)	202. (a)	203. (b)	204. (d)	205. (b)	206. (b)	207. (b)	208. (a)	209. (c)	210. (b)
211. (b)	212. (b)	213. (d)	214. (b)	215. (a)	216. (d)	217. (a)	218. (b)	219. (b)	220. (a)
221. (b)	222. (a)	223. (a)	224. (b)	225. (d)	226. (a)	227. (b)	228. (a)	229. (a)	230. (c)
231. (d)									

AIPMT Previous Year Questions

1. (b)	2. (b)	3. (a)	4. (b)	5. (b)	6. (a)	7. (b)	8. (d)	9. (c)	10. (a)
11. (d)	12. (c)	13. (b)	14. (d)	15. (b)	16. (a)	17. (a)	18. (a)	19. (d)	20. (d)
21. (c)	22. (c)	23. (a)	24. (c)	25. (c)	26. (d)	27. (d)	28. (a)	29. (d)	30. (b)
31. (b)	32. (d)	33. (a)	34. (c)	35. (c)	36. (b)				

CHAPTER 25

Human Reproduction

1. Humans are ____ and ____ organisms:
   (a) sexually reproducing, oviparous
   (b) asexually reproducing, ovoviviparous
   (c) asexually reproducing, viviparous
   (d) sexually reproducing, viviparous
2. The formation of gametes is termed as:
   (a) Gametogamy
   (b) Syngamy
   (c) Gametogenesis
   (d) Gestation
3. The transfer of sperms into the female genital tract is called:
   (a) Insemination
   (b) Gametogenesis
   (c) Fertilization
   (d) Gestation
4. The fusion of male and female gametes is known as:
   (a) Insemination
   (b) Fertilization
   (c) Implantation
   (d) Parturition
5. Match the following correctly.

Column-I	Column-II
1. Gestation	A. Fusion of male and female gametes
2. Parturition	B. Formation of gametes
3. Gametogenesis	C. Attachment to the uterine wall
4. Implantation	D. Delivery of the baby
	E. Embryonic development

   (a) 1:A, 2:C, 3:B, 4:D
   (b) 1:E, 2:D, 3:A, 4:C
   (c) 1:E, 2:D, 3:B, 4:C
   (d) 1:C, 2:D, 3:A, 4:C
6. The correct chronological order of the following events is:
   (a) Gametogenesis → Fertilization → Insemination → Gestation → Implantation → Parturition
   (b) Gametogenesis → Insemination → Fertilization → Impanation → Parturition → Gestation
   (c) Gametogenesis → Insemination → Fertilization → Implantation → Gestation → Parturition
   (d) None of these
7. Following statements are true except:
   (a) In an individual, reproductive changes occur after puberty.
   (b) Sperm formation occurs even in old men.
   (c) Formation of ovum continues in women after fifty years.
   (d) Humans are sexually producing and viviparous.

8. The testes are situated ____ the abdominal cavity within a pouch called ____.
(a) inside, testicular lobules
(b) outside, scrotum
(c) outside, vas deferens
(d) inside, scrotum

9. The scrotum helps in maintaining a temperature ____ lower than the internal body temperature.
(a) 1–1.5 °C
(b) 2–2.5 °C
(c) 3–3.5 °C
(d) 4–4.5 °C

10. An adult testes is oval in shape. Its width is about ____ and length is about ____ respectively
(a) 4–5 cm, 2–3 cm
(b) 2–5 cm, 1–3 cm
(c) 2–3 cm, 4–5 cm
(d) 2–5 cm, 4–7 cm

Figure given for questions 11 to 15.

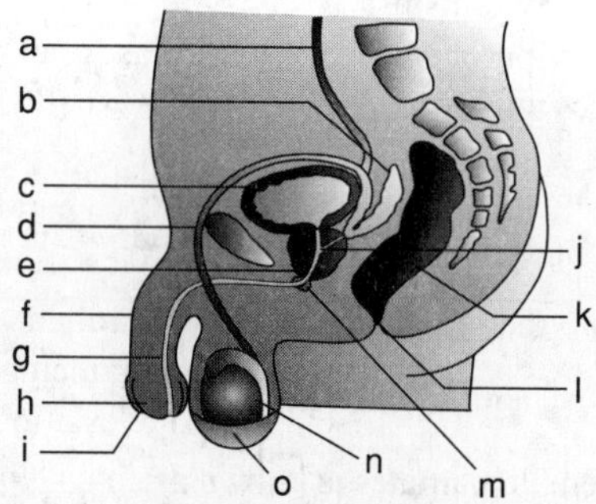

11. What does 'm' represent?
(a) Ureter
(b) Ejaculatory duct
(c) Bulbourethral gland
(d) Urethra

12. What is indicated by 'd' in the figure?
(a) Urethra
(b) Vas deferens
(c) Vasa efferentia
(d) Ureter

13. What does 'o' represent in the figure?
(a) Glans penis
(b) Scrotum
(c) Testis
(d) Epididy

14. What is indicated by 'h' in the figure?
(a) Penis
(b) Foreskin
(c) Glans penis
(d) Urethral meatus

15. What is indicated by 'b' in the figure?
(a) Prostate gland
(b) Bulbourethral gland
(c) Ureter
(d) Seminal vesicle

16. An adult tests bears ____ compartments called testicular lobules.
(a) 150
(b) 250
(c) 350
(d) 500

17. Each testicular lobule contains ____ seminiferous tubule.
(a) Only three
(b) Only one
(c) One to three
(d) More than three

18. Male germ cells are known as

(a) Sperms (b) Spermatogonia
(c) Spermatid (d) Sertoli cells

19. Seminiferous tubules contain ____ cells for providing nutrition to sperm cells.

(a) Leydig cells (b) Interstitial cell
(c) Sertoli cells (d) Germ cells

20. The cells which secrete androgens are:

(a) Spermatozoa (b) Interstitial cells
(c) Sertoli cells (d) Germ cells

21. Select the correct anatomical sequence.

(a) Seminiferous tubules → rete testis → Vasa efferentia → Vasa deferens → Epididymis
(b) Seminiferous tubules → rete testis → Vasa efferentia → Epididymis → Vasa deferens
(c) Seminiferous tubules → Vasa efferentia → rete testis → Vasa deferens → Epididymis
(d) None of the above

22. The enlarged end of penis is known as

(a) Glans (b) Foreskin
(c) Urethra (d) Prostate

23. If A stands for seminal vesicles, B stands for bulbourethral glands, C stands for prostate gland, then, which of the following is true?

(a) A and C occurs in pair (b) A and B occur in pair
(c) B and C occur in pair (d) None of the above

24. Seminal plasma is rich in which sugar?

(a) Sucrose (b) Glucose
(c) Fructose (d) Maltose

Figure given for questions 25 to 30.

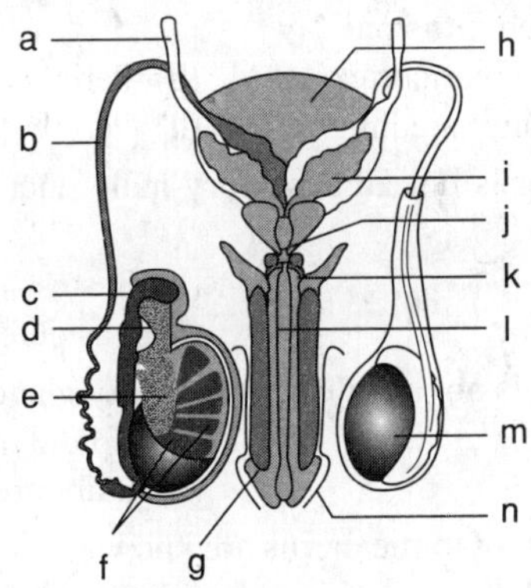

25. What is indicated by 'e' in the figure?

(a) Testicular lobule (b) Testis
(c) Vasa efferentia (d) Rete testis

26. What is indicated by 'c' in the figure?

(a) Vasa efferentia (b) Rete testis
(c) Epididymis (d) Vas deferens

27. What is indicated by 'i' in the figure?
(a) Prostate (b) Urinary bladder
(c) Seminal vesicle (d) Bulbourethral gland

28. What does 'k' represent?
(a) Prostate (b) Urinary bladder
(c) Seminal vesicle (d) Bulbourethral gland

29. What is indicated by 'l' in the figure?
(a) Vas deferens (b) Ureter
(c) Urethra (d) Ejaculatory duct

30. The secretion of which gland help in lubrication of penis?
(a) Seminal vesicle (b) Prostate
(c) Bulbourethral (d) Epididymis

31. Which is the primary female sex organ?
(a) Uterus (b) Ovaries
(c) Oviducts (d) Vagina

32. The ovaries are located
(a) One on each side of the upper abdomen (b) Two on each side of the lower abdomen
(c) Two on each side of the upper abdomen (d) One on each side of the lower abdomen

33. Which of the following statements about ovary is not true?
(a) Ovaries are responsible for production of several steroid hormones.
(b) Each ovary is about 4–6 cm in length.
(c) Ovary is connected to the pelvic wall.
(d) Ovary produces female gamete (Ovum).

34. Ovarian stroma is enclosed by ____.
(a) Endothelium (b) Epithelium
(c) Mesothelium (d) Ciliated epithelium

35. The ovarian stroma is divided into zones
(a) Peripheral medulla and inner cortex (b) Peripheral epithelia and inner endothelia
(c) Peripheral cortex and inner medulla (d) Peripheral endothelia and inner epithelia

36. Which one of the following is not an accessory male duct in context of male reproductive system?
(a) Rete testis (b) Testes
(c) Epididymis (d) Vas deferens

37. Which one of the following is not a male sex accessory gland?
(a) Seminal vesicle (b) Epididymis
(c) Prostate (d) bulbourethral

38. The tubes which conduct ovum to the uterus are known as
(a) Fallopian tube (b) Oviduct
(c) Cervical opening (d) Both (a) and (b)

39. Which one of the following is not a female accessory duct?
(a) Vagina (b) Uterus
(c) Oviduct (d) Ovary

40. Each oviduct is about ____ long.
(a) 5–6 mm (b) 10–12 cm
(c) 10–12 mm (d) 5–6 cm

Figure given for questions 41 to 44.

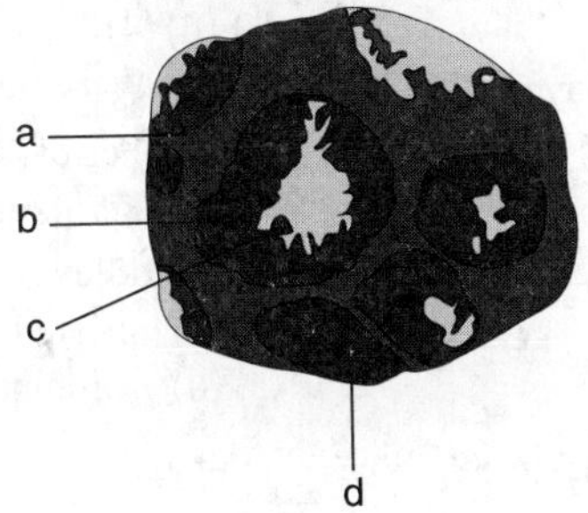

41. What is indicated by 'a' in the figure?
(a) Sertoli cells (b) Interstitial cells
(c) Spermatogonia (d) Spermatozoa

42. What is indicated by 'c' in figure?
(a) Spermatozoa (b) Spermatogonia
(c) Interstitial cells (d) Sertoli cells

43. What does 'b' in the figurerepresent?
(a) Interstitial cells (b) Sertoli cells
(c) Spermatogonia (d) Spermatozoa

44. What is indicated by 'd' in the figure?
(a) Sertoli cells (b) Spermatozoa
(c) Spermatogonia (d) Interstitial cells

45. The funnel shaped part of fallopian tube which traps ovum is known as
(a) Isthmus (b) Ampulla
(c) Infundibulum (d) Cervix

46. Isthmus a part of oviduct, is a narrow lumen and joins ____.
(a) Uterus (b) Ampulla
(c) Infundibulum (d) Both (a) and (b)

47. The anatomical structure which succeeds infundibulum is
(a) Isthmus (b) Ampulla
(c) Uterus (d) Ovary

48. Finger-like projection of infundibulum are known as
(a) Cilia (b) Flagella
(c) Fimbriae (d) None

49. Uterus is commonly known as
(a) Birth canal (b) Womb
(c) Primary female sex organ (d) Female external genitalia

50. The uterus opens into vagina through ____.
(a) ampulla (b) isthmus
(c) cervix (d) labia minora

51. Birth canal is formed by
(a) Cervical canal + uterus (b) Cervical canal + vagina
(c) Cervical canal + Isthmus (d) Cervical canal + Fallopian tube

52. The wall of uterus is made up of ____ layers of tissue.
(a) 2
(b) 3
(c) 1
(d) 4

53. External thin membranous layer of uterus is known as.
(a) Pleura
(b) Pericardium
(c) Perimetrium
(d) Periostium

54. Thick muscular layer of ____ muscle constitutes middle layer of uterus.
(a) smooth
(b) striated
(c) intercalated
(d) voluntary

Figure given for question 55 to 58.

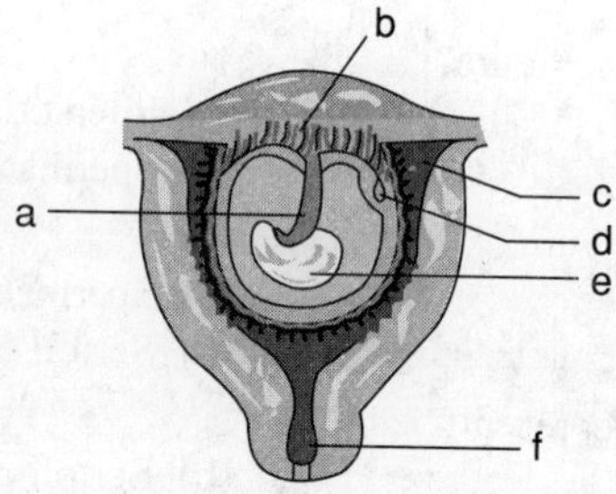

55. What is indicated by 'e' in the figure?
(a) Yolk sac
(b) Embryo
(c) Cavity of uterus
(d) Placental villi

56. What does 'a' represent in the figure?
(a) Umbilical cord
(b) Embryo
(c) Yolk sac
(d) Placental villi

57. What does 'd' represent in the figure?
(a) Embryo
(b) Umbilical cord
(c) Yolk sac
(d) Cavity of uterus

58. What does 'b' represent in the figure?
(a) Cavity of uterus
(b) Embryo
(c) Yolk sac
(d) Placental villi

59. Which layer of uterus undergoes cyclic changes during menstrual cycle?
(a) Mesoderm
(b) Myometrium
(c) Endothelium
(d) Endometrium

60. The layer of uterine tissues responsible for strong contractions during childbirth is
(a) Perimetrium
(b) Mesometrium
(c) Mesoderm
(d) Myocardium

61. Of the following statements, which one is true for Mons Pubis
(a) It is the region of pubic hair growth found in females as well as males.
(b) It is a cushion of proteins covered by skin and pubic hair.
(c) It is a cushion of fats covered by skin and pubic hair.
(d) It is a part of female internal genitalia

62. Clitoris lies at the junction of
(a) Labia Majora (b) Labia Minora
(c) Mons pubis (d) Pubis symphysis

63. The clitoris is a tiny ____ shaped structure which lies above the urethral opening
(a) flagellated (b) finger like
(c) bean shaped (d) pear

64. The only statement correct about hymen is
(a) It is an opening of cervix.
(b) It is a reliable indicator of virginity.
(c) It is always torn after first coitus.
(d) It can be broken by a sudden fall or jolt, insertion of vaginal tampon, cycling, etc.

65. Mammary lobes contain cluster of cells known as ____.
(a) mammary duct (b) alveoli
(c) ampulla (d) lactiferous duct

66. The terminal structure of the mammary glands through which milk is sucked out is known as
(a) Lumen of alveoli (b) Mammary duct
(c) Lactiferous duct (d) Mammary lobe

67. Several mammary ducts join to form
(a) Mammary lobe (b) Alveoli
(c) Mammary ampulla (d) Lactiferous duct

68. Immature male germ cells are known as
(a) Spermatid (b) Spermatozoa
(c) Spermatogonia (d) Sperm

69. Spermatogonium undergoes ____.
(a) reduction division (b) meiotic division
(c) mitotic division (d) none

Figure given for question 70 to 73.

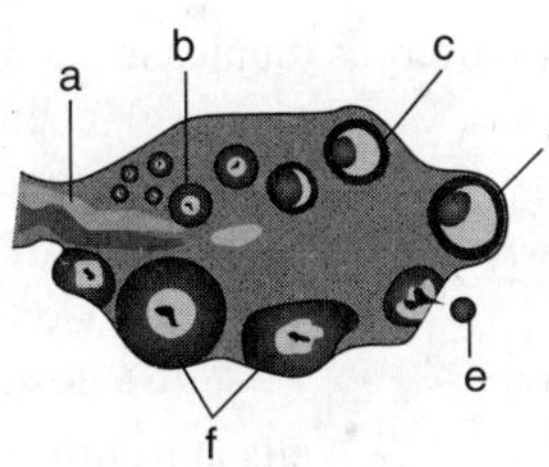

70. What does 'a' represent in the figure?
(a) Lymph vessels (b) Blood vessels
(c) Nerve fibres (d) Ligament

71. What is indicated by 'c' in the figure?
(a) Primary follicle (b) Second follicle
(c) Tertiary follicle (d) Graafian follicle

72. What does 'f' represent in the figure?
(a) Antrum (b) Corpus luteum
(c) Corpora cavernosa (d) Ovum

73. What does 'e' represent in the figure?
(a) Ovum (b) Oogonium
(c) Mature follicle (d) Zona pellucida

74. Each spermatogonium is ____ and has ____ number of chromosomes.
(a) n, 45 (b) 2n, 23
(c) 2n, 46 (d) n, 46

75. The spermatogonia which undergo meiosis are known as
(a) Sperm (b) Spermatid
(c) Secondary spermatocyte (d) Primary spermatocyte

76. The difference between primary and secondary spermatocyte lies in ____.
(a) presence/absence of a tail
(b) number of chromosomes
(c) being hormone producing/non-hormone producing
(d) Primary gamete/Secondary gamete in males

77. Secondary spermatocytes give rise to
(a) Diploid spermatids (b) Haploid sperm
(c) Diploid sperm (d) Haploid spermatid

78. Sperms are synonymous with
(a) Spermatid (b) Spermatogonia
(c) Primary spermatocyte (d) Spermatozoa

79. Spermiogenesis is
(a) Transformation of sperm into spermatids
(b) Transformation of spermatogonia into primary spermatocyte
(c) Transformation of secondary spermatocyte into spermatids
(d) Transformation of spermatid into spermatozoa

80. After spermiogenesis, the sperm head is embedded in the ____ cells.
(a) sertoli (b) leydig
(c) interstitial (d) both (a) and (b)

81. The release of sperms from seminiferous tubules is known as ____.
(a) ejaculation (b) copulation
(c) spermiation (d) none

82. Spermatogenesis starts at puberty due to the secretion of
(a) Luteinizing hormone (b) Gonadotropin releasing hormone
(c) Follicle stimulating Hormone (d) Testosterone

83. Luteinizing hormone (LH) acts on ____ cells and stimulates synthesis and secretion of ____.
(a) Leydig cells, FSH (b) interstitial cells, androgens
(c) Leydig cells, GnRH (d) none of these

84. Androgens stimulate ____.
(a) spermiation (b) insemination
(c) spermatogenesis (d) oogenesis

85. The function of FSH in male is
(a) Act on Leydig cells and stimulates secretion of factors responsible for spermiation
(b) Act on sertoli cells and stimulates secretion of factors responsible for spermatogenesis
(c) Act on interstitial cells and stimulates secretion of factors responsible for spermiogenesis
(d) Act on sertoli cells and stimulates secretion of factors responsible for spermiogenesis

86. The microscopic structure of sperm consists of
    (a) Head, Neck, Tail
    (b) Head, Neck, Middle piece, Tail
    (c) Head, Middle piece, Tail
    (d) Neck, Middle piece, Tail

Figure given for question 87 to 90.

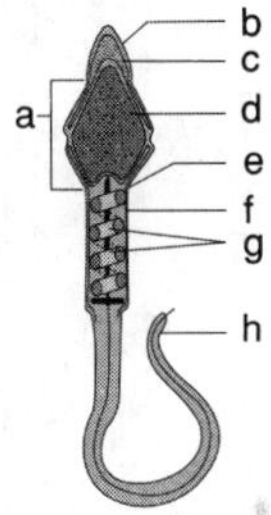

87. What is indicated by 'c' in the figure?
    (a) Ascosome
    (b) Acrosome
    (c) Nucleosome
    (d) Hyaluronidase
88. What does 'd' represent in the figure?
    (a) Nucleosome
    (b) Acrosome
    (c) Nucleus
    (d) Hyaluronidase
89. What does 'g' represent in the figure?
    (a) Middle piece
    (b) Mitochondria
    (c) Neck
    (d) Tail
90. What is indicated by 'b' in the figure?
    (a) Plasma membrane
    (b) Nuclear membrane
    (c) Acrosome
    (d) Hyaluronidase
91. The sperm head contains:
    (a) Antherosome
    (b) Acrosome
    (c) Arthosome
    (d) Ascosome
92. The function of acrosome is
    (a) Stimulates synthesis of ovum
    (b) Stimulates release of ovum
    (c) Stimulates fertilization of ovum
    (d) Stimulates degradation of ovum
93. The middle piece of sperm contains cell organelles like
    (a) Filaments
    (b) Mitochondria
    (c) Nucleus
    (d) Ribosomes
94. How many sperm cells are there in an average human ejaculation?
    (a) 200 to 300 billion
    (b) 200 to 300 million
    (c) 200 to 300 trillion
    (d) 200 to 300 lacs
95. For a normal male fertility, which of the following statements is correct?
    (a) 60% sperm must have normal motility and 40% must have normal shape
    (b) 60% sperm must have normal shape and 40% must have acrosome
    (c) 60% sperm must have normal shape and 40% must have vigorous motility
    (d) None of these

96. Semen consists of
(a) Seminal plasma + Spermatid (b) Seminal plasma + Spermatozoa
(c) Seminal plasma + Spermatogonia (d) None of these

97. The process of formation of mature female gamete is known as
(a) Gametogenesis (b) Spermatogenis
(c) Oogenesis (d) Morphogenesis

98. Oogenesis initiates after/at
(a) Fertilization (b) Puberty
(c) Embryonic development (d) Time of birth

99. Each female ovary consists of
(a) Millions of ova (b) Millions of primary oocytes
(c) Millions of oogonia (d) Millions of secondary oocytes

100. The primary oocytes are in which stage of cell division?
(a) Prophase – I of mitotic division (b) Prophase – I of meiotic division
(c) Prophase – II of meiotic division (d) Prophase – II of mitotic division

101. For the period of birth till puberty, which cells degenerate in ovary?
(a) Oogonia (b) Ova
(c) Secondary follicle (d) Primary follicle

102. The primary and secondary follicle are surrounded by cells known as
(a) Granulosa (b) Mucosa
(c) Serosa (d) Granuloma

103. The tertiary follicle in ovary is characterized by presence of
(a) Fundus (b) Antrum
(c) Vacuole (d) Cavity

104. The mature tertiary follicle is also known as
(a) Ovum (b) Oogonia
(c) Graafian follicle (d) Polar body

105. The membrane around Graafian follicle is known as
(a) Zona fasciculata (b) Zona musculauis
(c) Zona externa (d) Zona pellucida

Figure given for question 106 to 108.

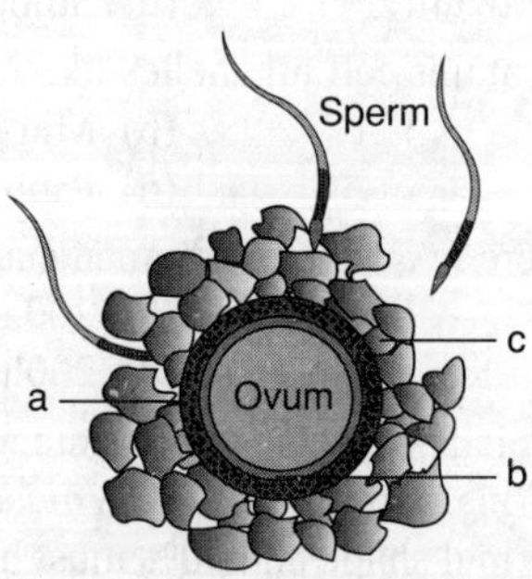

106. What is indicated by 'b' in the figure?
(a) Ovum (b) Cells of corona radiata
(c) Perivitelline space (d) Zone pellucida

107. What does ‘a’ represent in the figure?
(a) Cells of corona radiata (b) Sperm
(c) Perivitelline space (d) Zone pellucida

108. What does ‘c’ represent in the figure?
(a) Cells of corona radiata (b) Sperm
(c) Perivitelline space (d) Zone pellucida

109. The Graafian follicles release
(a) Secondary oocyte (b) Primary oocyte
(c) Ovum (d) Both (a) and (b)

110. The release of ovum from ovary is known as
(a) Ovulation (b) Oogenesis
(c) Parturition (d) Gametogenesis

111. How many total polar bodies are formed in oogenesis
(a) 2 (b) 1
(c) 3 (d) 0

112. The first menstruation which begins at puberty is called
(a) Menstrual cycle (b) Menarche
(c) Oogenesis (d) Ovulation

113. An average interval of menstrual cycle in females is about ____ days.
(a) 15/16 (b) 30/31
(c) 28/29 (d) 25/26

114. One ovum is released during the ____ of each menstrual cycle.
(a) initial (b) middle
(c) terminal (d) alternative

115. What does ‘a’ represent in this figure?

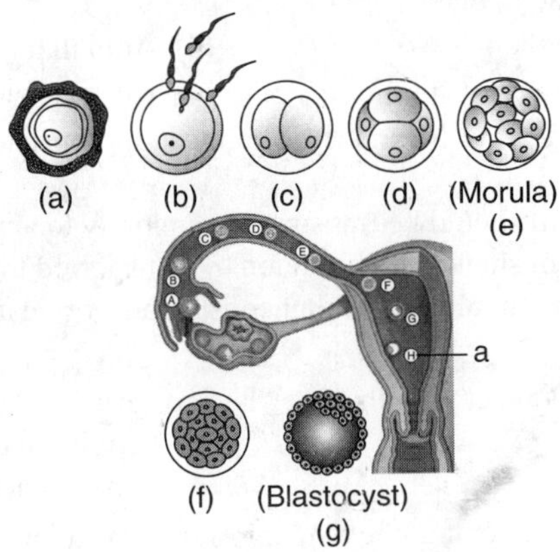

(a) Blastocyst (b) Blastocyst implantation
(c) Morula (d) Cells

116. The menstrual flow in menstrual cycle lasts for about
(a) 6–7 days (b) Almost 7 days
(c) 3–5 days (d) 1–2 days

117. Lack of menstruation may be indicative of
(a) Pregnancy (b) Routine work stress
(c) Poor health (d) All of the above

118. In females, gonadotropins attain a peak level at about the ____ day of the menstrual cycle.
(a) 15th (b) 14th
(c) 28th (d) 29th

119. LH surge causes
(a) Rupture of graafian follicle (b) Release of ovum
(c) Endometrial shedding (d) Both (a) and (b)

120. The ovulation phase is followed by ____ phase.
(a) Gestation (b) Luteal
(c) Menstrual (d) Oogenesis

121. After ovulation, Graafian follicle transforms into:
(a) Corpus cavernosa (b) Corpus pellucida
(c) Corpus luteum (d) Corpus metrium

122. Large amounts of progesterone is secreted by
(a) Corpus metvium (b) Corpus luteum
(c) Corpus cavernosa (d) Corpus pellucida

123. If fertilization does not occur corpus luteum ____.
(a) proliferates (b) degenerates
(c) regenerates (d) divides

124. The menstrual cycle ceases at the age of 50 in human females and is known as
(a) Ovopause (b) Menarche
(c) Menopause (d) Menstruation

125. Once the sperm is injected into the female genital tract, which junction is primarily concerned with meeting of sperm with ovum?
(a) Utero-ampullary junction (b) Ampullary-isthmic junction
(c) Isthmic-infundibullary junction (d) Uteri-carvical junction

126. All copulations do not lead to pregnancy. The most appropriate reason to support this statement is
(a) The ovum and sperm should be transported randomly to ampullary-isthmic junction.
(b) The ovum and sperm should be continuously transported to ampullary-isthmic junction.
(c) The ovum and sperm should be simultaneously transported to ampullary- isthmic junction.
(d) None of the above

127. The sperm comes into contact with the ____ layer of ovum to cause fertilization.
(a) Corona radiate (b) Perivitelline layer
(c) Zona pellucida (d) Zona fasciculate

128. Once a sperm fuses with an ovum, the remaining sperms cannot fertilize ovum. What changes are responsible for such phenomenon?
(a) Selective permeation through ovum
(b) Specific spatial arrangement of corona radiata cells
(c) Change in the membrane zona pellucida
(d) Ovum releases toxic substances thereby killing other sperms

129. After entry of sperm into cytoplasm of ovum following event takes place
(a) Mitotic division of secondary oocyte (b) Meiotic division of primary oocyte
(c) Mitotic division of secondary oocyte (d) Meiotic division of secondary oocyte

130. Human female has following sex chromosome pattern
(a) XX (b) YY
(c) XY (d) XYX

131. Human male has following sex chromosome pattern
(a) XYX (b) XY
(c) XX (d) YY

132. Female produces only
(a) One type of gamete Y (b) One type of gamete X
(c) Either X or Y type of gamete (d) All of above

133. Scientifically sex of the baby is determined by
(a) Only mother (b) Only father
(c) Either mother or father (d) Gestational phase

134. After formation of zygote, it cleaves into 2, 4, 8, 16 daughter cells called:
(a) Blastocyst (b) Morula
(c) Trophoblast (d) Blastomere

Figure given for question 135 to 138.

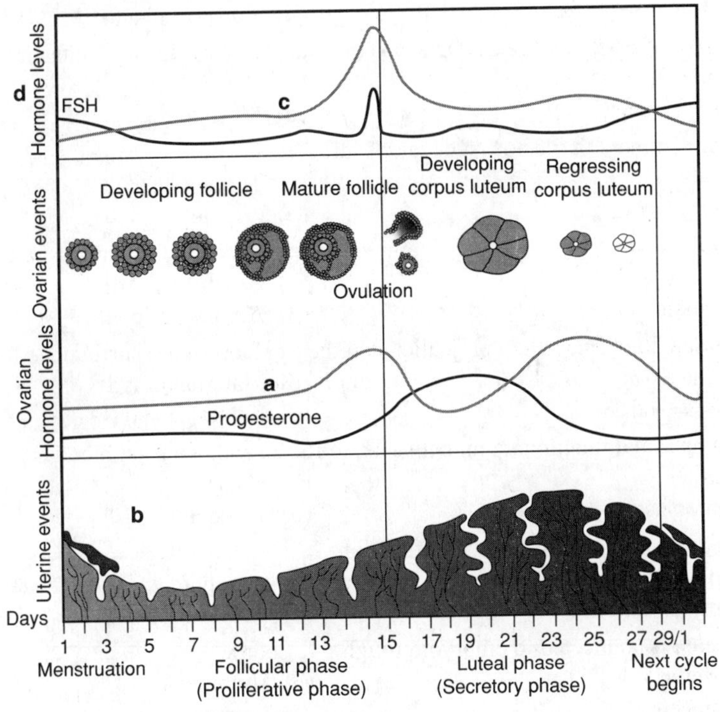

135. What does 'b' represent?
(a) LH
(b) Pituitary
(c) Menses
(d) Ovarian

136. What is indicated by 'd' in the figure?
(a) Estrogen
(b) Pituitary
(c) LH
(d) Menses

137. What does 'c' represent in the figure?
(a) LH
(b) Pituitary
(c) Menses
(d) Ovarian

138. What is indicated by 'a' in the figure?
(a) Estrogen
(b) Menses
(c) Pituitary
(d) progesterone

139. The embryo with 2^3 or 4^2 blastomeres is known as
(a) Blastocyst
(b) Morula
(c) Trophoblast
(d) Zygote

140. Morula divides and transforms into
(a) Inner cell mass
(b) Blastocyst
(c) Trophoblast
(d) Blastomere

141. The outer layer of blastocyst is known as
(a) Zona pellucida
(b) Trophoblast
(c) Blastomere
(d) Corona radiata

142. Which layer of blastocyst gets attached to the endometrium during implantation?
(a) Trophoblast
(b) Blastomere
(c) Inner cell mass
(d) Morula

143. The inner cell mass of blastocyst develops into
(a) Morula
(b) Trophoblast
(c) Embryo
(d) Zygote

144. After implantation finger-like projection which appears on the trophoblast are known as
(a) Intestinal villi
(b) Ampullary villi
(c) Chorionic villi
(d) Amniocentic villi

145. After implantation finger-like projections on the trophoblast are surrounded by
(a) Uterine tissue
(b) Maternal blood
(c) Both (a) and (b)
(d) Either (a) and (b)

146. The structural and functional unit between the foetus and maternal blood is known as
(a) Inner cell
(b) Placenta
(c) Trophoblast
(d) Chorionic villi

147. Placenta does not perform following function
(a) Supply of O_2
(b) Supply of excretory materials
(c) Supply of nutrients
(d) Removal of CO_2

148. The placenta is connected to embryo through ____ cord.
(a) Chorionic
(b) Umbilical
(c) Amniocentic
(d) Uterine

149. Placenta also acts as a/an ____ tissue.
(a) Endocrine
(b) Exocrine
(c) Paracrine
(d) Mepacrine

150. Which of the following hormone is released by placenta?
(a) FSH (b) HCG
(c) Relaxin (d) LH

151. Relaxin is secreted by
(a) Ovary (b) Uterus
(c) Cervix (d) Oviduct

152. How many germinal layers does embryo consist of initially, after implantation?
(a) 3 (b) 2
(c) 4 (d) 5

153. In human embryonic development, which layer develops between the ectoderm and endoderm?
(a) Mesothelium (b) Mesoderm
(c) Myoderm (d) Myometrium

154. In humans, the inner cell mass (embryo) contains certain cells called ____ cells which have the potential to give rise to all the tissues and organs.
(a) root (b) leaf
(c) stem (d) seed

155. The average time span of human gestation is
(a) 8 months (b) 9 months
(c) 10 months (d) 1 year

156. The pregnancy phase in humans is divided into how many trimesters?
(a) 2 (b) 4
(c) 3 (d) 5

157. After one month of pregnancy which vital organ is formed in the foetus?
(a) Brain (b) Heart
(c) Lungs (d) Liver

158. In a developing foetus, most of the major organ systems are developed by the end of ____ weeks.
(a) Fourteen (b) Twelve
(c) Ten (d) Sixteen

159. Foetal limbs and digits are formed in the ____ month of embryonic development.
(a) 4th (b) 2nd
(c) 3rd (d) 7th

160. The second trimester of human pregnancy is characterized by
(a) Appearance of heart and aorta
(b) Appearance of external genital organs
(c) Appearance of fine hair, eye-lashes on the eye-lids
(d) Appearance of limbs and digits

161. The scientific name of childbirth is
(a) Gestation (b) Parturition
(c) Implantation (d) Foetal development

162. During parturition, the mild uterine contractions which lead to expulsion of the foetus is known as
(a) Foetal ejection release (b) Foetal ejection reflex
(c) Foetal uterine reflex (d) Foetal placental reflex

163. Which hormone is responsible for severe uterine contractions during parturition?
(a) Estrogen (b) Oxytocin
(c) Progesterone (d) Relaxin

Figure given for question 164 to 167.

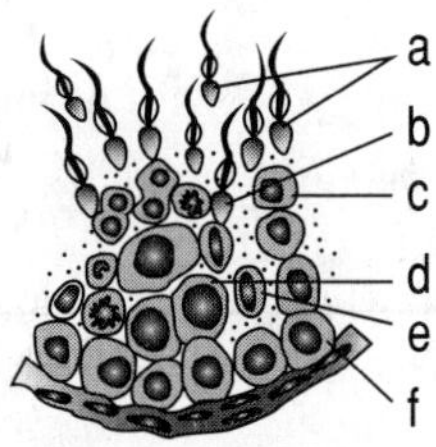

164. What does 'f' represent in the figure?
(a) Sertoli cell (b) Spermatogonium
(c) Spermatid (d) Primary spermatocyte

165. What is indicated by 'e' in the figure?
(a) Sertoli cell (b) Spermatogonium
(c) Spermatid (d) Primary spermatocyte

166. What does 'd' represent in the figure?
(a) Sertoli cell (b) Spermatogonium
(c) Spermatid (d) Primary spermatocyte

167. What is indicated by 'a' in the figure?
(a) Spermatid (b) Spermatozoa
(c) Secondary spermatocyte (d) Primary spermatocyte

168. After delivery of the foetus the following structure is also expelled out?
(a) Uterus (b) Corpus uterum
(c) Placenta (d) Ovary

169. The production of milk in mammary gland occurs:
(a) During parturition (b) After parturition
(c) Before embryogenesis (d) At the end of pregnancy

170. The milk produced during the initial days of lactation is called
(a) Menstrum (b) Colostrum
(c) Gynostrum (d) None of these

171. The first foetal movement is observed during the ____ month of embryonic development.
(a) 4th (b) 5th
(c) 3rd (d) 7th

172. Embryos with more than 8 blastomeres could be transferred into the ____.
(a) Uterus (b) Fallopian tube
(c) Placenta (d) Cervix

173. Transfer of an ovum from a donor to another female who can provide a suitable environment for fertilization is called
(a) ZIFT (b) GIFT
(c) ICSI (d) IUT

174. Intra cytoplasmic sperm injection is a specialized procedure in which the sperm is directly injected into the ____.
(a) Ovary (b) Fallopian tube
(c) Ovum (d) Uterus

175. In artificial insemination, the semen from husband/healthy donor is artificially introduced into the ____.
(a) Vagina (b) Oviduct
(c) Uterus (d) Both (a) and (c)

Figure given for question 176 to 180.

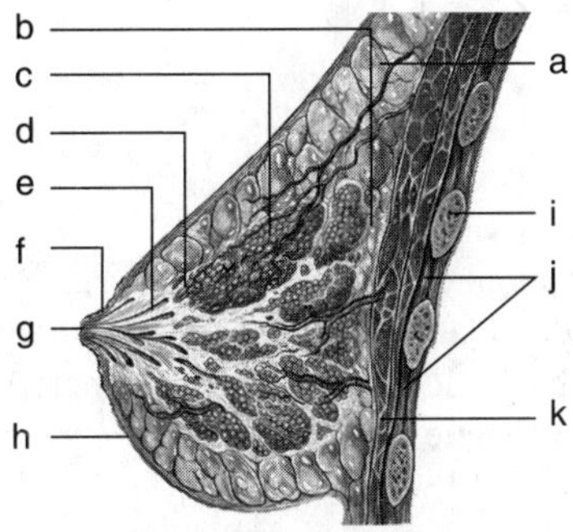

176. What is indicated by 'h' in the figure?
(a) Nipple (b) Areola
(c) Lacticiferous duct (d) Breast

177. What does 'e' represent in the figure?
(a) Lacticiferous duct (b) Ampulla
(c) Mammary duct (d) Areola

178. What does 'a' represent in the figure ?
(a) Mammary alveolus (b) Fat
(c) Proteins (d) Lacticiferous duct

179. What is indicated by 'j' in the figure?
(a) Cartilage between ribs (b) Ribs
(c) Sterum (d) Muscles between ribs

180. What does 'k' represent in the figure?
(a) Pectoral girdle (b) Rib cage
(c) Pectoralis major muscle (d) Pectoralis minor muscle

181. In an adult, each testis is ____ in shape, with a length of about ____ and a width of about ____.
(a) round, 4 to 5 cm, 2 to 3 cm (b) oval, 2 to 3 cm, 4 to 5 cm
(c) oval, 4 to 5 cm, 2 to 3 cm (d) round, 2 to 3 cm, 4 to 5 cm

182. Each testis has how many testicular tubules?
(a) 200 (b) 250
(c) 300 (d) 150

183. Male sex accessory ducts include
(i) Rele testis
(ii) Vasa efferenta
(iii) Epididymis
(iv) Vas deferens
(a) i, ii
(b) ii, iii
(c) i, ii, iii
(d) i, ii, iii, iv

184. Which of the following duct stores sperm?
(a) Vasa efferentia
(b) Rete testis
(c) Epididymis
(d) All of these

185. The female reproductive system along with a pair of mammary glands is integrated structurally and functionally to support process of
(a) Ovulation, fertilization
(b) Pregnancy and birth
(c) Child care
(d) All of these

186. Find out incorrect statement about ovaries.
(a) Each ovary is connected to the pelvic wall and uterus by ligaments.
(b) The ovarian stroma is divided into two zones a peripheral cortex and an inner medulla.
(c) Each ovary is covered by thick epithelium which encloses the ovarian stroma.
(d) Ovaries are the primary female sex organs

187. The fallopian tube is about _____ long.
(a) 10–12 cm
(b) 8–10 cm
(c) 12–14 cm
(d) 14–16 cm

188. The part of the fallopian tube closer to the ovary is:
(a) Infundibulum
(b) Ampulla
(c) Isthmus
(d) Womb

189. Which of the facts about the uterus (in human females) is true?
(a) Single
(b) Also called womb
(c) Inverted pear shape
(d) All of these

190. Birth canal is formed by:
(i) Uterus
(ii) Cervix
(iii) Vagina
(a) i and ii
(b) 1 and iii
(c) ii and iii
(d) iii only

191. Which statement is true about walls of the uterus?
(a) It has a thick membranous external wall called the perimetrium.
(b) It has a thin middle layer of smooth muscles called the myometrium.
(c) It has an inner glandular layer called the endometrium.
(d) All are true

192. The endometrium undergoes cyclical changes during the ____ cycle.
(a) menstrual
(b) oestrous
(c) thermal
(d) none

193. The opening of vagina is often covered partially by
(a) Mons pubis
(b) Labia majora
(c) Labia minora
(d) Hymen

194. Which of the facts is true about clitoris?
   (i) It is a tiny finger-like structure.
   (ii) It lies at upper junction of two labia minora.
   (iii) It lies at upper junction of two labia majora.
   (iv) It lies above utheral opening.
   (v) It lies below urethral opening.
   (a) i, ii, iii
   (b) i, ii, v
   (c) i, ii, iv
   (d) iii, v
195. Hymen can be torn or broken by
   (i) First coitus
   (ii) Sudden fall or jolt
   (iii) Horse riding
   (iv) Cycling
   (v) Insertion of a vaginal tampon
   (a) i, ii and iv only
   (b) iii, iv and v only
   (c) i, iv and v only
   (d) All
196. Select the true statement.
   (a) Presence of hymen is a reliable indicator of virginity.
   (b) Absence of hymen is a reliable indicator of sexual experience.
   (c) Presence of hymen is a reliable indicator of sexual experience.
   (d) Presence or absence of hymen is not a reliable indicator of virginity.
197. Which is the correct path for secretion and transport of milk in mammary gland?
   (a) Alveoli → Cavity of alveoli → Mammary tubule → Mammary duct → Mammary ampulla → Lactiferous duct
   (b) Mammary duct → Mammary tubule → Alveoli → Lactiferous duct → Mammary ampulla → Cavity of alveoli
   (c) Mammary duct → Cavity of alveoli → Lactiferous duct → Mammary ampulla → Mammary tubule → Alveoli
   (d) Alveoli → Mammary tubule → Mammary ampulla → Cavity of alveoli → Mammary duct → Lactiferous duct
198. Which fact about the mammary glands in humans is false?
   (a) A non-functional mammary gland is characteristic of all male mammals.
   (b) Mammary glands are paired structures.
   (c) It is a glandular tissue containing fixed amount of fat.
   (d) Glandular tissue of each breast is divided into 15-20 mammary lobes containing clusters of cells called alveoli.
199. Spermatogonia is
   (a) Immature male germ cells
   (b) Mature male germ cells
   (c) Immature male gamete
   (d) Mature male gamete
200. The spermatids are transformed into spermatozoa (sperm) by the process called
   (a) Spermatogenesis
   (b) Spermiogenesis
   (c) Spermiation
   (d) Capacitation

Figure given for question 201 to 206.

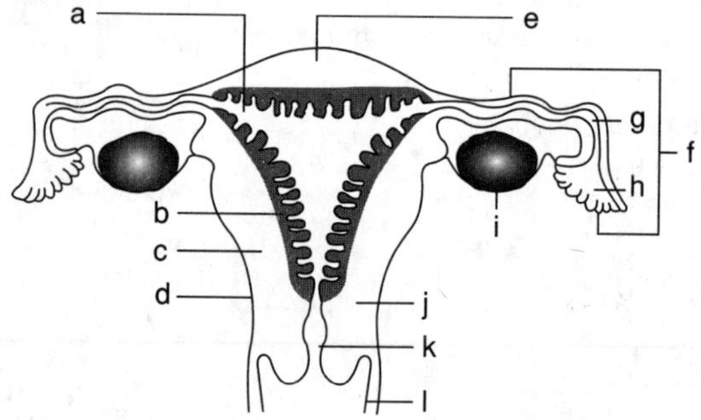

201. What is indicated by 'j' in the figure?
(a) Vagina
(b) Cervical canal
(c) Cervix
(d) Myometrium
202. What does 'h' represent in the figure?
(a) Fimbral
(b) Infundibulum
(c) Isthmus
(d) Ampulla
203. In the figure, Identify structure 'f' which consists of 'g' and 'h'.
(a) Ovary
(b) Fallopian tube
(c) Uterus
(d) Cervix
204. What does 'd' represent in the figure?
(a) Pericardium
(b) Perimetrium
(c) Peritoneum
(d) Epimetrium
205. What is indicated by 'b' in the figure?
(a) Villi
(b) Endothelium
(c) Endometrium
(d) Epithelium
206. What does 'e' represent in the figure?
(a) Uterus
(b) Isthmus
(c) Uterine fundus
(d) Uterine ampulla
207. Select the correct sequence:
(a) GnRH → LH → Leydig cells → Androgens → Spermatogenesis
(b) GnRH → FSH → Sertoli cells → Some factors → Spermiogenesis
(c) Both correct
(d) Both incorrect
208. Acrosome is modified
(a) Golgi body
(b) ER
(c) Vacuole
(d) Ribosome
209. Antrum is present in
(a) Primary follicle
(b) Secondary follicle
(c) Tertiary follicle
(d) All
210. Primary oocyte grows in size and completes its first meiotic division inside the:
(a) Primary follicle
(b) Secondary follicle
(c) Tertiary follicle
(d) All

211. Which of the following undergo unequal division?
(a) Primary oocyte
(b) Pollen grain of Angiosperm
(c) Yeast cell during bud formation
(d) All

212. Secondary oocyte develops zona pellucida around it in the ____.
(a) Primary follicle (b) Secondary follicle
(c) Tertairy follicle (d) Graafian follicle

213. Theca layer organized into theca interna and externa in which follicle
(a) 1° (b) 2°
(c) 3° (d) Mature follicle

214. How many ovum(s) is/are released in one menstruation?
(a) 1 (b) 2
(c) 3 (d) 4

215. Which of the facts is true about menstruation?
(a) It occurs only when the released ovum is not fertilized.
(b) It occurs due to breakdown of endometrial lining.
(c) Menstrual flow lasts for 3–5 days.
(d) All

216. Menopausal age in human being is
(a) 45 yr (b) 55 yr
(c) 50 yr (d) 60 yr

217. The time required to convert primary follicle into mature follicle:
(a) 4 days (b) 9 to 11 days
(c) 18–20 days (d) 2 days

218. Fertilization takes place at
(a) Isthumus (b) Ampulla
(c) Infundibulum (d) Ampullary-isthmic junction

219. Which part of the sperm helps in penetration into the ovum?
(a) Mitochondria (b) Acrosome
(c) Tail (d) All

220. Second Meiotic division in secondary oocyte is
(a) Unequal (b) Complete after sperm penetration
(c) Both (d) Equal

221. The embryo with 8 to 16 blastomeres is called
(a) Blastula (b) Gastrula
(c) Morula (d) None

222. Implantation leads to
(a) Formation of trophoblast in blastocyst
(b) Formation of inner cell mass in blastocyst
(c) Pregnancy
(d) All

223. Which of these hormones is/are produced in women during pregnancy?
(a) HCG (b) HPL
(c) Relaxin (d) All

224. Which of these statements is incorrect about embryo development?
(a) After one month of pregnancy the heart is formed.
(b) By the end of first trimester most of the major organ systems are formed.
(c) First movement of foetus observed in the seventh month.
(d) At the end of second trimester, the body is covered with fine hair, eye-lids separate and eye lashes are formed.

225. The process of delivery of foetus is called
(a) Parturition (b) Gestation
(c) Ejaculation (d) Capacitation

226. Find the false statement.
(a) A pair of seminal vesicles is present in human males.
(b) A pair of prostates is present in human males.
(c) Glans penis is covered by a loose fold of skin called foreskin.
(d) Each fallopian tube is about 10–12 cm long in a human female.

227. Ploidy of spermatogonia, primary spermatocyte, secondary spermatocyte and spermatid is
(a) 2n, 2n, 2n, n (b) n, 2n, 2n, n
(c) n, 2n, n, n (d) 2n, 2n, n, n

228. Stem cells which have the potential to produce all types of cells, tissues and organs are present in
(a) Ectoderm (b) Inner cell mass
(c) Throbhoblast (d) Endoderm

Figure given for question 229 to 233.

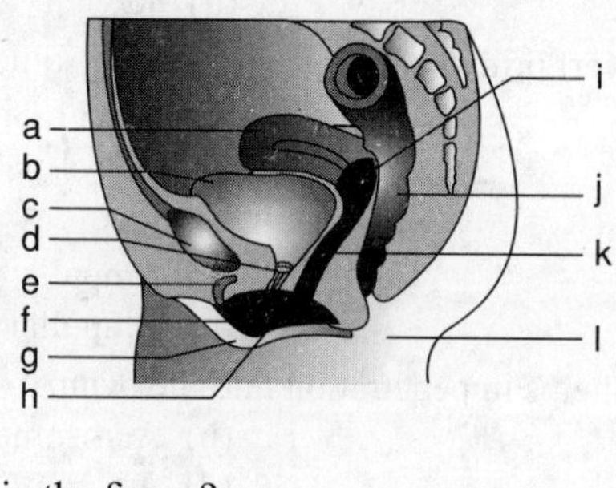

229. What is indicated by 'c' in the figure?
(a) Urethra (b) Ovary
(c) Clitoris (d) Public symphysis

230. What does 'f' represent in the figure?
(a) Clitoris (b) Labia majora
(c) Labia minora (d) Urethra

231. What is indicated by 'k' in the figure?
(a) Ovary (b) Cervix
(c) Vagina (d) Urethra

232. What is indicated by 'b' in the figure?
(a) Uterus (b) Vagina
(c) Public symphysis (d) Urinary bladder

233. What does 'd' represent in the figure?
(a) Vagina (b) Clitoris
(c) Urethra (d) Cervix

*Read the **assertion** and **reason** carefully to mark the correct option out of the options given below:*

(a) If both the assertion and the reason are true and the reason is a correct explanation of the assertion
(b) If both the assertion and reason are true but the reason is not a correct explanation of the assertion
(c) If the assertion is true but the reason is false
(d) If both the assertion and reason are false

234. Assertion: Testis are situated outside the abdominal cavity with in a pouch called scrotum.
Reason: Scrotum helps in maintain the low temperature of the testes necessary for spermatogenesis.

235. Assertion: Male germ cells undergo mitotic division finally leading to sperm formation.
Reason: Sertoli cells provide nutrition to Leydig cells

236. Assertion: Myometrium undergoes cyclical changes during menstrual cycle.
Reason: Myometrium's lines th uterine cavity

237. Assertion: Spermatogonia are haploid cells.
Reason: Spermatogonia multiply by binary fisision.

238. Assertion: Androgens stimulate the process of spermatogenesis.
Reason: FSH acts on sertoli cells and stimulate secretion of some factors which help in the process of spermiogenesis.

239. Assertion: Oogenesis is initiate during the embryonic development stage when a couple of million gamete mother cell (oogonia) are formed with in each foetal ovary.
Reason: No more oogonia are formed and added after birth.

240. Assertion: Rupture of Graffian follicle occur before 14th day of onset of next menstrual cycle.
Reason: LH level is maximum during mid of cycle i.e. (14th day).

241. Assertion: Only one sperm can fertilize ovum.
Reason: A sperm when come in contact with zona pellucida layer of the ovum, some changes occur in membrane that blocks the entry of other sperm.

242. Assertion: In human menopause occur at approx 50 year of age.
Reason: Cyclic menstruation is an indicator of abnormal reproductive phase.

243. Assertion: Mammary glands differentiate during pregnancy.
Reason: Mammary glands secretes milk after child birth.

AIPMT PREVIOUS YEAR QUESTIONS

1. Signals from fully developed foetus and placenta ultimately lead to a parturition which requires the release of

[AIPMT MAINS 2010]

(a) Estrogen from placenta (b) Oxytocin from maternal pituitary
(c) Oxytocin from foetal pituitary (d) Relaxin from placenta

2. Secretions from which one of the following are rich in fructose, calcium and some enzymes? [AIPMT MAINS 2010]

(a) Male accessory glands (b) Liver
(c) Pancreas (d) Salivary glands

3. In human female, the blastocyst [AIPMT MAINS 2010]

(a) Forms placenta even before implantation
(b) Gets implanted into uterus 3 days after ovulation
(c) Gets nutrition from uterine endometrial secretion only after implantation
(d) Gets implanted in endometrium by the trophoblast cells

4. Seminal plasma in human males is rich in: [AIPMT PRE 2010]

(a) Fructose and calcium (b) Glucose and calcium
(c) DNA and testosterone (d) Ribose and potassium

5. Sertoli cells are found in [AIPMT PRE 2010]

(a) Ovaries and secrete progesterone
(b) Adrenal cortex and secrete adrenalin
(c) Seminiferous tubules and provide nutrition to germ cells
(d) Pancreas and secrete cholecystokinin

6. Vasa efferentia are the ductules leading from: [AIPMT PRE 2010]

(a) Testicular lobules to rete testis (b) Rete testis to vas deferens
(c) Vas deferens to epididymis (d) Epididymis to urethra

7. The signals for parturition originate from: [AIPMT PRE 2010]

(a) Placenta only
(b) Placenta as well as fully developed foetus
(c) Oxytocin released from maternal pituitary
(d) Fully developed foetus only

8. The first movements of the foetus and appearance of hair on its head are usually observed during which month of pregnancy? [AIPMT PRE 2010]

(a) Fourth month (b) Fifth month
(c) Sixth month (d) Third month

9. The second maturation division of the mammalian ovum occurs [AIPMT PRE 2010]

(a) Shortly after ovulation before the ovum makes entry into the Fallopian tube
(b) Until after the ovum has been penetrated by a sperm
(c) Until the nucleus of the sperm has fused with that of the ovum
(d) In the Graafian follicle following the first maturation division

10. Which one of the following statements about human sperm is correct?

[AIPMT PRE 2010]

(a) Acrosome has a conical pointed structure used for piercing and penetrating the egg, resulting in fertilization
(b) The sperm lysins in the acrosome dissolve the egg envelope facilitating fertilization
(c) Acrosome serves as a sensory structure leading the sperm towards the ovum
(d) Acrosome serves no particular function

11. Which one of the following statements about morula in humans is correct?

[AIPMT PRE 2010]

(a) It has almost equal quantity of cytoplasm as an uncleaved zygote but much more DNA
(b) It has far less cytoplasm as well as less DNA than in an uncleaved zygote
(c) It has more or less equal quantity of cytoplasm and DNA as in uncleaved zygote
(d) It has more cytoplasm and more DNA than an uncleaved zygote

12. The part of fallopian tube closest to the ovary is

[AIPMT PRE 2010]

(a) Isthmus (b) Infundibulum
(c) Cervix (d) Ampulla

13. The figure given below depicts a diagrammatic sectional view of the female reproductive system of humans. Which one set of three parts out of A-F have been correctly identified?

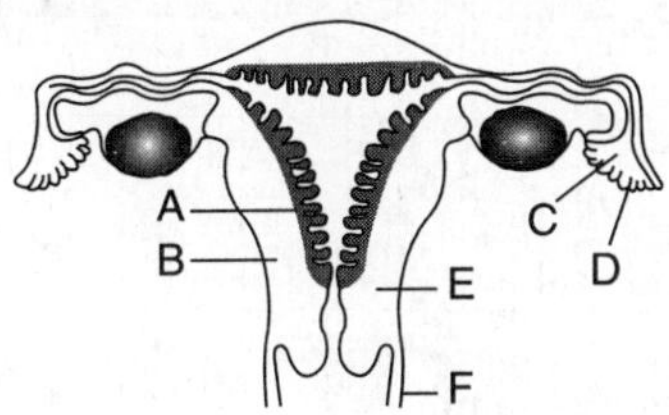

[AIPMT PRE 2011]

(a) C - Infundibulum, D - Fimbriae, E – Cervix
(b) D - Oviducal funnel, E - Uterus, F – Cervix
(c) A - Perimetrium, B - Myometrium, C - Fallopian tube
(d) B - Endometrium, C - Infundibulum, D - Fimbriae

14. The testes in humans are situated outside the abdominal cavity inside a pouch called scrotum. The purpose served is for:

[AIPMT PRE 2011]

(a) Escaping any possible compression by the visceral organs
(b) Providing more space for the growth of epididymis
(c) Providing a secondary sexual feature for exhibiting the male sex
(d) Maintaining the scrotal temperature lower than the internal body temperature

15. What happens during fertilization in humans after many sperms reach close to the ovum?

[AIPMT MAINS 2011]

(a) Secretions of acrosome helps one sperm enter cytoplasm of ovum through zona pellucida
(b) All sperms except the one nearest to the ovum lose their tails
(c) Cells of corona radiata trap all the sperms except one
(d) Only two sperms nearest the ovum penetrate zona pellucida

16. About which day in a normal human menstrual cycle does rapid secretion of LH(popularly called LH surge) normally occurs?

[AIPMT MAINS 2011]

(a) 14th day (b) 20th day
(c) 5th day (d) 11th day

17. The secretory phase in the human menstrual cycle is also called:

[AIPMT MAINS 2012]

(a) Follicular phase lasting for about 6 days
(b) Luteal phase and lasts for about 13 days
(c) Follicular phase and lasts for about 13 days
(d) Luteal phase and lasts for about 6 days

18. Identify the human development stage shown below as well as the related right place of its occurrence in a normal pregnant women and select the right option for the two together:

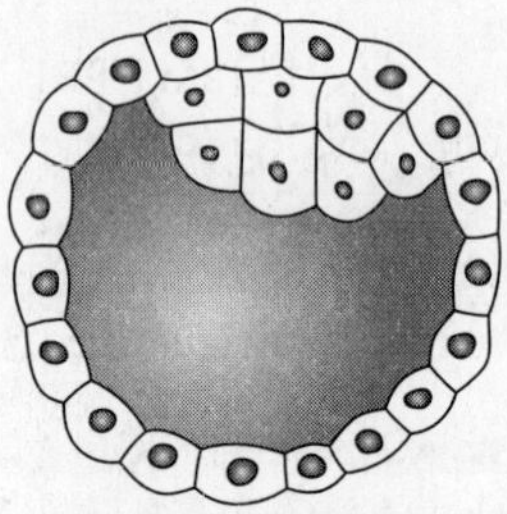

[AIPMT MAINS 2012]

Developmental stage	**Site of occurrence**
(a) Blastula	End part of fallopian tube
(b) Blastocyst	Uterine wall
(c) 8-celled morula	Starting point of fallopian tube
(d) Late morula	Middle part of fallopian tube

19. Which one of the following statements is false in respect of viability of mammalian sperm?

[AIPMT PRE 2012]

(a) Sperm is viable for only up to 24 hours
(b) Survival of sperm depends on the pH of the medium and is more active in alkaline medium
(c) Viability of sperm is determined by its motility
(d) Sperms must be concentrated in a thick suspension

20. Signals for parturition originate from:

[AIPMT PRE 2012]

(a) Both placenta as well as fully developed foetus
(b) Oxytocin released from maternal pituitary
(c) Placenta only
(d) Fully developed foetus only

21. In a normal pregnant woman, the amount of total gonadotropin activity was assessed. The result expected was.

[AIPMT PRE 2012]

(a) High level of circulating FSH and LH in the uterus to stimulate implantation of the embryo.
(b) High level of circulating HCG to stimulate endometrial thickening.
(c) High level of FSH and LH in uterus to stimulate endometrial thickening
(d) High level of circulating HCG to stimulate estrogen and progesterone synthesis.

22. What is the correct sequence of sperm formation?

[AIPMT 2013]

(a) Spermatid, spermatocyte, spermatogonia, spermatozoa
(b) Spermatogonia, spermatocyte, spermatozoa
(c) Spermatogonia, spermatozoa, spematocyte
(d) Spermatogonia, spermatocyte, spermatid, spermatozoa

23. Menstrual flow occurs due to lack of:

[AIPMT 2013]

(a) Progesterone (b) FSH
(c) Oxytocin (d) Vasopressin

24. Which one of the following is not the function of placenta? It:

[AIPMT 2013]

(a) Facilitates supply of oxygen and nutrients to embryo
(b) Secretes estrogen
(c) Facilitates removal of carbon dioxide and waste material from embryo.
(d) Secretes oxytocin during parturition

25. The shared terminal duct of the reproductive and urinary system in the human male is:

[AIPMT 2014]

(a) Urethra (b) Ureter
(c) Vas deferens (d) Vasa efferentia

26. The main function of mammalian corpus luteum is to produce:

[AIPMT 2014]

(a) Estrogen only (b) Progesterone
(c) Human chorionic gonadotropin (d) Relaxin only

27. Select the correct option describing gonadotropin activity in a normal pregnant female:

[AIPMT 2014]

(a) High level of FSH and LH stimulates the thickening of endometrium
(b) High level of FSH and LH facilitate implantation of the embryo
(c) High level of hCG stimulates the synthesis of estrogen and progesterone
(d) High level of hCG stimulates the thickening of endometrium

28. Capacitation refers to changes in the :

[AIPMT 2015]

(a) Sperm before fertilization (b) Ovum before fertilization
(c) Ovum after fertilization (d) Sperm after fertilization

29. Which of these is not an important component of initiation of parturition in humans?

[AIPMT 2015]

(a) Increase in estrogen and progesterone ratio
(b) Synthesis of prostaglandins
(c) Release of oxytocin
(d) Release of prolactin

30. Which of the following cells during gameto- genesis is normally diploid?

[AIPMT 2015]

(a) Primary polar body (b) Spermatid
(c) Spermatogonia (d) Secondary polar body

31. Hysterectomy is surgical removal of:

[AIPMT 2015]

(a) Uterus (b) Prostate gland
(c) Vas-deference (d) Mammary glands

32. Which of the following events is not associated with ovulation in human female?

[RE-AIPMT 2015]

(a) Full development of Graafian follicle (b) Release of secondary oocyte
(c) LH surage (d) Decrease in estradiol

33. Ectopic pregnancies are referred to as:

[RE-AIPMT 2015]

(a) Implantation of embryo sat side other than uterus
(b) Implantation of defective embryo in the uterus
(c) Pregnancies terminated due to hormonal imbalance
(d) Pregnancies with genetic abnormality

34. Which of the following layers in an antral follicle is acellular?

[RE-AIPMT 2015]

(a) Theca interna (b) Stroma
(c) Zona pellucida (d) Granulosa

35. In human female, meiosis-II is not completed until?

[RE-AIPMT 2015]

(a) Fertilization (b) Uterine implanation
(c) Birth (d) Puberty

Answer Keys

1. (d)	2. (c)	3. (a)	4. (b)	5. (c)	6. (c)	7. (c)	8. (b)	9. (b)	10. (c)
11. (c)	12. (b)	13. (b)	14. (c)	15. (d)	16. (b)	17. (c)	18. (b)	19. (c)	20. (b)
21. (b)	22. (a)	23. (b)	24. (c)	25. (d)	26. (c)	27. (c)	28. (d)	29. (c)	30. (c)
31. (b)	32. (d)	33. (b)	34. (b)	35. (c)	36. (b)	37. (b)	38. (d)	39. (d)	40. (b)
41. (b)	42. (a)	43. (c)	44. (a)	45. (c)	46. (d)	47. (b)	48. (c)	49. (b)	50. (c)
51. (b)	52. (b)	53. (c)	54. (a)	55. (b)	56. (a)	57. (c)	58. (d)	59. (d)	60. (b)
61. (c)	62. (b)	63. (b)	64. (d)	65. (b)	66. (c)	67. (c)	68. (c)	69. (c)	70. (b)
71. (c)	72. (b)	73. (a)	74. (c)	75. (d)	76. (b)	77. (d)	78. (d)	79. (d)	80. (a)
81. (c)	82. (b)	83. (b)	84. (c)	85. (d)	86. (b)	87. (b)	88. (c)	89. (b)	90. (a)
91. (b)	92. (c)	93. (b)	94. (b)	95. (c)	96. (b)	97. (c)	98. (c)	99. (c)	100. (b)
101. (d)	102. (a)	103. (b)	104. (c)	105. (d)	106. (c)	107. (d)	108. (a)	109. (a)	110. (a)
111. (a)	112. (b)	113. (c)	114. (b)	115. (b)	116. (c)	117. (d)	118. (b)	119. (d)	120. (b)
121. (c)	122. (b)	123. (b)	124. (c)	125. (b)	126. (c)	127. (c)	128. (c)	129. (d)	130. (a)
131. (b)	132. (b)	133. (b)	134. (d)	135. (c)	136. (b)	137. (a)	138. (a)	139. (b)	140. (b)
141. (b)	142. (a)	143. (c)	144. (c)	145. (c)	146. (b)	147. (b)	148. (b)	149. (a)	150. (b)
151. (a)	152. (b)	153. (b)	154. (c)	155. (b)	156. (c)	157. (b)	158. (b)	159. (b)	160. (c)
161. (b)	162. (b)	163. (b)	164. (b)	165. (a)	166. (d)	167. (b)	168. (c)	169. (d)	170. (b)

171. (b)	172. (b)	173. (b)	174. (c)	175. (d)	176. (b)	177. (b)	178. (b)	179. (d)	180. (c)
181. (c)	182. (b)	183. (d)	184. (d)	185. (d)	186. (c)	187. (a)	188. (a)	189. (d)	190. (c)
191. (c)	192. (a)	193. (d)	194. (c)	195. (d)	196. (d)	197. (a)	198. (c)	199. (a)	200. (b)
201. (c)	202. (b)	203. (b)	204. (b)	205. (c)	206. (a)	207. (c)	208. (a)	209. (c)	210. (c)
211. (d)	212. (d)	213. (c)	214. (a)	215. (d)	216. (c)	217. (b)	218. (d)	219. (b)	220. (c)
221. (c)	222. (c)	223. (d)	224. (c)	225. (a)	226. (b)	227. (d)	228. (b)	229. (d)	230. (c)
231. (c)	232. (d)	233. (c)	234. (a)	235. (d)	236. (d)	237. (d)	238. (b)	239. (b)	240. (a)
241. (a)	242. (c)	243. (b)							

AIPMT Previous Year Questions

1. (b)	2. (a)	3. (d)	4. (a)	5. (c)	6. (b)	7. (b)	8. (b)	9. (b)	10. (b)
11. (a)	12. (b)	13. (a)	14. (d)	15. (a)	16. (a)	17. (b)	18. (b)	19. (d)	20. (a)
21. (d)	22. (d)	23. (a)	24. (d)	25. (a)	26. (b)	27. (c)	28. (a)	29. (c)	30. (c)
31. (a)	32. (d)	33. (a)	34. (c)	35. (a)					

CHAPTER 26 Reproductive Health

1. What is the full form of WHO?
   (a) Ware House Organization
   (b) War and Health Organization
   (c) World Health Office
   (d) World Health Organization
2. What are the various aspects of reproduction covered by WHO?
   (a) Physical, Emotional, Behavioral
   (b) Physical, Emotional, Behavioral, Social
   (c) Physical, Emotional, Gestational, Social
   (d) Physical, Emotional, Social
3. Which was the first country in the world to initiate a nationwide programme for reproductive health?
   (a) China
   (b) USA
   (c) India
   (d) Russia
4. The figure indicates which contraceptive device?

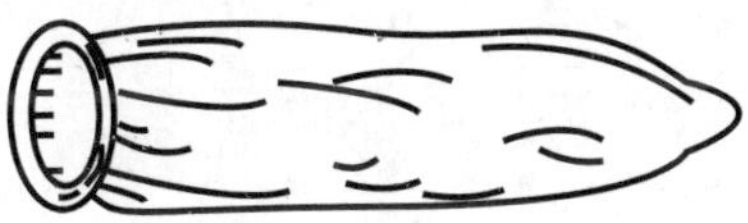

   (a) Condom for female
   (b) Condom for male
   (c) Diaphragm
   (d) Cervical cap
5. The programme of 'Family Planning' was initiated in the year ________.
   (a) 1950
   (b) 1947
   (c) 1949
   (d) 1951
6. The reproductive program RCH stands for:
   (a) Reproductive and Community Health Care
   (b) Restorative and Communal Health Care
   (c) Reproductive and Child Health Care
   (d) Reproductive and Congenital Health Care
7. In context of reproductive health, STD stands for:
   (a) Sexually Terminal Disease
   (b) Sexually Transmitted Disease
   (c) Sexually Transformed Disease
   (d) Sexually Transducted Disease

8. The fluid which envelops the developing foetus is called
(a) Chorionic fluid
(b) Placentae fluid
(c) Amniotic fluid
(d) Uterine fluid

9. Statutory ban has been laid on ________ to check female foeticide.
(a) choriocentesis
(b) aminocentesis
(c) uterocentesis
(d) embryocentesis

10. Amniocentesis test is based on ________ to determine sex of developing foetus.
(a) external genitalia
(b) secondary sexual characters
(c) chromosomal pattern
(d) embryonic enzymes

11. CDRI, Lucknow developed which new female contraceptive?
(a) 'Sakhi'
(b) 'Saheli'
(c) 'Saloni'
(d) 'Smiti'

12. CDRI stands for
(a) Contraceptive Drug Research Institute
(b) Central District Research Institute
(c) Central Drug Research Institute
(d) Central Dermatologic Research Institute

13. The world population was 2000 million in the year
(a) 1980
(b) 1970
(c) 1960
(d) 1990

14. Which IUD is shown in the given figure?

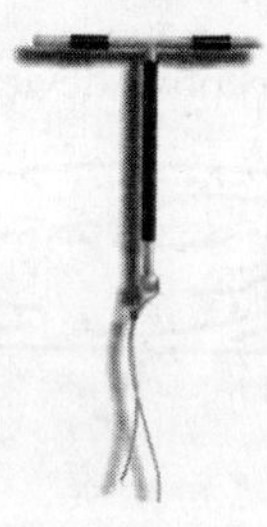

(a) Lippes loop
(b) Progestasert
(c) Copper T
(d) Multiload-375

15. By the year 2000, the world population rocketed to
(a) 6 million
(b) 6 billion
(c) 6 trillion
(d) 600 million

16. MMR stands for
(a) Magnetic Maxima Resonance
(b) Mortality Memorandum Rate
(c) Mortality Maternal Rate
(d) Maternal Mortality Rate

17. IMR stands for
(a) Indigenous Mortality Rate
(b) Infant Migratory Rate
(c) Infant Mortality Rate
(d) Infant Mitigation Rate

18. According to the census report of 2001, the population growth rate was
(a) 1.5%
(b) 1.7%
(c) 1.6%
(d) 2.1%

19. Smaller families can be encouraged by using various
(a) Educational methods
(b) Contraceptive methods
(c) Abortive methods
(d) Rhythm method

20. A wise way to encouraging small families is by raising marriageable age of female to ________ years and that of male to ________ years respectively.
(a) 16, 18
(b) 18, 20
(c) 18, 21
(d) 17, 22

21. Many couples in the urban working areas have adopted the ________ norm.
(a) Two child
(b) One child
(c) No child
(d) Three child

22. Identity the characteristic which an ideal contraceptive should NOT have
(a) Use friendly
(b) Easily available
(c) Non reversible
(d) Least side effect

23. A natural method of contraception, periodic abstinence is
(a) Abstaining from coitus from day 1–5 of the menstrual cycle
(b) Abstaining from coitus from day 17–22 of the menstrual cycle
(c) Abstaining from coitus from day 10–17 of the menstrual cycle
(d) Abstaining from coitus from day 5–10 of the menstrual cycle

24. Coitus interrupts/withdrawal method concerns with
(a) Withdrawal of penis from vagina before ejaculation
(b) Withdrawal of penis from vagina after ejaculation
(c) Prevention of coitus
(d) Alternate prevention of coitus

25. After parturition, which natural contraception way can be utilized?
(a) Lactational menorrhea
(b) Lactational amenorrhea
(c) Lactational deficiency
(d) Lactational prevention

26. The figure indicates which contraceptive device?

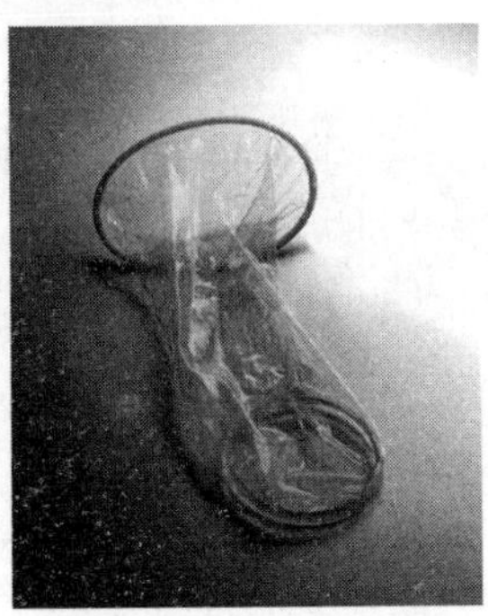

(a) Condom for female
(b) Condom for male
(c) Diaphragm
(d) Cervical cap

27. In lactational amenorrhea, which event does not occur in menstrual cycle?
(a) Menstrual flow
(b) Ovulation
(c) Fouicular phase
(d) Luteal phase

28. Lactational amenorrhea is effective only up to a maximum of ________ months.
(a) two (b) four
(c) six (d) eight

29. In the ________ method of contraception ovum and sperms are prevented from physically meeting by the use of a membranous sheath.
(a) Barrier (b) Sterilization
(c) Natural (d) Pillls

30. ________ is a popular brand of condom for males.
(a) 'Nishodh' (b) 'Nirodh'
(c) 'Nidosh' (d) 'Nirdosh'

31. Which of the following is not applicable to females for contraception?
(a) Diaphragms (b) Vasectomy
(c) Condoms (d) Cervical caps

32. Multiload 375 is an
(a) Disease resistant crop (b) New Viral Vector
(c) Intra Uterine Device (d) Biological Warfare Device

33. IUD stand for
(a) Intra Ureter Device (b) Intrinsic Uterine Device
(c) Intra Uterine Device (d) Intra Urinogenital Device

34. Lippes loop is a
(a) Structure associated with nephron
(b) Structure associated with male reproductive system
(c) Structure associated with ligamentous tissue
(d) A non-medicated IUD

35. Which of the following is a copper releasing IUD?
(a) CUT (b) Multiload 375
(c) Cu 7 (d) All of the above

36. Progestasert is a
(a) Oral contraceptive (b) Natural contraceptive
(c) Hormonal IUD (d) Implant contraceptive

37. LNG-20 is a
(a) Fuel (b) Modified crop
(c) Hormonal IUD (d) Cu releasing IUD

38. Which of the following is a most widely used contraceptive in India?
(a) IUD (b) Pills
(c) Barrier method (d) Natural method

39. Pills used by females to prevent conception contain
(a) Only estrogen (b) Only progestogen
(c) Combination of estrogen progestogen (d) Both (b) and (c)

40. 'Pills' have to be taken for contraception continuously for a period ________ days.
(a) 22 (b) 21
(c) 24 (d) 25

41. Oral pills work by
(a) Inhibiting ovulation
(b) Inhibiting implantation
(c) Altering the quality of mucus
(d) All of the above

Figure given for questions 42 – 43.

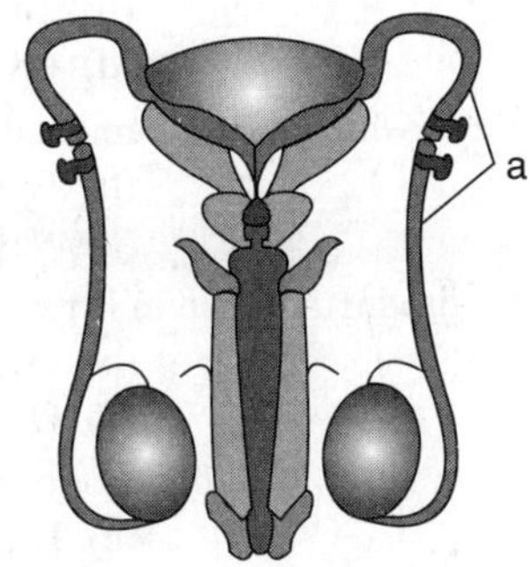

42. Which portion of male reproductive system has been cut and ligated in figure?
(a) Vasa efferentia
(b) Urethra
(c) Vas deferens
(d) Rete testis

43. The surgical procedure indicated in the figure is
(a) Tubectomy
(b) Hysterectomy
(c) Vasectomy
(d) Orchiectomy

44. 'Saheli', the new oral contraceptive for females, contains a ________ preparation.
(a) Steroidal
(b) Peptide
(c) Non steroidal
(d) Inorganic

45. 'Saheli' is a/an ________ contraceptive pill.
(a) Emergency
(b) One week
(c) 72 hr.
(d) One month

46. Apart from pills of progestogen alone or in combination with estrogen, which other means can be used for contraception?
(a) Implants
(b) Injections
(c) Syrups
(d) Both (a) and (b)

47. Emergency contraceptive should be under which of the following conditions
(a) Casual unprotected intercourse
(b) In conjunction with pills
(c) Rape
(d) Both (a) and (c)

48. Emergency contraceptive should be used within ________ hours of unprotected intercourse.
(a) 48
(b) 72
(c) 36
(d) 86

49. To prevent further pregnancies, a surgical method called ________ is advised for male/female partner as a means of contraception:
(a) radiation
(b) sterilization
(c) abortion
(d) neutralization

50. Surgical method for terminal contraception work on the following grounds:
(a) Block gamete transport
(b) Block gamete generation
(c) Alter biochemical nature of gamete
(d) Gamete destruction permanently

51. Sterilization procedure in males is known as:
(a) Tubectomy
(b) Vasectomy
(c) Testotomy
(d) Spermotomy

52. Sterilization procedure in females is known as
(a) Vasectomy
(b) Tubectomy
(c) Hysterectomy
(d) Ovotomy

53. In vasectomy, a small portion of which duct is removed and tied up?
(a) Testis
(b) Epididymis
(c) Vas deferens
(d) Vasa efferentia

54. In tubectomy, which part of reproductive system is removed and/or tied up?
(a) Cervix
(b) Oviduct
(c) Uterus
(d) Ovary

55. Which of the following is/are the ill-effect/effects of using contraceptives?
(a) Abdominal pain
(b) Breast cancer
(c) Irregular menstrual bleeding
(d) All of above

56. Intentional or voluntary termination of pregnancy before full term is called ________.
(a) Medical transformation of pregnancy
(b) Median Terminal pregnancy
(c) Medical Termination of Pregnancy
(d) Non of the above

57. Nearly ________ MTPs are preformed in a year all over the world.
(a) 45 to 50 billion
(b) 45 to 50 million
(c) 45 to 50 thousands
(d) 45 to 50 lac

58. Government of India legalized MTP in the year ________.
(a) 1970
(b) 1971
(c) 1972
(d) 1973

59. MTPs are considered relatively safe during ________ trimester of pregnancy.
(a) 1st
(b) 2nd
(c) 3rd
(d) None

60. MTPs are harmful to mother and foetus during ________ trimester of pregnancy.
(a) 1st
(b) 2nd
(c) 3rd
(d) None

61. Misuse of amniocentesis has led to misuse of ________.
(a) MTP
(b) STD
(c) RTI
(d) HIV

62. Sexually transmitted diseases are also known as
(a) Venereal disease
(b) Vulnerable diseases
(c) Reproductive tract infections
(d) Both (a) and (c)

Figure given for questions 63 – 64.

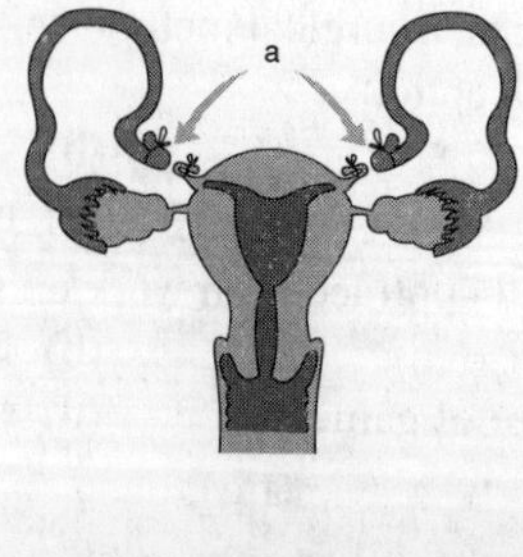

63. Which portion of the female reproductive system is cut and ligated in the figure?
(a) Uterus (b) Fallopian tubes
(c) Ovary (d) Cerrix

64. The surgical procedure indicated in the figure is
(a) Tubectomy (b) Hysterectomy
(c) Vasectomy (d) Orchidectomy

65. Which infections can be transmitted by sharing of injection needles, surgical instruments, etc., with infected persons; through transfusion of blood, or from an infected mother to the foetus?
(a) AIDS (b) Hepatitis B
(c) Genital herpes (d) Both (a) and (b)

66. Which of the following STD is not completely curable?
(a) Gonorrhoea (b) Genital warts
(c) Genital herpes (d) Chlamydiasis

67. Which of these options is correct with regards to statements X and Y?
Statement X: Some STDs do not show symptoms in females.
Statement Y: Some STDs in females may remain undetected for long time.
(a) Statement 'X' and 'Y' are correct and 'X' is the correct explanation for 'Y'.
(b) Only statement 'X' is correct.
(c) Only statement 'Y' is correct.
(d) Statement 'X' and 'Y' are correct.

68. Severe complications of STDs lead to further complications like
(a) Abortion (b) Still birth
(c) Ectopic pregnancy (d) All of the above

69. The age group of ________ years is quite vulnerable to STDs.
(a) 10–19 (b) 15–22
(c) 17–27 (d) 15–24

70. In order to prevent STDs, one of the following is NOT correct?
(a) Avoid sex with unknown partners/multiple partners.
(b) Go to an unqualified doctor at earliest instance of STD.
(c) Always use condoms during coitus.
(d) Participate in sex education sessions.

71. The reasons for infertility can be
(a) Physical (b) Diseases
(c) Psychological (d) All of the above

72. In India, which gender is generally wrongly blamed for being infertile?
(a) Woman (b) Man
(c) Either man or woman (d) Genetic factors

73. In India, most of the infertility cases are because of the
(a) Male (b) Female
(c) Either (a) and (b) (d) Hereditary disorders

74. In order to combat infertility, special techniques are used like ________.
(a) Stimulated Reproductive Technologies (b) Assisted Reproductive Technologies
(c) Fertile Reproductive Technologies (d) In-vitro fertilization

75. Fertilization outside the body in almost similar conditions as that in the body is termed as
(a) In-Vitro fertilization (b) Ex-Vivo fertilization
(c) In-Vivo fertilization (d) Ex-Vitro fertilization

76. Which of the following define Test Tube Baby correctly?
(a) Ova and sperms are collected and mixed in test tube to form zygote.
(b) Ova and sperms are centrifuged in test tube to form zygote.
(c) Ova and sperms are induced to form zygote under controlled condition.
(d) Embryogenesis is allowed to continue in test tube under controlled conditions.

77. Under ZIFT procedure, zygote or embryos, with up to 8 blastomeres, can be transferred into the
(a) Uterus (b) Placenta
(c) Fallopian tube (d) Cervix

78. WHO refers reproductive health as
(a) Physically healthy reproductive organ
(b) Functionally healthy reproductive organ
(c) Normal emotional and behavioural interaction among people in all sex-related aspect
(d) All of the above

79. Programme called family planning was initiated in ________.
(a) 1941 (b) 1951
(c) 1961 (d) 1971

80. What is shown in the figure?

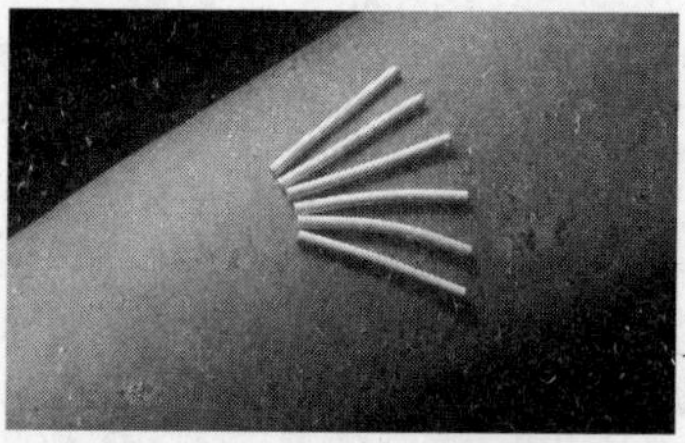

(a) Copper T (b) Implants
(c) Stents (d) Vault

81. Full form of RCH is
(a) Reproduction and Contraception Hazard (b) Reproductive and Child Health Care
(c) Research and Care Development (d) Reproductive Community Health Centre

82. 'Saheli', oral contraceptive for the females, was developed by which institute?
(a) CDRI, Lucknow (b) NBG, Lucknow
(c) Kazari, Jodhpur (d) NIV, Pune

83. Following are indicative signs which indicate improved reproductive health of society. Choose the correct combination.
(i) Better awareness about sex related problem
(ii) Better detection and cure of STDs
(iii) Better Postnatal care
(iv) Increased number of couples with large families
(a) i and iv only (b) ii, iii and iv only
(c) i and ii only (d) i, ii and iii only

84. Every ________ person in the world is an Indian.

(a) 4th (b) 6th
(c) 8th (d) 10th

85. India's population grew from 350 million to a billion in 2000 mainly due to

(i) Rapid decline in Death rate (MMR and IMR)
(ii) Increase in number of people in reproducecible age group
(iii) Increase in number of people in post re-productive age group

(a) (iii) only (b) (i) and (iii) only
(c) (i) and (ii) only (d) (i) only

86. Motivation for smaller families in India can be provided by

(a) Slogans like 'Hum Do Hamare Do'
(b) Raising marriageable age (female–18 years and male–21 years)
(c) Giving incentive to couples with small families
(d) All of the above

87. An ideal contraceptive should be

(A) User-friendly
(B) Easily available
(C) Effective and reversible
(D) With nor or least side-effects

(a) A, B and C only (b) A, D only
(c) B and C only (d) All

*Read the **assertion** and **reason** carefully to mark the correct option out of the options given below:*

(a) If both the assertion and the reason are true and the reason is a correct explanation of the assertion
(b) If both the assertion and reason are true but the reason is not a correct explanation of the assertion
(c) If the assertion is true but the reason is false
(d) If both the assertion and reason are false

88. **Assertion:** Statuary ban on amniocentesis for sex determination is done.

Reason: There is increase is female foeticides.

89. **Assertion:** There is decrease in maternal & infant mortality rates now a days.

Reason: Better awareness about sex related matter, increased number of medical assisted deliveries and better post-natal care leading to it.

90. **Assertion:** Couple avoid coitus from day 10 to 17 of the menstrual cycle is one of the method of contraception.

Reason: ovulation occur during these days (fertile period) so there is no chance of conception by abstaining from coitus during this period

91. **Assertion:** Barrier method one of the contraceptive method.

Reason: Barrier method prevent physical meeting of ovum & sperm.

92. **Assertion:** Spermicidal creams, jellies and foams are usually used along with nutrients.
Reason: All of above products increases their contraceptive efficiency.

93. **Assertion:** Copper releasing IUDs are used as contraceptives.
Reason: Cu ions releases form IUDs suppress sperm motility and the fertilizing capacity of sperms.

94. **Assertion:** Intentional or voluntary termination of pregnancy before full term is called MTP.
Reason: MTP has a insignificant role in decreasing the population.

95. **Assertion:** GIFT is gamete intra fallopian transfer.
Reason: ZIFT is zygote intra fallopian transfer.

96. **Assertion:** IUT is ART.
Reason: IVF embryo is transfer to uterus to Complete (more than 8 blastomere) its further development .

97. **Assertion:** In ability to conceive or produce children even after years of unprotected sexual cohabitation is called infertility.
Reason: ART is commonly used for such couples.

AIPMT PREVIOUS YEAR QUESTIONS

1. In vitro fertilization is a technique that involves transfer of which one of the following into the fallopian tube?

[AIPMT PRE 2010]

(a) Embryo only, upto 8 cell stage
(b) Either zygote or early embryo upto 8 cell stage
(c) Embryo of 32 cell stage
(d) Zygote only

2. The permissible use of the technique amniocentesis is for:

[AIPMT PRE 2010]

(a) Detecting sex of the unborn foetus
(b) Artificial insemination
(c) Transfer, of embryo into the uterus of a surrogate mother
(d) Detecting any genetic abnormality

3. Cu ions released from copper-releasing Intra Uterine Devices (IUDs):

[AIPMT PRE 2010]

(a) Make uterus unsuitable for implantation
(b) Increase phagocytosis of sperms
(c) Suppress sperm motility
(d) Prevent ovulation

4. Medical Termination of Pregnancy (MTP) is considered safe up to how many weeks pregnancy?

[AIPMT PRE 2011]

(a) Twelve weeks (b) Eighteen weeks
(c) Six weeks (d) Eight weeks

5. If for some reason, the vasa efferentia in the human reproductive system get blocked, the gametes will not be transported from

[AIPMT PRE 2011]

(a) Epididymis to vas deferens
(b) Ovary to uterus
(c) Vagina to uterus
(d) Testes to epididymis

6. Which one of the following is the most widely accepted method of contraception in India, as at present?

[AIPMT PRE 2011]

(a) Tubectomy
(b) Diaphragms
(c) IUDs (Intra Uterine Devices)
(d) Cervical caps

7. The technique called Gamete Intra Fallopian Transfer (GIFT) is recommended for those females

[AIPMT MAINS 2011]

(a) Who cannot produce an ovum
(b) Who cannot retain the foetus inside uterus
(c) Whose cervical canal is too narrow to allow passage for the sperms
(d) Who cannot provide suitable environment for fertilization

8. What is the figure given below showing in particular?

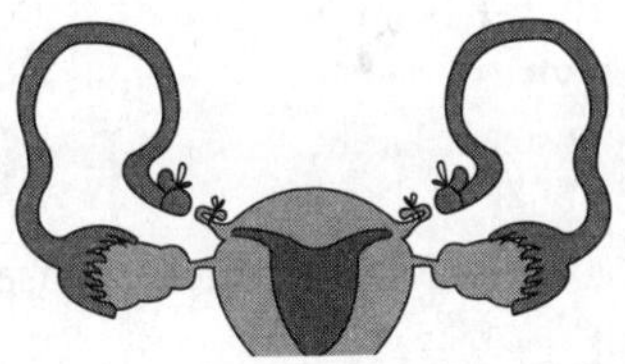

[AIPMT PRE 2012]

(a) Ovarian cancer
(b) Uterine cancer
(c) Tubectomy
(d) Vasectomy

9. One of the legal methods of birth control is:

[AIPMT 2013]

(a) Abortion by taking an appropriate medicine
(b) By abstaining from coitus from day 10 to 17 of the menstrual cycle
(c) By having coitus at the time of day break
(d) By a premature ejaculation during coitus

10. Which of the following cannot be detected in a developing foetus by amniocentesis?

[AIPMT 2013]

(a) Klinefelter syndrome
(b) Sex of the foetus
(c) Down syndrome
(d) Jaundice

11. Artificial insemination means:

[AIPMT 2013]

(a) Transfer of sperms of a healthy donor to a test tube containing ova
(b) Transfer of sperms of husband to a test tube containing ova
(c) Artificial introduction of sperms of a healthy donor into the vagina
(d) Introduction of sperms of a healthy donor directly into the ovary

12. Tubectomy is a method of sterilization in which:

[AIPMT 2014]

(a) Small part of the fallopian tube is removed or tied up
(b) Ovaries are removed surgically
(c) Small part of vas deferens is removed or tied up
(d) Uterus is removed surgically

13. Which of the following is a hormone releasing Intra Uterine Device (IUD)?

[AIPMT 2014]

(a) Multiload 375 (b) LNG – 20
(c) Cervical cap (d) Vault

14. Assisted reproductive technology, IVF involves transfer of:

[AIPMT 2014]

(a) Ovum into the fallopian tube
(b) Zygote into the fallopian tube
(c) Zygote into the uterus
(d) Embryo with 16 blastomeres into the fallopian tube

15. Which of the following viruses is not transferred through semen of an infected male?

[AIPMT 2015]

(a) Hepatitis B virus
(b) Human immunodeficiency virus
(c) Chikunguniya virus
(d) Ebola virus

16. Which of the following is not a sexually transmitted disease?

[AIPMT 2015]

(a) Syphilis
(b) Acquired Immuno Deficiency Syndrome disease (AIDS)
(c) Trichomoniasis
(d) Encephalitis

17. A childless couple can be assisted to have a child through a technique called GIFT. The full form of this technique is:

[RE-AIPMT 2015]

(a) Gamete intra fallopian transfer
(b) Gamete internal fertilization and transfer
(c) Germ cell internal fallopian transfer
(d) Gamete inseminated fallopian transfer

Answer Keys

1. (d)	2. (b)	3. (c)	4. (b)	5. (d)	6. (c)	7. (b)	8. (c)	9. (b)	10. (c)
11. (b)	12. (c)	13. (d)	14. (c)	15. (b)	16. (d)	17. (c)	18. (b)	19. (b)	20. (c)
21. (b)	22. (c)	23. (c)	24. (a)	25. (b)	26. (a)	27. (b)	28. (c)	29. (c)	30. (b)
31. (b)	32. (c)	33. (c)	34. (d)	35. (d)	36. (c)	37. (c)	38. (a)	39. (d)	40. (b)
41. (d)	42. (c)	43. (c)	44. (c)	45. (b)	46. (d)	47. (d)	48. (b)	49. (b)	50. (a)

51. (b)	52. (b)	53. (c)	54. (b)	55. (d)	56. (c)	57. (b)	58. (b)	59. (a)	60. (b)
61. (a)	62. (d)	63. (b)	64. (a)	65. (d)	66. (c)	67. (a)	68. (d)	69. (d)	70. (b)
71. (d)	72. (a)	73. (a)	74. (b)	75. (a)	76. (c)	77. (c)	78. (d)	79. (b)	80. (b)
81. (b)	82. (a)	83. (d)	84. (b)	85. (c)	86. (d)	87. (d)	88. (a)	89. (a)	90. (a)
91. (a)	92. (a)	93. (a)	94. (c)	95. (b)	96. (a)	97. (b)			

AIPMT Previous Year Questions

1. (b)	2. (d)	3. (c)	4. (a)	5. (d)	6. (c)	7. (a)	8. (c)	9. (a)	10. (d)
11. (c)	12. (a)	13. (b)	14. (b)	15. (c)	16. (d)	17. (a)			

Unit VII

Genetics and Evolution

This is the most important unit in this book and requires extra understanding from student. This unit is divided into three chapters—Principles of Inheritance and Variation, Molecular Basis of Inheritance and Evolution. Students are suggested to read '64' codon tables carefully, and learn the pneumonics form it. Diagrams related to evolution should be prioritized as these form an integral part in **AIPMT**.

CHAPTER

27

Principles of Inheritance and Variation

1. Mendel was born in
(a) 17th century
(b) 18th century
(c) 19th century
(d) 8th century

2. Mendel was the native of
(a) France
(b) Sweden
(c) India
(d) Austria

3. Mendel proposed which of the following terms for hereditary units?
(a) Factor (determiner)
(b) Genome
(c) Genetic particle
(d) None of the above

4. In genetics, the use of chequer board was done by
(a) Mendel
(b) Correns
(c) Punnet
(d) Darwin

5. In 1900 A.D., three biologists independently discovered Mendel's principles. They are
(a) De Vries, Correns and Tschermak
(b) Sutton, Morgan and Bridges
(c) Avery, McLeod and McCarthy
(d) Bateson, Punnet and Bridges

6. Which of the following has been used for genetic researches?
(a) Pisum
(b) Neurospora
(c) E. coli
(d) All of the above

7. Organism of pure line is that which produces individuals of
(a) Dominant characters
(b) Recessive characters
(c) Its own characters
(d) Intermediate type

8. Mendel is famous for his work on
(a) Pisum
(b) Drosophila
(c) Neurospora
(d) Oenothera

9. The main reason for the success of Mendel was
(a) Study of all the characters at the same time
(b) Study of one character at one time
(c) Study of all the plants at the same time
(d) Counting of plants

10. The alleles are
(a) A pair of genes governing a specific character such as tallness or dwarfness
(b) Multiple forms of genes
(c) Genes governing eye characters
(d) Genes present in allosomes

11. An allele is said to be dominant if
(a) It is expressed only in heterozygous combination
(b) It is expressed only in homozygous combination
(c) It is expressed in both homozygous and heterozygous condition
(d) It is expressed only in second generation

12. What is the correct sequence of the following events?
1. Formation of the chromosome theory of heredity
2. Experiments which proved that DNA is the hereditary material
3. Mendel's laws of inheritance—discovery
(a) 1, 3 and 2 (b) 1, 2 and 3
(c) 3, 1 and 2 (d) 2, 1 and 3

13. When a true breeding pea plant that has yellow seeds is pollinated by a plant that has green seeds, then all the F_1 plants have yellow seeds. This means that the allele for yellow is
(a) Heterozygous (b) Dominant
(c) Recessive (d) Lethal

14. An organism's genetic constitution is called its
(a) Genotype (b) Phenotype
(c) Holotype (d) None of these

15. An organism with two identical alleles for a given trait is
(a) Homozygous (b) Segregating
(c) Dominant (d) A hermaphrodite

16. What type of gametes will form by genotype RrYy
(a) RY, Ry, rY, ry (b) RY, Ry, ry, ry
(c) Ry, Ry, Yy, ry (d) Rr, RR, Yy, YY

17. Which genotype characterises an organism that is heterozygous for two genes
(a) RRYy (b) RrYY
(c) RRYY (d) RrYy

18. The dwarfness in plants of F_2 generation is
(a) Recessive (b) Dominant
(c) Both of the above (d) None of the above

19. When heterozygous tall plants are self-pollinated, then tall and dwarf plants are obtained. This explains
(a) Law of purity of gamete (b) Segregation of law
(c) Division in spores (d) Independent assortment

20. Mendel's principle of segregation was based on the separation of alleles in the garden pea during
(a) Pollination (b) Embryonic development
(c) Seed formation (d) Gamete formation

21. Which of the following is dominant character according to Mendel?
(a) Dwarf plant and yellow fruit (b) Terminal fruit and wrinkled seed
(c) White testa and yellow pericarp (d) Green coloured pod and rounded seed

22. In Mendelism, linkage was not observed due to
(a) Mutation (b) Independent assortment
(c) Synapsis (d) Crossing over

23. Mendel's law of heredity can be explained with the help of
(a) Mitosis (b) Meiosis
(c) Both mitosis and meiosis (d) None of the above

24. A cross between plants having RRYY and rryy composition will yield plants with
(a) Round and yellow seeds (b) Round and green seeds
(c) Wrinkled and yellow seeds (d) Wrinkled and green seeds

25. The genotype of an individual is Rr Bb. How many different types of gametes will it produce based on the law of independent assortment?
(a) 16 (b) 9
(c) 8 (d) 4

26. Which of the following is heterozygous for two pairs of alleles?
(a) TTRR (b) TrRR
(c) ttrr (d) TrtR

27. In Mendel's experiment, nature of seed coat, flower colour, position of flower, pod colour, stem height, etc., are referred to as
(a) Alleles (b) Genotypes
(c) Phenotypes (d) All of the above

28. A cross between a homozygous recessive and a heterozygous plant is called
(a) Monohybrid cross (b) Dihybrid cross
(c) Test cross (d) Back cross

29. Cross between F_1 plant and recessive female plant is called
(a) Back cross (b) Test cross
(c) Out cross (d) Mutation

30. In F_2 generation, a phenotypic ratio of 1:1:1:1 exhibits
(a) Back cross (b) Monohybrid test cross
(c) Lethality (d) Dihybrid test cross

31. Which of the following depicts the Mendel's dihybrid ratio?
(a) 3:1 (b) 9:3:3:1
(c) 9:7 (d) 15:1

32. In dihybrid cross, out of 16 plants obtained, the number of genotypes will be
(a) 4 (b) 9
(c) 16 (d) 12

33. Pure homozygous offsprings in a dihybrid cross in the F_2 generation will be
(a) 1/2 (b) 1/4
(c) 1/8 (d) 1/16

34. In hybridization, Tt × tt gives rise to the progeny of ratio
(a) 1:1 (b) 1:2
(c) 2:1 (d) 1:2:1

35. Self-pollination between Tt and Tt plants results into genotype ratio of
(a) 3:1 (b) 1:2:1
(c) 1:3 (d) 4:0

36. Mendel crossed a pure white-flowered recessive pea plant with a dominant pure red-flowered plant. The first generation of hybrids from the cross should show
(a) 50% white-flowered and 50% red-flowered plants
(b) All red-flowered plants
(c) 75% red-flowered and 25% white-flowered plants
(d) All white-flowered plants

37. If in a dihybrid cross, Mendel had used two such characters which have linked, he would have faced difficulty in explaining the results on the basis of his
(a) Law of segregation
(b) Law of multiple factor hypothesis
(c) Law of independent assortment
(d) Law of dominance

38. From a cross Aa BB × aa BB, following genotypic ratio will be obtained in F_1 generation
(a) 1 Aa BB:1 aa BB
(b) 1 Aa BB:3 aa BB
(c) 3 Aa BB:1 aa BB
(d) All Aa BB:No aa BB

39. A farmer crossed a walnut combed chicken with a single combed one and obtained all walnut combed chickens in F1. The genotype of the parents was
(a) Rr Pp × rr pp
(b) RR PP × rr pp
(c) RR pp × rr pp
(d) RR Pp × rr pp

40. In sweet peas, genes C and P are necessary for colour in flowers. The flowers are white in the absence of either or both the genes. What will be the percentage of coloured flowers in the offspring of the cross Cc pp × cc Pp
(a) 100%
(b) 75%
(c) 25%
(d) 50%

41. In a monohybrid cross, 120 plants are obtained. The ratio of homozygous and heterozygous will be
(a) 40:80
(b) 60:60
(c) 20:100
(d) 10:110

42. If Mendel had studied the seven traits using a plant with 12 chromosomes instead of 14, in what way would his interpretation have been different?
(a) He could have mapped the chromosome
(b) He would have discovered blending or incomplete dominance
(c) He would not have discovered the law of independent assortment
(d) He would have discovered sex linkage

43. How many different types of genetically different gametes will be produced by a heterozygous plant having the genotype AABbCc?
(a) Two
(b) Four
(c) Six
(d) Nine

44. Mendel's law of independent assortment is applicable for
(a) All genes in all organisms
(b) All genes of pea plant only
(c) All linked genes only
(d) All non-linked genes only

45. In a plant, red fruit (R) is dominant over yellow fruit (r) and tallness (T) is dominant over shortness (t). If a plant with RRTt genotype is crossed with a plant that is rrtt, then
(a) 75% will be tall with red fruit
(b) All the offspring will be tall with red fruit
(c) 25% will be tall with red fruit
(d) 50% will be tall with red fruit

46. When a tall plant with rounded seeds (TTRR) is crossed with a dwarf plant with wrinkled seeds (ttrr), then the generation consists of tall plants with rounded seeds. How many types of gametes a plant would produce?

(a) One (b) Three
(c) Four (d) Eight

47. Mendel did his experiment on

(a) Garden pea (Pisum sativum) (b) Snapdragon
(c) Drosophila (d) Lathyrus odaratus

48. How many contrasting traits are chosen by Mendel?

(a) 7 (b) 14
(c) 21 (d) 4

49. Mendel conducted experiment on garden pea for how many years?

(a) 7 (b) 10
(c) 4 (d) 15

50. Select incorrect matching

Characters **Dominant trait** **Recessive trait**

(a) Seed shape
(b) Seed colour
(c) Flower colour
(d) Pod shape

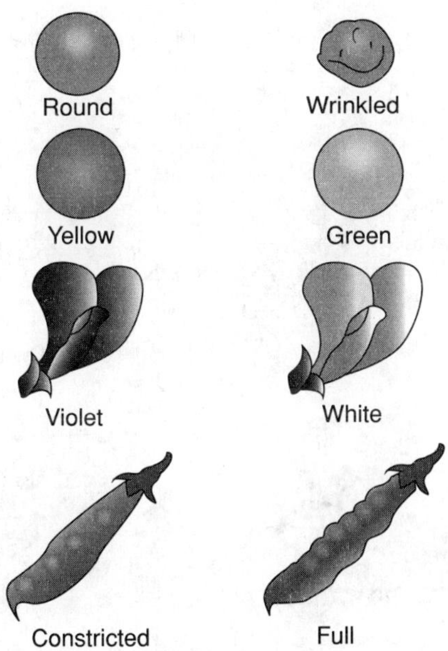

51. Mendel chose how many characters of flower of garden pea for his experiment?

(a) 1 (b) 2
(c) 3 (d) 4

52. Select false statement from the following:

(a) Mendel first time applied statistical analysis and mathematical logics to problem in biology
(b) Mendel's experiment had a large sampling size, which gave greater credibility to the data that he collected
(c) Mendel conducted artificial cross-pollination experiment using true-breeding pea lines
(d) Mendel selected 14 true-breeding pea plant varieties, as pairs which were similar except for two characters with contrasting traits

53. In Mendelian dihybrid cross, how many individuals are homozygous dominant for both the genes in F_2-generation?
(a) 1/16 (b) 2/16
(c) 4/16 (d) 6/16

54. In Mendelian dihybrid cross, how many individuals are homozygous recessive for one of the character only in F_2 generation?
(a) 1/16 (b) 2/16
(c) 3/16 (d) 6/16

55. In Mendelian dihybrid cross, how many individuals are heterozygous of both the character in F_2-generation?
(a) 1/16 (b) 2/16
(c) 3/16 (d) 4/16

56. In Mendelian dihybrid cross, how many of progeny in F_2-generation possess genotype rryy?
(a) 1/16 (b) 2/16
(c) 3/16 (d) 4/16

57. How many genotypes are formed in Mendelian dihybrid cross?
(a) 4 (b) 9
(c) 6 (d) 8

58. Above diagram shows:

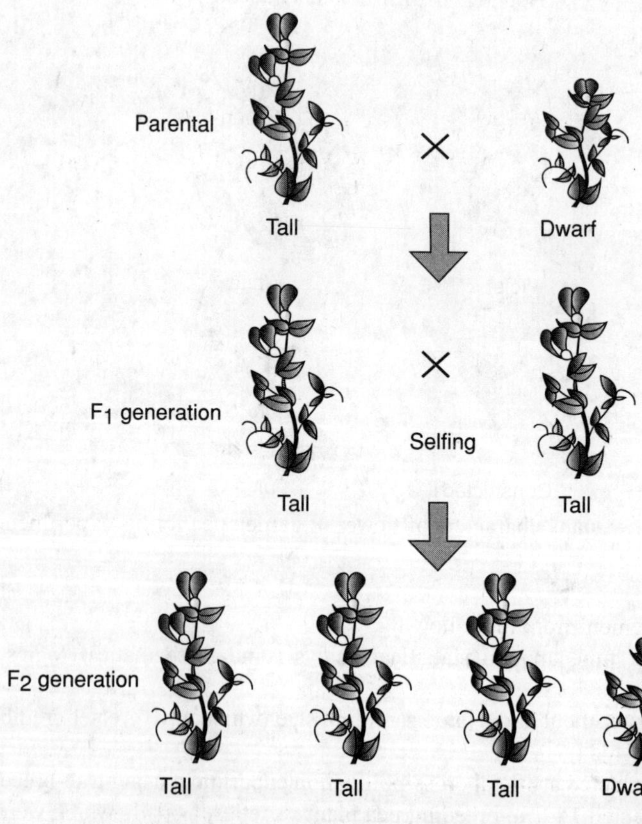

(a) Monohybrid cross
(b) Dihydrid cross
(c) Trihydrid cross
(d) All of the above

59. Above diagram represents

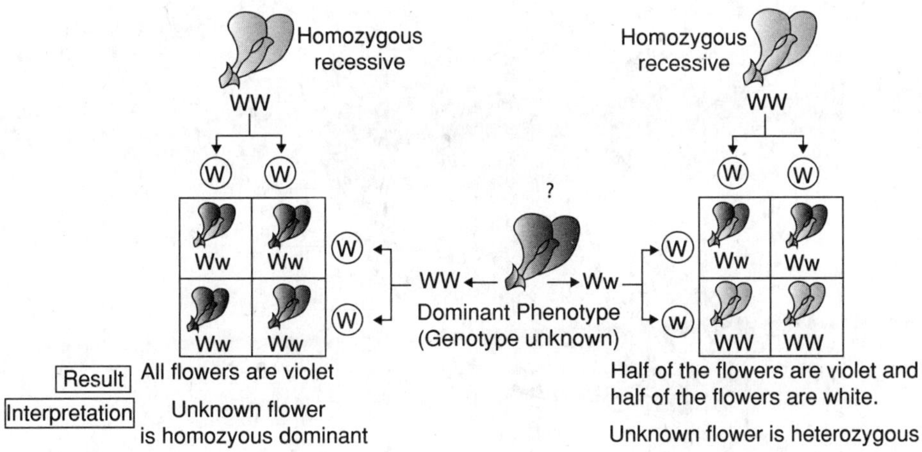

(a) Back cross
(b) Out cross
(c) Test cross
(d) Dihybrid cross

60. Above diagram represents

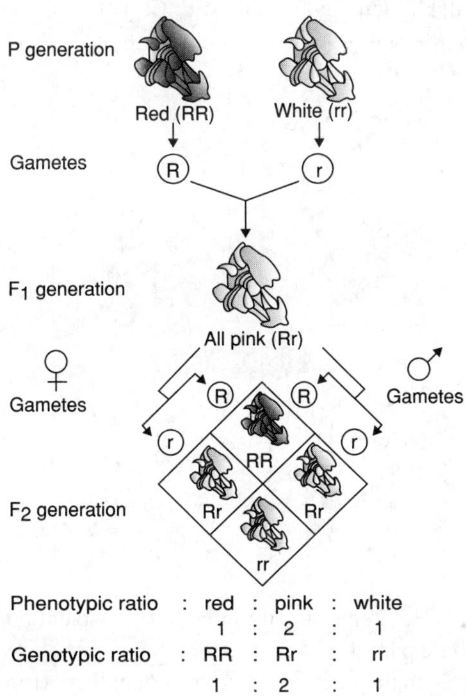

(a) Dominant epistasis
(b) Recessive epistasis
(c) Incomplete dominance
(d) Co-dominance

61. Identify A to E in this figure.

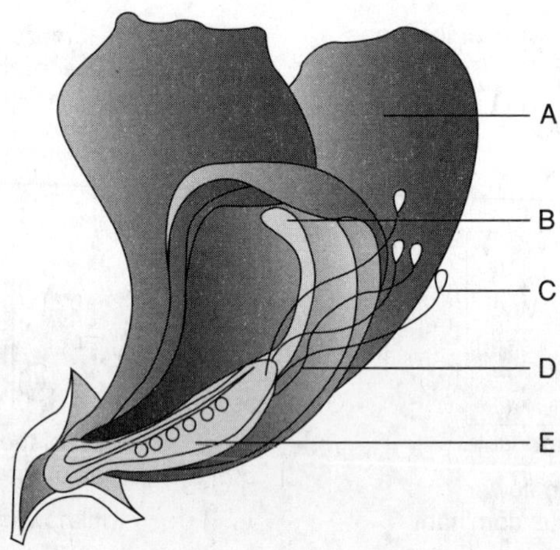

(a) A: Petal; B: Stigma; C: Anther; D: Stamen; E: Carpel
(b) A: Anther; B: Petal; C: Stigma; D: Carpel; E: Stamen
(c) A: Carpel; B: Stamen; C: Anther; D: Stigma; E: Petal
(d) A: Stigma; B: Petal; C: Stamen; D: Anther; E: Carpel

62. Identify A, B, C and D in this figure?

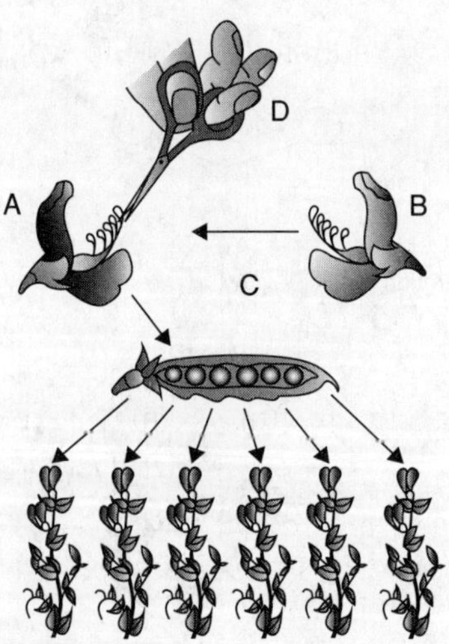

(a) A: Female parent; B: Removal of anthers (Emasculation); C: Transfer of pollen (Pollination); D: Male parent
(b) A: Male parent; B: Female parent; C: Removal of anthers (Emasculation); D: Transfer of pollen (Pollination)

(c) A: Removal of anthers (Emasculation); B: Female parent; C: Transfer of pollen (Pollination); D: Male parent
(d) A: Female parent; B: Male parent; C: Transfer of pollen (Pollination); D: Removal of anthers (Emasculation)

63. Inheritance of ABO blood group system is an example of
(a) Multiple allelism (b) Partial dominance
(c) Epistasis (d) Dominance

64. Genotype of blood group 'A' will be
(a) I^AI^A (b) I^BI^B
(c) I^AI^A or I^AI^O (d) I^AI^O

65. Blood group 'B' will have alleles
(a) ii (b) I^AI^A
(c) I^BI^B (d) I^AI^B

66. If one parent belongs to 'A' blood group and the other to 'O' blood group, their children possibly represent
(a) A and B groups only (b) AB only
(c) A and O groups only (d) All four groups

67. If a child has O type of blood group and the father has B type, the genotype of the father will be
(a) I^OI^O (b) I^AI^B
(c) I^OI^B (d) I^BI^B

68. A person with antigens 'B' in RBC and antibodies 'A' in the plasma belongs to the blood group
(a) A (b) B
(c) AB (d) O

69. Rh factor may be responsible for
(a) Turner's syndrome (b) AIDS
(c) Sickle-cell anaemia (d) Erythroblastosis foetalis

70. A human female with blood group 'A' has
(a) Antibody-anti-B in the red blood cells and antigen A in the serum
(b) Antigen A in the red blood cells and antibody-anti-B in the serum
(c) Antigen B in the red blood cells and antibody-anti-B in the serum
(d) Antigen A in the red blood cells and antibody-anti-A in the serum

71. Rh factor is named after
(a) Man (b) Rat
(c) Monkey (d) Chimpanzee

72. If one parent has blood group A and the other parent has blood group B, the offspring have which blood group?
(a) AB (b) O
(c) BO (d) A, B, AB, O

73. Mendel did not recognize the linkage phenomenon in his experiments because
(a) There were many chromosomes to handle
(b) Characters he studied were located on different chromosomes
(c) He did not have powerful microscope
(d) He studied only pure plants

74. Exchange of genetic material between chromatids of homologous chromosomes during meiosis is called
(a) Synapsis (b) Chiasmata
(c) Transformation (d) Crossing over

75. In maize, chromosome number is 2n = 20. The number of linkage groups in it will be
(a) 20 (b) 40
(c) 10 (d) 5

76. The map distance between genes A and B is 3 units, between B and C is 10 units and between C and A is 7 units. The order of the genes in a linkage map constructed on the above data would perhaps be
(a) A, B, C (b) A, C, B
(c) B, C, A (d) B, A, C

77. Crossing over in diploid organism is responsible for
(a) Dominance of genes (b) Linkage between genes
(c) Segregation of alleles (d) Recombination of linked allele

78. The percentage of crossing over will be more if
(a) Linked genes are located far apart from each other
(b) Linked genes are located close to each other
(c) Genes are not linked
(d) Genes are located in a different cell

79. Linkage was first observed in
(a) Field pea (b) Sweet pea
(c) Pea (d) Grass pea

80. Drosophila has four pairs of chromosomes. How many linkage groups does it have?
(a) Eight (b) Four
(c) One less than the pairs of chromosomes (d) One more than the pairs of chromosomes

81. Linkage in Drosophila was first discovered by
(a) Morgan (b) Bateson and Punnet
(c) Sturtevant (d) Bridges

82. Number of linkage group in Pisum sativum is
(a) 2 (b) 5
(c) 7 (d) 9

83. Who coined the term linkage?
(a) Mendel (b) Tshermak
(c) Sturtevant (d) TH. Morgan

84. In humans, chromosomal condition of male is
(a) 44 AA + XO (b) 44 AA + XX
(c) 44 AA + XY (d) 44 AA + XXY

85. Physical association of two genes is known as
(a) Heterozygosis (b) Linkage
(c) Recombination (d) Homozygosis

86. Find out incorrect statement

(a) Morgan carried out several dihybrid crosses in drosophila to study genes that were sex linked.

(b) Sturtevant used the frequency of recombination between gene pairs on the same chromosome as a measure of the distance between genes and mapped their position on chromosome.

(c) Henking gave the term X-body.

(d) Boveri united the knowledge of chromosomal segregation with Mendelian principles and called it the chromosomal theory of inheritance.

87. Which cross shows very tight linkage?

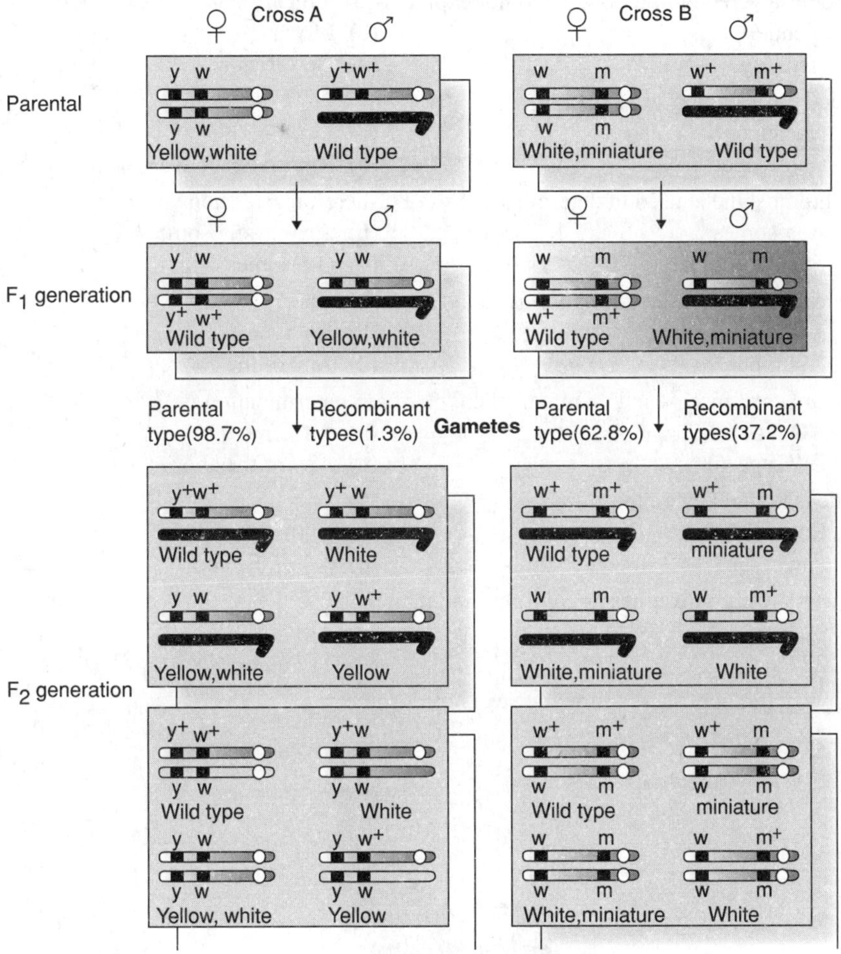

(a) Cross A
(b) Cross B
(c) Both (a) and (b)
(d) None of these

88. Why drosophila melanogaster is suitable for study of genetical variation?
(a) Could be grown on simple synthetic medium in laboratory
(b) Complete life cycle is 2 weeks and single mating produces a large number of progeny flies
(c) Clear sexual dimorphism is present and many types of heredity variation can be seen with low power microscope
(d) All of these

89. Cytological observation made in a many number of ________ led to the development of the concept of genetic/chromosomal basis of sex determination
(a) Mammals (b) Birds
(c) Humans (d) Insects

90. Who discovered X-body but could not explain its significance
(a) Mendel (b) Morgan
(c) Henking (d) De varies

91. X-body of Henking was
(a) Nucleus (b) Lipid
(c) Chromosome (d) Ribosomes

92. X-chromosome is used in determination of sex; therefore, it is known as
(a) Autosomes (b) Sex-chromosome
(c) Microsomes (d) Oxysomes

93. Which type of sex-determination is found in grasshopper?
(a) XO type (b) XY type
(c) ZW type (d) Any of the above

94. In number of insects and mammals the type of sex determination is
(a) XO type (b) XY type
(c) ZW type (d) Any of the above

95. Male is homogametic in
(a) Drosophila (b) Human
(c) Fowl (d) All of the above

96. How many chromosomes are present in human male?
(a) 22 Pairs + XX (b) 22 Pairs + YY
(c) 22 Pairs + XY (d) 21 Pairs + XY

97. Below diagram possess following sex chromosome

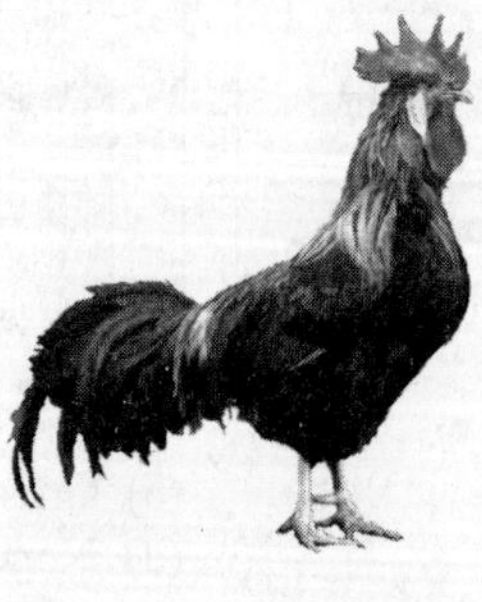

(a) XX (b) XY
(c) ZZ (d) ZW

98. Below diagram shows:

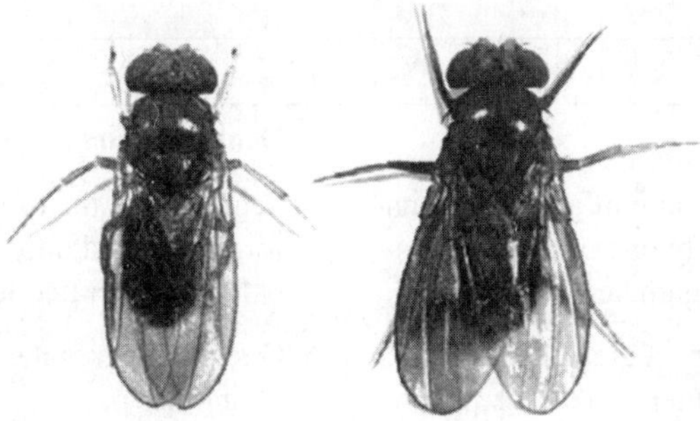

(a) M and F drosophila, respectively
(b) M and F housefly, respectively
(c) F and M drosophila, respectively
(d) F and M housefly, respectively

99. Which of the following is responsible for sex of the chicks?
(a) Sperm
(b) Egg
(c) Both (a) and (b)
(d) None of these

100. Find out the correct statement.
(a) Genetic makeup of the egg determines sex of the child in human
(b) Genetic makeup of the sperm determines sex of the child in human
(c) XO and XY type of sex determination is an example of female heterogamety
(d) Henking (1891) could trace a specific nuclear structure all through oogenesis of few insects

101. Female heterogamety is found in
(a) Human
(b) Drosophila
(c) Chicks
(d) All of the above

102. Why Mendel's work was not recognized till 1900?
(a) His work could not be widely published.
(b) His concept of factor (stable and discrete units that control expression of trait) was not accepted by his contemporaries.
(c) His approach of using mathematics to explain biological phenomenon was totally new and unacceptable by many of the biologist of his time.
(d) All of these

103. How many scientists rediscovered mendelism in 1900 independently?
(a) 1
(b) 2
(c) 3
(d) 4

104. Mendelian rediscoverers are
(a) Devries, Holland
(b) Correns, Germany
(c) Von Tschermak, Austria
(d) All of these

105. Who noted that behaviour of chromosomes was parallel to the behaviour of genes and use chromosome movement to explain Mendel's law?
(a) T.H. Morgan
(b) Hugo Devries
(c) Sutton and Boveri
(d) Beadle and Tatum

106. Which of the column A or B represents chromosome and which of the column represents gene?

A	B
1. Occur in pairs	2. Occur in pairs
3. Segregate at the time of gamete formation such that only one of each pair is transmitted to a gamete	4. Segregate at the time of gamete formation and only one of each pair is transmitted to a gamete
5. Independent pairs segregate independently of each other	6. One pair segregates independently of another pair

(a) A: Gene, B: Gene
(b) A: Chromosome, B: Chromosome
(c) A: Gene, B: Chromosome
(d) A: Chromosome. B; Gene

107. Which of the diagrams represents independent assortment?

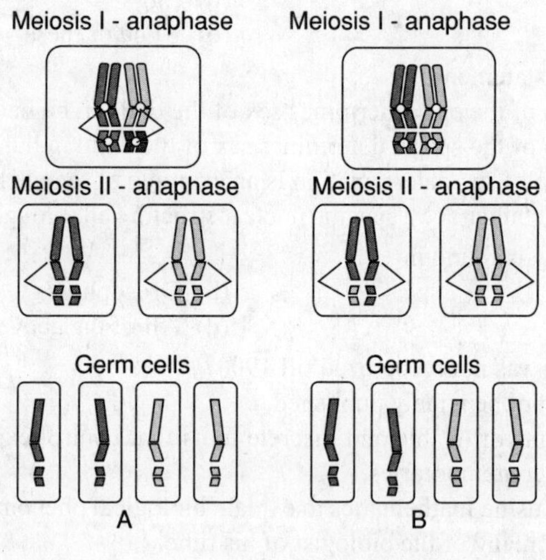

(a) A only
(b) B only
(c) Both (a) and (b)
(d) None of these

108. Identify A and B in this figure.

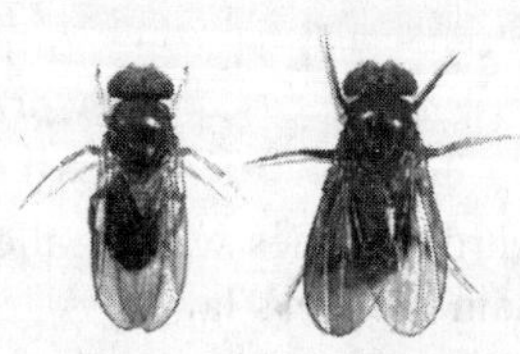

(a) A: Male, B: Female
(b) A: Female, B: Male
(c) A: Male, B: Male
(d) A: Female, B: Female

109. Method for analyzing inheritance pattern of traits in human being is

(a) DNA finger printing (b) Control cross
(c) Pedigree analysis (d) All of the above

110. Standard symbol used for consanguineous mating in pedigree analysis is

(a) 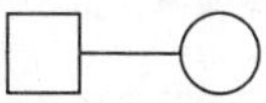 (b) 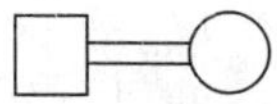

(c) 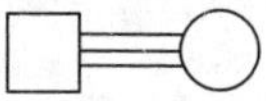 (d) 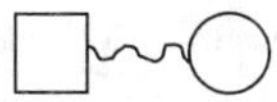

111. Select correct matching regarding standard symbol of pedigree analysis

Column–I	Column–II
(A) 	(1) Female
(B) 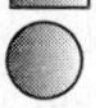	(2) Male
(C) 	(3) Mating
(D) 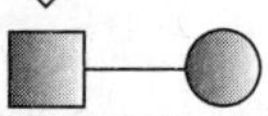	(4) Sex unspecified

(a) A:2, B:1, C:4, D:2 (b) A:2, B:1, C:2, D:4
(c) A:1, B:2, C:2, D:4 (d) A:1, B:2, C:4, D:2

112. Which symbol represents parents with male child affected with diseases?

(a) 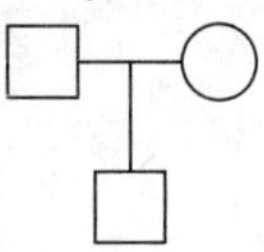 (b) 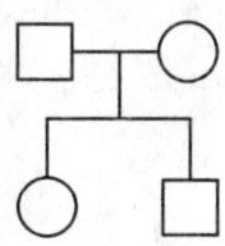

(c) 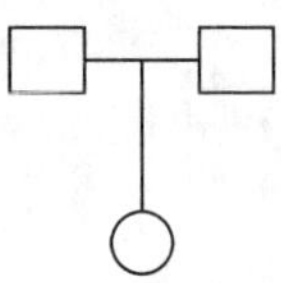 (d) 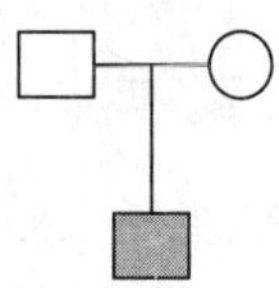

113. Which of the following symbol is not used in pedigree analysis?

(a) 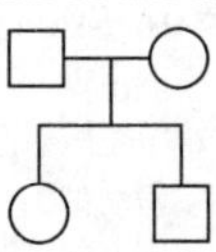 (b) 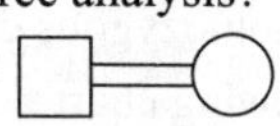

(c) 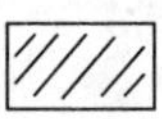 (d) 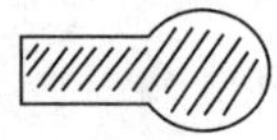

114. Following pedigree shows

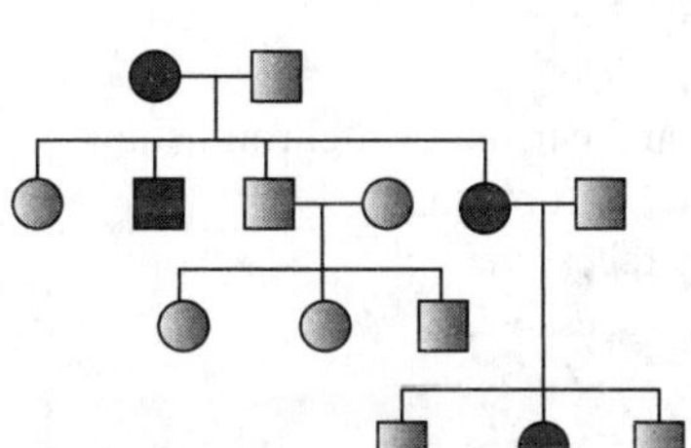

(a) Autosomal dominant trait (b) Autosomal recessive trait
(c) X-linked recessive trait (d) X-linked dominant trait

115. Following pedigree shows

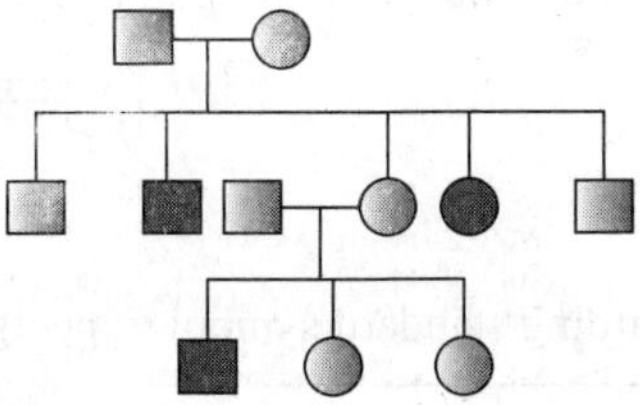

(a) Autosomal dominant trait (b) Autosomal recessive trait
(c) X-linked recessive trait (d) X-linked dominant trait

116. Given below is a pedigree chart of family with five children. It shows the inheritance of attached ear-lobes as opposed to the free ones. The squares represent the male individuals and circles the female individuals.

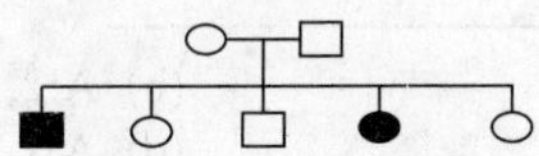

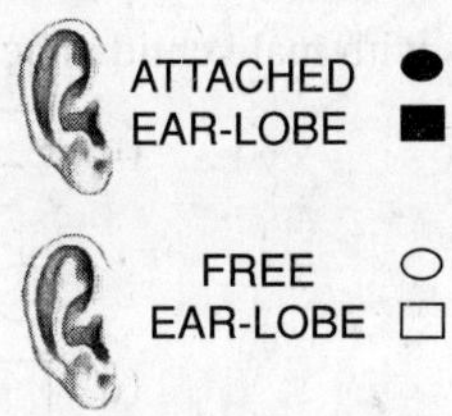

Which one of the following conclusions drawn is correct?
(a) The parents are homozygous recessive. (b) The trait is Y-linked.
(c) The parents are homozygous dominant. (d) The parents are heterozygous.

117. Predict from the following chart

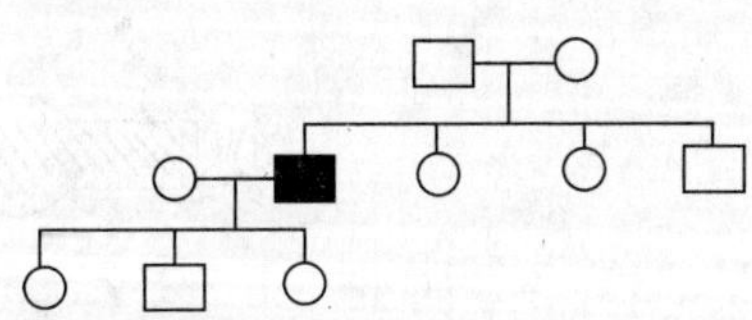

(a) Character is dominant and carried by x chromosome.
(b) Character is carried by y chromosome.
(c) Character is sex-linked recessive.
(d) Character is autosomal recessive.

118. The pedigree shows the occurrence of albinism which is a recessive trait. If person 4 is homozygous, the carrier for the trait is

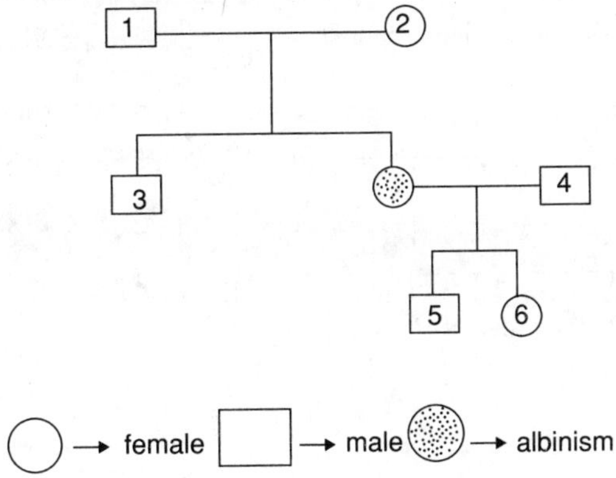

(a) 1, 4, 5 and 6
(b) 5 and 6
(c) 1, 2 and 3
(d) 1, 2, 5 and 6

119. This is pedigree for autosomal recessive disease albinism (aa). What is the probability of II-1 homozygous normal?

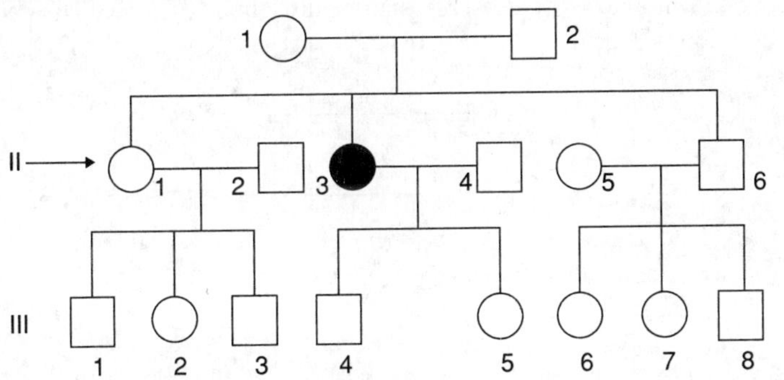

(a) 1/3
(b) 1/2
(c) 2/3
(d) 1/4

120. According to the given pedigree, the trait indicated

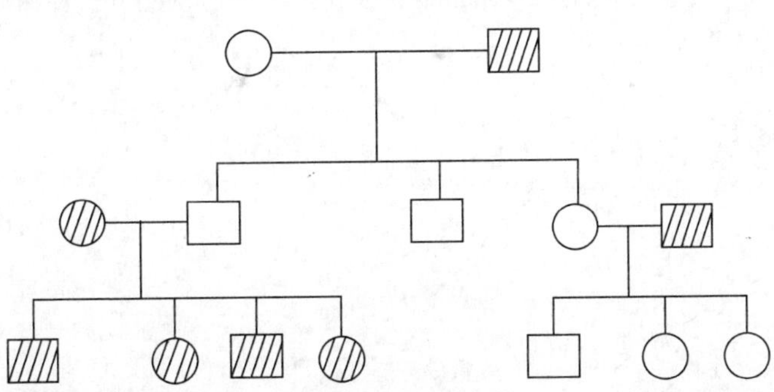

(a) Autosomal recessive ☐: Normal male (b) X-linked recessive ▨: Affected male

(c) Maternal imprinting ○: Normal female (d) Paternal imprinting ⊘: Affected female

121. Given pedigree shows inheritance of autosomal recessive gene. What is the genotype of given parents?

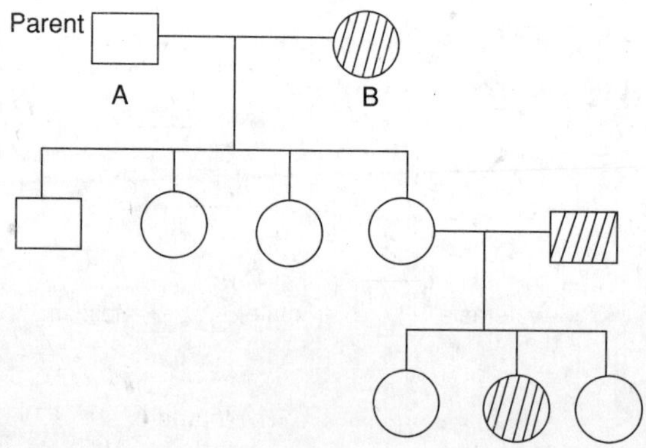

(a) AA, aa (b) Aa, AA
(c) aa, aa (d) Aa, Aa

122. A pedigree is shown below for a disease that is autosomal recessive. The genetic makeup of the first generation will be

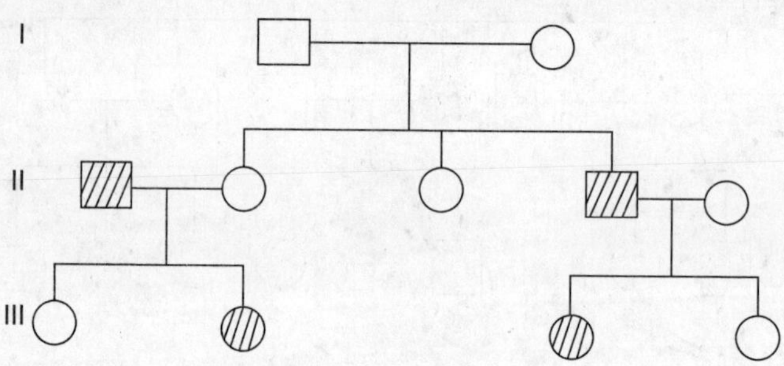

(a) AA, aa (b) Aa, Aa
(c) Aa, aa (d) aa, aa

123. 1:1:1:1 ratio of progenies can be obtained if the plants employed for crossing are:
(A) TTRR × ttRR
(B) TtRr × ttrr
(C) TtRR × ttrr
(D) Ttrr × ttRr

(a) A, C, D
(b) A, B, C, D
(c) B, D
(d) A, B

124. A pedigree is shown below for a disease that is autosomal dominant. The genetic makeup of the first generation is

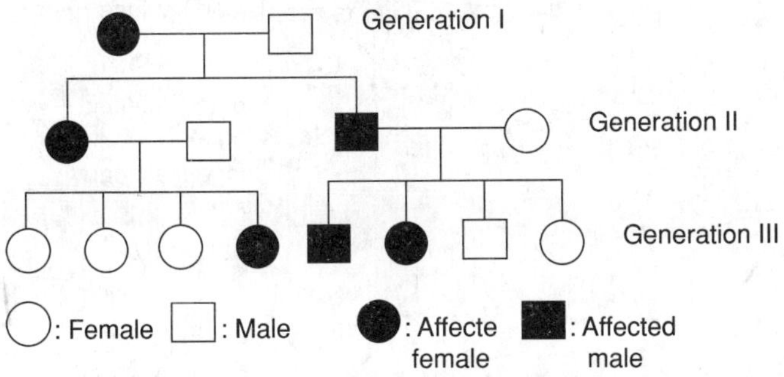

(a) AA, Aa (b) Aa, aa
(c) Aa, AA (d) Aa, Aa

125. Failure of segregation of chromatids during cell division cycles results in the gain or loss of a chromosome(s) called
(a) Anenploidy (b) Polyploidy
(c) Trisomy (d) Nullisomy

126. Down's syndrome occurs due to the gain in extra copy of
(a) Chromosome 19
(b) Chromosome 5
(c) Chromosome 21
(d) Chromosome 24

127. Turner's syndrome occurs due to loss of
(a) Chromosome 5
(b) Chromosome 21
(c) Chromosome 'X'
(d) Chromosome 'Y'

128. How many sex chromosomes are present in human cell?
(a) 1 pair (b) 2 pairs
(c) 3 pairs (d) 4 pairs

129. Gynaecomastia is seen in case of
(a) Down's syndrome (b) Klinefelter's syndrome
(c) Turner's syndrome (d) All of these

130. Following features belong to which syndrome?
(A) Furrowed tongue
(B) Palm is broad with characteristic palm crease
(C) Physical, psychomotor and mental retardation
(D) Short statured with small round head

(a) Down's syndrome (b) AIDS
(c) Turner's syndrome (d) Klinefelter's syndrome

131. Below diagram shows which type of syndrome

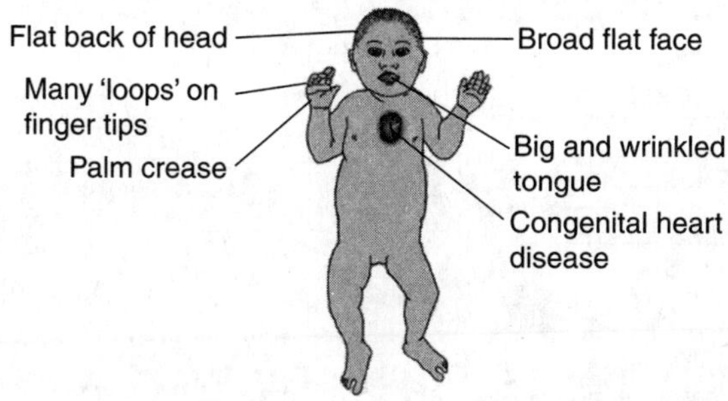

(a) Down's syndrome (b) Cri-du chat syndrome
(c) PKU (d) Turner's syndrome

132. Increase in a whole set of chromosome in an organism is known as
(a) Polyploidy (b) Aneuploidy
(c) Trisomy (d) Tetrasomy

133. Langdon down describe Down's syndrome in which year
(a) 1866 (b) 1890
(c) 1852 (d) 1953

134. Two allelic genes are located on
(a) The same chromosomes (b) Two homologous chromosomes
(c) Two non-homologous chromosomes (d) Any two chromosomes

135. In human beings, the colour of skin is controlled by
(a) Multiple alleles (b) Lethal genes
(c) Polygenic effect (d) None of these

136. Which of the following is genetically dominant in man?
(a) Colour blindness (b) Rh positive
(c) Haemophilia (d) Albinism

137. If a certain patient with blood group B requires immediate blood transfusion, the following type can be given to him
(a) O and B (b) O and AB
(c) A and AB (d) B and AB

138. Karyotype of Klinefelter's syndrome is
(a) 44 + XXY (b) 44 + XO
(c) 44 + XYY (d) 44 + XXXY

139. Which is not a character of Klinefelter's syndrome?
(a) Masculine development (b) Gynaecomastia
(c) Fertile individual (d) Sterile individual

140. All are characters of Down's syndrome except
(a) Congenital heart disease (b) Broad flat face
(c) Small and wrinkled tongue (d) Many 'loops' on finger tips

141. Identify syndrome of diagrams a and b, respectively.

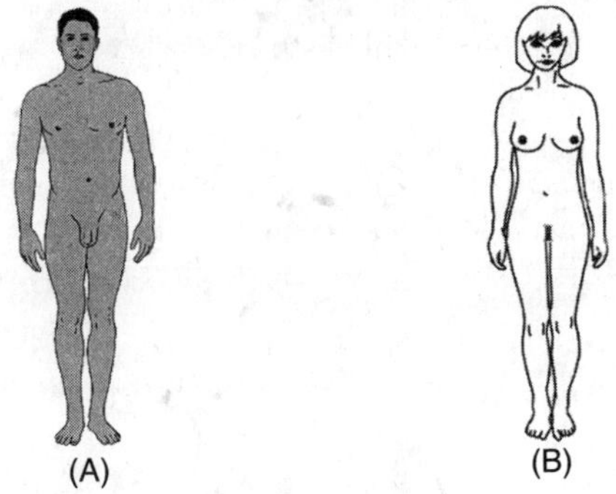

(a) A: Down's syndrome, B: Turner's syndrome
(b) A: Klinefelter's syndrome, B; Turner's syndrome
(c) A: Turner's syndrome, B: Klinefelter syndrome
(d) A: Turner's syndrome, B: Down's syndrome

142. Which karyotype present monosomy?
(a) 2n + 1 (b) 2n – 2
(c) 2n – 1 (d) 2n + 2

143. Which karyotype represents trisomy?
(a) 2n + 1 (b) 2n – 2
(c) 2n – 1 (d) 2n + 2

144. Find out total number of Mendelian disorder from the following:
Cystic Fibrosis, Haemophilia, Sickle cell anaemia, Colorblindness, Thalesemia, Phenyllketonuria
(a) 4 (b) 5
(c) 6 (d) 3

145. Which of the following is sex-linked recessive disorder?
(a) Myotonic dystrophy (b) Sickle-cell anaemia
(c) Haemophilia (d) Phenylketonuria

146. Following is autosomal dominant trait
(a) Phenylketonuria (b) Sickle-cell anaemia
(c) Haemophilia (d) Myotonic dystrophy

147. Queen Victoria was a carrier of which disease?
(a) Myotonic dystrophy (b) Sickle-cell anaemia
(c) Haemophilia (d) Phenylketonuria

148. Sickle cell anaemia caused by substitution of Glutamic acid (Glue) by ________ at the sixth position of the beta globin chain of the haemoglobin molecule.
(a) Asn (Aspargine) (b) Gly (Glycine)
(c) Arg (Argenine) (d) Val (Valine)

149. Which enzyme is defective in PKU?
(A) DOPA $\xrightarrow{\text{Enzyme(1)}}$ Melanin (B) Tyrosine $\xrightarrow{\text{Enzyme(2)}}$ Thyroxin
(C) Phenylalanine $\xrightarrow{\text{Enzyme(3)}}$ tyrosine (D) Tyrosine $\xrightarrow{\text{Enzyme(4)}}$ Homogentisic acid
(a) Enzyme (A) (b) Enzyme (B)
(c) Enzyme (C) (d) Enzyme (D)

150. True about Phenyllketonuria
(a) Metal retardation
(b) Accumulation of phenylalanine and phenyl pyruvic acid and other derivatives
(c) Autosomal recessive trait
(d) All of the above

151. The substitution of amino acid in the globin protein results due to the single bass substitution at the sixth codon of the beta globin gene from.
(a) GAG to GGG (b) CAG to GAG
(c) GAG to GUG (d) GGC to GGA

152. Which of the following amino acid not present in first six amino acids in affected β-chain of Haemoglobin?
(a) Val (b) Thr
(c) Glu (d) Leu

153. Identify A, B, C

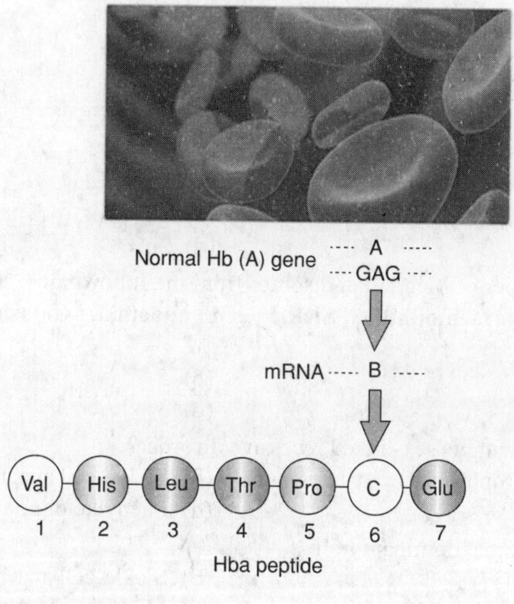

(a) A: CTC; B: GAG; C: Glu (b) A: GAG; B: CTC; C: Pro
(c) A: CTC; B: GAG; C: Thr (d) A: CTC; B: GAG; C: Leu

154. Identify A, B, C

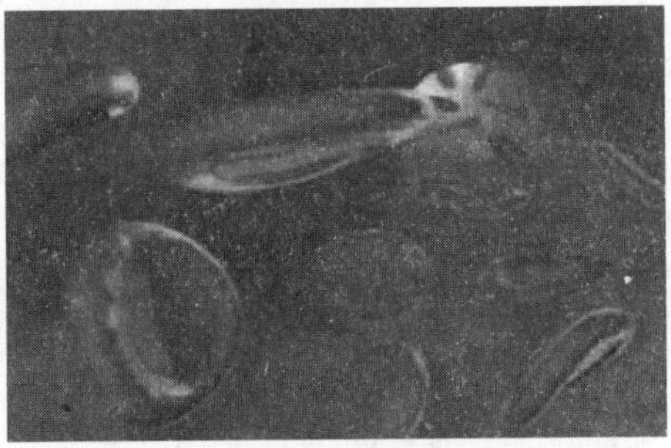

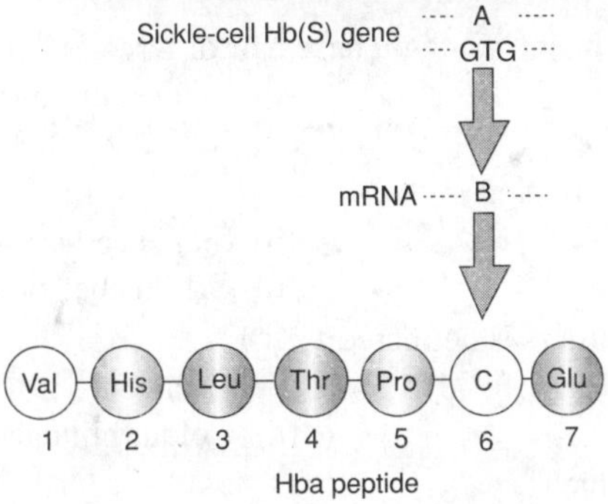

(a) A: CAC; B: GUG; C: Pro
(b) A: CAC; B: GUG; C: Val
(c) A: CTC, B: GUG, C: Leu
(d) A: GAC, B: GUG, C: His

155. Name the amino acid which has its 2 molecules present in the first 7 amino acid of β-chain of haemoglobin.
(a) Val
(b) His
(c) Leu
(d) Glu

156. Probability of which of the following is extremely rare?
(a) Carrier female in haemophilia
(b) Carrier male in haemophilia
(c) Affected male in haemophilia
(d) Affected female in haemophilia

157. In hemophilia how many proteins that is a part of the cascade of protein involved in clotting of blood affected?
(a) One
(b) Two
(c) Three
(d) Multiple/many

158. Diseased phenotype in sickle cell anaemia is shown by which of the following genotype?
(a) $Hb^A Hb^A$
(b) $Hb^S Hb^S$
(c) $Hb^A Hb^S$
(d) All of above

159. Variation in DNA is due to
(a) Mutation
(b) Recombination
(c) Both (a) and (b)
(d) None of these

160. Alteration in chromosome may be due to
(a) Deletion of a segment of DNA
(b) Addition of segment of DNA
(c) Duplication of segment of DNA
(d) Any of above

161. Deletion or insertion of base pairs of DNA causes
(a) Point mutation
(b) Frameshift mutation
(c) Transversion
(d) All of the above

162. Find out correct statement.
(a) UV radiation can cause mutation in organism
(b) Chromosomal aberration are commonly observed in cancer cells
(c) Mutation is a phenomenon which results in alteration of DNA sequences and results in changes in the genotype and the phenotype of an organism
(d) All of the above

163. Mutation arises due to the change in single base pair of DNA is known as
(a) Point mutation
(b) Frameshift mutation
(c) Silent mutation
(d) Recombination

164. Classical example of point mutation is
(a) Haemophilia
(b) Sickle cell anaemia
(c) Mangolism
(d) Cri-du chat syndrome

165. Which of the following disorders is not hereditary?
(a) Haemophilia
(b) Cataract
(c) Sickle-cell anaemia
(d) Colour blindness

166. A pleiotropic gene is one which
(a) Affects one character
(b) Affects more than one characters
(c) (a) and (b) both
(d) None of these

167. Phenyketonuria is a genetic disorder of
(a) Trisomic condition
(b) Monosomic condition
(c) Autosomal dominant gene
(d) Autosomal recessive gene
(e) X-linked

168. Which of the following is not X-linked recessive?
(a) Haemophilia-A
(b) Colour blindness
(c) BETA-Thalasemia
(d) G-6 PD deficiency

169. Monosomy and trisomy can be represented as
(a) $2n + 1, 2n + 3$
(b) $2n - 1, 2n - 2$
(c) $2n, 2n + 1$
(d) $2n - 1, 2n + 1$

170. Which result proved that there was no blending in Mendelian Cross?
(a) $Filial_1$ progeny of monohybrid cross
(b) $Filial_2$ progeny of dihybrid cross
(c) $Filial_1$ progeny of dihybrid cross
(d) All of the above

171. F_2-progeny of Mendelian monohybrid cross between Tall and Dwarf plant made up of
(a) Tall plant, identical to their parental type
(b) Dwarf plant, identical to their parental type
(c) Plant with intermediate light were produced
(d) Both (a) and (b)

172. Select incorrect statement
(a) Capital latter is used to denote dominant trait
(b) Small latter is used to denote recessive trait
(c) True breeding variety is represented by similar allele pair of gene
(d) Alleles are completely similar forms of the same genes

173. Punnett was
(a) Italian botanist (b) British geneticist
(c) American geneticist (d) Austrian geneticist

174. What genotype ratio of Mendelian monhybrid cross?
(a) 3:1 (b) 1:2:1
(c) 1:1 (d) 3:2

175. Mendel found that the F_1 always resembled either one of the parents and that the trait of the other parent was not seen in them. This is due to
(a) Segregation (b) Dominance
(c) Partial dominance (d) Unit factor

176. In monohybrid cross, proportion of 3:1 explains
(a) Dominance (b) Segregation
(c) Both (a) and (b) (d) Unit factor

177. In Morgan's experiment, what will be the percentage of recombination in case of body colour and eye colour?
(a) 37.2% (b) 1.3%
(c) 98.7% (d) 37.2%

178. Which symbol of pedigree is correctly matched?
(a) – Female 
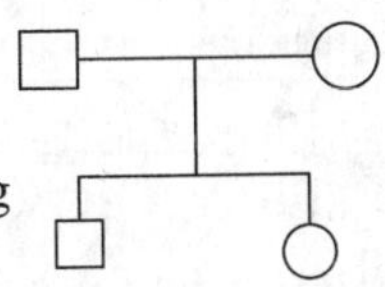
(b) – Affected offspring
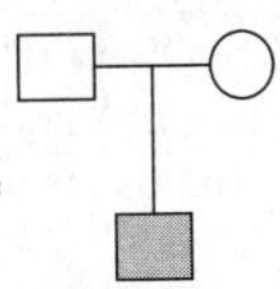
(c) – Affected male of autosomal recessive disease
(d) – Marriage between relatives 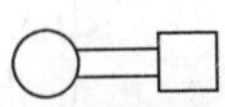

179. Which of the following was/were applied first time to problems in biology during Mendel's investigations into inheritance?
(a) Statistical analysis (b) Mathematical logic
(c) Computational devices (d) Both (a) and (b)

180. Mendel proposed how many general rules to consolidate his understanding of inheritance in monohybrid cross?
(a) One
(b) Two
(c) Three
(d) None of the rules, he proposed laws/principles

181. In the theoretical explanation of allelic interaction for dominant and recessive forms, the recessive trait is seen due to the production of
(a) Normal or less efficient enzyme (b) A non-functional enzyme
(c) No enzyme production (d) Either (b) or (c)

182. Genes responsible for ABO blood group determine which of the following biomolecules of RBC plasma membrane?
(a) Phospholipid (b) Proteins (c) Sugars (d) Cholesterols

183. Shape of seed depends on starch granules size; so inheritance of seed shape show ________ relationship, while inheritance of starch grains show ________.
(a) Dominant recessive, codominance
(b) Incomplete dominance, codominance
(c) Dominant-recessive, incomplete dominance
(d) Codominance, incomplete dominance

184. If yellow body, white eyed drosophila is crossed with wild brown body red eyes drosophila. Then what would be the frequency of recombinants in F_1 generation?
(a) 100% (b) 1.3% (c) 98.7% (d) 0%

185. Chromosomal aberrations are commonly observed in
(a) Germinal cells (b) Cancer cells (c) Nail base cells (d) Gametes

186. Which of the following cell cycle event is responsible for polyploidy phenomenon?
(a) Failure of karyokinesis (b) Failure of cytokinesis
(c) Failure of segregation (d) Failure of spindle apparatus

187. Match the following

Column – I	Column – II
A. Haemophilia	1. Board palm with characteristic palm creased
B. Down's syndrome	2. Delayed clotting of blood
C. Klinefelter's syndrome	3. However feminine development
D. Turner's Syndrome	4. Rudimentary ovaries

(a) A:1; B:3; C:2; D:4 (b) A:2; B:1; C:3; D:4
(c) A:4; B:2; C:1; D:3 (d) A:1; B:2; C:3; D:4

188. Mendel's Law of independent assortment holds good for genes situated on the
(a) non-homologous chromosomes (b) homologous chromosomes
(c) extra nuclear genetic element (d) same chromosome

189. Occasionally, a single gene may express more than one effect. The phenomenon is called
(a) Multiple allelism (b) Mosaicism
(c) Pleiotropy (d) Polygeny

190. In a certain taxon of insects, some have 17 chromosomes and the others have 18 chromosomes. The 17 and 18 chromosome-bearing organisms are
(a) Males and females, respectively (b) Females and males, respectively
(c) All males (d) All females

191. The inheritance pattern of a gene over generations among humans is studied by the pedigree analysis. Character studied in the pedigree analysis is equivalent to
(a) Quantitative trait (b) Mendelian trait
(c) Polygenic trait (d) Maternal trait

192. It is said that Mendel proposed that the factor controlling any character is discrete and independent. This proposition was based on the
(a) Results of F_3 generation of a cross
(b) Observations that the offsprings of a cross made between the plants having two contrasting characters show only one character without any blending
(c) Self-pollination of F_1 offsprings
(d) Cross-pollination of parental generations

193. Two genes 'A' and 'BA' are linked. In a dihybrid cross involving these two genes, the F_1 heterozygote is crossed with homozygous recessive parental type (aa bb). What would be the ratio of offspring in the next generation?
(a) 1:1:1:1
(b) 9:3:3:1
(c) 3:1
(d) 1:1

194. In the F_2 generation of a Mendelian dihybrid cross, the number of phenotypes and genotypes are
(a) phenotypes-4; genotypes-16
(b) phenotypes-9; genotypes-4
(c) phenotypes-4; genotypes-8
(d) phenotypes-4; genotypes-9

195. Mother and father of a person with '0' blood group have 'A' and 'B' blood group, respectively. What would be the genotype of both mother and father?
(a) Mother is homozygous for 'A' blood group and father is heterozygous for 'B'
(b) Mother is heterozygous for 'A' blood group and father is homozygous for 'B'
(c) Both mother and father are heterozygous for 'A' and 'B' blood group, respectively
(d) Both mother and father are homozygous for 'A' and 'B' blood group, respectively

*Read the **assertion** and **reason** carefully to mark the correct option out of the options given below:*

(a) If both the assertion and the reason are true and the reason is a correct explanation of the assertion
(b) If both the assertion and reason are true but the reason is not a correct explanation of the assertion
(c) If the assertion is true but the reason is false
(d) If both the assertion and reason are false

196. Assertion: Gregor Mendel, conducted hybridisation experiment on garden peas and proposed the laws of inheritance in living organism.
Reason: Mendel selected 7 true-breeding pea plant varieties.

197. Assertion: In a monohybrid cross F_1 generation indicate recessive characters.
Reason: Dominance occurs only in homozygous state.

198. Assertion: Gene which code for a pair of contrasting traits are known alleles.
Reason: Alleles are slightly different forms of the same gene.

199. Assertion: The law of dominance is used to explain the expression of only one of the parental character is a monohybrid cross in the F_1- generation.
Reason: The law of dominance explain the propportion of 3 : 1 obtained at the F_2 – generation.

200. Assertion: Deletions & insertions of base pairs of DNA, causes frame – shift mutation.
Reason: A classical example of frame –shift mutation is sickle cell anaemia.

201. Assertion: Increase in a whole set of chromosome in an organism is known as polyploidy
Reason: Failure of cytokinesis after telophase stage of cell division results in polyploidy

202. Assertion: Test cross is a back cross.
Reason: In test cross, F_1 – individual is crossed with recessive parents.

203. Assertion: Inheritance of holandric gene are always from father to son.
Reason: Holandric genes are found on Y- chromosome

204. Assertion: In humans, the gamete contributed by the male determines whether the child produced will be male or female
Reason: Sex in human is a polygenic trait depending upon a cumulative effect of some gene on X-chromosome and some on Y-chromosome.

205. Assertion: In birds, the chromosomes composition of the sperm determines the sex.
Reason: Male birds are heterogametic.

AIPMT PREVIOUS YEAR QUESTIONS

1. Study the pedigree chart of a certain family given in figure and select the correct conclusion which can be drawn for the character.

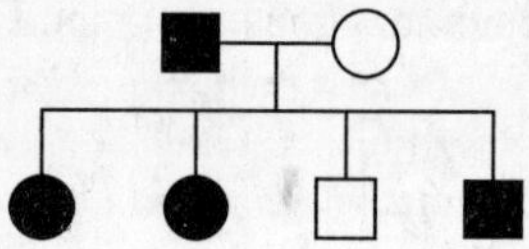

[AIPMT MAINS 2010]

(a) The female parent is heterozygous
(b) The parents could not have had a normal daughter for this character
(c) The trait under study could not be colour blindness
(d) The male parent is homozygous dominant

2. In Antirrhinum two plants with pink flowers were hybridized. The F_1 plants produced red, pink and white flowers in the proportion of 1 red, 2 pink and 1 white. What could be the genotype of the two plants used for hybridization Red flower colour is determined by RR, and white by rr genes.

[AIPMT MAINS 2010]

(a) rrrr (b) RR
(c) Rr (d) rr

3. A cross in which an organism showing a dominant phenotype is crossed with the recessive parent in order to know its genotype is called

[AIPMT MAINS 2010]

(a) Monohybrid cross (b) Back cross
(c) Test cross (d) Dihybrid cross

4. ABO blood grouping is controlled by gene I which has three alleles and show co-dominance. There are six genotypes. How many phenotypes in all are possible?

[AIPMT MAINS 2010]

(a) Six (b) Three
(c) Four (d) Five

5. The fruit fly Drosophila melanogaster was found to be very suitable for experimental verification of chromosomal theory of inheritance by Morgan and his colleagues because: [AIPMT MAINS 2010]

(a) It reproduces parthenogenetically
(b) A single mating produces two young flie
(c) Smaller female is easily recognisable from larger male
(d) It completes life cycle in about two weeks

6. The fruit fly, drosophila melanogaster was found to be very suitable for experimental verification of chromosomal theory of inheritance by Morgan and his colleagues because: [AIPMT MAINS 2010]

(a) It reproduces parthenogenetically
(b) A single mating produces two young flies
(c) Smaller female is easily recognisable from larger male
(d) It completes life cycle in about two weeks

7. Which one of the following cannot be explained on the basis of Mendel's Law of Dominance? [AIPMT PRE 2010]

(a) The discrete unit controlling a particular character is called a factor
(b) Out of one pair of factors one is dominant, and the other recessive
(c) Alleles do not show any blending and both the characters recover as such in F_2 generation
(d) Factors occur in pairs

8. The genotype of a plant showing the dominant phenotype can be determined by: [AIPMT PRE 2010]

(a) Test cross (b) Dihybrid cross
(c) Pedigree analysis (d) Back cross

9. ABO blood groups in humans are controlled by the gene I. It has three alleles - 1^A, I^B and i. Since there are three different alleles, six different genotypes are possible. How many phenotypes can occur? [AIPMT PRE 2010]

(a) Three (b) One
(c) Four (d) Two

10. Select the correct statement from the ones given below with respect to dihybrid cross. [AIPMT PRE 2010]

(a) Tightly linked genes on the same chromosome show higher recombinations
(b) Genes far apart on the same chromosome show very few recombinations
(c) Genes loosely linked on the same chromosome show similar recombinations as the tightly linked ones
(d) Tightly linked genes on the same chromosome show very few recombinations

11. Which one of the following symbols and its representation, used in human pedigree analysis is correct? [AIPMT PRE 2010]

(a) □=○ = Mating between relatives
(b) ○ = Unaffected male
(c) □ = Unaffected female
(d) ◈ = Male affected

12. Which one of the following conditions correctly describes the manner of determining the sex in the given example?

[AIPMT PRE 2011]

(a) XO type of sex chromosomes determine male sex in grasshopper
(b) XO condition in humans as found in Turner syndrome, determines female sex
(c) Homozygous sex chromosomes (XX) produce male in Drosophila
(d) Homozygous sex chromosomes (ZZ) determine female sex in birds

13. A collection of plants and seeds, having diverse alleles of all the genes of a crop, is called

[AIPMT PRE 2011]

(a) Germplasm
(b) Gene library
(c) Genome
(d) Herbarium

14. When two unrelated individuals or lines are crossed, the performance of F_1 hybrid is often superior to both its parents. This phenomenon is called:

[AIPMT PRE 2011]

(a) Transformation
(b) Splicing
(c) Metamorphosis
(d) Heterosis

15. Test cross in plants or in Drosophila involves crossing

[AIPMT MAINS 2011]

(a) Between two genotypes with recessive trait
(b) Between two F_1 hybrids
(c) The F_1 hybrid with a double recessive genotype
(d) Between two genotype with dominant trait

16. Which one of the following conditions of the zygotic cell would lead to the birth of a normal human female child?

[AIPMT MAINS 2011]

(a) Two X chromosome
(b) Only one Y chromosome
(c) Only one X chromosome
(d) One X and one Y chromosome

17. Read the following four statements (A - D):

[AIPMT MAINS 2012]

(A) In transcription, adenosine pairs with uracil
(B) Regulation of lac operon by repressor is referred to as positive regulation
(C) The human genome has approximately 50,000 genes
(D) Haemophilia is a sex-linked recessive disease

How many of the above statements are right?

(a) 3
(b) 4
(c) 1
(d) 2

18. A test cross is carried out to:

[AIPMT MAINS 2012]

(a) Predict whether two traits are linked
(b) Assess the number of alleles of a gene
(c) Determine whether two species or varieties will breed successfully
(d) Determine the genotype of a plant at F_2

19. Represented below is the inheritance pattern of the certain type of traits in humans. Which one of the following conditions could be an example of this pattern?

[AIPMT MAINS 2012]

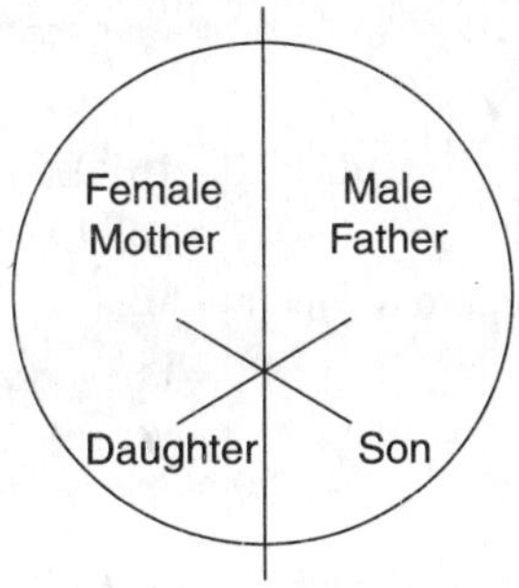

(a) Sickel cell anaemia (b) Haemophilia
(c) Thalassemia (d) Phenylketonuria

20. A normal-visioned man whose father was colour-blind, marries a women whose father was also colour-blind. They have their first child as a daughter. What are the chances that this child would be colour-blind".

[AIPMT PRE 2012]

(a) 100% (b) Zero percent
(c) 25% (d) 50%

21. F_2 generation in a Mendelion cross showed that both genotypic and phenotypic rations are same as 1:2:1. It represents a case of:

[AIPMT PRE 2012]

(a) Co-dominance
(b) Dihybrid cross
(c) Monohybrid cross with complete dominance
(d) Monohybrid cross with incomplete dominance

22. Which of the following statements is not true of two genes that shows 50% recombination frequency?

[AIPMT 2013]

(a) The genes may be on different chromosomes
(b) The genes are tightly linked
(c) The genes show independent assortment
(d) If the genes are present on the same chromosome, they undergo more than one crossovers in every meiosis

23. Variation in gene frequencies within populations can occur by change rather than by natural selection. This is referred to as:

[AIPMT 2013]

(a) Genetic flow (b) Genetic drift
(c) Random mating (d) Genetic load

24. If two persons with 'AB' blood group marry and have sufficiently large number of children, these children could be classified as 'A' blood group: 'AB' blood group: 'B' blood group in 1:2:1 ratio. Modern technique of protein electrophoresis reveals presence of both 'A' and 'B' type proteins in 'AB' blood group individuals. This is an example of:

[AIPMT 2013]

(a) Codominance (b) Incomplete dominance
(c) Partial dominance (d) Complete dominance

25. Which Mendelian idea is depicted by a cross in which the F_1 generation resembles both the parents?

[AIPMT 2013]

(a) Incomplete dominance (b) Law of dominance
(c) Inheritance of one gene (d) Co–dominance

26. The incorrect statement with regard to Haemophilia is:

[AIPMT 2013]

(a) It is a sex – linked disease
(b) It is a recessive disease
(c) It is a dominant disease
(d) A single protein involved in the clotting of blood is affected

27. If both parents are carriers for the thalessemia, which is an autosomal recessive disorder, what are the chances of pregnancy resulting in an affected child?

[AIPMT 2013]

(a) No chance (b) 50%
(c) 25% (d) 100%

28. Fruit colour in squash is an example of:

[AIPMT 2014]

(a) Recessive epistasis (b) Dominant epistasis
(c) Complementary genes (d) Inhibitory genes

29. A man whose father was colour blind marries a woman who had a colour blind mother and normal father. What percentage of male children of this couple will be colour blind?

[AIPMT 2014]

(a) 25% (b) 0%
(c) 50% (d) 75%

30. In a population of 1000 individuals 360 belong to genotype AA, 480 to Aa and the remaining 160 to aa. Based on this data, the frequency of allele A in the population is:

[AIPMT 2014]

(a) 0.4 (b) 0.5
(c) 0.6 (d) 0.7

31. A human female with Turner's syndrome:

[AIPMT 2014]

(a) Has 45 chromosomes with XO
(b) Has one additional X chromosome
(c) Exhibits male characters
(d) Is able to produce children with normal husband

32. How many pairs by contrasting characters in pea plants was studied by Mendel in his experiments?

[AIPMT 2015]

(a) Five (b) Six
(c) Eight (d) Seven

33. The movement of a gene from one linkage group to another is called:

[AIPMT 2015]

(a) Inversion (b) Duplication
(c) Translocation (d) Crossing over

34. Multiple alleles are present:

[AIPMT 2015]

(a) On different chromosomes
(b) At different location the same chromosome
(c) At the same locus of the chromosome
(d) On non sister chromatids

35. An abnormal human baby with 'XXX' sex chromosomes was born due to:

[AIPMT 2015]

(a) Formation of abnormal sperms in the father
(b) Formation of abnormal ova in the mother
(c) Fusion of two ova and one sperm
(d) Fusion two sperms and one ovum

36. Alleles are :

[AIPMT 2015]

(a) Different phenotype
(b) True breeding homozygotes
(c) Different molecular forms of a gene
(d) Heterozygotes

37. A man with blood group 'A' marries a woman with blood group 'B'. which are all the possible blood groups of their offsprings?

[AIPMT 2015]

(a) A and B only
(b) A, B and AB only
(c) A, B, AB and O
(d) O only

38. In his classic experiments on pea plants, Mendel did not use.

[RE-AIPMT 2015]

(a) Pod length
(b) Seed shape
(c) Flower position
(d) Seed colour

39. A pleiotropic gene:

[RE-AIPMT 2015]

(a) Is a gene evolved during Pliocene
(b) Controls a trait only in combination with another gene
(c) Controls multiple traits in an individual
(d) Is expressed only in primitive plants

40. A gene showing codominance has:

[RE-AIPMT 2015]

(a) Alleles tightly linked on the same chromosome
(b) Alleles that are recessive to each other
(c) Both alleles independently expressed in the heterozygote
(d) One allele dominant on the other

41. A colour blind man marries a woman with normal sight who has no history of colour blindness in her family. What is the probability of their grandson being colour blind?

[RE-AIPMT 2015]

(a) 1
(b) Nil
(c) 0.25
(d) 0.5

42. The term "linkage" was coined by:

[RE-AIPMT 2015]

(a) T. Boveri
(b) G. Mendel
(c) W. Sutton
(d) T.H. Morgan

43. In the following human pedigree, the filled symbols represent the affected individual. Identify the type of given pedigree.

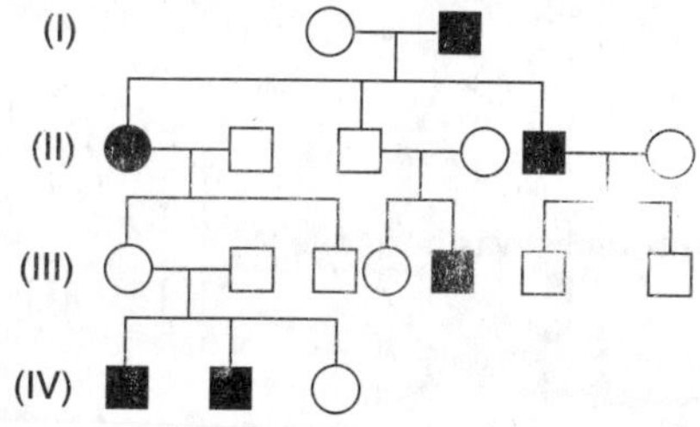

[RE-AIPMT 2015]

(a) X-linked recessive
(b) Autosomal recessive
(c) X-linked dominant
(d) Autosomal dominant

Answer Keys

1. (c)	2. (d)	3. (a)	4. (c)	5. (a)	6. (d)	7. (c)	8. (a)	9. (b)	10. (b)
11. (c)	12. (c)	13. (b)	14. (a)	15. (a)	16. (a)	17. (d)	18. (a)	19. (b)	20. (d)
21. (d)	22. (b)	23. (b)	24. (a)	25. (d)	26. (a)	27. (c)	28. (c)	29. (d)	30. (d)
31. (b)	32. (b)	33. (b)	34. (a)	35. (b)	36. (b)	37. (c)	38. (a)	39. (b)	40. (c)
41. (b)	42. (c)	43. (b)	44. (d)	45. (d)	46. (a)	47. (a)	48. (b)	49. (a)	50. (d)
51. (b)	52. (d)	53. (a)	54. (d)	55. (d)	56. (a)	57. (b)	58. (a)	59. (c)	60. (c)
61. (a)	62. (d)	63. (a)	64. (c)	65. (c)	66. (c)	67. (c)	68. (b)	69. (d)	70. (b)
71. (c)	72. (d)	73. (b)	74. (d)	75. (c)	76. (d)	77. (d)	78. (a)	79. (b)	80. (b)
81. (a)	82. (c)	83. (d)	84. (c)	85. (b)	86. (d)	87. (a)	88. (d)	89. (d)	90. (c)
91. (c)	92. (b)	93. (a)	94. (b)	95. (c)	96. (c)	97. (c)	98. (a)	99. (b)	100. (b)
101. (c)	102. (d)	103. (c)	104. (d)	105. (c)	106. (c)	107. (c)	108. (a)	109. (c)	110. (b)
111. (a)	112. (d)	113. (d)	114. (a)	115. (b)	116. (d)	117. (c)	118. (d)	119. (a)	120. (c)
121. (a)	122. (b)	123. (c)	124. (b)	125. (a)	126. (c)	127. (c)	128. (a)	129. (b)	130. (a)
131. (a)	132. (a)	133. (a)	134. (b)	135. (c)	136. (b)	137. (a)	138. (a)	139. (c)	140. (c)
141. (b)	142. (c)	143. (a)	144. (c)	145. (c)	146. (d)	147. (c)	148. (d)	149. (c)	150. (d)
151. (c)	152. (c)	153. (a)	154. (b)	155. (d)	156. (d)	157. (a)	158. (b)	159. (c)	160. (d)
161. (b)	162. (d)	163. (a)	164. (b)	165. (b)	166. (b)	167. (d)	168. (c)	169. (d)	170. (d)
171. (d)	172. (d)	173. (b)	174. (b)	175. (b)	176. (b)	177. (b)	178. (d)	179. (d)	180. (c)
181. (d)	182. (c)	183. (c)	184. (d)	185. (b)	186. (b)	187. (b)	188. (a)	189. (c)	190. (a)
191. (b)	192. (b)	193. (a)	194. (d)	195. (c)	196. (c)	197. (d)	198. (a)	199. (b)	200. (c)
201. (b)	202. (a)	203. (a)	204. (b)	205. (d)					

AIPMT Previous Year Questions

1. (a)	2. (c)	3. (c)	4. (c)	5. (d)	6. (d)	7. (c)	8. (a)	9. (c)	10. (d)
11. (a)	12. (a)	13. (a)	14. (d)	15. (c)	16. (a)	17. (d)	18. (a)	19. (b)	20. (b)
21. (d)	22. (b)	23. (b)	24. (a)	25. (d)	26. (c)	27. (c)	28. (b)	29. (c)	30. (c)
31. (a)	32. (d)	33. (c)	34. (c)	35. (b)	36. (c)	37. (c)	38. (a)	39. (c)	40. (c)
41. (b)	42. (d)	43. (d)							

CHAPTER 28

Molecular Basis of Inheritance

Figure given for questions 1 and 2.

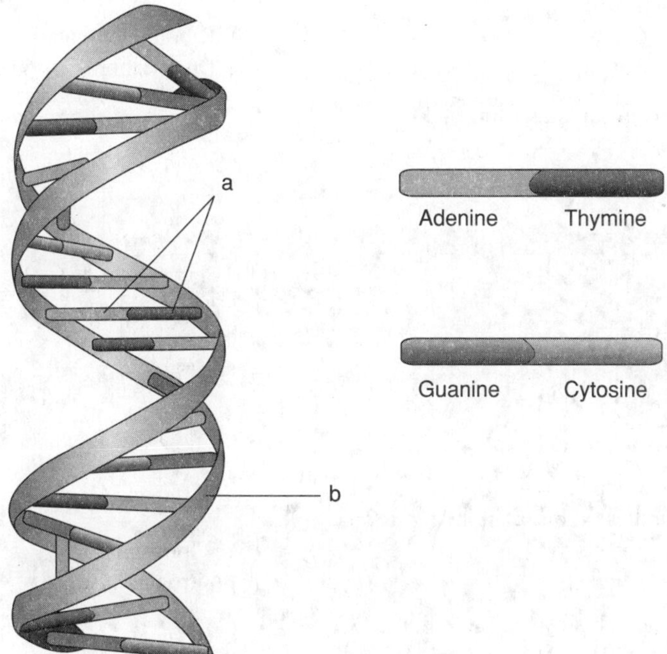

1. What is indicated by 'a' in the figure?
   (a) Sugar
   (b) Phosphate
   (c) Base pairs
   (d) Singular bases
2. What is indicated by 'b' in the figure?
   (a) Base pair end
   (b) Only sugar backbone
   (c) Only phosphate backbone
   (d) Both (b) and (c)
3. How many types of nucleic acids are found in living systems?
   (a) Three
   (b) One
   (c) Two
   (d) Four

4. Which nucleic acid, in some viruses, can also act as genetic material?
(a) DNA (b) RNA
(c) mRNA (d) tRNA

5. The process of making RNA from DNA is termed as
(a) Transaction (b) Transformation
(c) Transcription (d) Transduction

6. The genetic code
(a) is a sequence of nucleotides on rRNA
(b) determines the sequence of amino acid in proteins
(c) is universal in biological systems
(d) none of the above

7. The process of protein synthesis in biological systems is termed as
(a) Transaction (b) Transcription
(c) Translation (d) Transformation

8. DNA is a polymer of
(a) Nucleotides (b) Ribonucleotides
(c) Nucleosides (d) Deoxyribonucleotides

Figure given for questions 9–11.

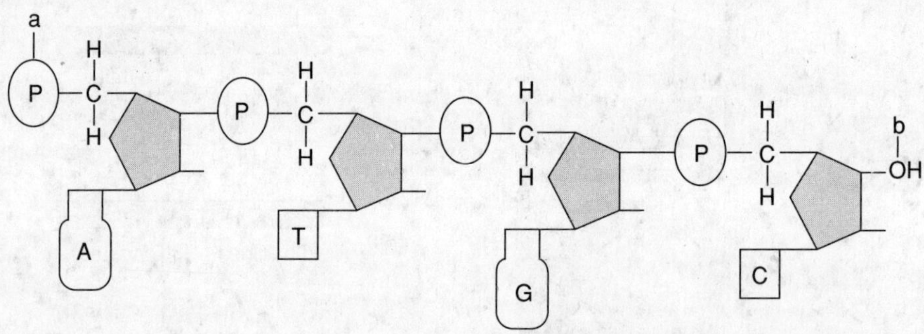

9. What is indicated by 'a' in the figure?
(a) 5' phosphate (b) 3' phosphate
(c) Ribose sugar (d) nitrogen base

10. What is indicated by 'b' in the figure?
(a) 5' phosphate (b) 3' hydroxyl
(c) Ribose sugar (d) nitrogen base

11. What does the figure represent?
(a) Polysaccharide (b) Polynucleoside
(c) Polynucleotide (d) Polyamine

12. The length of DNA is defined in terms of
(a) No. of nucleotides (b) Base pairs
(c) Both (a) and (b) (d) μm

13. A bacteriophage φ × 174 has
(a) 5836 base pairs (b) 5683 nucleotides
(c) 5386 nucleotides (d) 5638 base pairs

14. Bacteriophage lambda has ________ base pairs in nucleic acid (genetic material).
   (a) 48205
   (b) 5386
   (c) 48502
   (d) 45802
15. Which of the following holds true for Escherichia coli?
   (a) E. coli has roughly 40 minutes of doubling time.
   (b) E. coli is a parasite in human digestive tract.
   (c) E. coli has 4.6×10^9bp long genetic material.
   (d) E. coli has 4.6×10^6bp long genetic material.
16. A nucleotide has the following components
   (a) A phosphate group, nitrogenous base, a hexose sugar
   (b) A phosphorous base, nitrogenous group, a ribose sugar
   (c) A nitrogenous base, phosphate group, a ribose sugar
   (d) A nitrogenous base, phosphate group, a hexose sugar
17. Which of the following is not a pyrimidine?
   (a) Thymine
   (b) Uracil
   (c) Adenine
   (d) Cytosine
18. What is represented by the figure?

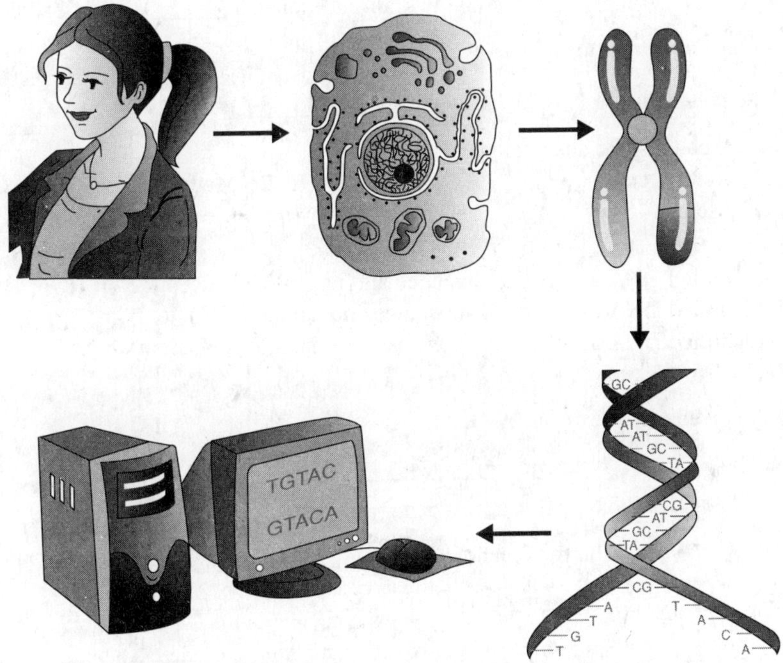

   (a) Criminal/Suspect identification
   (b) Human genome project
   (c) Recombinant DNA technology
   (d) Development of Bioinformatics
19. ________ is present in DNA only and ________ is present in RNA only
   (a) Cytosine, thymine
   (b) Thymine, uracil
   (c) Uracil, thymine
   (d) Thymine, cytosine

20. A nitrogenous base is linked to the pentose sugar through
(a) Phosphoester linkage
(b) O-Glycosidic linkage
(c) Phosphodiester linkage
(d) N-glycosidic linkage

21. In context of genetic material: Base + Sugar ⟶
(a) Nucleotide
(b) Nucleoside
(c) Nucleic acid
(d) Nuclein

22. In the context of genetic material, nucleotide consists of
(a) N-base, Ribose sugar, Phosphate group
(b) N-base, Hexose sugar, Phosphate group
(c) Nucleoside + Phosphate
(d) Both (a) and (c)

23. Uracil is associated with which sugar?
(a) Generally Deoxyribose
(b) Sometimes Ribose
(c) Only ribose
(d) Hexose

24. 5 - end of ribose sugar bears
(a) N-base
(b) Deoxyribose
(c) Phosphate group
(d) Hydroxyl group

25. 3′ end of the polynucleotide chain bears
(a) Phosphate group
(b) Hydroxyl group
(c) Methyl group
(d) Nitro group

26. In RNA, every nucleotide residue has an additional ________ group present at ________ position of ribose
(a) PO_4^{3-}, 3′
(b) OH^-, 3
(c) OH^-, 2
(d) OH^-, 2′

27. Thymine can also be designated as
(a) 3 - Methyl uracil
(b) 2 - Methyl uracil
(c) 4 - Methyl uracil
(d) 5 - Methyl Uracil

28. Friedrich Miescher
(a) Identified DNA as a basic substance and named it 'Nucleotide' in 1896
(b) Identified DNA as an acidic substance and named it 'Nuclein' in 1896
(c) Identified DNA as an acidic substance and named it 'Nuclein' in 1869
(d) None of the above

Figure given for questions 29–32.

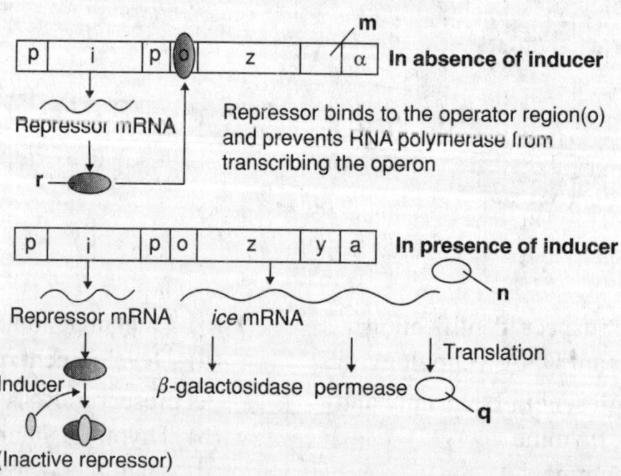

29. What is indicated by 'm' in the figure?
(a) y gene
(b) o gene
(c) z gene
(d) a gene

30. What is indicated by 'r' in the figure?
(a) Suppresor
(b) Operator
(c) Repressor
(d) Inducer

31. What is indicated by 'n' in the figure?
(a) Induction
(b) Replication
(c) Transcription
(d) Derepression

32. What is indicated by 'q' in the figure?
(a) Lactase
(b) Transacetylase
(c) β-galactosidase
(d) Permease

33. J.D. Watson and F.H. Crick utilized X-ray diffraction data produced by
(a) Rosalind Wilkins and Maurice Franklin
(b) Maurice Wilkins and Rosalind Franklin
(c) Sutton and Boveri
(d) None of the above

34. Erwin Chargaff found that
(a) Ratios of adenine and cytosine and thymine and guanine are constant.
(b) Ratios of adenine and thymine and guanine and cytosine are constant.
(c) Ratios of adenine and guanine and thymine and cytosine are constant.
(d) Ratios of adenine – guanine and thymine – cytosine are constant.

35. DNA has two strands which are ________ to each other.
(a) supplementary
(b) complementary
(c) opposite
(d) perpendicular

Figure given for questions 36–37.

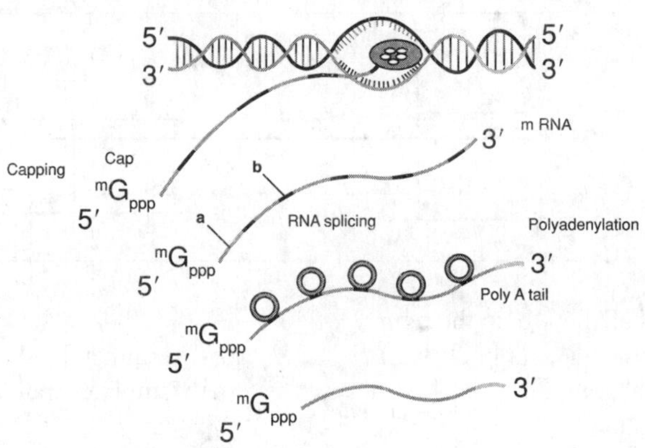

Messenger RNA (m RNA)

36. What is indicated by 'a' in the figure?
(a) Extron
(b) Intron
(c) Intein
(d) Exon

37. What does 'b' represent in the figure?
(a) Extron
(b) Intron
(c) Intein
(d) Exon

38. The backbone of DNA double helix consists of
(a) Sugar-Base
(b) Sugar-Phosphate
(c) Sugar-Hydroxyl group
(d) Sugar-Methyl group
39. Anti-parallel polarity is exhibited by
(a) RNA
(b) t-RNA
(c) mRNA
(d) DNA
40. Which of the following holds true in case of DNA?
(a) A = T
(b) Adenine forms two H-bond with thymine
(c) Adenine forms one π bond with thymine
(d) Both (a) and (b)
41. Three H-bcnds is exhibited by which DNA bases in double helix structure?
(a) Adenine, Guanine
(b) Guanine, Cytosine
(c) Cytosine, Thymine
(d) Adenine, Thymine
42. Double helix model of DNA has a pitch of
(a) 0.34 nm
(b) 3.4 nm
(c) 34 Å
(d) Both (b) and (c)
43. Double helix model of DNA proposed by Watson and Crick has how many base pairs in one turn?
(a) 9
(b) 11
(c) 12
(d) 10
44. What confers additional stability to double helix model of DNA apart from the H-bond?
(a) One base pair provides inductive effect to the other.
(b) One base pair is stacked over the other.
(c) One base pair is perpendicular to another.
(d) One base pair interacts with another base pair via steric hindrance.

Figure given for questions 45–49.

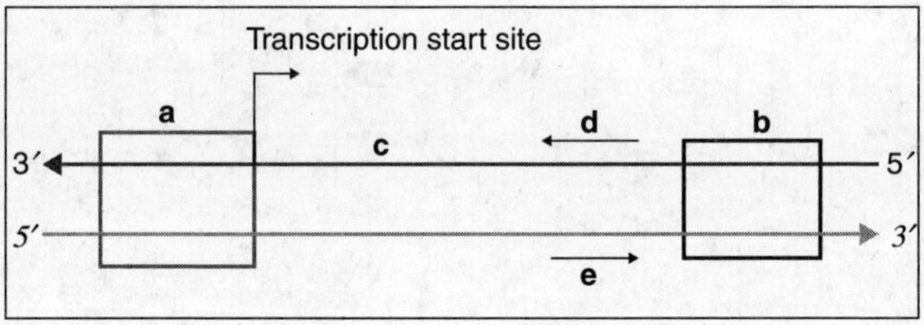

45. What is indicated by 'b' in the figure?
(a) Promoter
(b) Terminator
(c) Structural gene
(d) Template strand
(e) Coding strand
46. What is indicated by 'e' in the figure?
(a) Terminator
(b) Structural gene
(c) Coding strand
(d) Promoter
(e) Template strand
47. What does 'd' represent in the figure?
(a) Template strand
(b) Promoter
(c) Terminator
(d) Structural gene
(e) Coding strand

48. What is indicated by ‘a’ in the figure?
    (a) Promoter
    (b) Terminator
    (c) Structural gene
    (d) Template strand
    (e) Coding strand
49. What does ‘c’ represent in the figure?
    (a) Coding strand
    (b) Template strand
    (c) Promoter
    (d) Terminator
    (e) Structural gene
50. Central dogma in molecular biology was independently proposed by
    (a) Wilkins
    (b) Crick
    (c) Watson
    (d) Franklin
51. Correct representation of central dogma is as follows
    (a) DNA $\xrightarrow{\text{Transcription}}$ mRNA $\xrightarrow{\text{Transformation}}$ Protein
    (b) DNA $\xrightarrow{\text{Transcription}}$ $\circlearrowleft$ mRNA $\xrightarrow{\text{Translation}}$ Proteins
    (c) Replication $\circlearrowleft$ DNA $\xrightarrow{\text{Transcription}}$ mRNA $\xrightarrow{\text{Transformation}}$ Proteins
    (d) Replication $\circlearrowleft$ DNA $\xrightarrow{\text{Transcription}}$ mRNA $\xrightarrow{\text{Translation}}$ Proteins
52. Which of the unusual metabolic process is shown by viruses?
    (a) DNA to RNA
    (b) RNA to DNA
    (c) Proteins to RNA
    (d) None of these
53. RNA $\longrightarrow$ DNA is termed as
    (a) Reverse translation
    (b) Reverse replication
    (c) Reverse transcription
    (d) Reverse transformation
54. The length of human DNA is approximately
    (a) 2.2 meters considering all cells of body
    (b) 3.1 meters considering only one cell
    (c) 2.2 meters considering only one cell
    (d) None of the above
55. DNA is held together by which proteins in prokaryotes?
    (a) Negatively charged proteins
    (b) Positively charged proteins
    (c) Amphoteric proteins
    (d) Histone proteins
56. Which statement is true in the context of histones?
    (a) They are positively charged acidic proteins
    (b) They are positively charged amphoteric protein
    (c) They are positively charged basic proteins
    (d) None of the above
57. In a nucleosome, histones are organized in which structure?
    (a) Octamer
    (b) Hexamer
    (c) Decamer
    (d) Septamer

58. The initial structure formed at the beginning of coiling of DNA around histones is
(a) Nuclein (b) Solenoid
(c) Nucleosome (d) Chromatin

59. Histones are rich in which amino acid?
(a) Methionine, Arginine (b) Lysine, Arginine
(c) Lysine, Proline (d) Methionine, Lysine

60. Typically a nucleosome consists of how many base pairs?
(a) 190 (b) 200
(c) 300 (d) 310

61. Chromatin is made up of
(a) Centromere (b) Nucleoid
(c) Centrosome (d) Nucleosome

Figure given for questions 62–65.

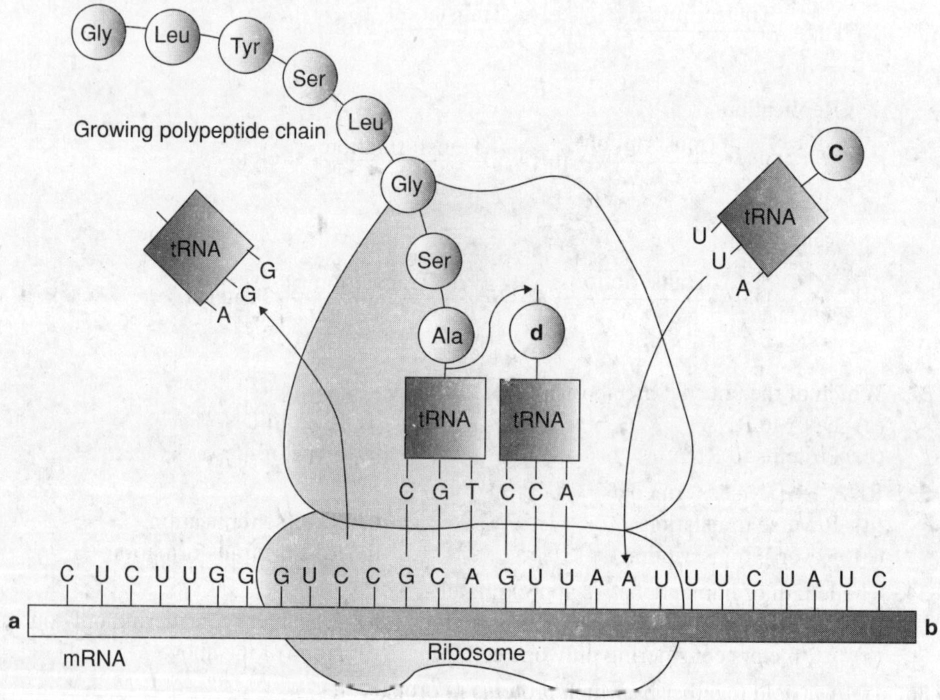

62. Which end of mRNA is shown by 'a' in the figure?
(a) 3′ (b) 3
(c) 5′ (d) 5

63. Which end of mRNA is shown by 'b' in the figure?
(a) 5′ (b) 5
(c) 3 (d) 3′

64. Which amino acid is shown by 'c' in the figure?
(a) Aspartic acid (b) Asparagine
(c) Alanine (d) Valine

65. Which amino acid is indicated by 'd' in the figure?
 (a) Glycine (b) Methionine
 (c) Alanine (d) Valine
66. 'Beads-on-string' structure can be viewed under:
 (a) Light microscope (b) Compound microscope
 (c) Confocal Laser microscope (d) Electron microscope
67. 'Beads-on-string' structure in chromatin is packaged to form ________.
 (a) Nucleosomes (b) Solenoids
 (c) Chromatin fibres (d) Chromatids
68. Chromatin fibres coil and condense at ________ stage of cell division to form ________.
 (a) prophase, nucleosomal (b) telophase, solenoid
 (c) metaphase, chromosome (d) anaphase, chromatid
69. Apart from histones, chromatin at higher level of coiling requires which proteins?
 (a) Neo Histone complex proteins (b) None Histone chromatic proteins
 (c) Non histone chromosomal proteins (d) None of the above

Figure given for questions 70–71.

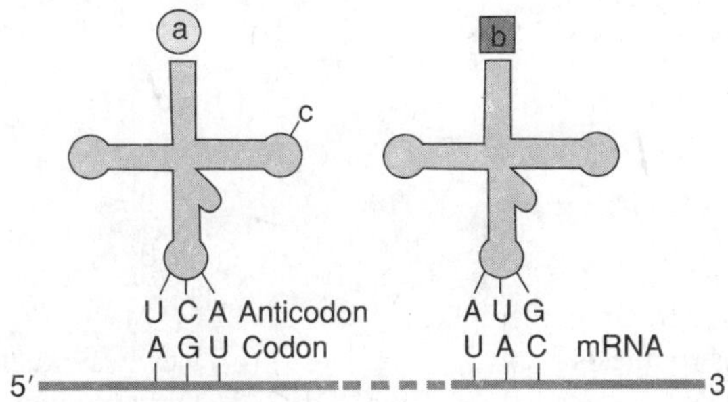

70. Which protein is indicated by 'a' in the figure?
 (a) Threonine (b) Serine
 (c) Tyrosine (d) Methionine
71. Which protein is indicated by 'b' in the figure?
 (a) Threonine (b) Serine
 (c) Tyrosine (d) Methionine
72. In the nucleus, the region of chromatin which is loosely packed is known as
 (a) Heterochromatin (b) Chromatin fibres
 (c) Euchromatin (d) Chromosome
73. Which is true about the structure of Heterochromatin?
 (a) Loosely packed; Stain light (b) Loosely packed; Stain dark
 (c) Densely packed; Stain light (d) Densely packed; Stain dark
74. Transformation experiments in search of genetic material were performed by
 (a) G.J. Mandel (b) T.H. Morgan
 (c) F. Griffith (d) F.H. Crick
75. Griffith carried out his experiments on mice using which pathogenic bacterium?
 (a) Haemophilus influenza (b) Corynebacterium diphtheria
 (c) Streptococcus pneumoniae (d) Yersinia pestis

76. In Griffith's experiment, heat killed S-strain when injected into mice resulted in ________.
(a) diseased condition only
(b) death only
(c) no disease or death
(d) Hybrid formation

77. The transforming principle in Griffith's experiment was detected
(a) When live S-strain of S. pneumoniae were injected in R stain
(b) When live R-strain of S. pneumoniae were injected in S-strain
(c) When heat killed R-strain of S. pneumoniae were injected in S-strain
(d) When heat killed S-strain of S. pneumonia were injected in R-strain

78. Oswald Avery, Colin MacLeod and Maclyn Mc Carty (1933 – 44) worked to determine the ________ nature of 'transforming principle' in Griffith's experiment.
(a) physical
(b) morphological
(c) structural
(d) biochemical

Figure given for questions 79–82.

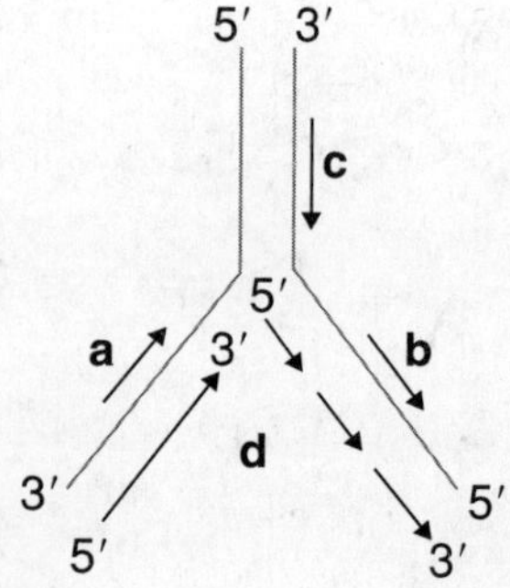

79. What is indicated by 'd' in the figure?
(a) Continuous synthesis
(b) Newly synthesised strands
(c) Template DNA
(d) Discontinuous synthesis

80. What does 'b' represent in figure?
(a) Template DNA
(b) Continuous synthesis
(c) Discontinuous synthesis
(d) Newly synthesised strands

81. What is indicated by 'a' in the figure?
(a) Newly synthesised strands
(b) Discontinuous synthesis
(c) Template DNA
(d) Continuous synthesis

82. What does 'c' represent in the figure?
(a) Template DNA
(b) Continuous synthesis
(c) Discontinuous synthesis
(d) Newly synthesised strands

83. RNA digesting enzymes are commonly known as
(a) Ribozymes
(b) Ribosomes
(c) RNases
(d) Ribulose

84. What is the difference between DNAs and DNase?
(a) Genetic material—DNA digesting enzyme
(b) DNA digesting enzyme—Genetic material
(c) Protein—Peptide
(d) None of the above

85. The experiment which provides unequivocal proof that DNA is genetic material came from the experiment of:
(a) Watson and Crick
(b) Wilkins and Franklin
(c) Hershey and Chase
(d) Avery, MacLeod and Maclyn Mc Carty

86. In the Hershey–Chase experiments the following isotopes were used
(a) ^{32}S, ^{30}P (b) ^{31}S, ^{29}P
(c) ^{35}S, ^{32}P (d) ^{34}S, ^{33}P

87. The Hershey–Chase experiments show the following steps chronologically:
(a) Blending, Infection, Centrifugation (b) Centrifugation, Infection, Blending
(c) Infection, Centrifugation, Blending (d) Infection, Blending, Centrifugation

88. In Hershey–Chase experiments, ^{35}S labelled ________ and ^{32}P labelled ________ respectively.
(a) Bacteria, DNA (b) DNA, Protein
(c) Protein, DNA (d) DNA, mRNA

89. DNA is a preferred genetic material over RNA due to one of the following reasons
(a) Bases are arranged linearly in a single strand.
(b) Bases show less propensity of mutation.
(c) 2' OH group in RNA is more liable.
(d) None of the above

90. Which was the first genetic material?
(a) DNA (b) RNA
(c) Proteins (d) None

91. 'It has not escaped our notice that the specific pairing we have postulated immediately suggests a possible copying mechanism for the genetic material.'This was a statement of
(a) Wilkins and Franklin (b) Hershey and Chase
(c) Avery, McLeod, McCarty (d) Watson and Crick

Figure given for questions 92–95.

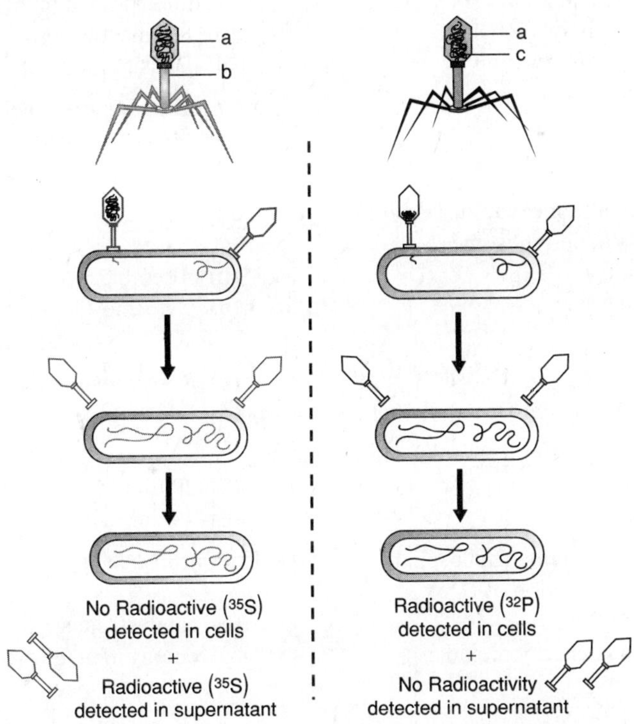

92. Which experiment is shown in the figure?
(a) Griffith's experiment
(b) Avery, MacLeod and Mc Carty
(c) Hershey-Chase experiment
(d) Meselson and Stahl experiment

93. What is indicated by 'a' in the figure?
(a) Bacteriophage
(b) Bacterium
(c) Lichen
(d) Fungus

94. What is indicated by 'b' in the figure?
(a) ^{35}S
(b) ^{32}S
(c) ^{30}P
(d) ^{32}P

95. What is indicated by 'c' in the figure?
(a) ^{35}S
(b) ^{32}S
(c) ^{30}P
(d) ^{32}P

96. After replication, each DNA molecule has one parental and one newly synthesized strand. This scheme is referred to as
(a) Fully conservative
(b) Mutation
(c) Crossing over
(d) Semiconservative

97. Semiconservative replication of DNA was demonstrated by
(a) Meselson and Stahl
(b) Watson and Crick
(c) Hershey and Chase
(d) Wilkins and Franklin

98. In Meselson and Stahl experiment, E. coli was grown in a medium containing
(a) ^{40}KCL
(b) $^{24}NaCl$
(c) $^{15}NH_4Cl$
(d) CsCl

99. In Meselson and Stahl experiment, ^{15}N can only be differentiated on the basis of
(a) Radioactivity
(b) Radioactive t ½
(c) Physical observation
(d) Density gradient

100. Taylor and his colleagues used which plant to detect distribution of newly synthesized DNA?
(a) Pisum sativum
(b) Mirabilis jalapa
(c) Vicia faba
(d) Triticum aestivum

101. Taylor and his colleagues used which radioactive probe to detect distribution of newly synthesized DNA in chromosomes?
(a) Thymine
(b) Ademine
(c) Guanine
(d) Cytosine

102. The process of replication of DNA in E. coli requires an enzyme referred to as
(a) RNA dependent DNA polymerase
(b) RNA polymerase
(c) DNA dependent DNA polymerase
(d) DNA ligase

103. E. coli completes replication in approximately
(a) 15 min
(b) 20 min
(c) 38 min
(d) 40 min

104. Deoxyribonucleotide triphosphate serves the dual purpose of ________ and ________ in the process of replication of DNA.
(a) enzyme, substrate
(b) catalyst, substrate
(c) substrate, energy provider
(d) energy, mutage provider

105. The average rate of polymerization of deoxyribonucleotides in E. coli DNA replication process is

(a) 2500 bp/s (b) 2000 bp/s
(c) 3000 bp/s (d) 3500 bp/s

106. DNA dependent DNA polymerase catalyses polymerization in _______ direction only (in terms of newly synthesized strands).

(a) $5 \longrightarrow 3$ (b) $3' \longrightarrow 5'$
(c) $5' \longrightarrow 3'$ (d) $3 \longrightarrow 5$

Figure given for questions 107–112.

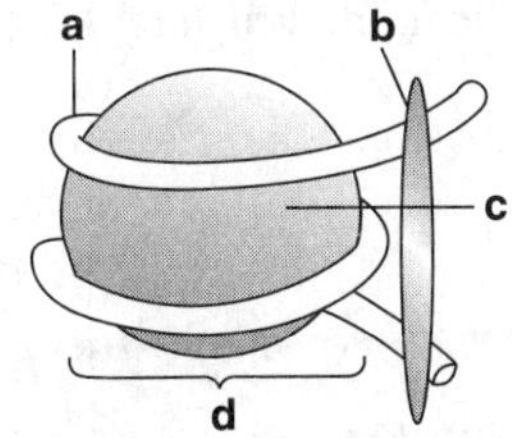

107. The figure shows an essential biomolecule associated with which cell organelle?

(a) Endoplasmic reticulum (b) Ribosome
(c) Nucleus (d) Golgi complex

108. What is indicated by 'a' in the figure?

(a) RNA (b) DNA
(c) Histone octamer (d) H1 histone

109. What is indicated by 'b' in the figure?

(a) RNA (b) DNA
(c) Histone octamer (d) H1 histone

110. What is indicated by 'd' in the figure?

(a) Core of Histone molecule (b) Part of Histone molecule
(c) Histone octamer (d) DNA

111. What is indicated by 'c' in the figure?

(a) Core of Histone molecule (b) Part of Histone molecule
(c) Histone octamer (d) DNA

112. The whole structure indicated in the figure is of ________.

(a) Chromosome (b) Nucleolus
(c) Nucleosome (d) Proteosome

113. Discontinuously synthesized strands of DNA adjacent to ________ DNA template are joined together by ________.

(a) $5 \longrightarrow 3$, DNA endonucleace (b) $3' \longrightarrow 5'$, DNAase
(c) $5' \longrightarrow 3'$, DNA ligase (d) $5 \longrightarrow 3$, DNA ligase

114. During which phase of the cell cycle does replication of DNA takes place in eukaryotes?

(a) G_1 (b) G_0
(c) S (d) G_2

115. The process of copying genetic information from DNA to RNA is known as
(a) Translation (b) Transduction
(c) Transcription (d) Transformation

116. The product of transcription process is in fact
(a) Entire segment of DNA copied to RNA (b) Only segment of DNA copied to RNA
(c) Both (a) and (b) (d) None of these

117. In the process of transcription, the strand of DNA with polarity ________ acts as a ________ strand.
(a) $5' \rightarrow 5'$, Coding strand (b) $3' \rightarrow 5'$ Template strand
(c) $3' \rightarrow 3'$, Coding strand (d) $5' \rightarrow 3'$, Template strand

118. The promoter and ________ flank the structural gene in a transcription unit.
(a) structure (b) regulator
(c) operator (d) terminator

119. A segment of DNA coding for a polypeptide is termed as:
(a) Intron (b) Exon
(c) Cistron (d) Distron

Figure given for questions 120–124.

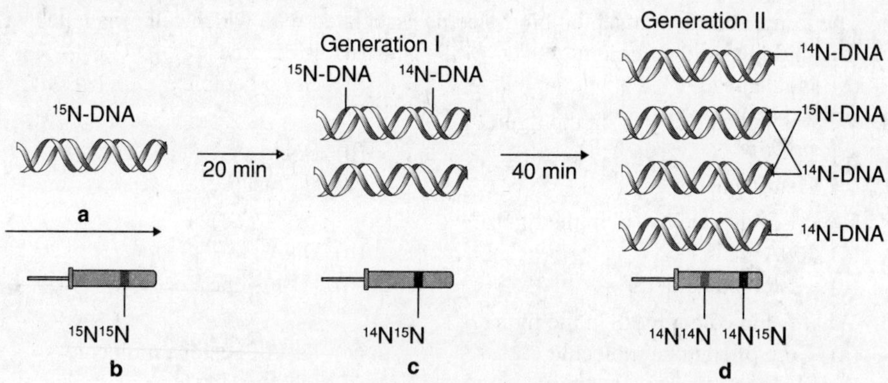

(Separation of DNA by Centrifugation)

120. Which experiment is shown in the figure?
(a) Griffith's experiment (b) Hershay and Chase experiment
(c) Meselson and Stahl experiment (d) Wastson and Crick experiment

121. What is indicated by 'a' in the figure?
(a) Centrifugal force (b) Centripetal force
(c) Gravitational force (d) Radioactive force

122. What is indicated by 'b' in the figure?
(a) Heavy (b) Hybrid
(c) Light (d) Heavy hybrid

123. What is indicated by 'c' in the figure?
(a) Heavy (b) Hybrid
(c) Light (d) Heavy hybrid

124. What is indicated by 'd' in the figure?
(a) Hybrid
(b) light and hybrid
(c) Heavy and hybrid
(d) Heavy and Light

125. The coding sequences of DNA are known as ________ and the intervening sequences are known as ________ respectively.
(a) exon, intron
(b) intron, exon
(c) cistron, exon
(d) exon, cistron

126. In bacteria, which of the following plays a structural and catalytic role in the translation process?
(a) mRNA
(b) rRNA
(c) tRNA
(d) DNA

127. What are the components required for the initiation of transcription in bacteria?
(a) RNA polymerase only
(b) Promoter, RNA polymerase and ρ–factor
(c) ρ factor only
(d) σ factor only

128. **ρ**-factor in the process of transcription in bacteria is also known as
(a) Initiation factor
(b) Elongation factor
(c) Termination factor
(d) Vital factor

129. In bacteria, in context of mRNA, which of the following is not true?
(a) Transcription and translation takes place in different compartment.
(b) Post-transcriptional modifications are required like splicing.
(c) Translation occurs only after transcription.
(d) All of these.

130. Total number of RNA polymerase found in eukaryotes is
(a) 3
(b) 4
(c) 2
(d) 5

131. Which of the following RNA is transcribed by RNA polymerase II in eukaryotes?
(a) tRNA
(b) rRNA
(c) snRNA
(d) hn RNA

132. RNA polymerase I transcribes ________ in eukaryotes.
(a) t RNA
(b) r RNA
(c) sn RNA
(d) hn RNA

133. In eukaryotes, RNA polymerase III is responsible for synthesis of
(a) 28 S RNA, 18 S RNA and 5.8 S RNA
(b) tRNA, hnRNA, rRNA
(c) tRNA, 5sRNA, snRNA
(d) hnRNA, tRNA, rRNA

134. The intervening sequences in the primary transcript of mRNA are removed by
(a) Recombination
(b) Linkage
(c) Capping
(d) Splicing

135. Additional post-transcriptional processing like capping and tailing is characteristic to
(a) rRNA
(b) hnRNA
(c) snRNA
(d) tRNA

136. Which classical model proposed by Watson and Creek is represented by this figure?

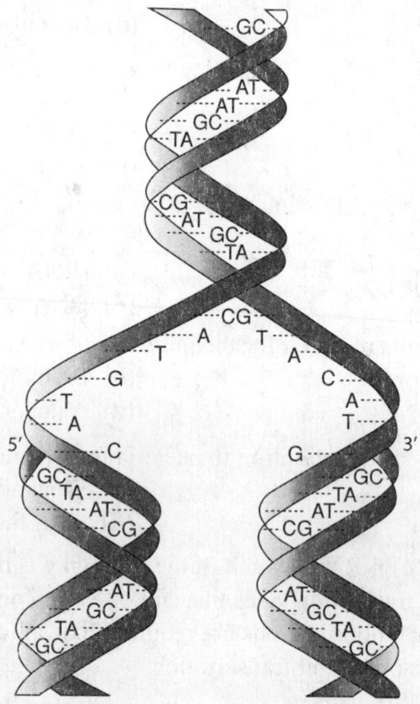

(a) Fully conservative DNA transcription
(b) Semi-conservative RNA replication
(c) Semi-conservative DNA replication
(d) Non-Conservative DNA replication

137. In a post-transcriptional modification, capping adds an unusual nucleotide like
(a) Guanosine triphosphate
(b) Methyl gunanine triphosphate
(c) Methyl guanosine triphosphate
(d) Adenosine triphosphate

138. In a post-transcriptional modification called tailing, ________ residues are added at the ________ of mRNA.
(a) Adenylate, 5′- end
(b) Guanylate, 3′- end
(c) Adenylate, 3′- end
(d) Guanylate, 5'- end

139. mRNA is in fact
(a) Unprocessed rRNA
(b) Unprocessed hnRNA
(c) Processed hnRNA
(d) Processed mRNA itself

140. A physicist, George Gamow, argued that genetic code is a combination of ________ nucleotides.
(a) three
(b) two
(c) four
(d) one

141. Humans requires ________ codons to synthesize 20 amino acids.
(a) 64 codons
(b) 61 codons
(c) 62 codons
(d) 60 codons

142. The chemical method developed by ________ was instrumental in synthesizing RNA molecules with defined combination of bases.
(a) Marshal Nirenberg
(b) George Gamow
(c) Har Gobind Khorana
(d) F.H.C. Crick

143. ________ cell-free system for protein synthesis finally helped the genetic code to be deciphered.
(a) George Gamow's (b) Marshall Nirenberg's
(c) Har Gobind Khorana's (d) J.D. Watson's

144. Some amino acids are coded by more than one codon. Hence the genetic code exhibits
(a) Specificity (b) Selectivity
(c) Degeneracy (d) Regenerancy

145. The codon AUG has dual function as it codes for ________ and also acts as a ________ codon.
(a) phenylalanine, initiator (b) methionine, terminator
(c) methionine, regulator (d) methionine, initiator

146. Sickle cell anaemia is a classic example of
(a) Frame shift mutation (b) Point mutation
(c) Deletion mutation (d) Duplication mutation

147. In sickle cell anaemia, which amino acid modification occurs in the ⊠-chain of amino acid?
(a) Valine → Glutamate (b) Threonine → Valine
(c) Tyrosine → Glutamate (d) Glutamate → Valine

148. tRNA was earlier called
(a) Adapter molecule (b) Special RNA
(c) Protein carrying RNA (d) Soluble RNA

149. For the initiation of translation process, specific tRNAs involved are known as
(a) Helper t-RNA (b) Assistor t-RNA
(c) Initiator t-RNA (d) Terminal t-RNA

Figure given for questions 150 and 151.

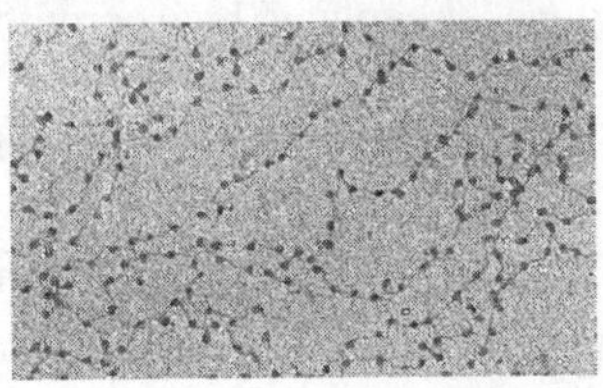

150. The picture is taken using ________ microscope.
(a) Phase contrast (b) Electron
(c) Bright field (d) Fluorescence

151. The picture shows characteristic coiling of DNA known as ________.
(a) Strings-on-beads (b) beads-on-strings
(c) Nanobead coiling (d) None of the above

152. The process of polymerization of amino acids to polypeptide is known as
(a) Pepto-polymerization (b) Transcription
(c) Translation (d) Transformation

153. Charging of tRNA is also known as
(a) Acylation (b) Transmination
(c) Amino allylation (d) Amino acylation

154. tRNA for serine bears anticodon ________.
(a) AUG (b) UAC
(c) UCA (d) UGA

155. The structure of tRNA resembles which leaf?
(a) Olive (b) Neem
(c) Clove (d) Clover

156. Ribosomes are the cellular factory for synthesis of ________.
(a) Carbohydrates (b) Enzymes
(c) Proteins (d) Lipids

157. Ribozyme in bacteria is ________ rRNA.
(a) 30 S (b) 32 S
(c) 23 S (d) 21 S

158. Additional sequences on mRNA referred to as ________ are not translated.
(a) Variable number tandem repeats (b) Non coding sequence
(c) Untranscribed regions (d) Untranslated regions

159. In Eukaryotes, which of the following mechanisms is not correct in terms of regulation of gene expression?
(a) Transcription
(b) Splicing
(c) Transport of mRNA from cytoplasm to nucleus
(d) Translation

160. β-galactosidase is synthesized by E. coli to catalyze hydrolysis of ________ into ________ and glucose.
(a) galactose, lactose (b) galactose, glucose
(c) lactose, galactose (d) maltose, galactose

161. Lac operon was elucidated by
(a) Watson, Crick (b) Jacob, Monod
(c) Johannson (d) Meischer

162. A polycistronic structural gene is regulated by a common promoter and regulator gene in bacteria and is commonly termed as
(a) Codon (b) Operon (c) Genetic code (d) None

163. Regulatory gene 'I' in lac operon is
(a) Inducer (b) Inhibitor (c) Structure (d) Initiator

Figure given for questions 164–166.

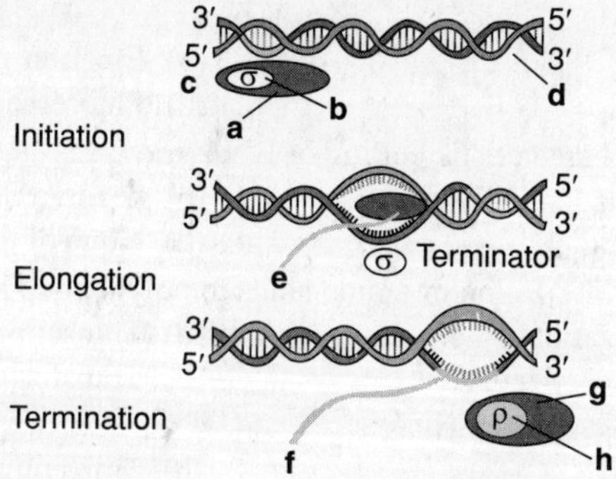

164. What is indicated by 'd' in the figure?
(a) RNA polymerase (b) DNA helix
(c) Sigma factor (d) Promoter

165. What is indicated by 'b' in the figure?
(a) Sigma factor (b) RNA
(c) DNA helix (d) Promoter

166. What does 'h' represent in the figure?
(a) RNA Polymerase (b) RNA
(c) Promoter (d) Rho factor

167. Out of the 3 structural genes z, y and a, the gene (s) which gene of E. coli lac Operon code for permease.
(a) z (b) s
(c) y (d) Both (b) & (c)

168. Repressor protein in lac operon concept binds to which gene?
(a) d (b) i (c) o (d) z

169. In lac operon, the inducer binds to ________ to initiate synthesis of enzymes responsible for lactose metabolism.
(a) i gene (b) Repressor (c) O gene (d) Z gene

170. Lac operon operates in E. Coli ________.
(a) occasionally (b) frequently
(c) all time (d) sometimes

171. Generally regulation of lac operon by repressor is referred to as ________ regulation.
(a) positive (b) negative
(c) feedback (d) both (b) and (c)

172. Considering cost of sequencing 1 bp to be US 3$, 4 the approximate cost of HGP (Human Genome Project) would come out to be ________.
(a) 3 billion (b) 9 million (c) 9 billion (d) 3 million

Figure given for questions 173 and 174.

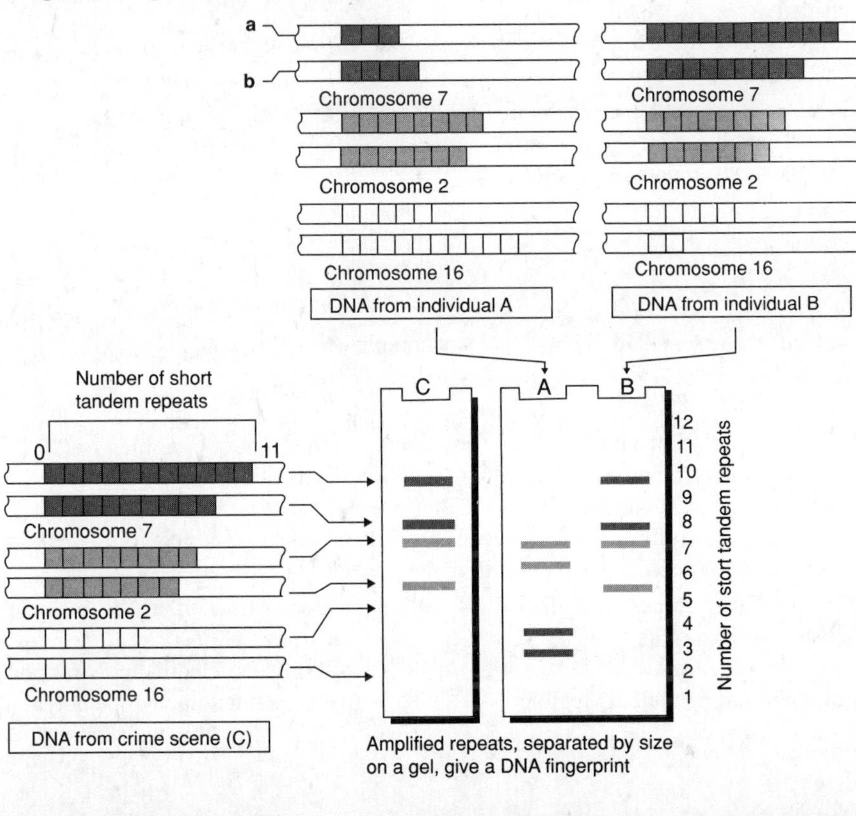

173. What is indicated by 'a' in the figure?
(a) Maternal Chromosome (b) Paternal Chromosome
(c) Foetal Chromosome (d) Sister Chromosome

174. What is indicated by 'b' in the figure?
(a) Maternal Chromosome (b) paternal Chromosome
(c) Foetal Chromosome (d) Sister Chromosome

175. HGP was closely associated with the rapid development of ________.
(a) Chemo informatics (b) Modern genetics
(c) Pharmaco informatics (d) Bioinformatics

176. Human Genome project was a __X__ year long project starting from __Y__ to __Z__.
(a) X = 13, Y = 1980, X = 1993 (b) X = 12, Y = 1990, Z = 2002
(c) X = 13, Y = 1990, Z = 2003 (d) X = 14, Y = 1990, Z = 2004

177. ELSI strands for:
(a) Ethical, Logical and Society Issues (b) Ethical, Legal and Society Issues
(c) Ethical, Logical and Social Issues (d) Ethical, Legal and Social Issues

178. Caenorhabditis elegans is a free-living non-pathogenic ________.
(a) Annelid (b) Nematode
(c) Crustocean (d) Mammal

179. Expressed sequence tags (ESTs) is an approach practised in ________.
(a) DNA fingerprinting (b) DNA sequencing
(c) DNA replicating (d) DNA transformation

180. Sequencing the whole genome of an organism into coding and non-coding sequences is termed as
(a) Sequence determination (b) Sequence detection
(c) Sequence annotation (d) Sequence completion

181. BAC, a vector used in biotechnology for cloning, stands for
(a) Bacterial Actual Chromosome (b) Bacterial Artificial Chromosome
(c) Bacterial Annoted Chromosome (d) None of the above

182. The credit for developing a method for determination of DNA as well as protein sequence goes to
(a) Sanger (b) Watson
(c) Taylor (d) Monod

183. In HGP, the chromosome ________ was completed in May 2006.
(a) 2 (b) 1
(c) 3 (d) 4

184. Which of the following is NOT a salient feature of the Human Genome Project?
(a) The human genome contains 3614.7 million nucleotide bases
(b) Less than 2% genome codes for proteins
(c) Over 50% of the genes discovered are yet to be investigated regarding their functions.
(d) Chromosome Y has the fewest of genes.

185. Under HGP, scientists have located 1.4 million locations where difference in single DNA base exists. It is termed as
(a) Microsatellites (b) Single nucleotide polymorphism
(c) Polymorphonucleuar regions (d) Sequential nucleotide polymorphis

186. DNA fingerprinting is based on the principle of identifying ________ sequences of DNA.
(a) satellite (b) variable
(c) mutated (d) repetitive

187. Variations at genetic level in nucletodies is termed as
(a) Allotropy (b) Polymorphism
(c) Isomerism (d) Tautomerism

188. If inheritable mutation is observed in a population at high frequency, it is termed as
(a) DNA mutation (b) DNA isomerism
(c) DNA polymorphism (d) None

189. The technique of ________ was discovered by Alec Jeffreys.
(a) DNA culture (b) DNA modification
(c) DNA mutation (d) DNA fingerprinting

190. A well-known technique to amplify a small protein of DNA is termed as
(a) PCR (b) VNTR
(c) UTR (d) EST

191. VNTRs vary in size from ________ to ________.
(a) 0.1 to 20 bases (b) 0.1 to 20 kilobases
(c) 0.1 to 20 hectobases (d) 0.1 to 20 decabses

192. Similar DNA finger printing is obtained for
(a) Dizygotic twins (b) Monozygotic twins
(c) Polyzytotic twins (d) None

193. In DNA fingerprinting, the hybridised strands are detected by
(a) Radiometery (b) Radioscopy
(c) Auto radiography (d) Scintillation counter

194. Under HGP, the largest known human gene was of
(a) Somatotrophin (b) Dystrophin
(c) Lactrophin (d) Somatostain

195. What is indicated by 'a' in figure?

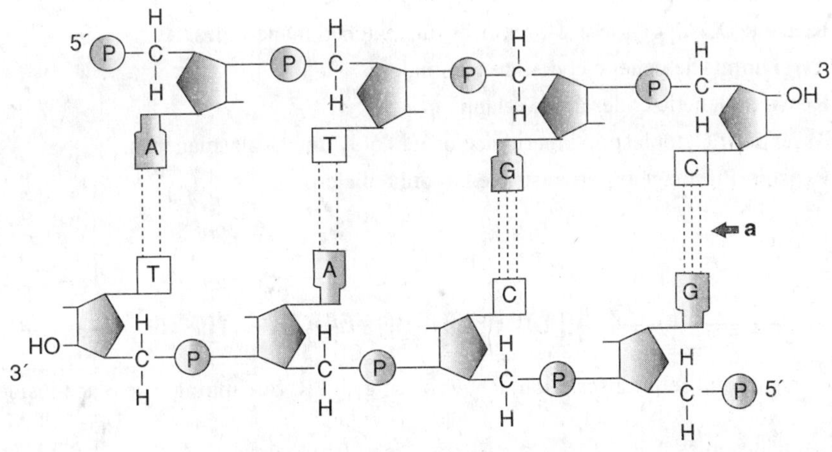

(a) H-bond (b) Ionic bond
(c) Covalent bond (d) van der Waals' bond

*Read the **assertion** and **reason** carefully to mark the correct option out of the options given below:*

(a) If both the assertion and the reason are true and the reason is a correct explanation of the assertion

(b) If both the assertion and reason are true but the reason is not a correct explanation of the assertion

(c) If the assertion is true but the reason is false

(d) If both the assertion and reason are false

196. Assertion: DNA act as the genetic material in most of the organisms.
Reason: DNA is chemically & structurally a stable molecule; has power of replication.

197. Assertion: In RNA the uracil is found at the place of thymine.
Reason: 5 – methyl uracil is chemical name for thymine

198. Assertion: There is uniform distance between two strands of DNA.
Reason: Purine always comes opposite to pyrimidine.

199. Assertion: Chargaff rule is applicable to RNA.
Reason: RNA is double standard molecule.

200. Assertion: Viruses having shorter life span, mutate & evolve faster.
Reason: Viruses have generally RNA genome.

201. Assertion: RNA was first genetic material.
Reason: Essential life processes (such as metabolism, translation, splicing etc.) evolve around RNA.

202. Assertion: UTRs are present at both 5' end and 3'end in m-RNA.
Reason: UTRs are required for efficient translation process.

203. Assertion: DNA polymerase-I acts as proofreader.
Reason: DNA polymerase-I removes mismatched nucleotides.

204. Assertion: The genetic codes are commaless.
Reason: Genetic codes are overlapping.

205. Assertion: Cytoplasmic inheritance occurs only due to plasmagenes.
Reason: Plasmagenes are restricted to only nucleus.

AIPMT PREVIOUS YEAR QUESTIONS

1. In eukaryotic cell transcription, RNA splicing and RNA capping take place inside the [AIPMT MAINS 2010]
(a) Ribosomes (b) Nucleus
(c) Dictyosomes (d) ER

2. Which one of the following statements about the particular entity is true? [AIPMT MAINS 2010]
   (a) Centromere is found in animal cells, which produces aster during cell division
   (b) The gene for producing insulin is present in everybody cell
   (c) Nucleosome is formed of nucleotides
   (d) DNA consists of core of eight histones
3. The lac operon consists of [AIPMT MAINS 2010]
   (a) Four regulatory genes only
   (b) One regulatory gene and three structural genes
   (c) Two regulatory genes and two structural genes
   (d) Three regulatory genes and three structural genes
4. The 3' – 5' phosphodiester linkages inside a polynucleotide chain serve to join [AIPMT MAINS 2010]
   (a) One DNA strand with the other DNA strand
   (b) One nucleoside with another nucleoside
   (c) One nucleotide with another nucleotide
   (d) One nitrogenous base with pentose sugar
5. Select the two statements out of the four (1- 4) given below about lac operon. [AIPMT PRE 2010]
   (1) Glucose or galactose may bind with the repressor and inactivate it
   (2) In the absence of lactose, the repressor binds with the operator region
   (3) The z-gene codes for permease
   (4) This was elucidated by Francois Jacob and Jacques Monod
   The correct statements are
   (a) (3) and (3)
   (b) (1) and (3)
   (c) (2) and (4)
   (d) (1) and (2)
6. The one aspect which is not a salient feature of genetic code is its being: [AIPMT PRE 2010]
   (a) Degenerate
   (b) Ambiguous
   (c) Universal
   (d) Specific
7. Satellite DNA is useful tool in: [AIPMT PRE 2010]
   (a) Organ transplantation
   (b) Sex determination
   (c) Forensic science
   (d) Genetic engineering
8. Which one of the following does not follow the central dogma of molecular biology? [AIPMT PRE 2010]
   (a) Pea
   (b) Mucor
   (c) Chlamydomonas
   (d) HIV
9. What are those structures that appear as 'beads-on-string' in the chromosomes when viewed under electron microscope? [AIPMT PRE 2011]
   (a) Nucleotides
   (b) Nucleosomes
   (c) Base pairs
   (d) Genes

10. Which one of the following also acts as a catalyst in a bacterial cell? [AIPMT PRE 2011]

(a) sn RNA
(b) hn RNA
(c) 23 S rRNA
(d) 5 S rRNA

11. The unequivocal proof of DNA as the genetic material came from the studies on a: [AIPMT MAINS 2011]

(a) Bacterium
(b) Fungus
(c) Viroid
(d) Bacterial virus

12. In history of biology, human genome project led to the development of: [AIPMT MAINS 2011]

(a) Biotechnology
(b) Biomonitoring
(c) Bioinformatics
(d) Biosystematics

13. What is it that forms the basis of DNA Fingerprinting? [AIPMT MAINS 2012]

(a) The relative difference in the DNA occurrence in blood, skin and saliva
(b) The relative amount of DNA in the ridges and grooves of the fingerprints
(c) Satellite DNA occurring as highly repeated short DNA segments
(d) The relative proportions of purines and pyrimidines in DNA

14. Companion cells are closely associated with: [AIPMT PRE 2012]

(a) Sieve elements
(b) Vessel elements
(c) Trichomes
(d) Guard cells

15. Removal of RNA polymerase III from nucleoplasm will affect the synthesis of: [AIPMT PRE 2012]

(a) t RNA
(b) hn RNA
(c) m RNA
(d) r RNA

16. PCR and Restriction Fragment Length Polymorphism are the methods for: [AIPMT PRE 2012]

(a) Study of enzymes
(b) Genetic transformation
(c) DNA sequencing
(d) Genetic Fingerprinting

17. Which one of the following is not a part of a transcription unit in DNA? [AIPMT PRE 2012]

(a) The inducer
(b) A terminator
(c) A promoter
(d) The structural gene

18. A single strand of nucleic acid tagged with a radioactive molecule is called: [AIPMT PRE 2012]

(a) Vector
(b) Selectable market
(c) Plasmid
(d) Probe

19. If one strand of DNA has the nitrogenous base sequence as ATCTG, what would be the complementary RNA strand sequence? [AIPMT PRE 2012]

(a) TTAGU
(b) UAGAC
(c) AACTG
(d) ATCGU

20. Removal of introns and joining of exons in a defined order during transcription is called: [AIPMT PRE 2012]

(a) Looping (b) Inducing
(c) Slicing (d) Splicing

21. The diagram shows an important concept in the genetic implication of DNA. Fill in the blanks A to C

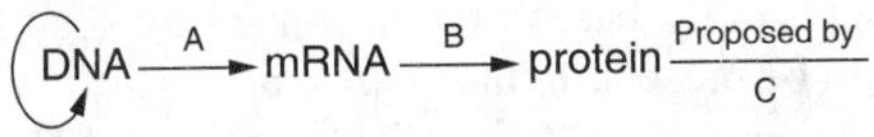

[AIPMT 2013]

(a) A: transcription B: protein C: James Watson
(b) A: translation B: transcription C: Erevin Chargaff
(c) A: transcription B: translation C: Francis Crick
(d) A: translation B: Extension C: Rosalind Franklin

22. Which enzyme/s will be produced in a cell in which there is a nonsense mutation in the lac Y gene? [AIPMT 2013]

(a) β-galactosidase (b) Lactose permease
(c) Transacetylase (d) Lactose permease and transacetylase

23. Which one of the following is wrongly matched? [AIPMT 2014]

(a) Transcription – Writing information from DNA to t – RNA
(b) Translation – Using information in m-RNA to make protein
(c) Repressor protein – Binds to operator to stop enzyme synthesis
(d) Operon – Structural genes, operator and promoter

24. Transformation was discovered by: [AIPMT 2014]

(a) Meselson and Stahl (b) Hershey and Chase
(c) Griffith (d) Watson and Crick

25. An analysis of chromosomal DNA using the Southern hybridization technique does not use [AIPMT 2014]

(a) Electrophoresis (b) Blotting
(c) Autoradiography (d) PCR

26. Select the correct option: (A: Direction RNA synthesis, B: Direction of reading of the template DNA strand) [AIPMT 2014]

(a) 5' ----- 3' 3' ------ 5'
(b) 3' ----- 5' 5' ------ 3'
(c) 5' ----- 3' 5' ------ 3'
(d) 3' ----- 5' 3' ------ 5'

27. Commonly used vectors for human genome sequencing are: [AIPMT 2014]

(a) T – DNA (b) BAC and YAC
(c) Expression Vectors (d) T/Cloning Vectors

28. Gene regulation governing lactose operon of E. coli that involves the lacI gene product is: [AIPMT 2015]

(a) Positive and inducible because it can be induced by lactose
(b) Negative and inducible because repressor protein prevents transcription
(c) Negative and repressible because repressor protein prevents transcription
(d) Feedback inhibition because excess of β galactosidase can switch off transcription.

29. In sea urchin DNA, which is double stranded, 17% of the bases were shown to be cytosine. The percentages of the other three bases expected to be present in this DNA are : [AIPMT 2015]

(a) G 34%, A 24.5%, T 24.5%
(b) G 17%, A 16.5%, T 32.5%
(c) G 17%, A 33%, T 33%
(d) G 8.5%, A 50%, T 24.5%

30. Which one of the following is not applicable to RNA? [RE-AIPMT 2015]

(a) 5' phosphoryl and 3'hydroxyl ends
(b) Heterocyclic nitrogeneous bases
(c) Chargaff's rule
(d) Complementary base pairing

31. Identify the correct order of organization of genetic material from largest to smallest: [RE-AIPMT 2015]

(a) Genome, chromosome, nucleotide, gene
(b) Genome, chromosome, gene, nucleotide
(c) Chromosome, genome, nucleotide, gene
(d) Chromosome, gene, genome, nucleotide

32. Balbiani rings are sites of [RE-AIPMT 2015]

(a) Nucleotide synthesis
(b) Polysaccharide synthesis
(c) RNA and protein synthesis
(d) Lipid synthesis

33. Satellite DNA is important because it: [RE-AIPMT 2015]

(a) Shows high degree of polymorphism in population and also the same degree of polymorphism in an individual, which is heritable from parents to children
(b) Does not code for proteins and is same in all members of the population
(c) Codes for enzymes needed for DNA repletion
(d) Codes for proteins needed in cell cycle.

Answer Keys

1. (c)	2. (d)	3. (c)	4. (b)	5. (c)	6. (b)	7. (c)	8. (d)	9. (a)	10. (b)
11. (c)	12. (c)	13. (c)	14. (c)	15. (d)	16. (c)	17. (c)	18. (b)	19. (b)	20. (d)
21. (b)	22. (d)	23. (c)	24. (c)	25. (b)	26. (d)	27. (d)	28. (c)	29. (a)	30. (c)
31. (c)	32. (b)	33. (b)	34. (b)	35. (b)	36. (d)	37. (b)	38. (b)	39. (d)	40. (d)
41. (b)	42. (d)	43. (d)	44. (b)	45. (b)	46. (c)	47. (a)	48. (a)	49. (e)	50. (b)
51. (d)	52. (b)	53. (c)	54. (c)	55. (b)	56. (c)	57. (a)	58. (c)	59. (b)	60. (b)
61. (d)	62. (c)	63. (d)	64. (b)	65. (d)	66. (d)	67. (c)	68. (c)	69. (c)	70. (b)
71. (c)	72. (c)	73. (d)	74. (c)	75. (c)	76. (c)	77. (d)	78. (d)	79. (b)	80. (c)

81. (d)	82. (a)	83. (c)	84. (a)	85. (c)	86. (c)	87. (d)	88. (c)	89. (c)	90. (b)
91. (d)	92. (c)	93. (a)	94. (a)	95. (d)	96. (d)	97. (a)	98. (c)	99. (d)	100. (c)
101. (a)	102. (c)	103. (c)	104. (c)	105. (b)	106. (c)	107. (c)	108. (b)	109. (d)	110. (a)
111. (c)	112. (c)	113. (c)	114. (c)	115. (c)	116. (b)	117. (b)	118. (d)	119. (c)	120. (c)
121. (c)	122. (a)	123. (b)	124. (b)	125. (a)	126. (b)	127. (b)	128. (c)	129. (d)	130. (b)
131. (d)	132. (b)	133. (c)	134. (d)	135. (b)	136. (c)	137. (c)	138. (c)	139. (c)	140. (a)
141. (b)	142. (c)	143. (b)	144. (c)	145. (d)	146. (b)	147. (d)	148. (d)	149. (c)	150. (b)
151. (b)	152. (c)	153. (d)	154. (c)	155. (d)	156. (c)	157. (c)	158. (d)	159. (c)	160. (c)
161. (b)	162. (b)	163. (b)	164. (b)	165. (a)	166. (d)	167. (c)	168. (c)	169. (b)	170. (c)
171. (b)	172. (c)	173. (b)	174. (a)	175. (d)	176. (c)	177. (d)	178. (b)	179. (b)	180. (c)
181. (b)	182. (a)	183. (b)	184. (a)	185. (b)	186. (d)	187. (b)	188. (c)	189. (d)	190. (a)
191. (b)	192. (b)	193. (c)	194. (b)	195. (b)	196. (a)	197. (b)	198. (a)	199. (d)	200. (a)
201. (a)	202. (a)	203. (a)	204. (c)	205. (c)					

AIPMT Previous Year Questions

1. (a)	2. (b)	3. (b)	4. (c)	5. (c)	6. (b)	7. (c)	8. (d)	9. (b)	10. (c)
11. (d)	12. (c)	13. (c)	14. (a)	15. (a)	16. (d)	17. (a)	18. (d)	19. (b)	20. (d)
21. (c)	22. (a)	23. (a)	24. (c)	25. (d)	26. (a)	27. (b)	28. (b)	29. (c)	30. (c)
31. (b)	32. (c)	33. (a)							

CHAPTER

29

Evolution

1. Evolutionary biology is related to the:
   (a) Origin of universe
   (b) Origin of earth
   (c) Study of history of life forms on earth
   (d) Origin of stars
2. Stellar distances are measured in:
   (a) km
   (b) m
   (c) Light year
   (d) pm
3. How old is the universe?
   (a) 10 billion years
   (b) 20 billion years
   (c) 5 billion years
   (d) 15 billion years
4. Galaxies contain:
   (a) Stars
   (b) Clouds of gas and dust
   (c) Both
   (d) None
5. Select the false statement from the following.
   (a) Big bang theory is used to explain the origin of the universe.
   (b) Expansion of the universe after the explosion lead to a decrease in temperature
   (c) Hydrogen and helium had formed before the explosion.
   (d) Gases condensed under gravitation and formed galaxies.
6. Earth was formed ________ billion years back.
   (a) 4.5
   (b) 5.5
   (c) 3.5
   (d) 1.5
7. Molten mass on early earth produced:
   (a) Water vapour and CH_4
   (b) CO_2
   (c) NH_3
   (d) All
8. Which part of solar radiation can break H_2O?
   (a) V.R.
   (b) U.V. radiation
   (c) Infrared
   (d) None of above
9. Life appeared ________ years after the formation of earth.
   (a) 1000 million
   (b) 100 million
   (c) 10 million
   (d) 500 million
10. Which of the following is related to the origin of life on earth?
    (a) Panspermia
    (b) Theory of spontaneous generation
    (c) Chemical evolution
    (d) All

11. Who proposed the theory of chemical evolution for the first time?
(a) Oparin and Haldane
(b) Miller
(c) Louis pesteur
(d) Darwin

12. Identify the parts A, B, C and D of the figure.

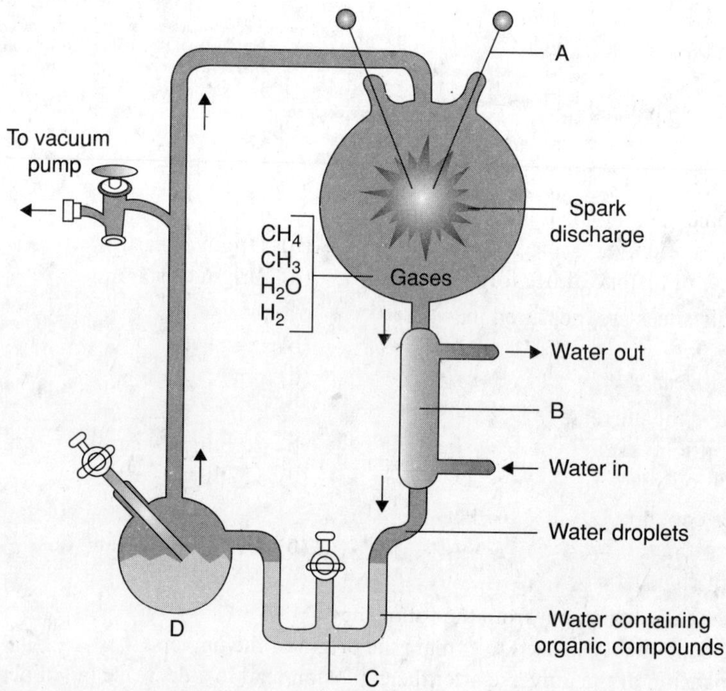

(a) A: Liquid water in trap, B: Electrode, C: Boiling water, D: Condenser
(b) A: Boiling water, B: Condenser, C: Electrode, D: Liquid water in trap
(c) A: Electrode, B: Condenser, C: Liquid water in trap, D: Boiling water
(d) A: Condenser, B: Liquid water in trap, C: Boiling water, D: Electrode

13. Miller simulated early Earth conditions in a laboratory by passing electric discharge through a closed flask raising its temperature to 800°C and containing:
(a) CH_4 and H_2
(b) NH_3
(c) Water vapour
(d) All

14. The first non-cellular form of life could have originated ________ billion years back.
(a) 1
(b) 2
(c) 3
(d) 4

15. Which of the given statement is wrong as per the 'Theory of Special Creation'?
(a) All living organism created as such.
(b) Diversity change as time changes.
(c) Earth is about 4000 years old.
(d) All are correct.

16. The fitness referred to in Darwin's theory is:
(a) Physical fitness
(b) Mental fitness
(c) Reproductive fitness
(d) All

17. Evidence of evolution from fossils is known as:
(a) Paleontological evidence (b) Embryological evidence
(c) Physiological evidence (d) Biochemical evidence

18. Find out the correct statement from the following.
(A) According to Darwin there is a gradual evolution of life forms.
(B) Darwin travelled around the world in a sail ship named H.M.S. Beagle.
(C) Alfred Wallace worked in Malay Archipelago.
(D) Fossils are remains of life forms which have become hard and turned into rock.
(a) A and B only (b) B only
(c) C only (d) All are correct

19. Homologous organ represents:
(a) Convergent evolution (b) Divergent evolution
(c) Anthropogenic evolution (d) Genetic drift

20. Analogous organs represent:
(a) Convergent evolution (b) Divergent evolution
(c) Anthropogenic evolution (d) Genetic drift

21. Which of the following shows analogy?
(a) Eye of octopus and mammals
(b) Vertebrate hearts
(c) Thorn of Bougainvillea and tendril of Cucurbita
(d) Vertebrate brains

22. Which of the following shows convergent evolution?
(a) Mouse and Marsupial mouse (b) Bobcat and Spotted cuscus
(c) Anteater and Marsupial mole (d) Lemur and Tasmanian wolf

23. Which of the following is an example of anthropogenic evolution?
(a) Selection of resistant varieties due to herbicides
(b) Selection of resistant varieties due to pesticides
(c) Industrial melanism
(d) All

24. Dryopithecus and Ramapithecus existed ________ mya.
(a) 5 (b) 10
(c) 15 (d) 25

25. Select false statements.
(A) Dryopithecus was more Ape-like.
(B) Ramapithecus was more Man-like.
(C) Dryopithecus and Ramapithecus both were hairy and walked like gorillas and chimpanzees.
(D) Australopithecines lived in the East African grasslands probably 3–4 mya.
(a) B only (b) B and C only
(c) D only (d) All are correct

26. Which statement is true about Australopithecines?
(a) They hunted with stone weapons.
(b) They ate fruit.
(c) Two mya they lived in the East African grasslands.
(d) All

27. Homo habilis had a cranial capacity of nearly:
(a) 650–800 cc (b) 900 cc
(c) 1400 cc (d) 1500 cc

28. Which is true about Homo erectus?
(a) Brain capacity is 900 cc approx (b) Ate meat
(c) Found in java and exist 1.5 mya (d) All of the above

29. What does this diagram show?

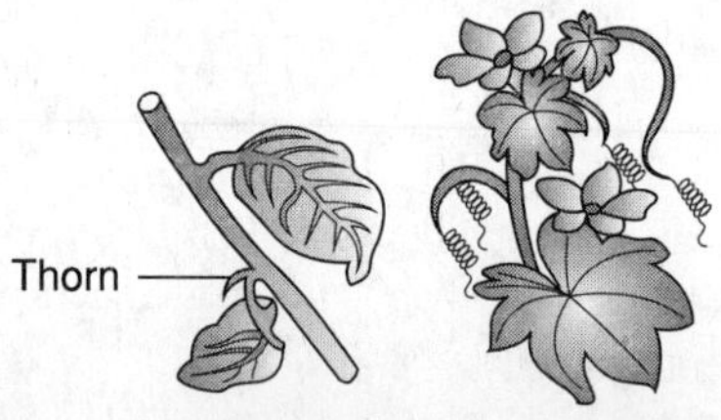

(a) Convergent evolution (b) Divergent evolution
(c) Homologous organ (d) Both (b) and (c)

30. All these facts are true about the Neanderthal man except:
(a) Brain size 1400 cc
(b) Used hides to protect their bodies
(c) Lived in east and central Asia between 1,00,000–40,000 years back
(d) Their fossils discovered in Java in 1891

31. All these facts are true about Homo sapiens except:
(a) Arose 75,000–10,000 years ago (b) Arose in Africa
(c) Brain capacity is 1400 cc (d) They developed into distinct races.

32. Arrange the following in the order of their evolution.
(a) Homo habilis → Ramapithecus→Homo erectus→ Dryopithecus → Homo sapiens → Australopithecines → Neanderthal man
(b) Dryopithecus→ Ramapithecus→ Australopithecus → Homo habilis→ Homo erectus→ Neanderthal man→ Homo sapiens
(c) Australopithecines→Homo sapiens→Ramapithecus→Dryopithecus→Homo habilis→Homo erectus→Neanderthal man
(d) Neanderthal man → Australopithecines → Homo sapiens → Homo erectus →Homo hab ilis→Ramapithecus→Dryopithecus

33. Match the columns.

Column-I	Column-II
(A) Homo habilis	(1) 650–800 cc
(B) Homo erectus	(2) 900 cc
(C) Neanderthal man	(3) 1400 cc

(a) A:1, B:2, C:3 (b) A:2, B: 1, C:3
(c) A:2, B:3, C:1 (d) A:3, B:2, C:1

34. Match the columns.

(1) Pre-historic cave art	(A) 10,000 years back
(2) Agriculture	(B) 18,000 years back
(3) Neanderthal man	(C) 1.5 mya
(4) Homoerectus	(D) 40,000 - 1,00,000 years back

(a) 1:A, 2:C, 3:B, 4:D
(b) 1:D, 2:B, 3:C, 4:A
(c) 1:B, 2:A, 3:D, 4:C
(d) 1:C, 2:A, 3:D, 4:B

35. Who buried their dead?
(a) Java men
(b) Homo habilis
(c) Homo erectus
(d) Neanderthal man

36. First cellular form of life appeared ________ mya.
(a) 1000
(b) 2000
(c) 3000
(d) 4000

37. Match the columns.

(A) Invertebrates	(1) 500 mya
(B) Jawless fish	(2) 320 mya
(C) Seaweeds	(3) 350 mya
(D) Dryopithecus and Ramapithecus	(4) 15 mya

(a) A:2, B:1, C:4, D:3
(b) A:1, B:3, C:2, D:4
(c) A:1, B:4, C:2, D:3
(d) A:4, B:3, C:1, D:2

38. The first organisms that invaded land were:
(a) Animals
(b) Plants
(c) Amphibians
(d) Reptiles

39. Which of the following is a lobe finned fish?
(a) Coelacanth
(b) Hippocampus
(c) Catla
(d) Pteropus

40. Amphibians evolved from:
(a) Synapsids
(b) Sauropside
(c) Lobed fin fishes
(d) Cycads

41. Which of these is a direct ancestor of turtles?
(a) Sauropsids
(b) Synapsids
(c) Pelycosaurs
(d) Thecodonts

42. Find out total number of correct statements from the following:
(A) Pteridophytes forms coal deposits.
(B) Fishlike reptiles (Ichthyosaurs) evolved 200 mya.
(C) About 65 mya dinosaurs suddenly disappeared from earth.
(D) Tyrannosaurus rex was biggest dinosaurs about 20 feet in height.
(E) Because of continental drift, pouched mammals of Australia survived as there was a lack of competition from any other mammals.
(a) 2
(b) 3
(c) 4
(d) 5

43. Which of these is/are aquatic mammals?
(a) Whale (b) Dolphin
(c) Seals and Sea cows (d) All

44. Find the total number of organisms evolved from Psilophyton in the following.
Bryophytes, Herbaceous lycopods, Sphenopsids, Ferns, Ginkgos, Conifers, Gnetales, Arborescent lycopods
(a) 2 (b) 3
(c) 5 (d) 6

45. All these are animals except:
(a) Synapsids (b) Therapsids
(c) Sphenopsids (d) Sauropsids

46. Seed fern evolved into:
(a) Cycads (b) Dicot
(c) Monocot (d) All

47. Following were extinct in the Permian period?
(a) Ferns (b) Cycads
(c) Arborescent lycopodus (d) Bryophytes

48. Bryophytes evolved in which of these periods?
(a) Carboniferous (b) Permian
(c) Triassic (d) Cretaceous

49. What does this diagram show?

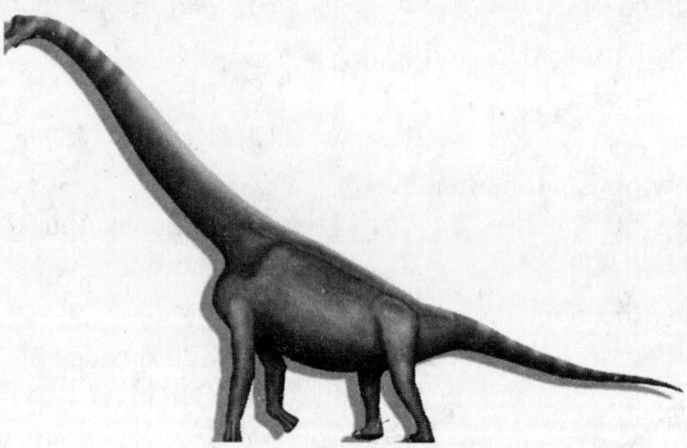

(a) Brachiosaurus (b) Stegosaurus
(c) Triceratops (d) Tyrannosaurus

50. How many of these periods belong to the paleozoic era?
Cretaceous, Jurrasic, Triassic, Permian, Carboniferous, Devonian, Silurin
(a) 1 (b) 2
(c) 3 (d) 4

51. Synapsids existed:
(a) 300 mya (b) 150 mya
(c) 350 mya (d) 50 mya

52. Zosterophyllum belonged to which period?
(a) Silurian (b) Devonian
(c) Carboniferous (d) Permian

53. Which of the following was/were most abundant in cenozoic era?
(a) Angiosperm (b) Cycads
(c) Conifers (d) Ginkgos

54. Which of these features belong/s to mammals?
(a) Viviparous, avoid danger (b) More intelligent in sensing
(c) Both (d) None

55. What can be said to be the success story of man in evolution?
(a) Language skills (b) Self-consciousness
(c) Increase cranial capacity (d) All

56. Conifers were most abundant in:
(a) Paleozoic era (b) Mesozoic era
(c) Coenozoic era (d) All eras

57. Seed ferns evolved from:
(a) Cycads (b) Gnetales
(c) Conifers (d) Progymnosperm

58. This diagram shows:

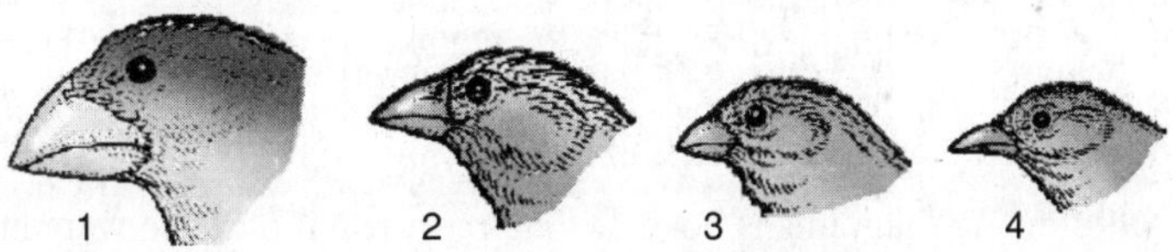

(a) Adaptive radiation (b) Genetic drift
(c) Founder effect (d) Mutation

59. Arrange ascending order of extinction (reptiles):
(a) Pelycosaurs, thecodonts, therapside, Dinosaurs
(b) Thecodonts, Dinosaurs, pelycosaurs, therapside
(c) Dinosaurs, therapside, thecodonts, Pelycosaurs
(d) Therapside, thecodonts, pelycosaurs, dinosaurs

60. When a given population is in genetic equilibrium, then:
(a) Gene pool remains constant.
(b) Allele frequencies in population is constant from generation to generation.
(c) Sum total of all allelic frequencies is 1.
(d) All

61. How many factors affect the Hardy–Weinberg equilibrium?
(a) 1 (b) 3
(c) 4 (d) 5

62. Factors affecting genetic equilibrium are the following except:
(a) Gene flow (b) Mutation
(c) Somatic variation (d) Genetic recombination

63. Five factors affecting genetic equilibrium are:
(a) Gene flow, genetic drift (b) Mutation, genetic recombination
(c) Natural selection (d) All of the above

64. Natural selection is of following types:
(a) Stabilising
(b) Disruptive
(c) Directional
(d) Any of the above

65. Variation may be due to:
(a) Mutation
(b) Genetic recombinant during gametogenesis
(c) Gene flow or genetic drift
(d) All of the above

66. Hugo de Vries, based on his work on ________ , brought forth the idea of mutations.
(a) Pisum, sativum
(b) Lathyrus odoratus
(c) Evening primrose
(d) Lathyms sativus

67. Mutations are:
(a) Directionless and random
(b) Random and directional
(c) Small variations and directional
(d) Not responsible for evolution

68. Select the false statement from the following:
(a) Darwinian variations are small and directional.
(b) Saltation is a single large step mutation.
(c) Branching descent and natural selection are the two key concepts of Darwinian theory of evolution.
(d) Mutation is random and progressive in nature.

69. Which of the following diagrams is not a correct representation of convergent evolution?

(a) 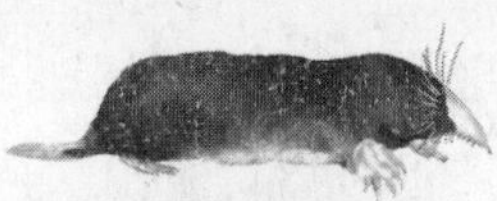 — 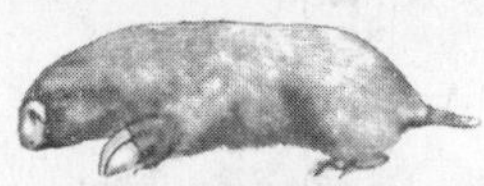

(b) 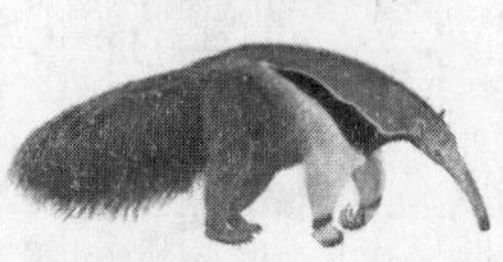 — 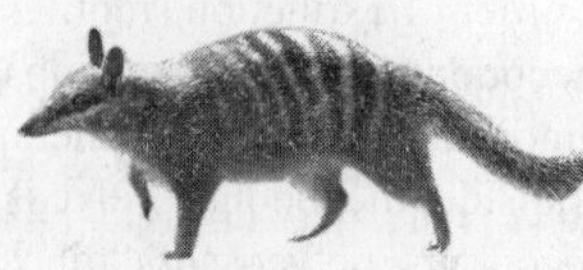

(c) 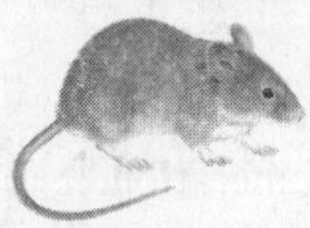 — 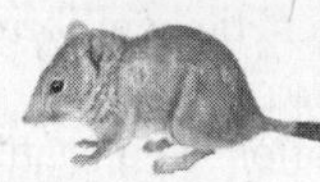

(d) 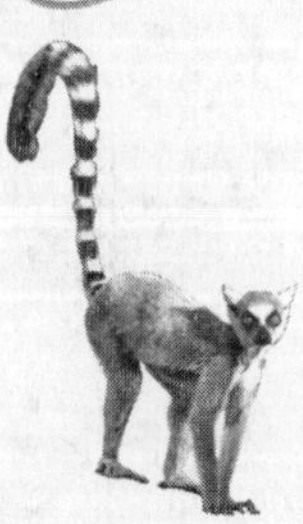 — 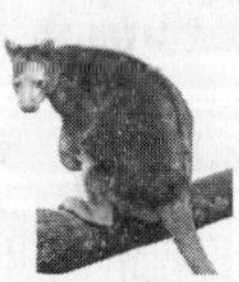

70. Abiogenesis means:
(a) Spontaneous generation
(b) Origin of viruses and microbes
(c) Origin of life from living organisms
(d) Origin of life from nonliving organisms

71. Pasteur's experiments and similar ones that followed convinced most people that spontaneous generation of life did not happen because:
(a) Pasteur was extremely meticulous.
(b) Pasteur did not boil his flask for a long time.
(c) Pasteur used very fine mesh screens to cover his flask.
(d) Pasteur's swan-necked flasks ruled out the objection that spoiled air could have contaminated his experiments.

72. The early belief of the spontaneous origin of life was disproved by:
(a) Lederberg (b) Robert Koch
(c) Louis Pasteur (d) Charles Darwin

73. Who said that organisms develop from pre-existing organisms?
(a) Aristotle (b) Louis Pasteur
(c) Alexander Oparin (d) Thomas Hunt Morgan

74. The idea that life originates from pre-existing life is referred to as:
(a) Biogenesis theory (b) Abiogenesis theory
(c) Extraterrestrial theory (d) Special creation theory

75. Life was created by some supernatural power. This theory is:
(a) Abiogenesis (b) Spore theory
(c) Special creation theory (d) Spontaneous generation

76. Life came from outer space—This theory is:
(a) Spore theory (b) Naturalistic theory
(c) Special creation theory (d) Spontaneous generation

77. About how long ago was the Earth formed?
(a) 3.0 billion years ago (b) 10 billion years ago
(c) 4.6 billion years ago (d) 20 billion years ago

78. 'Modern theory of origin of life' was propounded by:
(a) Oparin (b) Miller
(c) Darwin (c) Khorana

79. A. I. Oparin was a:
(a) Polish biologist (b) Russian biochemist
(c) Belgian nutritionist (d) Swedish cosmologist

80. Oparin's theory of 'Origin of life' is based on:
(a) Chemical evolution (b) Cosmic evolution
(c) Artificial synthesis (d) Organic evolution

81. According to Oparin, which one of the following was not present in the primitive atmosphere of the Earth?
(a) Oxygen (b) Methane
(c) Hydrogen (d) Water vapour

82. The basic components of atmosphere of primitive Earth were:
(a) Ammonia, methane and water (b) Methane, ozone, nitrogen and water
(c) Hydrogen, nitrogen, methane and water (d) Ammonia, methane, hydrogen and water

83. Which of the following is a true statement?
(a) The primitive atmosphere had 20% oxygen, just like it is today.
(b) The reducing primitive atmosphere contributed to the origin of life, and the oxidizing one today would hinder it
(c) The primitive atmosphere was an oxidizing one and today's is a reducing one, making photosynthesis possible.
(d) It took so long for prokaryote evolution because the primitive atmosphere screened out the ultraviolet radiation from the sun.

84. Life originated in:
(a) Air (b) Water
(c) Land (d) All of these

85. Stanley Miller proposed origin of life by:
(a) Biogenesis (b) Abiogenesis
(c) Chemical synthesis (d) None of these

86. The first experiment on chemical evolution and origin of life was carried out by:
(a) Watson and Crick (b) Miller and Urey
(c) Beadle and Tatum (d) Darwin and Wallace

87. The spark-discharge apparatus to test chemical evolution of life was designed by:
(a) Urey and Miller (b) Dixon and Jolley
(c) Jacob and Monod (d) Oparin and Haldane

88. The diagram represents Miller's experiment. Choose the correct combination of labelling:

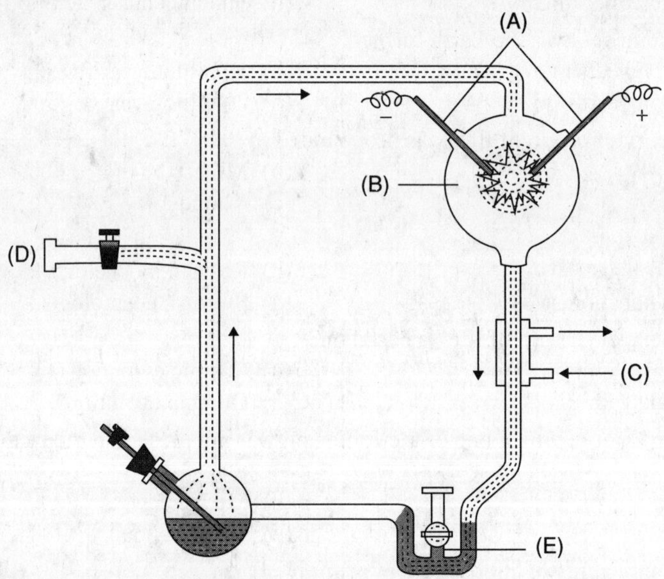

(a) A: Electrodes, B: $NH_3 + H_2 + H_2O + CH_4$, C: Hot water, D: Vacuum, E: U trap
(b) A: Electrodes, B: $NH_3 + H_2O$, C = Hot water, D = Tap, E: U trap
(c) A: Electrodes, B: $NH_3 + H_2 + H_2O$, CH_4, C: Cold water, D: Vacuum, E: U trap
(d) A: Electrodes, B: $NH_3 + H_2 + H_2O + CH_4$, C: Steam, D: Vacuum, E: U Trap
(e) A: Electrodes, B: $NH_3 + CH_4$, C: Cold water, D: Sink, E: U trap

89. Findings of Miller's experiment on origin of life have provided evidence for:
(a) Theory of biogenesis (b) Oparin-Haldane theory
(c) Theory of special creation (d) Theory of organic evolution

90. The category of molecules produced by the Miller–Urey experiment was:
(a) Organic polymers (b) Inorganic polymers
(c) Organic monomers (d) inorganic monomers

91. Stanley Miller who is famous for 'simulation experiments' belonged to:
(a) USA (b) UK
(c) USSR (d) Canada

92. Stanley Miller conducted his experiments and produced animo acids by electric discharge passed through NH_3, H_2O, CH_4 and ________.
(a) Oxygen (b) Hydrogen
(c) Nitrogen (d) Carbon dioxide

93. This diagram shows:

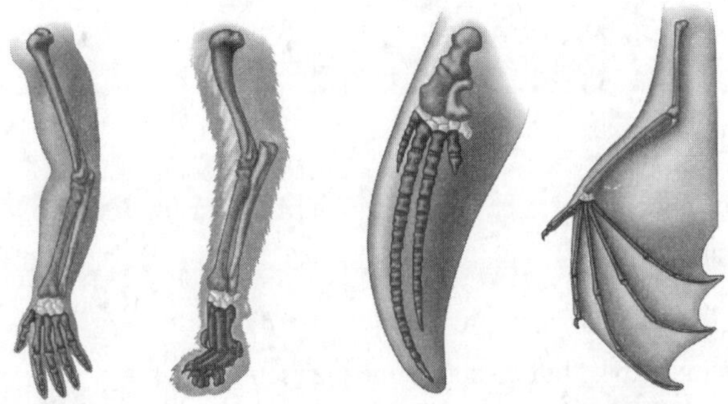

(a) Convergent evolution (b) Divergent evolution
(c) Homologus organ (d) Both (b) and (c)

94. The energy used in the Miller–Urey experiment was:
(a) Photo energy (b) Electric spark
(c) Atomic radiation (d) Mechanical energy

95. Earliest life forms on the earth were:
(a) Autotrophs (b) Cyanobacteria
(c) Photoautotrophs (d) Chemoheterotrophs

96. The concept of chemical evolution is based on:
(a) Crystallization of chemicals
(b) Effect of solar radiation on chemicals
(c) Interaction of water, air and clay under intense heat
(d) Possible origin of life by combination of chemicals under suitable environmental conditions

97. Which one of the following is incorrect about the characteristic of protobionts (coacervates and microspheres) as envisaged in abiogenic origin of life?
(a) They were able to reproduce.
(b) They could maintain an internal environment.
(c) They were partially isolated from the surroundings.
(d) They could separate combination of molecule from the surroundings.

98. Biologists define evolution as:
(a) Heritable change in a line of descent over generations
(b) Inheritance of characteristics acquired by the individual
(c) The origin of species
(d) None of the above

99. Which of the following diagram does not correctly represent the convergent evolution?

(a) 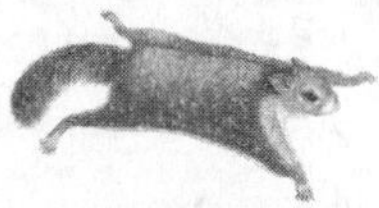 — 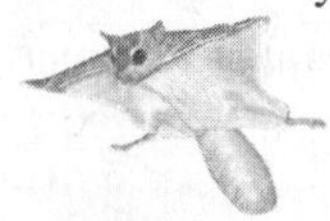

(b) 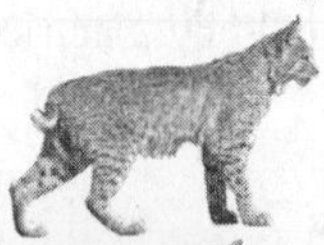 — 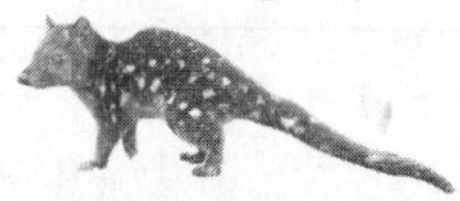

(c) 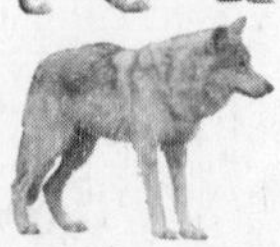 — 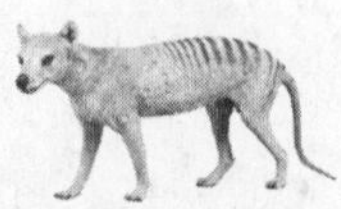

(d) None of these

100. Basic idea of evolution is:
(a) Cosmic evolution
(b) Special creation
(c) Spontaneous generation
(d) Descent with modification

101. Process of evolution is:
(a) Continuous
(b) Discontinuous
(c) Continuous in the past but discontinuous presently
(d) Discontinuous in the past but continuous presently

102. Concept of evolution is an excellent working hypothesis to approach the problem of:
(a) Matter, energy and life
(b) Environmental conditions
(c) Prodigality in reproduction
(d) Diversity of organisms upon earth

103. Darwin's finches provide excellent evidence in favour of evolution. This evidence comes from the field of:
(a) Anatomy
(b) Biogeography
(c) Embryology
(d) Palaeontology

104. The evolution of numerous species, such as Darwin's finches from a single ancestor is called:
(a) Gradualism
(b) Adaptive radiation
(c) Sympatric speciation
(d) Geographical isolation

105. Darwin's finches discovered from the Galapagos Islands serve as a good example of:
(a) Mimicry
(b) Camouflage
(c) Seasonal migration
(d) Biogeographical evidence of evolution

106. The classical example of adaptive radiation in development of new species is:
(a) Darwin's finches
(b) Marsupials of Australia
(c) Both of these
(d) None of these

107. The organs of different species that are related to each other through common descent though becomes functionally different are called:
(a) Vestigial
(b) Analogous
(c) Homologous
(d) None of these

108. Organs which have the same fundamental structure but different in functions are called:
(a) Vestigial organs (b) Analogous organs
(c) Homoplastic organs (d) Homologous organs

109. Homology does not refer to:
(a) Divergent evolution (b) Common descent
(c) Convergent evolution (d) Adaptive radiation

110. The homologous organs are wings of:
(a) Pigeon and bat (b) Butterfly and bat
(c) Sparrow and honeybee (d) Parrot and limbs of man

111. Which of the following are not homologous?
(a) Insect mouthparts (b) Insect legs
(c) Vertebrate forelimbs (d) Bird and insect wings

112. Which of the following is a set of homologous organs?
(a) Wings of grasshopper, flippers of whale (b) Wings of birds, front feet of horse
(c) Wings of housefly, wings of birds (d) None of the above

113. Name the organism represented by A to F in the illustration.

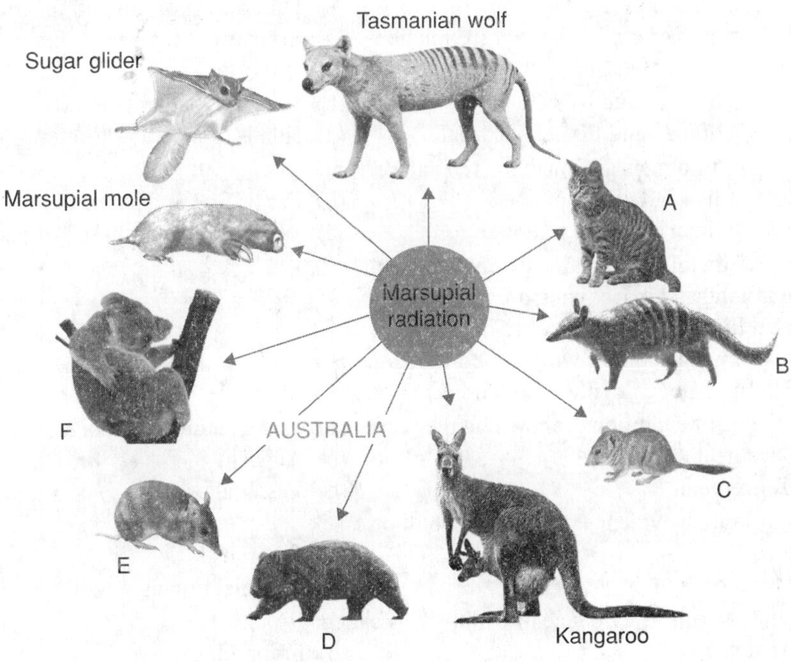

(a) A: Tigercat, B: Banded anteater, C: Marsupial rat, D: Wombat, E: Bandicoot, F: Koala
(b) A: Bandicoot, B: Wombat, C: Marsupial rat, D: Koala, E: Tigercat, F: Banded anteater
(c) A: Koala, B: Banded anteater, C: Tigercat, D: Bandicoot, E: Marsupial rat, E: Wombat
(d) A: Wombat, B: Tigercat, C: Koala, D: Bandicoot, E: Banded anteater, F: Marsupial rat

114. Which group includes homologous organs?
(a) Wings of butterfly, flying fish and bird
(b) Tentacles of Hydra and arms of starfish
(c) Fins of seal, wings of birds and forelimbs of man
(d) Horns of cattle, tail of horse and teeth of mammals

115. Which of the following are homologous organs?
(a) Hand of man, wings of bat
(b) Eyes of man, eyes of squid
(c) Gills of fish, lungs of man
(d) Leaf of moss, frond of fern

116. Thorn of Bougainvillea and tendril of cucurbita are examples of:
(a) Vestigial organs
(b) Analogous organs
(c) Homologous organs
(d) Retrogressive evolution

117. Although all mammals whale, dolphin, bat, monkey and horse have some important common characters, but they also show conspicuous differences. This is due to the phenomenon of:
(a) Divergence
(b) Genetic drift
(c) Convergence
(d) Normalization

118. Which of the following are homologous organs?
(a) Wings insects and bats
(b) Fins of fishes and flippers of whale
(c) Fins of fishes and forearms of human
(d) Forearm of human, bat's wings and whale's flippers

119. Analogous structures are:
(a) Similar in origin and function
(b) Different in origin and function
(c) Different in origin but similar in function
(d) Similar in origin but different in function

120. Analogy is found between:
(a) Wings of birds and bats
(b) Wings of bat and butterfly
(c) Hands of man and flippers of whale
(d) Hands of man and forelimbs of horse

121. Which pair of organs are analogous in nature?
(a) Gill of fish and gill of prawn
(b) Ear of frog and ear of rabbit
(c) Arm of man and limb of horse
(d) Wing of bat and flipper of seal

122. Which of the following pairs are correct?
(a) Bat wing and insect wing are analogous
(b) Seal flippers and bat paw are homologous
(c) Insect wing and bird wing are homologous
(d) Thorn of Bougainvillea and tendril of pea are analogous

123. Which type of evolution is shown by the wings of bats, mosquitoes and pigeons?
(a) Divergent
(b) Atavism
(c) Convergent
(d) Vestigial organs

124. The most direct evidence of organic evolution is:
(a) Fossils
(b) Embryos
(c) Morphology
(d) Vestigial organs

125. The study fossils as evidence of evolution is called:
(a) Anatomy
(b) Embryology
(c) Palaeontology
(d) Biogeography

126. The fossils are preserved in:
(a) Sedimentary rocks
(b) Igneous rocks
(c) Metamorphic rocks
(d) None of these

127. Fossil X is older than fossil Y because:
(a) Fossil Y was found in deeper sedimentation.
(b) Fossil X was found in deeper sedimentation.
(c) Fossil Y has some vestigial organs functional in X.
(d) Fossil Y has homologous and analogous organs of X.

128. Our best estimate for the age of Earth, which is 4.5 billion years, is supported by:
(a) Gradualism (b) Big bang theory
(c) Assumption of uniformitarianism (d) Radioactive dating of the oldest rocks found

129. Correct order is:
(a) Palaeozoic → Mesozoic → Coenozoic
(b) Mesozoic → Archaeozoic → Proterozoic
(c) Palaeozoic → Archaeozoic → Coenozoic
(d) Archaeozoic → Palaeozoic → Proterozoic

130. The largest subdivision in geological time-scale is:
(a) Era (b) Period
(c) Epoch (d) Century

131. Which of the following is called 'age of fish'?
(a) Silurian (b) Permian
(c) Devonian (d) Cretaceous

132. Carboniferous period of coal deposition was:
(a) 50 million years ago (b) 300 million years ago
(c) 500 million years ago (d) 2000 million years ago

133. What is A, B, C and D in the diagram?

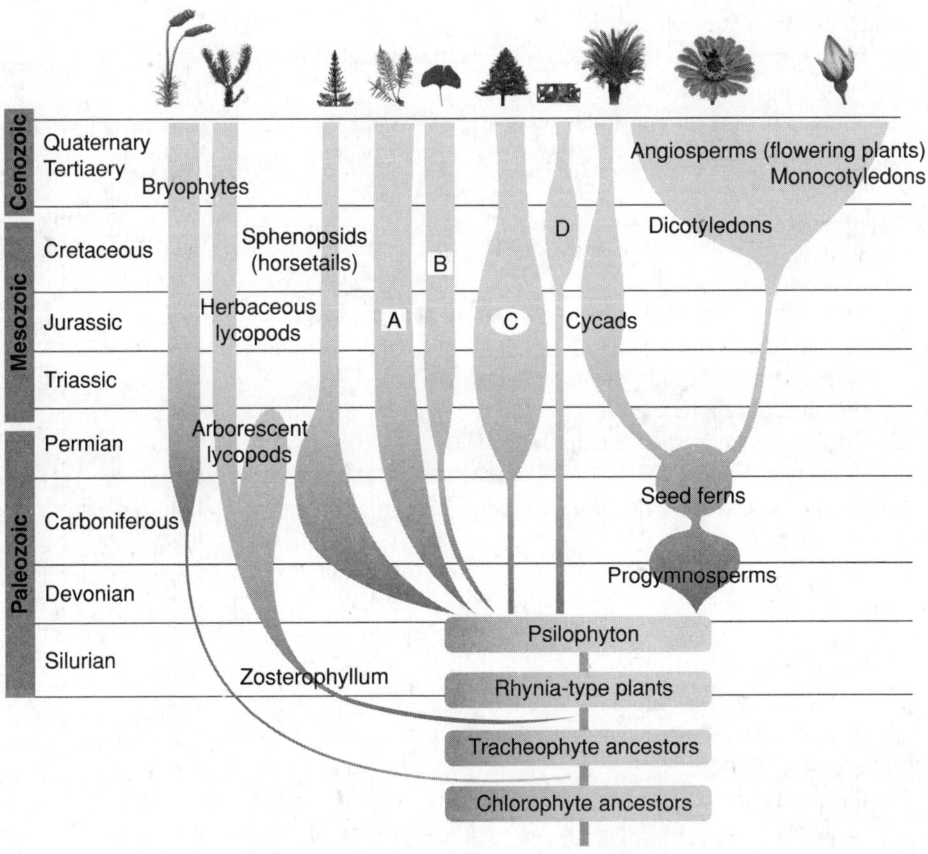

(a) A: Conifers, B: Ginkgos, C: Ferns, D: Gnetales
(b) A: Ferns, B: Ginkgos, C: Conifers, D: Gnetales
(c) A: Gnetales, B: Conifers, C: Ginkgos, D: Ferns
(d) A: Ginkgos, B: Gnetales, C: Ferns, D: Conifers

134. Mesozoic era is the age of:
(a) Birds (b) Fishes
(c) Reptiles (d) Mammals

135. Dinosaurs were the:
(a) First mammals (b) Extinct reptiles
(c) Giant mammals (d) First amphibians

136. If you want to see a dinosaur, it would be best to set the controls of your time machine for the:
(a) Mesozoic era (b) Precambrian era
(c) Palaeozoic era (d) Pleistocene period

137. Dinosaurs became extinct during:
(a) Jurassic (b) Triassic
(c) Permian (d) Cretaceous

138. Which era was dominated by reptiles?
(a) Mesozoic era (b) Coenozoic era
(c) Palaeozoic era (d) Archaeozoic era

139. Golden age of reptile was:
(a) Mesozoic era (b) Coenozoic era
(c) Palaeozoic era (d) Proterozoic era

140. The Jurassic period belongs to the era:
(a) Coenozoic (b) Mesozoic
(c) Palaeozoic (d) Archaeozoic

141. Evolution of unique groups of mammals in South America, Africa and Australia is an evidence supporting:
(a) Continental drift (b) Glaciation
(c) Crustal movement (d) Geographical juxtaposition

142. Occurrence of endemic species in South America and Australia is due to:
(a) Progressive evolution
(b) Continental separation
(c) Absence of terrestrial route to these places
(d) Extinction of these species in other regions

143. The first attempt to solve the problem of mechanism of organic evolution was made by:
(a) Oparin (b) Darwin
(c) Wallace (d) Lamarck

144. Lamarck was a:
(a) French naturalist (b) German biologist
(c) British evolutionist (d) American biochemist

145. Lamarck's theory of evolution is called:
(a) Inheritance of acquired characters (b) Theory of special creation
(c) Survival of fittest (d) None of the above

146. The theory of use and disuse of organs was given by:
(a) Lamarck (b) Darwin
(c) Weismann (d) Hugo de Vries

147. The most important theory of evolution was proposed by:
(a) Beadle and Tatum (b) Watson and Crick
(c) Darwin and Wallace (d) Mendel and Morgan

148. The concepts of natural selection in evolution were proposed by:
(a) Hugo de Vries (b) Charles Darwin
(c) August Weismann (d) Jean Baptiste de Lamarck

149. Darwin travelled in which ship?
(a) H.N.S. Eagle (b) Titanic
(c) H.M.S. Beagle (d) D. Matrica

150. The main point of Darwin's theory is:
(a) Variation (b) Mutation
(c) Enormous fertility (d) Natural selection

151. Survival of fittest is possible due to:
(a) Overproduction (b) Favourable variations
(c) Environmental changes (d) Inheritance of acquired characters

152. What is A, B, C and D in this figure?

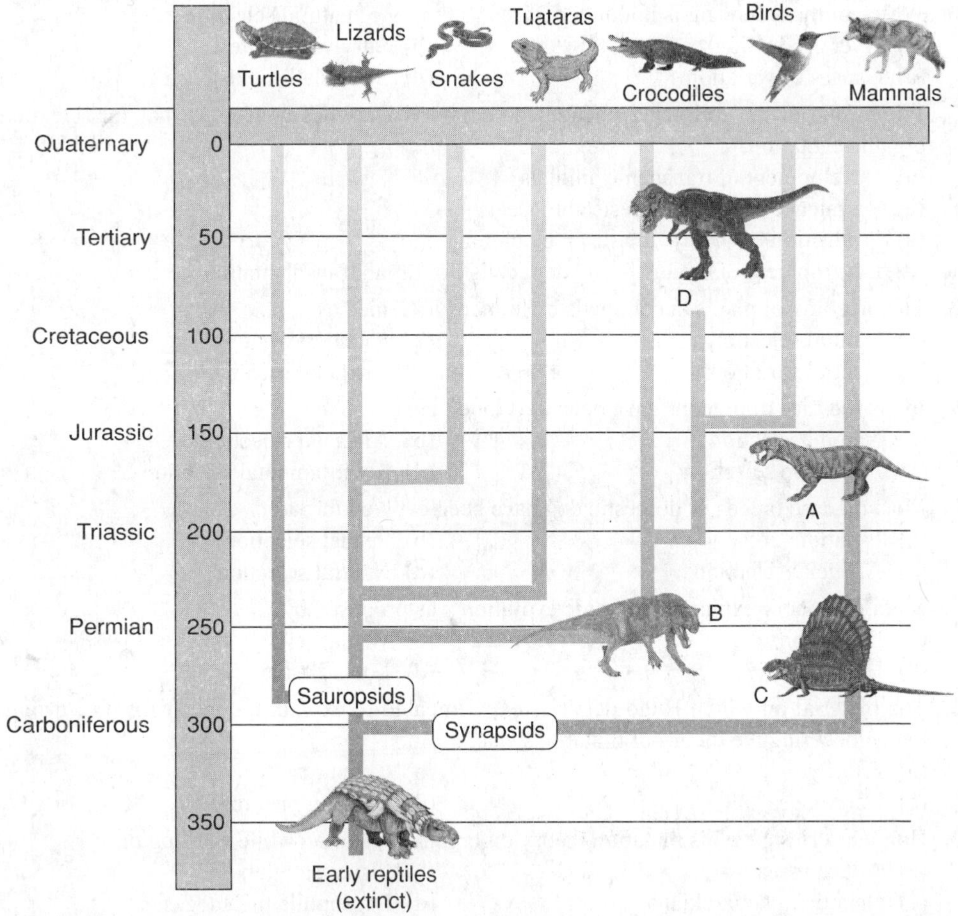

(a) A: Therapsids, B: Thecodonts, C: Pelycosaurs, D: Dinosaurs
(b) A: Thecodonts, B: Dinosarus, C: Therapsids, D: Pelycosaurs
(c) A: Dinosaurs, B: Pelycosaurs, C: Thecodonts, D: Therapsids
(d) A: Pelycosaurs, B: Therapsids, C: Dinasours, D: Thecodonts

153. The theory of natural selection of Darwin:
(a) Does not explain fossils
(b) Is completely changed
(c) Has the first theory of organic evolution
(d) Has failed in explaining origin of variations

154. Darwin was influenced by reading the essays of:
(a) Wallace (b) Spencer
(c) Mendel (d) Malthus

155. Which one provides correct sequence of events in origin of species according to Darwinism?
(A) Natural selection (B) Variations and their inheritance
(C) Survival of fittest (D) Struggle for existence
(a) A, B, C, D (b) B, D, C, A
(c) D, B, C, A (d) B, C, A, D

156. Which of the following is not under Darwin's theory of natural selection?
(a) Over production (b) Survival of fittest
(c) Causes of variation (d) Struggle for existence

157. Which one of the following phenomena supports Darwin's concept of natural selection in organic evolution?
(a) Development of transgenic animals
(b) Prevalence of pesticide resistant insects
(c) Production of 'Dolly' the sheep by cloning
(d) Development of organs from 'stem cells' for organ transplantation

158. The breeding of plants and animals by humans is termed as:
(a) Natural selection (b) Founder effect
(c) Neutral variation (d) Artificial selection

159. Improved race of pigeons have been developed by:
(a) Natural selection (b) Artificial selection
(c) Protective selection (d) Environmental selection

160. Most modern breeds of domestic dog have been evolved through:
(a) Isolation (b) Sexual selection
(c) Artificial selection (d) Natural selection

161. Mutation theory explaining organic evolution was proposed by:
(a) E. Darwin (b) W. Harvey
(c) Hugo de Vries (d) Louis Pasteur

162. The material on which Hugo de Vries experimented to explain the mechanism of evolution thus pioneering the theory of mutations was:
(a) Fruitfly (b) China rose
(c) Garden pea (d) Evening primrose

163. Hugo de Vries gave his mutation theory on organic evolution while working on:
(a) Althea rosea (b) Pisum sativum
(c) Oenothera lamarckiana (d) Drosophila melanogaster

164. For natural selection the important factor is:
(a) Disuse (b) Variation
(c) Catastrophe (d) Special creation

165. In which condition does the gene ratio remain constant for any species?
(a) Mutation (b) Gene flow
(c) Sexual selection (d) Random mating

166. Initiating force of evolution is:
(a) Variation (b) Adaptation
(c) Competition (d) Natural selection

167. The raw material for organic evolution is:
(a) Asexual reproduction (b) Mutation
(c) Nutritive substances (d) Effect of hormones

168. Lederberg replica experiment explains:
(a) Mutation theory (b) Darwin's theory
(c) Lamarck's theory (d) None of these

169. Some bacteria are able to grow in streptomycin containing medium due to:
(a) Genetic drift (b) Natural selection
(c) Induced mutation (d) Reproductive isolation

170. Sum of all the genes in a population is called:
(a) Genome (b) Gene pool
(c) Germplasm (d) Gene bank

171. At a particular locus, frequency of 'A' allele is 0.6 and that of 'a' is 0.4. What would be the frequency of heterozygotes in a random mating population at equilibrium?
(a) 0.36 (b) 0.48
(c) 0.16 (d) 0.24

172. Genetic drift operates in:
(a) Large isolated population (b) Small isolated population
(c) Fast reproductive population (d) Slow reproductive population

173. Match the following concepts of evolution in List-I with List-II and select the correct answer using the codes given below the lists:

List-I	List-II
(A) Mutation	(1) Changes in population's allele frequencies due to chance alone
(B) Gene flow	(2) Differences in survival and reproduction among variant individuals
(C) Natural selection	(3) Immigration, emigration change allele frequencies
(D) Genetic drift	(4) Source of new alleles

(a) A:1, B:2, C:3, D:4 (b) A:4, B:2, C:3, D:1
(c) A:3, B:1, C:4, D:2 (d) A:4, B:3, C:2, D:1

174. Which of the following concepts is known as the Sewall Wright effect?
(a) Genetic drift (b) Isolation
(c) Gene pool (d) Gene flow

175. Which of the following would stop evolution by A barring the occurrence of the natural selection?
(a) If humans became extinct because of a disease or epidemic.
(b) If ozone depletion led to increased ultraviolet radiation which caused many new mutations.
(c) If a thermonuclear war killed most living organisms and changed the environment drastically.
(d) If genetic recombination, sexual reproduction and mutation stopped so that all offspring of all organisms were exact copies of their parents.

176. Directional selection ________.
(a) works against adaptive traits
(b) favours intermediate forms of a trait
(c) eliminates uncommon forms of alleles
(d) shifts allele frequencies in a steady, consistent direction

177. Disruptive selection ________.
(a) eliminates uncommon forms of alleles
(b) does not favour intermediate forms of a trait
(c) shifts allele frequencies in a steady, consistent direction
(d) all of the above

178. Which of these is a correct match?

(a) 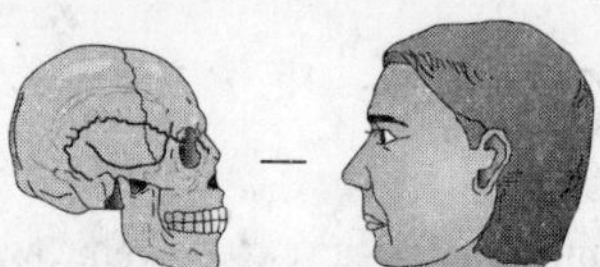

(b) 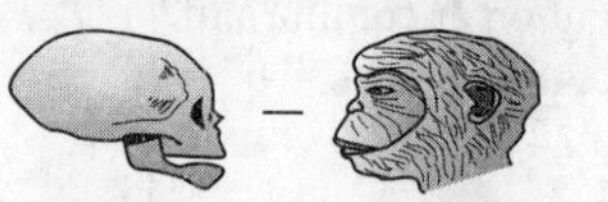

(c) 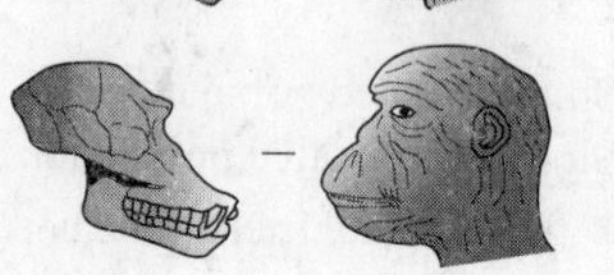

(d) All of the above

179. The processes of ________ and ________ generate variation and ________ produces adaptation to the environment.
(a) sexual selection, natural selection, mutation
(b) mutation, sexual recombination, genetic drift
(c) genetic drift, mutation, sexual recombination
(d) mutation, sexual recombination, natural selection

180. Industrial melanism was highlighted by:
(a) Polar bear
(b) Rock python
(c) Mimosa pudica
(d) Biston betularia

181. The phenomenon of 'Industrial melanism' demonstrates:
(a) Natural selection
(b) Induced mutation
(c) Reproductive isolation
(d) Geographical isolation

182. The change of the lighter coloured variety of peppered moth, Biston betularia, to its darker variety (carbonaria) is due to:
(a) Deletion of a segment of genes due to industrial pollution
(b) Mutation of single Mendelian gene for survival in smoke laden industrial environment
(c) Industrial carbon deposited on the wings of the moth resulting in darker variety
(d) Translocation of a block of genes in chromosomes in response to heavy carbons

183. Speciation usually occurs:
(a) Suddenly
(b) By genetic drift
(c) When populations are geographically isolated
(d) When populations are not geographically isolated

184. Which is basis of evolution?
(a) Cell (b) Species
(c) Individual (d) Population

185. The classical example of adaptive radiation in development of new species is:
(a) Darwin finches (b) Marsupials of Australia
(c) Giant turtles (d) All of these

186. The spread of genes from one breeding population to another by migration which may result in change in gene frequency is:
(a) Gene flow (b) Genetic drift
(c) Gene frequency (d) None of these

187. Arrange the periods of Palaeozoic era in ascending order in a geological time scale:
(a) Cambrian → Ordovician → Silurian → Devonian → Carboniferous → Permian
(b) Cambrian → Devonian → Ordovician → Silurian → Carboniferous → Permian
(c) Cambrian → Ordovician → Devonian → Silurian → Carboniferous → Permian
(d) Silurian → Devonian → Cambrian → Ordovician → Permian → Carboniferous

188. Presence of recessive trait is 16%. The frequency of dominant allele in population is:
(a) 0.6 (b) 0.32
(c) 0.84 (d) 0.92

189. Frequency of an autosomal lethal gene is 0.4. The frequency of carrier in a population of 200 individual is:
(a) 72 (b) 96
(c) 104 (d) 36

190. Darwin's finches are found in:
(a) Tahiti (b) Tundra
(c) Galapagos Island (d) None of these

191. In the developmental history of mammalian heart, it is observed that it passes through a two-chambered fishlike heart, three chambered frog-like heart and finally four-chambered stage. To which hypothesis can this above cited statement be approximated?
(a) Biogenetic law (b) Lamarck's principle
(c) Hardy-Weinberg law (d) Mendelian principles

192. Darwin's finches are an excellent example of:
(a) Connecting links (b) Brood parasitism
(c) Adaptive radiation (d) Seasonal migration

193. Sweet potato and potato are examples of:
(a) Homologous structures (b) Analogous structures
(c) Both (a) and (b) (d) None of these

194. The principle that gives the geneticists a tool to determine when evolution is occurring is:
(a) Hardy–Weinberg principle (b) Chemiosmotic theory
(c) Malthusian principle (d) Cloning theory

195. Which of the following defines Hardy–Weinberg's law?
(a) $p^2 + 2pq + q^2 = 0$ (b) $q^2 + p^2 + 2pq = 0$
(c) $p^2 + 2pq + q^2 = 1$ (d) $p^2 + 3pq + q^2 = 1$

196. Hardy–Weinberg equilibrium is known to be affected by gene flow, genetic drift, mutation, genetic recombination and ________.
(a) saltation (b) evolution
(c) limiting factors (d) natural selection

197. In this figure, which kind of selection does A, B and C represent respectively?

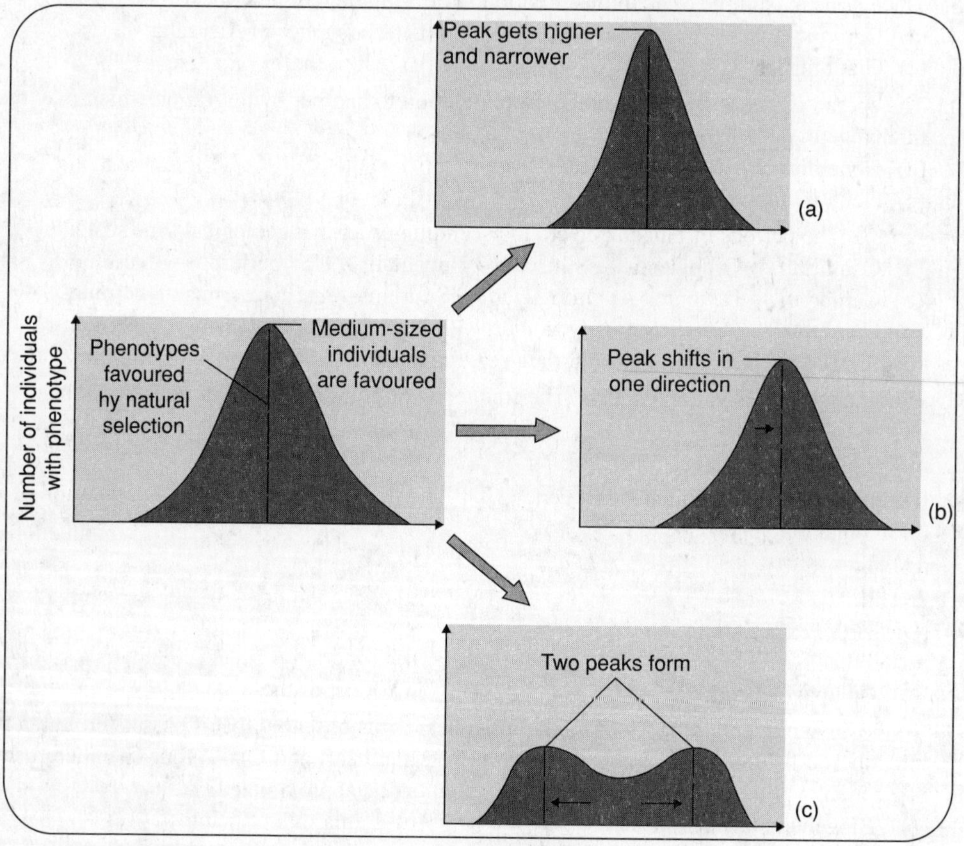

(a) A: Stabilising, B: Disruptive, C: Directional
(b) A: Stabilising, B: Directional, C: Disruptive
(c) A: Disruptive, B: Stabilising, C: Directional
(d) A: Directional, B: Disruptive, C: Stabilising

Read the ***assertion*** *and* ***reason*** *carefully to mark the correct option out of the options given below:*

(a) If both the assertion and the reason are true and the reason is a correct explanation of the assertion
(b) If both the assertion and reason are true but the reason is not a correct explanation of the assertion
(c) If the assertion is true but the reason is false
(d) If both the assertion and reason are false

198. **Assertion:** The Big bang theory attempts to explain to us the origin of universe.
Reason: It talks of a singular huge explosion unimaginable in physical terms.

199. **Assertion:** Natural selection is mechanism of evolution.
Reason: Those who are better fit in an environment, leave more progeny than other, therefore will survive more and hence selected by nature.

200. **Assertion:** Homologous organ represent divergent evolution.
Reason: Homology indicate common ancestry.

201. **Assertion:** Single step large mutation is called saltation.
Reason: Mutation is responsible for speciation.

202. **Assertion:** Homo erectus probably ate meat.
Reason: Homo erectus had a large brain around 900 cc.

203. **Assertion:** Pouched mammals of Australia survived by continental drift.
Reason: It is because of lack of competition from any other mammals.

204. **Assertion:** Agriculture came around 18,000 years ago.
Reason: Pre-historic cave art developed about 10000 years ago.

205. **Assertion:** Dryopithecus was more man-like.
Reason: Ramapithecus was more ape – like.

206. **Assertion:** Comparative biochemistry provides strong evidence in favor of common ancestry of living beings.
Reason: Genetic code in universal.

207. **Assertion:** Human losses gene for tail.
Reason: Lamarck's theory of evolution is known as theory of continuity of germplasm.

AIPMT PREVIOUS YEAR QUESTIONS

1. The most apparent change during the evolutionary history of Homo sapiens is raced in [AIPMT MAINS 2010]

(a) Loss of body hair
(b) Walking upright
(c) Shortening of the jaws
(d) Remarkable increase in the brain size

2. Given below are four statements (A-D) each with one or two blanks. Select the option which correctly fills up the blanks in two statements.

Statements:

(A) Wings of butterfly and birds look alike and are the results of ____ evolution

(B) Miller showed that CH_4, H_2, NH_3 and ____ when exposed to electric discharge in a flask resulted in formation of ____.

(C) Vermiform appendix is a ____ organ and are ____ evidence of evolution.

(D) According to Darwin evolution took place due to ____ and ____ of the fittest.

[AIPMT MAINS 2010]

(a) (D) – (i) small variations, (ii) survival, (A) – (i) convergent
(b) (A) – (i) convergent, (B) – (i) oxygen, (ii) nucleosides
(c) (B) – (i) water vapour, (ii) amino acids (C) – rudimentary, (ii) anatomical
(d) (C) – (i) vestigial, (ii) anatomical (D) – (i) mutations, (ii) multiplication

3. Darwin's finches are a good example of

[AIPMT PRE 2010]

(a) Industrial melanism
(b) Connecting link
(c) Adaptive radiation
(d) Convergent evolution

4. What was the most significant trend in the evolution of modem man (Homo sapiens) from his ancestors?

[AIPMT PRE 2011]

(a) Shortening of jaws
(b) Binocular vision
(c) Increasing brain capacity
(d) Upright posture

5. Mutations can be induced with:

[AIPMT PRE 2011]

(a) IAA
(b) Ethylene
(c) Gamma radiations
(d) Infra red radiations

6. Sweet potato is homologous to

[AIPMT MAINS 2011]

(a) Potato
(b) Colocasia
(c) Ginger
(d) Turnip

7. The idea of mutations was brought forth by:

[AIPMT MAINS 2012]

(a) Gregor Mendel, who worked on pisum sativum
(b) Hardy Weinberg, who worked on allele frequencies in a population
(c) Charles Darwin, who observed a wide variety of organisms during sea voyage
(d) Hugo de Vries, who worked on evening primrose

8. Which one of the following sets of items in the option 1–4 are correctly categorized with one exception in it?

[AIPMT MAINS 2012]

Items	Category	Exception
(a) Kangaroo, Koala, Wombat	Australian marsupials	Wombat
(b) Plasmodium, Cuscuta, Trypanosoma	Protozoan para sites	Cusscuta
(c) Typhoid, Pneumonia, Diphtheria	Bacterial diseases	Diphtheria
(d) UAA, UAG, UGA	Stop codons	UAG

9. Which one of the following is a wrong statement regarding mutations? [AIPMT MAINS 2012]
   (a) Cancer cells commonly show chromosomal aberrations
   (b) UV and Gamma rays are mutagens
   (c) Change in a single base pair of DNA does not cause mutation
   (d) Deletion and insertion of base pairs cause frame-shift mutations

10. Evolution of different species in a given area starting from a point and spreading to other geographical areas is known as: [AIPMT PRE 2012]
   (a) Adaptive radiation (b) Natural selection
   (c) Migration (d) Divergent evolution

11. Which one of the following options gives one correct example each of convergent evolution and divergent evolution? [AIPMT PRE 2012]

	Convergent evolution	Divergent evolution
(a)	Eyes of octopus and mammals	Bones of forelimbs of vertebrates
(b)	Thorns of bougainvillea cucurbita	Wings of butterflies and birds
(c)	Bones of forelimbs if vertebrates	Wings of butterfly and birds
(d)	Thorns of bougainvillea and tendrils of cucurbita	Eyes of octopus and mammals

12. What was the most significant trend in the evolution of modern man (Homo sapiens) from his ancestors? [AIPMT PRE 2012]
   (a) Shortening of jaws (b) Binocular vision
   (c) Increasing cranial capacity (d) Upright posture

13. The extinct human who lived 1,00,000 to 40,000 years ago, in Europe, Asia and parts of Africa, with short stature, heavy eye brows, retreating fore heads, large jaws with heavy teeth, stocky bodies, a lumbering gait and stooped posture was: [AIPMT PRE 2012]
   (a) Homo hibilis (b) Neanderthal human
   (c) Cro-magnan human (d) Ramapithecus

14. The process by which organisms with different evolutionary history evolve similar phenotypic adaptations in response to a common environmental challenge, is called: [AIPMT 2013]
   (a) Natural selection (b) Convergent evolution
   (c) Non-random evolution (d) Adaptive radiation

15. The tendency of population to remain in genetic equilibrium may be disturbed by: [AIPMT 2013]
   (a) Random mating (b) Lack of migration
   (c) Lack of mutations (d) Lack of random mating

16. The eye of octopus and eye of cat show different patterns of structure, yet they perform similar function. This is an example of: [AIPMT 2013]
   (a) Homologous organs that have evolved due to convergent evolution
   (b) Homologous organs that have evolved due to divergent evolution
   (c) Analogous organs that have evolved due to convergent evolution
   (d) Analogous organs that have evolved due to divergent evolution

17. According to Darwin, the organic evolution is due to:

[AIPMT 2013]

(a) Intraspecific competition
(b) Interspecific competition
(c) Competition within closely related species
(d) Reduced feeding efficiency in one species due to the presence of interfering species.

18. Forelimbs of cat, lizard used in walking; forelimbs of whale used in swimming and forelimb of bats used in flying are an example of:

[AIPMT 2014]

(a) Analogous organs
(b) Adaptive radiation
(c) Homologous organs
(d) Convergent evolution

19. Which one of the following are analogous structures?

[AIPMT 2014]

(a) Wings of Bat and Wings of Pigeon
(b) Gills of Prawn and Lungs of Man
(c) Thorns of Bougainvillea and Tendrils of Cucurbita
(d) Flippers of Dolphin and Legs of Horse

20. Which is the most common mechanism of genetic variation in the population of the sexually reproducing organism?

[AIPMT 2015]

(a) Transduction
(b) Chromosomal aberrations
(c) Genetic drift
(d) Recombination

21. Which of the following had the smallest brain capacity?

[AIPMT 2015]

(a) Homo erectus
(b) Homo sapiens
(c) Homo neanderthalensis
(d) Homo habilis

22. A population will not exist in Hardy-Weinberg equilibrium if:

[AIPMT 2015]

(a) Individuals mate selectively
(b) There are no mutations
(c) There is no migration
(d) The population is large

23. Industrial melanism is an example of:

[RE-AIPMT 2015]

(a) Natural selection
(b) Mutation
(c) Leo Lamarckism
(d) Neo Darwinism

24. The wings of a bird and the wings of an insect are:

[RE-AIPMT 2015]

(a) Analogous structures and represent convergent evolution
(b) Phylogenetic structures and represent divergent evolution
(c) Homologous structures and represent convergent evolution
(d) Homologous structures and represent divergent evolution

Answer Keys

1. (c)	2. (c)	3. (b)	4. (c)	5. (c)	6. (a)	7. (d)	8. (b)	9. (d)	10. (d)
11. (a)	12. (c)	13. (d)	14. (c)	15. (b)	16. (c)	17. (a)	18. (d)	19. (b)	20. (a)
21. (a)	22. (a)	23. (d)	24. (c)	25. (c)	26. (d)	27. (a)	28. (d)	29. (d)	30. (d)
31. (c)	32. (b)	33. (a)	34. (c)	35. (d)	36. (b)	37. (b)	38. (b)	39. (a)	40. (c)
41. (a)	42. (d)	43. (d)	44. (c)	45. (c)	46. (d)	47. (c)	48. (a)	49. (a)	50. (d)
51. (a)	52. (a)	53. (a)	54. (c)	55. (d)	56. (b)	57. (d)	58. (a)	59. (a)	60. (d)
61. (d)	62. (c)	63. (d)	64. (d)	65. (d)	66. (c)	67. (a)	68. (d)	69. (c)	70. (a)
71. (d)	72. (c)	73. (b)	74. (a)	75. (c)	76. (a)	77. (c)	78. (a)	79. (b)	80. (a)
81. (a)	82. (d)	83. (b)	84. (b)	85. (c)	86. (b)	87. (a)	88. (c)	89. (b)	90. (c)
91. (a)	92. (b)	93. (d)	94. (b)	95. (d)	96. (d)	97. (a)	98. (a)	99. (d)	100. (d)
101. (a)	102. (d)	103. (b)	104. (b)	105. (d)	106. (c)	107. (c)	108. (d)	109. (c)	110. (d)
111. (d)	112. (b)	113. (a)	114. (c)	115. (a)	116. (c)	117. (a)	118. (d)	119. (c)	120. (b)
121. (a)	122. (a)	123. (c)	124. (a)	125. (c)	126. (a)	127. (b)	128. (d)	129. (a)	130. (a)
131. (c)	132. (b)	133. (b)	134. (c)	135. (b)	136. (a)	137. (d)	138. (a)	139. (a)	140. (b)
141. (a)	142. (b)	143. (d)	144. (a)	145. (a)	146. (a)	147. (c)	148. (b)	149. (c)	150. (d)
151. (b)	152. (a)	153. (d)	154. (d)	155. (c)	156. (c)	157. (b)	158. (d)	159. (b)	160. (c)
161. (c)	162. (d)	163. (c)	164. (b)	165. (d)	166. (a)	167. (b)	168. (b)	169. (b)	170. (b)
171. (b)	172. (b)	173. (d)	174. (a)	175. (d)	176. (d)	177. (b)	178. (d)	179. (d)	180. (d)
181. (a)	182. (b)	183. (c)	184. (b)	185. (a)	186. (a)	187. (a)	188. (a)	189. (b)	190. (c)
191. (a)	192. (c)	193. (b)	194. (a)	195. (c)	196. (d)	197. (b)	198. (b)	199. (a)	200. (a)
201. (b)	202. (b)	203. (a)	204. (d)	205. (d).	206. (b)	207. (d)			

AIPMT Previous Year Questions

1. (d)	2. (a)	3. (c)	4. (c)	5. (c)	6. (d)	7. (d)	8. (b)	9. (c)	10. (a)
11. (a)	12. (c)	13. (b)	14. (b)	15. (d)	16. (c)	17. (b)	18. (c)	19. (b)	20. (d)
21. (d)	22. (a)	23. (a)	24. (a)						

Unit

VIII

Biology in Human Welfare

This unit is divided into three chapters—Human Health and Disease, Strategies for Enhancement in Food Production and Microbes in Human Welfare. Out of all the chapters, Chapter 8 (Human health and Disease) is very important. Also, in Chapters 9 and 10, the given examples are very important.

CHAPTER 30

Human Health and Disease

1. Which scientist, along with Norman Borlaug, brought 'Green Revolution' to India?
   (a) Kartikeyan
   (b) Murlidharan
   (c) Swaminanthan
   (d) Khurana
2. ________ varieties of wheat brought 'Green Revolution' to India.
   (a) American
   (b) Mexican
   (c) Peruvian
   (d) Chilean
3. Greeks like Hippocrates and Indian Ayurveda system considered health as ________.
   (a) imbalance of certain 'humors'
   (b) absence of certain 'humors'
   (c) balance of certain 'humors'
   (d) presence of certain 'humors'
4. People with ________ were believed to have hot personality and would have fevers.
   (a) black bile
   (b) yellow bile
   (c) green bile
   (d) brown bile
5. Who discovered blood circulation?
   (a) William Harvey
   (b) Land Steiner
   (c) J.F. Watson
   (d) Edison
6. Which device was used by William Harvey to disprove 'good humor' hypothesis of health?
   (a) Cardiograph
   (b) Sphygmomanometer
   (c) Thermometer
   (d) Barometer
7. Which system of the human body is actually responsible for maintaining health?
   (a) Neuronal system
   (b) Circulatory system
   (c) Endocrine system
   (d) Immune system
8. Health is affected by
   (a) Genetic disorders
   (b) Infections
   (c) Life style
   (d) All
9. A state of complete physical, mental and social well-being is termed as
   (a) Disease
   (b) Comfort
   (c) Health
   (d) Hygiene
10. Good health can be maintained by
    (a) Balanced diet
    (b) Personal hygiene
    (c) Regular exercise
    (d) All
11. ________ has been practised since time immemorial to achieve physical and mental health
    (a) Sports
    (b) Yoga
    (c) Aerobics
    (d) Gym

12. Which disease is shown in the figure?

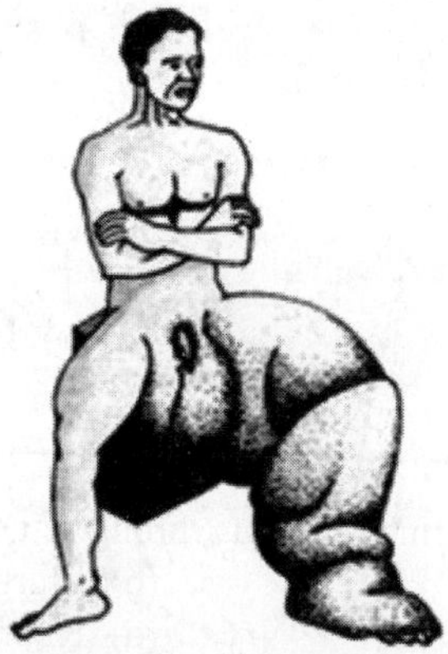

(a) Malaria (b) Kala azar
(c) Filariasis (d) Ascariasis

13. Diseases which are transmitted from person to person are called
(a) Non-infections (b) Genetic
(c) Infectious (d) Deadly

14. An infectious disease which is fatal is
(a) Cold (b) Conjunctivitis
(c) AIDS (d) Cholera

15. Disease causing organisms are known as
(a) Vectors (b) Pathogens
(c) Carriers (d) Parasites

16. Pathogens have to ________ within the environment of the host.
(a) adapt to attach (b) adapt to only body temperature
(c) adapt to life (d) adapt to mutation

17. Typhoid fever in humans is caused by
(a) Rotavirus (b) Salmonella typhi
(c) Escherichia coli (d) Amoeba

18. Salmonella *typhi* generally enters which part of the alimentary canal?
(a) Stomach (b) Large intestine
(c) Small intestine (d) Mouth

19. S. *typhi* spreads through
(a) Air (b) Sexual contact
(c) Contaminated food and water (d) Physical touch

20. Sustained high fever (39° to 40° C) and intestinal perforation in severe cases is a symptom of which disease?
(a) Malaria (b) Typhoid
(c) Cholera (d) Common cold

21. Which test is performed to confirm typhoid fever?
(a) ELISA test (b) Widal test
(c) Biopsy (d) Schick test

22. I was a cook by profession and spread typhoid through the food I used to cook.
(a) Madam Curie (b) Mary Mallon
(c) Rosalin Franklin (d) G.J Mendel

23. What is shown in the figure?

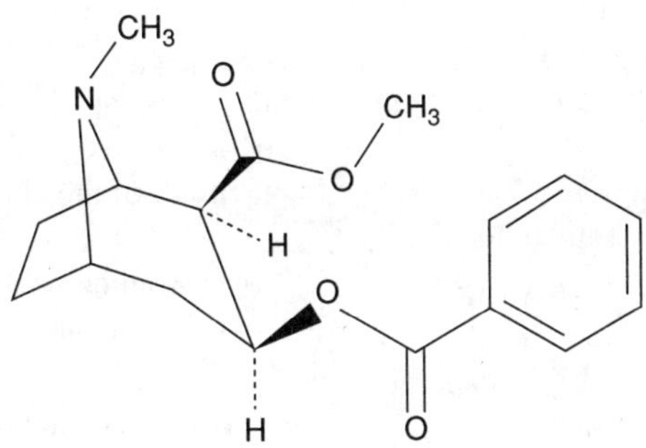

(a) Cannabinoid molecule (b) Morphine
(c) Nicotine (d) Lobeline

24. Pneumonia is caused by
(a) Streptococcus pneumonia (b) Pneumococcus pneumonia
(c) Haemophilus influenza (d) All of the above

25. Which part of the lungs is infected in pneumonia?
(a) Alveoli (b) Trachea
(c) Bronchus (d) Terminal bronchioles

26. In which disease, lips and fingernails turn gray and in severe cases bluish?
(a) Jaundice (b) Pneumonia
(c) Typhoid (d) Malaria

27. Which of the following is not a bacterial disease?
(a) Dysentery (b) Plague
(c) Polio (d) Diphtheria

28. Pneumonia is spread by
(a) Inhaling droplets/aerosols (b) Mosquito
(c) Reusing syringes (d) Genetic disease

29. Common cold is caused by
(a) Tobacco mosaic virus (b) Rhino virus
(c) Rota virus (d) Adeno virus

30. In common cold, which part of respiratory system is not infected?
(a) Nose (b) Respiratory passage
(c) Lungs (d) All of the above

31. What is the one thing that is common between common cold and pneumonia?
(a) Both are caused by same pathogen.
(b) Both are caused by same vector.
(c) Both are caused by droplet infection.
(d) Both are incurable.

32. Malaria is caused by which species of plasmodium?
(a) P. vivax
(b) P. malaria
(c) P. falciparum
(d) All of the above

33. Plasmodium is a
(a) Bacterium
(b) Virus
(c) Protozoan
(d) Fungi

34. The most serious form of malaria, malignant malaria, is caused by
(a) P. falciparum
(b) P. vivax
(c) P. malarial
(d) All of the above

35. Plasmodium enters the human body as ________.
(a) Merozoite
(b) Trophozoie
(c) Hypnozoite
(d) Sporozoite

36. The vector of plasmodium is
(a) Male anopheles mosquito
(b) Female anopheles mosquito
(c) Aedes egypti
(d) Sand worm

37. In malaria, fever and chills occur every 3 to 4 days due to rupture of RBCs and release of which toxic substance?
(a) Haemophilia
(b) Hematocrit
(c) Haemozoin
(d) Haemoglobin

38. Sporozoites in mosquitoes are stored in
(a) Intestine
(b) Mouth
(c) Salivary glands
(d) Proboscis

39. Malarial parasites require two hosts. They are
(a) Humans, female anopheles mosquito
(b) Humans, Aedes Egypti
(c) Cattle, female anopheles mosquito
(d) Cattle, Aedes Egypti

40. After the injection of sporozoites in the blood of humans, which organ do they travel initially?
(a) Lymph nodes
(b) Brain
(c) Lungs
(d) Liver

41. The plasmodium parasite reproduces in liver by ________ and in blood by ________.
(a) sexual reproduction, asexual reproduction
(b) asexual reproduction, sexual reproduction
(c) spore formation, sexual reproduction
(d) sexual reproduction, spore formation

42. Entamoeba histolytica causes ________ in humans.
(a) histolysis
(b) amoebiasis
(c) catharsis
(d) sporogenesis

43. Stool with excess of mucous and blood clots is known as
(a) Diarrhoea
(b) Dysentery
(c) Both (a) and (b)
(d) None

44. Carrier for amoebiasis is
(a) Entamoebia histolytica
(c) Mosquito
(c) House flies
(d) Plasmodium vivax

Figure given for questions 45–47.

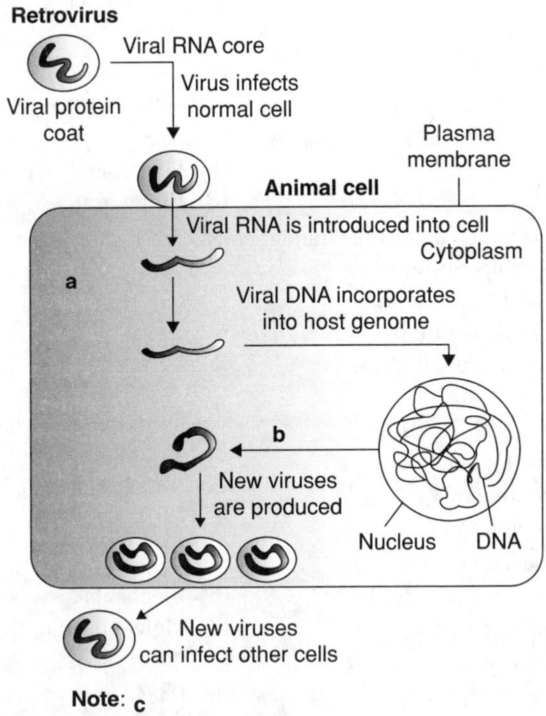

45. What is indicated by 'a' in the figure?
(a) Viral RNA produced by RNA polymerase
(b) Viral DNA produced by DNA polymerase
(c) Viral DNA produced by Reverse transcriptase
(d) Viral RNA produced by reverse transcriptase

46. What is indicated by 'b'?
(a) New viral RNA (b) New viral DNA
(c) New viral Proteins (d) New viral Cell

47. What is indicated by 'c' in the figure?
(a) Infected cell survives (b) Infected cell dies
(c) Virus being replicated (d) Both (a) and (c)

48. Ascaris is also known as
(a) Common round worm (b) Common whip worm
(c) Common thread worm (d) Common pin worm

49. In humans, ascaris causes
(a) Filariasis (b) Ascites
(c) Ascariasis (d) Malaria

50. Symptoms like internal bleeding, muscular pain, fever, anaemia, and blockage of intestinal passage occur in which disease?
(a) Typhoid (b) Ascariasis
(c) Malaria (d) Pneumonia

51. Contaminated water, vegetables and fruits with eggs of round worm causes
(a) Filariasis (b) Ascariasis
(c) Malaria (d) Pneumonia

52. Filariasis is also known as
(a) Ascariasis (b) Elephantiasis
(c) Ringworm (d) Amoebiasis

53. Wuchereria causes which disease in humans
(a) Amoebiasis (b) Filariasis
(c) Ascariasis (d) Ringworm

54. W. bancrofti infects which part of the human body?
(a) Blood vessels of upper limbs
(b) Lymph vessels of lower limb
(c) Blood vessels of lower limb
(d) Lymph vessels of upper limb

55. Wuchereria causes
(a) Acute inflammation
(b) Chronic inflammation
(c) Bacterial inflammation
(d) Viral inflammation

56. Elephantiasis is caused by the bite of
(a) W. malayi (b) Elephants
(c) Female mosquito (d) Male mosquito

57. Ringworm is caused by
(a) Round worm (b) Bacteria
(c) Fungi (d) Virus

58. Which fungal genera are not responsible for causing ringworm?
(a) Megasporum (b) Trichophyton
(c) Epidermophyton (d) None

59. Which are the main symptoms of ringworm?
(a) Appearance of worms on skin
(b) Appearance of dry scaly lesions
(c) Inflammation of limbs
(d) Fever and chills

60. Which factors are necessary for the growth of the fungi?
(a) Moisture and sebum (b) Heat and Hair
(c) Body odour (d) Heat and moisture

61. In ringworm which parts of the body are usually affected?
(a) Skin, hair and scalp
(b) Skin, nails and hands
(c) Skin, hair and lips
(d) Skin, nails and scalp

62. Combs of individuals infected with ________ can transmit the disease.
(a) sebborhitis (b) dermatitis
(c) ringworm (d) dandruff

Figure given for questions 63–65.

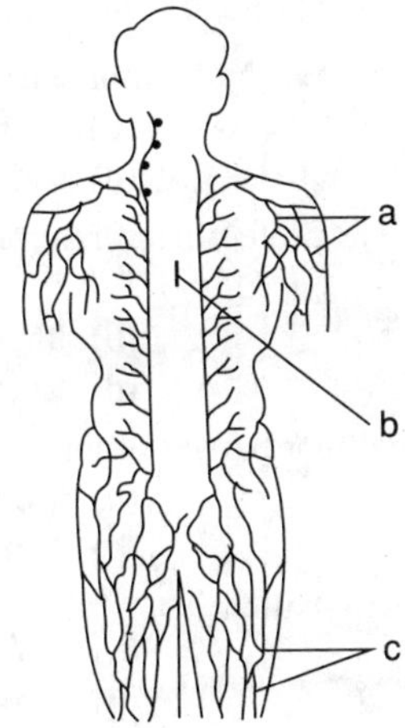

63. What is indicated by 'a' in the figure?
(a) Lymph Vessels (b) Lymph nodes
(c) Lymph valves (d) Tonsilar carpsale

64. What is indicated by 'c' in the figure?
(a) Lymph Vessels (b) Lymph nodes
(c) Lymph valves (d) Tonsilar carpsale

65. What does 'b' represent in the figure?
(a) Thyroid (b) Tonsil
(c) Thymus (d) Trachea

66. Ringworms are generally acquired from
(a) Water (b) Air
(c) Soil (d) Food

67. The mosquito larvae are fed upon by
(a) Ambrosia (b) Gambusia
(c) Mosquito repellent (d) Turtles

68. Dengue is caused by which vector?
(a) Anopheles mosquito (b) Aedes mosquito
(c) Apollo mosquito (d) Plasmodium

69. A deadly disease, small pox, has been eradicated through
(a) Antiserum (b) Vaccination
(c) Cauterisation (d) Antidote

70. Chikungunya is spread by the vector
(a) Fungal spores (b) Housefly
(c) Mosquito (d) Reptiles

71. Every day our body is exposed to a large number of infectious agents. But all are not capable of causing disease. This is due to
(a) Decreased virulence of pathogen (b) Immunity of an individual
(c) Genotype of an individual (d) Lifestyle of an individual

72. Innate immunity is a ________ type of defense mechanism.
(a) specific (b) non specific
(c) congenital (d) both (b) and (c)

73. Skin and mucus is which type of barrier under innate immunity?
(a) Physiological (b) Morphological
(c) Physical (d) Cellular

74. Saliva in mouth and tears from eye protect from microbial infection. This type of barrier is known as
(a) Cellular (b) Physical
(c) Physiological (d) Cytokine

75. Which of the following is not a cellular barrier of innate immunity?
(a) PMNL-Neutrophils (b) Monocytes
(c) Lymphocytes (d) Thrombocytes

76. Virus infected cells secrete a protein called ________ to protect other non-infected cells.
(a) cytokine (b) immunoglobulin
(c) interferon (d) clotting factors

77. Acquired immunity is
(a) Pathogen specific (b) Pathogen non specific
(c) Congenital (d) Non effective

78. Acquired immunity has one of the following features
(a) Non specific (b) Memory
(c) Anti-cancer (d) Congenital

79. When a pathogen comes in contact with body for the first time, it causes a ________ response of low intensity
(a) anamnestic (b) anaphylactic
(c) primary (d) secondary

Figure given for questions 80–200.

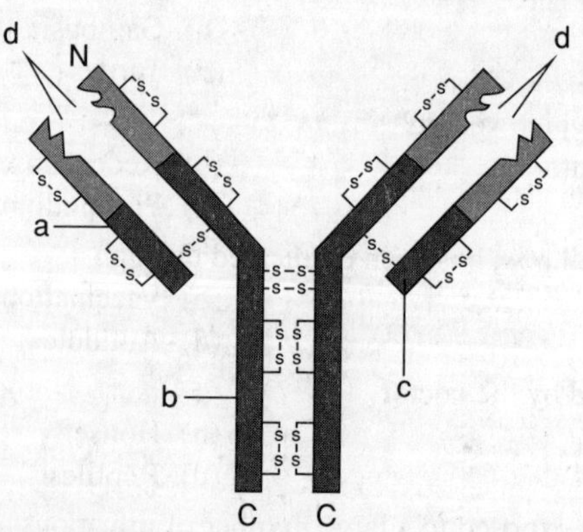

80. What is indicated by 'd' in the figure?
(a) Light chain (b) Heavy chain
(c) Antigen binding site (d) CMI

81. What does 'a' represent in the figure?
(a) Light chain (b) Heavy chain
(c) Antigen binding site (d) CMI

82. What is indicated by 'b' in the figure?
(a) CMI (b) Heavy chain
(c) Light chain (d) Antigen binding site

83. If a pathogen gains access to the body the second time then a highly intensified response called ________ may occur.
(a) analgesia (b) anamnestic
(c) anthropologic (d) arthus reaction

84. The army of proteins produced by B-lymphocytes is called
(a) Antigen (b) Interferons
(c) Cytokines (d) Antibodies

85. The two types of lymphocytes responsible for immune response are
(a) A-type (b) B-type
(c) T-type (d) Both (b) and (c)

86. The immunity conferred by B-lymphocytes is also known as
(a) Immediate (b) Histological
(c) Humoral (d) Cell-mediate

87. Which lymphocytes help B-cells to secrete antibodies?
(a) Nature killer (b) Macrophage
(c) T-cells (d) Monocytes

88. An antibody has ________ heavy chains and ________ light chains respectively.
(a) 2, 4 (b) 4, 2
(c) 2, 2 (d) 1, 2

89. An antibody is represented as
(a) $H_1 L_2$ (b) $H_2 L_2$
(c) $H_4 L_1$ (d) $H_4 L_4$

90. Select the correct option
(a) Ig A, Ig G, Ig E, Ig D, Ig I
(b) Ig G, Ig A, Ig G, Ig H, Ig J
(c) Ig A, Ig G, Ig E, Ig D, Ig M
(d) Ig M, Ig A, Ig E, Ig I, Ig G

91. The chains of antibodies are held together by
(a) Dihydrogen (b) Covalent
(c) Disulfide (d) Ionic

92. The immunity conferred by T-lymphocyte is known as
(a) Humoral mediated (b) Tissue mediated
(c) Cell mediated (d) Neural mediated

93. After any graft/transplant which medications does a patient have to take all his/her life?
(a) Immuno modulators (b) Immuno suppressants
(c) Immuno Competors (d) Immuno depressants

94. Before any graft/organ transplant, which procedure should be performed?
(a) Tissue matching (b) Pedigree analysis
(c) CT scan (d) X-ray

95. What is shown in the figure?

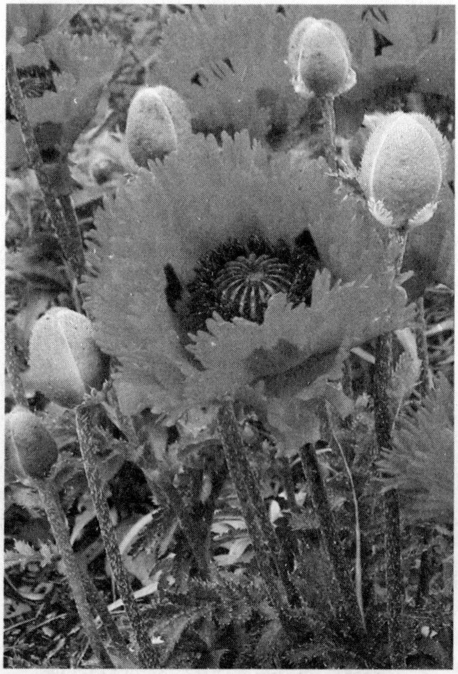

(a) Sunflower plant (b) Poppy plant
(c) Datura plant (d) Tobacco plant

96. Which immune response makes graft rejection obvious?
(a) Humoral mediated (b) Innate immunity
(c) Cell mediated (d) Acquired immunity

97. Which immunity is slow and takes time for full effective response?
(a) Active (b) Passive
(c) Acquired (d) Innate

98. When a host is exposed to antigens, antibodies are produced in the host body. This type of immunity is known as ________.
(a) Passive (b) Active
(c) Innate (d) Cell mediated

99. Active immunity is induced by
(a) Injecting prepared antibodies (b) Injecting live infectious microbes
(c) Injecting dead microbes or proteins (d) Injecting vaccine

100. When readymade antibodies are given to protect the body against foreign agents, it is called ________ immunity
(a) passive (b) active
(c) innate (d) humoral

101. In initial days of lactation, the mother's milk 'Colostrum' is rich in which antibody?
(a) Ig A (b) Ig E
(c) Ig M (d) Ig G

102. Foetus receives ________ from mother through the placenta during pregnancy.
(a) antigens (b) antibodies
(c) t-cells (d) b-cells

103. Principle of ________ is based on the property of 'memory' of the immune system.
(a) passive immunity (b) antigen antibody
(c) immunisation (d) agglutinisation

104. Immunisation is also known as
(a) Passive immunity (b) Innate immunity
(c) Vaccination (d) Resistance

105. A vaccine is
(a) Prepared antigenic proteins
(b) Inactivated/weakened pathogen
(c) Live pathogens
(d) Both (a) and (b)

106. When a quick immune response is required, we can
(a) Directly inject weakened pathogen at time of emergency
(b) Directly inject preformed antigens
(c) Directly inject preformed antibodies
(d) Directly inject immuno depressants

107. In Tetanus case we inject
(a) Antigenic proteins (b) Antibodies
(c) Weakened pathogen (d) Saline

108. When a person is bitten by snake, we inject antitoxin in the patient. This type of immunity is known as
(a) Active immunisation
(b) Passive immunisation
(c) Innate immunisation
(d) Humoral immunity

109. Antigenic polypeptides of pathogen has been produced on a large scale. This is due to ________ technology.
(a) Polymerase Chain Reaction
(b) DNA fingerprinting
(c) Recombinant DNA technology
(d) In-vitro fertilization

110. By using recombinant DNA technology, hepatitis B vaccine is produced from ________.
(a) bacteria (b) yeast
(c) fungi (d) lichen

111. A sudden episode of sneezing-wheezing when you travel to a new place is due to ________ response.
(a) inflammation (b) allergic
(c) auto-immune (d) cell mediated immunity

112. Substances which cause allergy are known as
(a) Mutagens (b) Irritants
(c) Allergens (d) Agglutinogens

Figure given for questions 112–116.

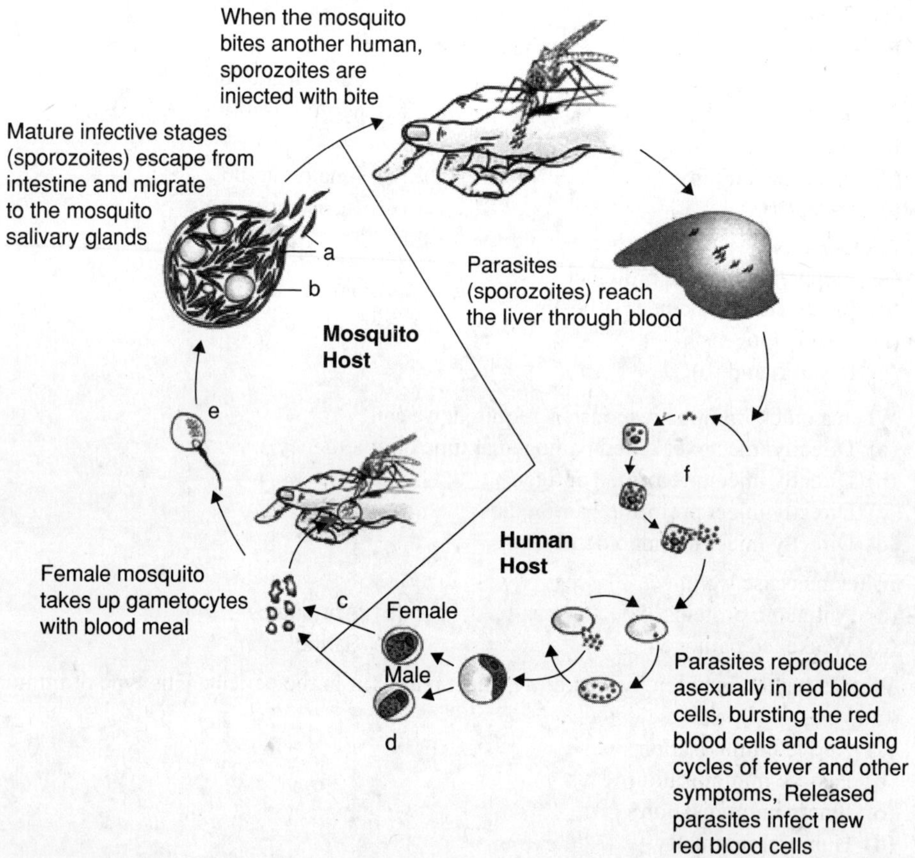

113. Which life cycle is indicated in the figure?
(a) Plasmozoa (b) Plasmodium
(c) Paramoecium (d) Filarial parasite

114. What is indicated by 'a' in the figure ?
(a) Merozoites (b) Hypnozoites
(c) Sporozoites (d) Gametocytes

115. What is indicated by 'b' in the figure?
(a) Gametocyte (b) Salivary gland
(c) Proboscis (d) Merozoites

116. Gametes are developing in which cells as shown by phase 'd' in the figure?
(a) WBC (b) RBC
(c) Lymphocytes (d) Hepatocyte

117. Which cells is bursting as shown by phase 'f' in the figure?
(a) WBC (b) RBC
(c) Lymphocytes (d) Hepatocyte

118. The antibodies primarily participating in allergic response are
(a) Ig A (b) Ig E
(c) Ig G (d) Ig M

119. Which of the following is an allergen?
(a) Dust (b) Pollen
(c) Animal dander (d) All of above

120. Which of the following is not an allergic reaction symptom?
(a) Sneezing (b) Watery eyes
(c) Difficulty in breathing (d) Hiccups

121. Which cells actively participate in allergic reaction?
(a) Mast cell (b) Monocytes
(c) Lymphocytes (d) macrophages

122. In an allergic reaction, which chemicals are released by the mast cells?
(a) Histamine and Serotonin (b) Histamine and Secretin
(c) Serotonin and Adrenalin (d) Serotonin and Nor-adrenalin

123. In case of allergy, which drugs reduce the symptoms?
(a) Anti-histamine (b) Adrenalin
(c) Steroids (d) All of above

124. In auto-immune disorders, the cells
(a) Produce more antibodies (b) Produce less antibodies
(c) Start attacking other body cells (d) Have exaggerated immune response

125. Which is of the following is in an example of auto-immune disease?
(a) Tetanus (b) Allergy
(c) Rheumatoid Arthritis (d) Asthma

126. Which of the following is a primary lymphoid organ?
(a) Thymus (b) Spleen
(c) Tonsils (d) Lymph nodes

127. Immature lymphocytes differentiate in
(a) Liver, Spleen (b) Bone morrow and Thyroid
(c) Thymus and Bone marrow (d) Spleen, Thymus

128. Which of the following is a secondary lymphoid organ?
(a) Brunner's gland (b) Peyer's patches
(c) Crypts of leiberkuhn (d) Glison's capsule

129. Which structure of the lymph system keeps degenerating from birth to puberty?
(a) Spleen (b) Tonsils
(c) Peyer's patches (d) Thymus

130. The spleen is
(a) Butterfly shaped (b) Bean shaped
(c) Button shaped (d) Wedge shaped

131. Thymus is responsible for maturation of which cells?
(a) Tendons (b) B-cells
(c) T-cells (d) Mast cells

132. Which organ act as filter of the blood by trapping blood borne micro-organisms?
(a) Spleen (b) Liver
(c) Tonsils (d) Bone marrow

133. Respiratory, digestive and urogenital tract has a lining of mucus along with lymph. This lining is known as
(a) Mucosa associated tissue
(b) Mucosa assisted lymphoid tissue
(c) Mucosa associated lymphoid tissue
(d) Mucosa assisted tissue

134. Which disease is indicated in the figure ?

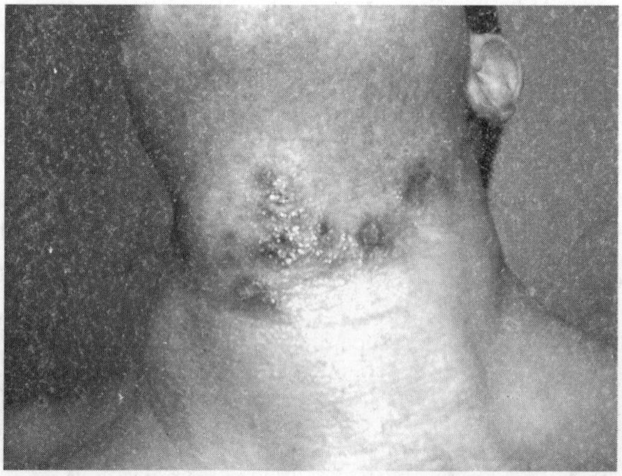

(a) Facial palsy
(b) Dermatitis
(c) Ringworm
(d) Round worm

135. In context of lymphoid tissue, MALT constitutes about ________% of all the lymphoid tissue in human body.
(a) 25%
(b) 60%
(c) 50%
(d) 90%

136. A group of symptoms is known as
(a) Infection
(b) Syndrome
(c) Disease
(d) Collection

137. AIDS was first reported in the year ________.
(a) 1971
(b) 1981
(c) 1991
(d) 1960

138. The death toll due to AIDS has crossed ________ globally.
(a) 2.5 billion
(b) 2500 million
(c) 25 million
(d) 250 million

139. AIDS is caused due to
(a) HIV
(b) DNA virus
(c) TMV
(d) Bacteriophage

140. HIV belongs to a group of viruses known as
(a) Inverto virus
(b) Retro virus
(c) Metro virus
(d) Flavo virus

141. Retro virus causing AIDS has which kind of genome?
(a) DNA
(b) RNA
(c) m-RNA
(d) Proteins

142. Which of the following is not a means of transmission of AIDS?
(a) Sexual contact with uninfected person (b) Transfusion of contaminated blood
(c) Sharing infected needles (d) Child born to an HIV infected mother

143. Time lag between infection and appearance of AIDS symptoms can be few months to ________ years.
(a) 2–3 (b) 5–10
(c) >15 (d) 1–2

144. Retro virus contains an enzyme to carry out biochemical activities in host. Name the enzyme.
(a) Polymerase (b) Exonuclease
(c) Reverse transcriptase (d) Ligase

145. The virus responsible for causing AIDS primarily infects?
(a) Monocytes (b) Mast cells
(c) Macrophages (d) Mucosal cells

146. What is shown in the figure?

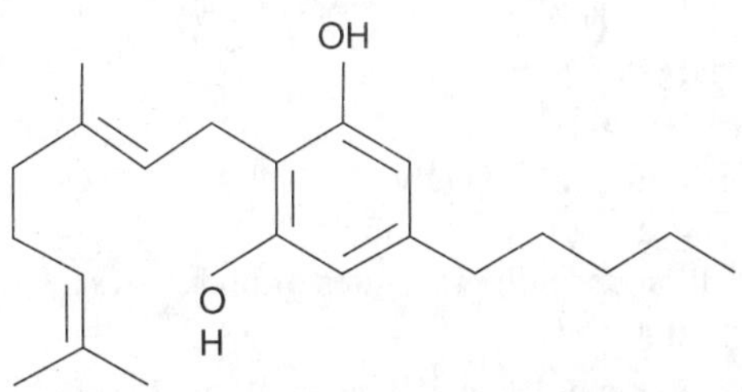

(a) Cannabinoid molecule (b) Morphine
(c) Nicotine (d) Lobeline

147. HIV enters which T-cells
(a) Helper (T_H) (b) Promoter (T_P)
(c) Suppressor (T_S) (d) Cytotoxic (T_C)

148. Death in AIDS is due to
(a) Aggravated immune response (b) Due to opportunistic infections
(c) Due to inflammation of genitilia (d) Due to diarrhoea and fever

149. AIDS can be detected by which diagnostic test?
(a) Widal (b) ELISA
(c) SGPT (d) Blood cell count

150. The organisation in India which is spreading awareness and educating people regarding AIDS is
(a) Gramin Yojna (b) Health Ministry
(c) National AIDS Control Organisation (d) None of the above

151. NGO stands for
(a) Non Governing Organisation (b) Non Governmental Organization
(c) Non Guaranteed Object (d) Non Granted Organisation

152. Normal cells in our body inhibit the uncontrolled growth of cells which they are in contact with. This is known as
(a) Cell–cell contact (b) Cell cycle Regulation
(c) Contact inhibition (d) Contact response

153. Tumour is an abnormal mass of
(a) Muscles
(b) Cells
(c) Inorganic salts
(d) Cartilagenous membrane

154. The tumour which does not spread to other parts of body is known as ________.
(a) benign (b) malignant
(c) neoplastic (d) lymphoma

155. The cancerous cells which have the ability to proliferate and cause cancer in new locations of the body are known as
(a) Benign (b) Lymphoma
(c) Leukaemia (d) Malignant

156. Cancer cells actively divide and grow due to
(a) Competition for vital nutrients with normal cells
(b) Competition for space with normal cells
(c) Competition for only support
(d) Excess food materials stored in body

157. Metastasis is
(a) Normal equilibrium condition of body
(b) Morphological changes from larva to adult
(c) Generation of new tumour in different sites of body
(d) Abnormal growth of the body muscles

158. The agents which can cause neoplastic cell generation are
(a) Gamma rays (b) X-rays
(c) UV rays (d) All of above

159. Which radiations can cause cancer?
(a) Visible light (b) UV rays
(c) Infra red light (d) Microwaves

160. Cancer causing viruses are known as
(a) Retro virus (b) Oncogenic virus
(c) Flavo virus (d) Adeno virus

161. The genes present in normal cells of the body which can cause cancer are known as
(a) Oncogenes (b) Carcinogenes
(c) Neogenes (d) Tumerogenes

162. Proto-oncogenes are also abbreviated as
(a) p-onc (b) c-onc
(c) p-con (d) c-con

163. Blood and bone marrow tests are usually performed to detect
(a) Anaemia (b) Leukaemia
(c) Thrombocytopenia (d) Filariasis

164. In case of ________, a piece of suspected tissue is cut into thin sections, stained and examined under microscope.
(a) Post mortem (b) Biopsy
(c) DNA fingerprinting (d) Pedigree analysis

165. Cancers of internal organs can be detected by
(a) Radiography (b) CT
(c) MRI (d) All of these

166. In which technique 3-D image of the internals of an objected are generated?
(a) Electron microscopy
(b) Radiography
(c) Computed Tomography
(d) Magnetic Resonance Imaging

167. MRI uses strong magnetic field and ________ radiations to detect pathological and physiological changes.
(a) ionising (b) non-ionising
(c) LASER (d) x-ray

168. Tobacco smoke primarily causes
(a) Mouth cancer (b) Lung cancer
(c) Breast cancer (d) Desophaleol cancer

169. Common approaches for treatment of cancer are
(a) Surgery (b) Radiation therapy
(c) Immuno therapy (d) All of above

170. Anti cancer drugs have the following side effects
(a) Hair loss (b) Anaemia
(c) Vomiting (d) All of these

171. For the treatment of cancer, biological response modifiers such as ________ are given.
(a) β-interferons (b) γ-interferons
(c) α-interferons (d) δ-interferons

172. Heroine is locally known as ________.
(a) smack (b) angel dust
(c) coke (d) marijuana

173. Smack is chemically
(a) Dicetyl morphine (b) Diacetyl morphine
(c) Dimethye morphile (d) Dihydro morphine

174. Morphine is obtained from
(a) Erythroxylum coca (b) Atropa belladonna
(c) Connabis sativa (d) Papaver somniferum

175. Heroin is a ________ drug.
(a) excitatory (b) depressant
(c) hallucinogenic (d) euphoric

176. Morphine is extracted from ________ of poppy plant
(a) leaf (b) latex
(c) fruit (d) flower

177. Cannabinoids are obtained from ________, ________ and ________ of cannabis sativa.
(a) leaves, flowers, fruits
(b) leaves, flower tops, resin
(c) leaves, flowers, latex
(d) flower, seed, tannins

178. What is shown in the figure?

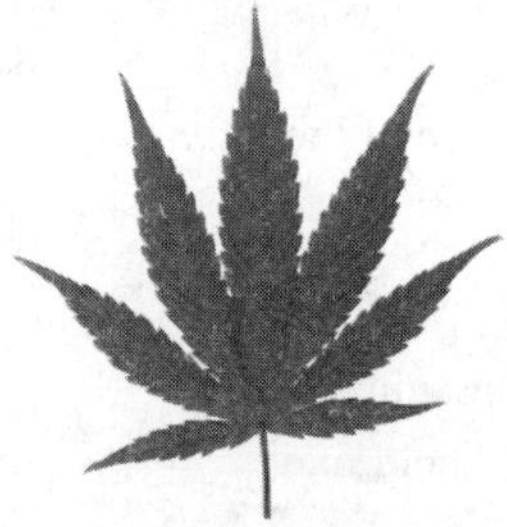

(a) Opium (b) Datura
(c) Cannabis (d) Tobacco

179. Cannabinoids are mainly known to effect?
(a) Cardio vascular system (b) Nervous system
(c) Sensory system (d) Excretory system

180. Charas, ganja, hashish and marijuana are all
(a) Opioids (b) Cannabinoids
(c) Coca alkaloids (d) Barbiturates

181. Cocaine is obtained from
(a) Erythroxylum coca (b) Paper somniferum
(c) Atropa belladonna (d) Connalris sativa

182. Coca plant is native to
(a) North America (b) South America
(c) South Africa (d) Australia

183. Cocaine is commonly known as
(a) Smack (b) Coke
(c) Crack (d) Both (b) and (c)

184. Cocaine produces a sense of ________.
(a) euphoria (b) dysphoria
(c) depression (d) androgenic effects

185. Excessive dosage of cocaine causes ________.
(a) cvs collapse (b) hallucinations
(c) nerve damage (d) vomiting

186. Atropa belladonna is
(a) Ornamental plant (b) Hallucinogenic plant
(c) Immunomodulator plant (d) Depressant plant

187. Generally, cannabinoids are taken by
(a) Intravenously (b) Intramuscularly
(c) Through oral route (d) Through Implants

188. LSD is
(a) Lauric Acid Dimethyl Amide (b) Lysergic Acid Dimethyl Amide
(c) Lysergic Acid Diethyl Amide (d) Lysergic Acid Diethyl amine

189. ________ a is very effective pain-killer and sedative used for patients who have undergone surgery.
(a) Paracetamol (b) Morphine
(c) LSD (d) Barbiturate

190. Datura is a ________ plant.
(a) sedative
(b) hallucinogenic
(c) excitatory
(d) health tonic

191. AIDS do Not spread by
(a) Sexual contact
(b) Body Fluids
(c) Physical touch
(d) Blood transfusion

192. Treatment of AIDS with anti-retro viral drugs is
(a) Not at all effective
(b) Fully effective
(c) Partially effective
(d) Leads to secondary infections

193. When plants having hallucinogenic properties are administered in more than required amount/frequency, it causes
(a) Addiction
(b) Drug abuse
(c) Cancer
(d) Both (a) and (b)

194. Barbiturates and Benzodiazepines are used in clinical conditions like
(a) Cancer and its prevention
(b) Euphoria and sense of well-being
(c) Depression and insomnia
(d) Increasing body strength and vigour

195. Tobacco has been used by human beings for more than ________ years
(a) 400 millions
(b) 40 millions
(c) 4000 millions
(d) 400

196. Tobacco contains an alkaloid known as ________.
(a) morphine
(b) piperine
(c) nicotine
(d) anabasine

197. Nicotine stimulates which gland primarily?
(a) Salivary
(b) Pancreas
(c) Spleen
(d) Adrenal

198. What is the effect of nicotine?
(a) Relieves stress and anxiety
(b) It gives a sense of well-being and happiness
(c) It raises blood pressure and heart rate
(d) It causes excess of acidity

199. Smoking increases the content of which compound in blood?
(a) CO_2
(b) CO
(c) H_2CO_3
(d) H_2O_2

200. Adolescence period ranges from ________ years.
(a) 10–16
(b) 12–18
(c) 13–19
(d) 11–20

201. Adolescence is a bridge linking ________ and ________.
(a) Teenage and Marriage
(b) Childhood and Adulthood
(c) Teenage and Adulthood
(d) Birth and Adulthood

202. ________ is a psychological attachment to certain effects like euphoria associated with drugs and alcohol?
(a) Hallucinations
(b) Addiction
(c) Delusion
(d) Ilusion

203. If regular dose of drugs/alcohol is abruptly discontinued it causes ________.
(a) hallucinations
(b) withdrawal syndrome
(c) diversion to criminal activities
(d) severe depression

204. Death in case of overdose of drugs occurs due to
(a) Respiratory failure (b) Heart failure
(c) Cerebral hemorrhage (d) All of the above

205. Drug abusers can suffer from infections like
(a) Hepatitis (b) Depression
(c) Euphoria (d) Cirrhosis

206. Chronic alcoholism damages which vital organ of the body?
(a) Heart (b) Kidney
(c) Liver (d) Brain

207. Generally sportsmen abuse which categories of drugs?
(a) Immuno modulators (b) Anabolic steroids
(c) Cannabinoids (d) Potent pain killers

208. Which categories of drugs are used by sportsmen?
(a) Certain hormones (b) Anabolic steroids
(c) Diuretics (d) All of above

209. Liver damage is termed as
(a) Leeching (b) Cirrhosis
(c) Aplasia (d) Haemorrhage

210. If females are administered anabolic steroids, following symptoms are observed
(a) Abnormal menstruation (b) Excessive hair growth
(c) Enlargement of clitoris (d) All of the above

*Read the **assertion** and **reason** carefully to mark the correct option out of the options given below:*

(a) If both the assertion and the reason are true and the reason is a correct explanation of the assertion
(b) If both the assertion and reason are true but the reason is not a correct explanation of the assertion
(c) If the assertion is true but the reason is false
(d) If both the assertion and reason are false

211. Assertion: Health means absence of disease.
Reason: Health can be defined as a state of complete physical well being only.

212. Assertion: Infectious diseases are very common.
Reason: These diseases are easily transmitted from one person to another.

213. Assertion: Chill & high fever occur in malaria.
Reason: Release of toxin, haemozoin from ruptured RBCs in malaria.

214. Assertion: Ringworms generally occur in skin fold. Such as groin or between toes.
Reason: Heat & moisture help fungi to grow.

215. Assertion: Saliva in mouth is physiological barriers.
Reason: Interferon are cytokine barriers.

216. **Assertion:** Yellowish fluid colostrum secreted by mother during the initiated days of lactation is protective for infant.
Reason: Colostrum contain abundant Ig A antibodies.

217. **Assertion:** Rheumatoid arthritis is an auto-immune disease.
Reason: Body attack self-cells in Rhematoid arthritis.

218. **Assertion:** HIV enters in macrophages only in human body.
Reason: In macrophages RNA genome of virus get incorporated into host cell DNA as such.

219. **Assertion:** Cancer cells shows uncontrolled growth.
Reason: Cancer cells losses property of contact inhibition.

220. **Assertion:** Crack is potent stimulant of CNS, producing sense of euphoria and increased energy.
Reason: It interfere with the transport of neurotransmitter dopamine.

AIPMT PREVIOUS YEAR QUESTIONS

1. Fastest distribution of some injectible material/ medicine and with no risk of any kind can be achieved by injecting it into the
[AIPMT MAINS 2010]
(a) Muscles (b) Arteries
(c) Veins (d) Lymph vessels

2. Which one of the following techniques is safest for the detection of cancers?
[AIPMT MAINS 2010]
(a) Magnetic resonance imaging (MRI) (b) Radiography (X-ray)
(c) Computed tomography (CT) (d) Histopathological studies

3. A person suffering from a disease caused by Plasmodium, experiences recurring chill and fever at the time when?
[AIPMT MAINS 2010]
(a) The sporozoites released from RBCs are being rapidly killed and broken down inside spleen
(b) The trophozoites reach maximum growth and give out certain toxins
(c) The parasite after its rapid multiplication inside RBCs ruptures them, releasing the stage to enter fresh RBCs
(d) The microgametocytes and megagametocytes are being destroyed by the WBCs

4. Select the correct statement from the ones given below
[AIPMT PRE 2010]
(a) Barbiturates when given to criminals make them tell the truth
(b) Morphine is often given to persons who have under gone surgery as a pain killer
(c) Chewing tobacco lowers blood pressure and heart rate
(d) Cocaine is given to patients after surgery as it stimulates recovery

5. Ringworm in humans is caused by
[AIPMT PRE 2010]
(a) Bacteria (b) Fungi
(c) Nematodes (d) Viruses

6. Widal test is used for the diagnosis of:

[AIPMT PRE 2010]

(a) Malaria
(b) Pneumonia
(c) Tuberculosis
(d) Typhoid

7. Which one of the following statements is correct with respect to AIDS?

[AIPMT PRE 2010]

(a) The HIV can be transmitted through eating food together with an infected person
(b) Drug addicts are least susceptible to HIV infection
(c) AIDS patients are, being fully cured cent percent with proper care and nutrition
(d) The causative HIV retrovirus enters helper T-lymphocytes thus reducing their numbers

8. Consider the following four statements (1- 4) regarding kidney transplant and select the two correct ones out of these.

[AIPMT PRE 2010]

(A) Even if a kidney transplant is proper the recipient may need to take immune suppresants for a long time
(B) The cell-mediated immune response is responsible for the graft rejection
(C) The B-lymphocytes are responsible for rejection of the graft
(D) The acceptance of rejection of a kidney transplant depends on specific interferons

The two correct statements are

(a) (B) and (C)
(b) (C) and (D)
(c) (A) and (C)
(d) (A) and (B)

9. A certain patient is suspected to be suffering from acquired immuno deficiency syndrome. Which diagnostic technique will you recommend for its detection?

[AIPMT PRE 2011]

(a) MRI
(b) Ultra Sound
(c) WIDAL
(d) ELISA

10. At which stage of HIV infection does one usually shows symptoms of AIDS?

[AIPMT PRE 2011]

(a) When viral DNA is produced by reverse transcriptase
(b) When HIV replicates rapidly in helper T Iymphocytes and damages large number of these
(c) With 15 days of sexual contact with an infected person
(d) When the infecting retrovirus enters host cells

11. Which one of the following acts as a physiological barrier to the entry of microorganisms in human body?

[AIPMT PRE 2011]

(a) Tears
(b) Monocytes
(c) Skin
(d) Epithelium of urogenital tract

12. Where will you look for the sporozoites of the malarial parasite?

[AIPMT PRE 2011]

(a) Red blood corpuscles of humans suffering from malaria
(b) Spleen of infected humans
(c) Salivary glands of freshly moulted female anopheles mosquito
(d) Saliva of infected female Anopheles Mosquito

13. The pathogen Microsporum responsible for ringworm disease in humans belongs to the same kingdom of organisms as that of

[AIPMT MAINS 2011]

(a) Taenia, a tapeworm
(b) Wuchereria, a filarial worm
(c) Rhizopus, a mould
(d) Ascaris, a round worm

14. Which one of the following options gives the correct matching of a disease with its causative organism and mode of infection? (A: Typhoid, B: Causative organism, C: Mode of infection)

[AIPMT MAINS 2011]

(a) A: Typhoid, B: Salmonella typhi, C: With inspired air
(b) A: Pneumonia, B: Streptococcus pneumonia, C: Droplet infection
(c) A: Elephantiasis, B: Wuchereria bancrofti, C: With infected water and food
(d) A: Malaria, B: Plasmodium vivax, C: Bite of male Anopheles mosquito

15. Common cold is not cured by antibiotics because it is

[AIPMT MAINS 2011]

(a) Caused by a virus
(b) Caused by a Gram-positive bacterium
(c) Caused by a Gram-negative bacterium
(d) Not an infectious disease

16. Select the correct statement with respect to diseases and immunisation.

[AIPMT MAINS 2011]

(a) If due to some reascn B and T lymphocytes are damaged, the body will not produce antibodies against a pathogen.
(b) Injection of dead/inactivated pathogens causes passive immunity.
(c) Certain protozoans have been used in mass production of hepatitis B vaccine.
(d) Injection of snake antivenom against snake bite is an example of active immunisation.

17. Which one of the following human organs is often called the "graveyard" of RBCs?

[AIPMT MAINS 2012]

(a) Kidney
(b) Spleen
(c) Liver
(d) Gall bladder

18. Identify the molecules (a) and (b) shown below and select the right option giving their source and use

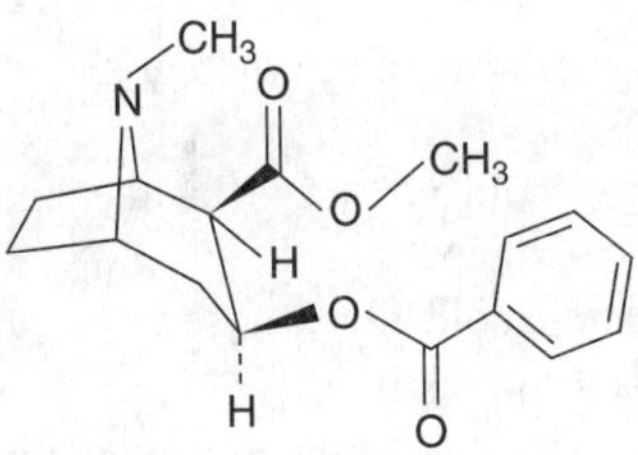

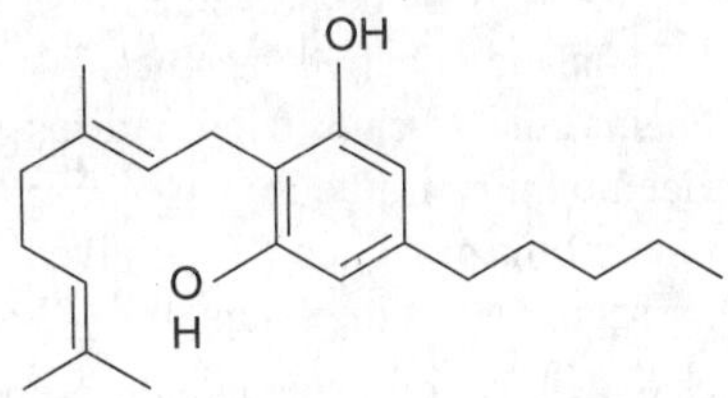

[AIPMT MAINS 2012]

Options:

	Molecule	Source	Use
(a)	(b) Heroin	Cannabis sativai	Depressant and slows down body functions
(b)	(b) Annabinoid	Atropa belladonna	Produces hallucinations
(c)	(a) Morphine	Papaver somniferum	Sedative and pain killer
(d)	(a) Coacine	Erythroxylum coca	Accelerates the transport of dopamine

19. Which one of the following organisms is scientifically correctly named, correctly printed according to the International Rules of Nomenclature and correctly described?

[AIPMT MAINS 2012]

(a) Plasmodium falciparum – a protozoan pathogen causing the most serious type of malaria
(b) Felis tigris – The Indian tiger, well protected in Gir forests
(c) E.Coli – Full name Entamoeba coli, a commonly occurring bacterium in human intestine
(d) Musca domestica – The common house lizards, a reptile

20. Which one of the following statements is correct with respect to immunity?

[AIPMT MAINS 2012]

(a) The antibodies against small pox pathogen are produced by T-lymphocytes
(b) Antibodies are protein molecules each of which has four light chains
(c) Rejection of a kidney graft is the function of B-lymphocytes
(d) Preformed antibodies need to be injected to treat the bite by a viper snake

21. The first clinical gene therapy was given for treating:

[AIPMT MAINS 2012]

(a) Chicken pox (b) Rheumatoid arthritis
(c) Adenosine deaminase deficiency (d) Diabetes mellitus

22. Motile zygote of Plasmodium occurs in:

[AIPMT PRE 2012]

(a) Gut of female Anopheles (b) Salivary glands of Anopheles
(c) Human RBCs (d) Human liver

23. Widal test is carried out to test:

[AIPMT PRE 2012]

(a) Malaria (b) Diabetes mellitus
(c) HIV/AIDS (d) Typhoid fever

24. Common cold differs from pneumonia in, that:

[AIPMT PRE 2012]

(a) Pneumonia is a communicable disease whereas the common cold is a nutritional deficiency disease
(b) Pneumonia can be prevented by a live attenuated bacterial vaccine whereas the common cold has no effective vaccine
(c) Pneumonia is caused by a virus while the common cold is caused by the bacterium Haemophilus influenza
(d) Pneumonia pathogen infects alveoli whereas the common cold affects nose and respiratory passage but not the lungs.

25. Which one of the following in not a property of cancerous cells whereas the remaining three are?

[AIPMT PRE 2012]

(a) They compete with normal cells for vital nutrients
(b) They do not remain confined in the area of formation
(c) They divide in an uncontrolled manner
(d) They show contact inhibition

26. Cirrhosis of liver is caused by the chronic intake of:

[AIPMT PRE 2012]

(a) Opium (b) Alcohol
(c) Tobacco (chewing) (d) Cocaine

27. In which one of the following options the two examples are correctly matched particular type of immunity?

[AIPMT PRE 2012]

	Examples	Type of immunity
(a)	Polymorpho nuclear leukocytes and monocytes	Cellular barriers
(b)	Anti-tetanus and anti-snake bite injections.	Active immunity
(c)	Saliva in mouth and tears in eyes	Physical barriers
(d)	Mucus coating of epithelium lining the urinogenital tract and the HCl in stomach	Physiological barriers

28. Infection of Ascaris usually occurs by:

[AIPMT 2013]

(a) Drinking water containing eggs of Ascaris
(b) Eating imperfectly cooked pork
(c) Tse – tse fly
(d) Mosquito bite

29. The cell – mediated immunity inside the human body is carried out by?

[AIPMT 2013]

(a) T – lymphocytes (b) B – lymphocytes
(c) Thrombocytes (d) Erythrocytes

30. Which is the particular type of drug that is obtained from the plant whose one flowering branch is shown below?

[AIPMT 2014]

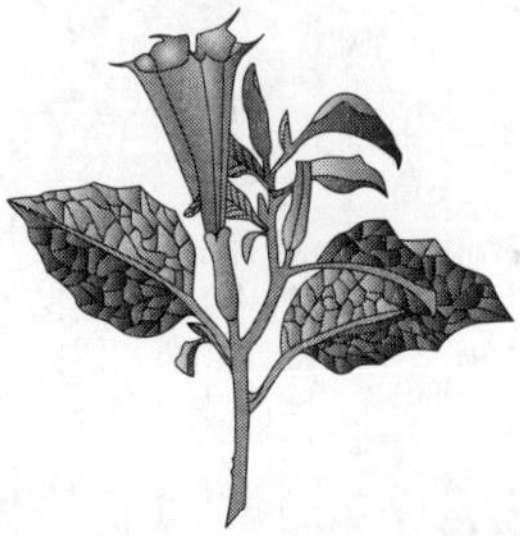

(a) Hallucinogen (b) Depressant
(c) Stimulant (d) Pain-killer

31. At which stager HIV infection does one usually show symptoms of AIDS?

[AIPMT 2014]

(a) Within 15 days of sexual contact with an infected person
(b) When the infected retro virus enters host cells
(c) When HIV damages large number of helper T-Lymphocytes
(d) When the viral DNA is produced by reverse transcriptase

32. Which of the following endoparasites of humans does show viviparity?

[AIPMT 2015]

(a) Ancylostoma duodenale (b) Enterobius vermicularis
(c) Trichimella spiralis (d) Ascaris lumbricoides

33. Match each disease with its correct type of vaccine:

(a) tuberculosis — (i) harmless virus
(b) whooping cough — (ii) inactivated toxin
(c) diphtheria — (iii) killed bacteria
(d) polio — (iv) harmless bacteria

[AIPMT 2015]

	(a)	(b)	(c)	(d)
(a)	(ii)	(i)	(iii)	(iv)
(b)	(iii)	(ii)	(iv)	(i)
(c)	(iv)	(iii)	(ii)	(i)
(d)	(i)	(ii)	(iv)	(iii)

34. HIV that causes AIDS, first starts destroying:

[AIPMT 2015]

(a) B-Lymphocytes (b) Leucocytes
(c) Helper T-Lymphocytes (d) Thrombocytes

35. The active form of *Entamoeba histolytica* feeds upon:

[AIPMT 2015]

(a) Erythrocytes, mucosa and submucosa of colon
(b) Mucosa and submucosa colon only
(c) food in intestine
(d) blood only

36. Which of the following immunoglobulins does constitute the largest percentage in human milk?

[RE-AIPMT 2015]

(a) Ig M (b) Ig A
(c) Ig G (d) Ig D

37. If you suspect major deficiency of antibodies in a person, to which of the following would you look for confirmatory evidence?

[RE-AIPMT 2015]

(a) Serum albumins (b) Haemocytes
(c) Serum globulins (d) Fibrinogin in plasma

38. Grafted kidney may be rejected in a patient due to

[RE-AIPMT 2015]

(a) Cell-mediated immune response (b) Passive immune response
(c) Innate immune response (d) Humoral immune response

Answer Keys

1. (c)	2. (b)	3. (c)	4. (a)	5. (a)	6. (c)	7. (d)	8. (d)	9. (c)	10. (d)
11. (b)	12. (c)	13. (c)	14. (c)	15. (b)	16. (c)	17. (b)	18. (c)	19. (c)	20. (b)
21. (b)	22. (b)	23. (b)	24. (d)	25. (a)	26. (b)	27. (c)	28. (a)	29. (b)	30. (c)
31. (c)	32. (d)	33. (c)	34. (a)	35. (d)	36. (b)	37. (c)	38. (c)	39. (a)	40. (d)
41. (b)	42. (b)	43. (b)	44. (c)	45. (c)	46. (a)	47. (a)	48. (a)	49. (c)	50. (b)
51. (b)	52. (b)	53. (b)	54. (b)	55. (b)	56. (c)	57. (c)	58. (a)	59. (b)	60. (d)
61. (d)	62. (c)	63. (b)	64. (a)	65. (c)	66. (c)	67. (b)	68. (b)	69. (b)	70. (c)
71. (b)	72. (d)	73. (c)	74. (c)	75. (d)	76. (c)	77. (a)	78. (b)	79. (c)	80. (c)
81. (a)	82. (b)	83. (b)	84. (d)	85. (d)	86. (c)	87. (c)	88. (c)	89. (b)	90. (c)
91. (c)	92. (c)	93. (b)	94. (a)	95. (b)	96. (c)	97. (a)	98. (b)	99. (c)	100. (a)
101. (a)	102. (b)	103. (c)	104. (c)	105. (d)	106. (c)	107. (b)	108. (b)	109. (c)	110. (b)
111. (b)	112. (c)	113. (b)	114. (c)	115. (b)	116. (b)	117. (d)	118. (b)	119. (d)	120. (d)
121. (a)	122. (a)	123. (d)	124. (c)	125. (c)	126. (a)	127. (c)	128. (b)	129. (d)	130. (b)
131. (c)	132. (a)	133. (c)	134. (c)	135. (c)	136. (b)	137. (b)	138. (c)	139. (a)	140. (b)
141. (b)	142. (a)	143. (b)	144. (c)	145. (c)	146. (a)	147. (a)	148. (b)	149. (b)	150. (c)
151. (b)	152. (c)	153. (b)	154. (a)	155. (d)	156. (a)	157. (c)	158. (d)	159. (b)	160. (b)
161. (a)	162. (b)	163. (b)	164. (b)	165. (d)	166. (c)	167. (b)	168. (b)	169. (d)	170. (d)
171. (c)	172. (a)	173. (b)	174. (d)	175. (b)	176. (b)	177. (b)	178. (c)	179. (a)	180. (b)
181. (a)	182. (b)	183. (d)	184. (a)	185. (b)	186. (b)	187. (c)	188. (c)	189. (b)	190. (b)
191. (c)	192. (c)	193. (d)	194. (c)	195. (d)	196. (c)	197. (d)	198. (c)	199. (b)	200. (b)
201. (b)	202. (b)	203. (b)	204. (d)	205. (a)	206. (c)	207. (b)	208. (d)	209. (b)	210. (d)
211. (d)	212. (a)	213. (a)	214. (a)	215. (b)	216. (a)	217. (a)	218. (d)	219. (a)	220. (a)

AIPMT Previous Year Questions

1. (c)	2. (a)	3. (c)	4. (b)	5. (b)	6. (d)	7. (d)	8. (d)	9. (d)	10. (c)
11. (a)	12. (d)	13. (c)	14. (b)	15. (a)	16. (a)	17. (b)	18. (c)	19. (a)	20. (d)
21. (c)	22. (a)	23. (d)	24. (d)	25. (d)	26. (b)	27. (a)	28. (a)	29. (a)	30. (a)
31. (c)	32. (c)	33. (c)	34. (c)	35. (a)	36. (b)	37. (a)	38. (a)		

CHAPTER

31

Strategies for Enhancement in Food Production

1. Following techniques/processes are used to enhance food production
   (a) Embryo transfer technology
   (b) Tissue culture technology
   (c) Animal husbandry and plant breeding
   (d) All of the above
2. Find out the incorrect statement.
   (a) Animal husbandry is the agricultural practice of breeding and raising livestock.
   (b) More than 70% of the world's livestock population is in India and China.
   (c) Dairying is the management of animals for milk and its products for human consumption.
   (d) Hisardale is a new breed of sheep developed in Punjab by crossing Bikaneri rams and Marino ewes.
3. Animal husbandry deals with the care and breeding of livestock like
   (a) Buffaloes and cows
   (b) Pig and horses
   (c) Sheep, camel and goat
   (d) All of the above
4. Fisheries include rearing, catching and selling of following organisms
   (a) Fish
   (b) Molluscs (shell-fish)
   (c) Crustaceans (prawn, crab)
   (d) All of the above
5. In dairy-farm management, we deal with processes and systems that are responsible for
   (a) Increase in yield of milk
   (b) Improvement in quality of milk
   (c) Both (a) and (b)
   (d) None
6. Good breeds should have
   (a) High yielding potential under climatic conditions of the area
   (b) Resistance to disease
   (c) Improved quality of the yield
   (d) All of the above
7. For realizing good yielding potential the following are required
   (a) Animal should be housed well and provided with adequate water
   (b) Maintain disease-free animals
   (c) Feeding should be in scientific manner along with good quality and quantity of fodder
   (d) All of the above
8. The word 'poultry' is used to refer meat of
   (a) Chicken and ducks
   (b) Turkey
   (c) Geese
   (d) All of these

9. How can we prevent the spreading of the flu in case some chicken are infected in poultry form
   (a) Select these chickens
   (b) Kill selected chicken and burn them
   (c) Kill selected chickens and burried them deep inside earth
   (d) All of the above

10. 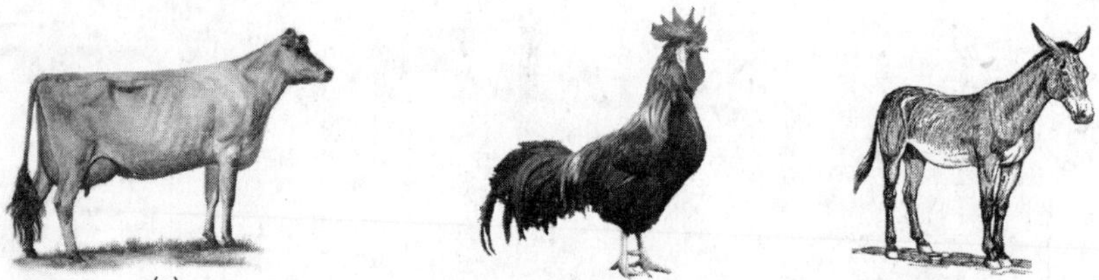

(a) (b) (c)

   (a) A-Improved breed of cattle—Jersey
   (b) B-Improved breed of chickens—Leghorn
   (c) C-Sterile—Mule
   (d) All are correct

11. The term 'breed' means
   (a) A group of animals related by descent and similar in most characters like general appearance, feature, size and configurations
   (b) A group of animals which are depend on each other
   (c) A group of animals living in a same habitat
   (d) A group of animals which can't reproduce with each other

12. Select the incorrect combination
   (a) Class of domesticated fowl (birds) used for food and eggs—Poultry
   (b) Breeding between animals of the same breed—Inbreeding
   (c) Breeding between different breeds—Outbreeding
   (d) Keeping honeybees for the production of honey—Pisciculture

13. Bee-keeping is known as
   (a) Pisciculture
   (b) Silviculture
   (c) Apiculture
   (d) Aquaculture

14. Following are freshwater fishes except
   (a) Catla
   (b) Rohu
   (c) Common carp
   (d) Mackerl

15. Following are marine water fishers except
   (a) Hilsa
   (b) Sardines
   (c) Pomfrets
   (d) Rohu

16. The following points are important for successful bee-keeping
   (a) Knowledge of nature and habits of bees
   (b) Catching and hiving of swarms (group of bees)
   (c) Management of beehives during different seasons
   (d) All of the above

17. Keeping beehives in crop fields during flowering period causes
   (a) Increased pollination efficiency
   (b) Increased in yield of crop
   (c) Increased in yield of honey
   (d) All of the above

18. Example of interspecific hybridization
   (a) Hisardale
   (b) Mule
   (c) Jersey
   (d) Leghorn

19. In MOET ________ cell stage, fertilized egg are recovered non-surgically and transferred to surrogate mothers.
(a) 8–32 (b) 2–4
(c) 6–8 (d) 4–6

20. Hisardale is a new breed of sheep developed in Punjab by crossing
(a) Bikaneri ewes and Marino rams (b) Dolly and Marino rams
(c) Ajmeri ewes and Marino rams (d) Jersey and Bikaneri ewes

21. Mule is produced by cross-breeding
(a) Male horse and female horse (b) Male donkey and female horse
(c) Female donkey and male horse (d) Male donkey and female donkey

22. Green revolution was dependent to a large extent on plant breeding techniques for development of high yielding and disease resistant verities in
(a) Wheat (b) Maize
(c) Rice (d) All

23. Which of the following is the most important character or trait that the breeders have tried to incorporate in plants first?
(a) Resistance to pathogens (virus, fungi and bacteria)
(b) Increase tolerance to insect pest
(c) Increased tolerance to environmental stress
(d) Increased crop yield

24. The entire collection (of plants/seeds) having all the diverse allele for all genes in a given crop is called
(a) Gene bank (b) Tissue culture
(c) Genetic engineering (d) Germplasm collection

25. Which process of plant breeding technique is the most time-consuming and tedious?
(a) Collection of variability
(b) Cross hybridization among the selected parents
(c) Evaluation and selection of parents
(d) Selection and testing of superior recombinants

26. Self-pollination for several generations create
(a) Heterozygosity (b) Homozygosity
(c) Hemizygosity (d) Aneuploidy

27. Which is not a step in breeding a new genetic variety of crop?
(a) Collection of variability
(b) Evaluation and selection of parent
(c) Self hybridization among the selected parents
(d) Selection and testing of superior recombinants

28. Testing, release and commercialization of new cultivar include
(a) Evaluation in research field
(b) Recoding performance of cultivar under ideal fertilizer application, irrigation and crop management practice
(c) Evaluation in farmer's field for at least three growing seasons at several locations in a country
(d) All of the above

29. In India agriculture accounts for approx ________ % of India's GDP and employs nearly ________ % of the population.
(a) 33, 62
(b) 62, 33
(c) 50, 50
(d) 60, 40

30. P1542 is a hybrid variety of
(a) Maize
(b) Wheat
(c) Rice
(d) Garden pea

31. Which of the following plant hybrids are successfully developed in India?
(a) Maize
(b) Jowar
(c) Bajara
(d) All of these

32. The development of several high yielding varieties of wheat and rice in the mid ________ through plant breeding techniques lead to the Green Revolution in India.
(a) 1950s
(b) 1960s
(c) 1970s
(d) 1980s

33. In 1963 several variety of wheat such as ________ and ________, which were high yielding and disease resistance, were introduced all over the wheat growing belt of India.
(a) Sonalika, Kalyan sona
(b) Sonalika, IR – 8
(c) Sonalika, Taichung Native-I
(d) Kalyan sona, Jaya

34. Semi-dwarf varieties of rice developed in India are
(a) Sonalika and Kalyan sona
(b) IR–8 and Taichung Native–I
(c) Jaya and Ratna
(d) Altas 66 and Himgiri

35. Semi-dwarf varieties of rice were derived from
(a) Sonalika and Kalyan sona
(b) IR – 8 and Taichung Native–I
(c) Jaya and Ratna
(d) Altas 66 and Himgiri

36. Taichung Native I variety of rice were from which country?
(a) India
(b) Philippines
(c) Taiwan
(d) Japan

37. All of the given options are true about Saccharum barberi except
(a) Grown in nNorth India
(b) Poor yield
(c) Poor sugar content
(d) High sugar content

38. All of the given options are true about Saccharum officinarum except
(a) Grown in South India
(b) Thicker stem
(c) High sugar content
(d) Grow well in North India

39. Match the column-I (Plant) with Column-II (Variety)

Column-I	Column-II
1. Wheat	A. Altas – 66
2. Sugar cane	B. Saccharum barberi
3. Okra	C. Pusa A – 4
4. Chilli	D. Pusa Vadabahar
5. Rice	E. Jaya

(a) 1-A, 2-B, 3-C, 4-D, 5-E
(b) 1-B, 2-D, 3-A, 4-E, 5-C
(c) 1-D, 2-A, 3-E, 4-C, 5-B
(d) 1-C, 2-E, 3-B, 4-A, 5-D

40. Select the incorrect match.
(a) SCP—Single Cell Protein
(b) IRRI—International Rice Research Institute
(c) MOET—Multiple Ovulation Embryo Transfer Technology
(d) IUCN—International Union for Conservation of Nation

41. Select the correct match.
(a) Plant breeding—Purposeful manipulation of plant species in order to create desired plant types that are better suited for cultivation gives better yield and are disease resistance
(b) Gene bank—The entire collection of plant/seeds having all the diverse alleles for all genes in a given crop
(c) Fishery—Industry devoted to the catching, processing or selling of fish only
(d) MOET—It is used for herd improvement. In this method, a cow is administered hormones, with LH-like activity, which lead to super-ovulation (i.e., produce 6 – 8 eggs/cycle)

42. Which combination of qualities is first priority of plant breeder?
(A) Increased yield
(B) Increased quality of food
(C) Increased resistance to pathogens
(D) Increased tolerance to environmental stresses
(a) A and B only
(b) C and D only
(c) All A, B, C, D
(d) A, B, and C only

43. Fill in the blanks Column-I (Crop), Column-II (Variety), Column-III (Resistance to disease).

Column-I	Column-II	Column-III
Wheat	A	Lear and strip rust
Brassica	B	C
Cowpea	Pusa komal	D
Chilli	E	Chilli mosaic virus, Tobacco mosaic virus and leaf curl

(a) A-Karan rai, B-Himgiri, C-Bacterial blight, D-White rust, E-Pusa swarnim
(b) A-Himgiri, B-Karan rai, C-White rust, D-Bacterial blight, E-Pusa sadabahar
(c) A-Pusa sadabahar, B-Himgiri, C-White rust, D-Pusa swarnim, E-White rust
(d) A-Bacterial blight, B-White rust, C-Karan rai, D-Himgiri, E-Pusa sadabahar

44. Following are varieties of Wheat except
(a) Altas–66
(b) Himgiri
(c) I R–8
(d) Sonalika

45. Which of the following is/are variety/varieties of cauliflower?
(a) Pusa shubhra
(b) Pusa komal
(c) Pusa snowball K-1
(d) Both (a) and (c)

46. In which plant, resistance to yellow mosaic virus and powdery mildew were induced by mutations?
(a) Flat bean
(b) A. esculentus
(c) Mung bean
(d) Pusa A–4

47. Resistance to _________ in bhindi was transferred from a wild species and resulted in a new variety of A. esculentus called _________.
(a) Yellow mosaic virus, pusa gaurav
(b) Chilly mosaic virus, pusa sadabahar
(c) Yellow mosaic virus, parbhani Kranti
(d) Whist rust, pusa swarnim

48. Find out the incorrect statement.
(a) Conventional breeding is often constrained by the availability of limited number of disease resistance genes.
(b) Transfer of resistance gene is achieved by sexual hybridization between the target and source plant.
(c) Inducing mutations in plant through various means and then screening the plant materials for resistance sometimes leads to desirable genes being identified.
(d) It is not possible to induce mutations artificially through use of chemicals or radiation like gamma radiation.

49. Maize offers resistance to maize stem borers by
(a) High aspartic acid
(b) Low nitrogen content
(c) Low sugar content
(d) All of the above

50. Match column-I (Plant Part) with Column-II (Insect Resistance).

Column-I	Column-II
1. Hairy leaves	A. Resistance to jassids in cotton
2. Solid stem	B. Resistance to Cereal leaf beetle in wheat
3. Smooth leaf and less nectar	C. Resistance to Stem sawfly in wheat
	D. Resistance to Bollworm in cotton

(a) 1-A, 2-B and C, 3-D
(b) 1-A and B, 2-C, 3-D
(c) 1-D, 2-C, 3-A and B
(d) 1-A and C, 2-B, 3-C

51. How many of the given names are various types of Brassica?
Pusa komal, Pusa sem 2, Pusa sem 3, Pusa gaurav, Pusa swarnim, Pusa sawami, Pusa shubhra
(a) 1
(b) 2
(c) 3
(d) 4

52. Fill in the blanks.

Column-I Crop	Column-II Variety	Column-III Insect Pests
Brassica (rapeseed mustard)	A	Aphids
Flat bean	Pusa sem 2, Pusa sem 3	B, Aphids and fruit borer
D	Pusa sawani Pusa A-4	C

(a) A-Pusa swarnim, B-Shoot borer, C-Jassids, D-Okra
(b) A-Pusa gaurav, B-Jassids, C-Shoot and fruit borer, D-Okra
(c) A-Okra, B-Jassids, C-Fruit borer, D-pusa komal
(d) A-Himgiri, B-Jassids, C-Shoot and fruit borer, D-Okra

53. Source of pest resistance gene may be
(a) Cultivated varieties
(b) Germplasm collection of the crop
(c) Wild relatives
(d) All of the above

54. Which brassica variety is resistant to white rust?
(a) Pusa sawani (b) Pusa komal
(c) Pusa swarnim (d) Pusa sadabahar

55. Which of the following pair are varieties of okra (A. esculentus)?
(a) Pusa sem 2 and Pusa sem 3 (b) Pusa shubhra and Pusa snowball K – I
(c) Pusa sawani and Pusa A–4 (d) Pusa swarnim and Pusa gaurav

56. Which of the following pair are varieties of cauliflower?
(a) Pusa sem 2 and Pusa sem 3 (b) Pusa shubhra and Pusa snowball K – I
(c) Pusa sawani and Pusa A – 4 (d) Pusa swarnim and Pusa gaurav

57. Match the column-I (Causative agent) with Column-II (Disease).

Column-I	Column-II
1. Virus	A. Brown rust of wheat
2. Bacteria	B. Red rot of sugar cane
3. Fungi	C. Late blight of potato
	D. Black rot of crucifer
	E. Tobacco mosaic
	F. Turnip mosaic

(a) 1-E, F ; 2-D; 3-A, B, C (b) 1-E; 2-D, F; 3-A, B, C
(c) 1-A, B, C; 2-D, E; 3-F (d) 1-A, B; 2-C, D; 3-E, F

58. Sequential steps for breeding are
(A) Screening germplasm for resistance sources
(B) Selection and Evaluation of hybrid
(C) Hybridization of selected parents
(D) Testing and release of new varieties
(a) D, C, B, A (b) A, B, C, D
(c) A, C, B, D (d) A, C, D, B

59. Breeding for improved nutritional quality is undertaken with objective of improving all of these except
(a) Protein content and Quality (b) Oil content and Quality
(c) Vitamin micronutrient and mineral content (d) Senescence of plant

60. In 2000 a new maize hybrid was developed, which was rich in the following amino acids
(a) Lysine and Glycine (b) Tryptophan and Glutamic acid
(c) Lysine and tryptophan (d) Glycine and Glutamic acid

61. From the following, how many are varieties of wheat?
Atlas 66, Himgiri, Sonalika, Kalyan sona, Jaya, Ratna
(a) 3 (b) 2
(c) 4 (d) 5

62. Iron fortified rice variety is ________ times richer in iron than the commonly used varieties.
(a) two (b) three
(c) four (d) five

63. Wheat variety Atlas 66 is rich in
(a) Lipid content (b) Water content
(c) Protein content (d) Mineral content

64. IARI, New Delhi released several vegetable crops that are rich in vitamins and mineral. With respect to that select the correct match.

Column-I	Column-II
1. Vitamin A	A. Correct, spinach, pumpkin
2. Vitamin C	B. Bitter gourd, bathua, mustard, tomato
3. Fe and Ca	C. Spinach and bathua
4. Protein	D. road bean, lablab, French and garden peas

(a) A-2, B-3, C-1, D-4 (b) A-1, B-2, C-3, D-4
(c) A-4, B-1, C-2, D-3 (d) A-3, B-4, C-1, D-2

65. Diet deficient in essential micro nutrients like Iron, Vitamin A, iodine and Zinc is responsible for
(a) Increase risk of disease (b) Reduce life span
(c) Reduce mental abilities (d) All of the above

66. Select the wrong combination.
(a) SCP–Single Cell Protein
(b) IRRI–International Rice Research Institute
(c) MOET–Multiple Ovulation Embryo Transfer Technology
(d) IARI–Indian Agro Revolution Institute

67. _________ kg of grains produces _________ kg of meat by animal farming.
(a) 3–10, 2 (b) 3–10, 10
(c) 3–10, 1 (d) 3–10, 5

68. What percentage of human population is suffering from hunger?
(a) >25% (b) >70%
(c) >80% (d) >90%

69. Which has high rate of biomass production?
(a) Cow (b) Buffalow
(c) Methylophilus methylotrophus (d) Pavo-cristatus

70. Spirulina can be grown easily on
(a) Waste water from potato processing plant (b) Straw and molasses
(c) Animal manure and sewage (d) All of the above

71. _________ of a micro-organism like Methylophilus methylotrophus, because of its high rate of biomass production and growth, can be expected to produce _________ of protein.
(a) 250 gm, 25 tonnes (b) 50 gm, 25 tonnes
(c) 20 gm, 25 kg (d) 25 gm, 250 gm

72. Following organism can be used as food
(a) Mushroom (b) Spirulina
(c) Chlorella (d) All

73. One of the alternate sources of proteins for animal and human nutrition is
(a) ROP (b) SCP
(c) GIP (d) BCG

74. The shift from grain to meat diet creates more demand for cereals as it takes _________ kg of grain to produce _________ kg of meat by animal farming.
(a) 1, 1 (b) 2, 2
(c) 3–10, 1 (d) 1, 3–10

75. In tissue culture, any part of a plant is taken out and grown in a test tube under sterile conditions in a special nutrient medium to regenerate whole plant. Part of plant used for this purpose is known as
(a) Somaclone (b) Embryo
(c) Explant (d) Zygote

76. Capacity to regenerate whole plant from plant cell or explant is known as
(a) Totipotency (b) Pleuripotency
(c) Metaplasia (d) Atrophy

77. Method of producing thousands of plants through tissue culture is called
(a) Explant (b) Totipotency
(c) Somaclone (d) Micro-propagation

78. Following plants have been produced by tissue culture method on commercial scale
(a) Tomato (b) Banana
(c) Apple (d) All

79. Scientists have succeeded in culturing meristems of which of the following plants?
(a) Banana (b) Sugarcane
(c) Potato (d) All of them

80. Part of virus infected plant used for tissue culture, free from viruses is
(a) Flower (b) Leaf
(c) Apical meristem (d) All of them

81. Protoplast from two different varieties of plants, each having a desirable character, can be fused by a process known as
(a) Somatic hybridization (b) Monohybrid cross
(c) Tissue culture (d) Embryo culture

82. Tomato and potato protoplast is fused to form
(a) Topoto (b) Pomato
(c) Totato (d) Tomapo

83. Find out the incorrect statement
(a) Virus free plant can be obtained by meristem culture.
(b) In micro-propagation soma clones are produced.
(c) Plant cell without cell wall is known as protoplast.
(d) Pomato (Somatic hybrid) has all the desired combinations of characteristics for its commercial utilization.

84. In tissue culture, nutrient medium should contain
(a) Carbon source, eg., Sucrose
(b) Inorganic salt, vitamin and amino acid
(c) Growth regulators like auxins and cytokinins
(d) All of the above

85. Find out total number of marine fishes from the following.
Hilsa, Sardines, Mackerel, Pomfrets, Catla, Rohu, Common carp
(a) 4 (b) 5
(c) 6 (d) 7

86. Which of the following are types of outbreeding?
(a) Out-crossing (b) Cross breeding
(c) Interspecific hybridization (d) All of the above

87. Match the columns.

Column-I	Column-II
A. White revolution	1. Increase in milk production
B. Green revolution	2. Increase in crop production
C. Blue revolution	3. Increase in fish production

(a) A-1, B-2, C-3 (b) A-2, B-3, C-1
(c) A-3, B-2, C-1 (d) A-1, B-3, C-2

88. Aquaculture means
(a) Production of aquatic animals (b) Production of aquatic plant
(c) Both 1 and 2 (d) None of the above

89. Interspecific hybridization means
(a) Mating of animals within the same breed
(b) Superior male of one breed mated with superior female of another breed
(c) Male and female animals of two different related species are mated
(d) All of the above

90. Which of the statements are true?
(a) Bee wax is a by-product of honey. (b) Honeybees are potent pollinators.
(c) Honey is a food of high nutritional value. (d) All of the above

91. Which of the following is a variety of rice?
(a) Atlas-66 (b) Himgiri
(c) Sonalika (d) Ratna

92. Which of the following diseases is caused by bacteria?
(a) Red rot of sugarcane (b) Powdery mildew
(c) Black rot of crucifer (d) Late blight of potato

93. In biofortification the objective is to improve quality as well as content of
(a) Micronutrient (b) Vitamin
(c) Oil (d) All of the above

94. Objectives of animal breeding are
(a) Increasing the quantity of yield (b) Improving the quality of the product
(c) Resistance to various diseases (d) All of the above

95. The father of Green Revolution is
(a) Norman E. Burlough (b) Panchanan Maheshwari
(c) Dr. Verghese Kurien (d) M.S. Swaminathan

96. Which are the advantages of SCP?
(a) Rich in high quality protein and poor in fat content
(b) Production is based on industrial effluents so helps to minimize environmental pollution
(c) It can be produced in laboratories throughout the year.
(d) All of the above

97. Disease resistance in plants can be induced by
(a) Mutation (b) Proper manuring
(c) Breeding with wild relatives (d) Early sowing

98. Variations in plants produced by tissue culture is known as
(a) Androgenic variation (b) Somaclonal variation
(c) Cybridization (d) Induced variation

99. Green revolution has been possible due to development of high yielding variety of
(a) Wheat and rice (b) Apples and pears
(c) Jowar and bajra (d) Sugarcane and grams

100. Somatic hybridization is a technique of
(a) Natural breeding (b) Natural pollination
(c) Artificial pollination (d) Somatic cell hybridization

101. Somaclonal variations appear in plants
(a) Growing in polluted soil or water
(b) Exposed to gamma rays
(c) Raised in tissue culture
(d) Transformed by recombinant DNA technology

102. In crop improvement programme, virus free clones can be obtained through
(a) Embryo culture (b) Shoot apex culture
(c) Grafting (d) Hybridization

103. Pollen grains of a plant, where 2n = 28, are cultured to get callus by tissue culture method. What would be the number of chromosomes in the cells of the callus?
(a) 14 (b) 56
(c) 28 (d) 21

104. By which of the following methods, new and better varieties of plants can be formed?
(a) Selection (b) Grafting
(c) Hybridization (d) Hybridization followed by selection

Read the ***assertion*** *and* ***reason*** *carefully to mark the correct option out of the options given below:*

(a) If both the assertion and the reason are true and the reason is a correct explanation of the assertion
(b) If both the assertion and reason are true but the reason is not a correct explanation of the assertion
(c) If the assertion is true but the reason is false
(d) If both the assertion and reason are false

105. **Assertion:** Inbreeding increases heterozygosity.
Reason: Continous inbreeding usually enhance fertility and even productivity.

106. **Assertion:** Mule is an examle of interspecific hybrid.
Reason: Mule produce by cross between male donkey and female horse.

107. **Assertion:** Mung beans are resistant to yellow mosaic virus.
Reason: Resistance is induced by mutation.

108. Assertion: Shoot-tip culture is used to raise virus free clones.
Reason: Other explants can equally give rise to virus free clones.

109. Assertion: Somatic hybridisation is fusion of potoplast of two different varieties of plants.
Reason: Somatic hybridisation is type of sexual reproduction.

110. Assertion: Hisardale is new breed of sheep.
Reason: Developed by crossing between Marino ewes and Bikaneri rams.

111. Assertion: Multiplication of plants in invitro condition from the explants is called micropropagation.
Reason: Micropropagation occurs either in the form of multiple shoot formation or somatic embryos.

112. Assertion: Hairy leaves in several plants are associated with resistance to insect pests.
Reason: Nectar less cotton varieties do not attract bollworms.

113. Assertion: Beeswax is an animal product produced by honeybee.
Reason: Honey contains only sugar, nothing else.

114. Assertion: Cattle breeds can be improved by superovulaton and embryo transplantaion.
Reason: Superovulation in high milk-yielding cows is induced by hormonal injection.

AIPMT PREVIOUS YEAR QUESTIONS

1. Black (stem) rust of wheat is caused by [AIPMT MAINS 2010]
(a) Alternaria solani (b) Ustilago nuda
(c) Puccinia graminis (d) Xanthomonas oryzae

2. Breeding of crops with high levels of minerals, vitamins and proteins is called [AIPMT 2010 PRE]
(a) Somatic hybridization (b) Biofortification
(c) Biomagnification (d) Micropropagation

3. An improved variety of transgenic basmati rice [AIPMT PRE 2010]
(a) Does not require chemical fertilizers and growth hormones
(b) Gives high yield and is rich in vitamin-A
(c) Is completely resistant to all insect pests and diseases of paddy
(d) Gives high yield but has no characteristic aroma

4. 'Jaya' and 'Ratna' developed for green revolution in India are the varieties of: [AIPMT PRE 2011]
(a) Rice (b) Wheat
(c) Bajra (d) Maize

5. 'Himgiri' developed by hybridisation and selection for disease resistance against rust pathogens is a variety of: [AIPMT PRE 2011]
(a) Maize (b) Sugarcane
(c) Wheat (d) Chilli

6. Consider the following statements (A-D) about organic farming:

(A) Utilizes genetically modified crops like Bt cotton
(B) Uses only naturally produced inputs like compost
(C) Does not use pesticides and urea
(D) Produces vegetables rich in vitamins and minerals

[AIPMT MAINS 2011]

(a) B, C, and D
(b) C and D only
(c) B and C only
(d) A and B only

7. Consider the following four statements (a-d) and select the option which includes all the correct ones only:

(A) Single cell Spirulina can produce large quantities of food rich in protein, minerals, vitamins etc.
(B) Body weight-wise the microorganisms Methylophilus methylotrophus may be able to produce several times more proteins than the cow per day
(C) Common button mushrooms are a very rich source of vitamin C
(D) A rice variety has been developed which is very rich in calcium

[AIPMT MAINS 2012]

Options:

(a) Statements (A), (C) and (D)
(b) Statements (B), (C) and (A)
(c) Statements (A), (B)
(d) Statements (C), (D)

8. Green revolution in India occurred during:

[AIPMT MAINS 2012]

(a) 1970's
(b) 1980's
(c) 1950's
(d) 1960's

9. Consumption of which one of the following foods can prevent the kind of blindness associated with vitamin 'A' deficiency?

[AIPMT PRE 2012]

(a) 'Flaver Savr' tomato
(b) Canolla
(c) Golden rice
(d) Bt-Brinjal

10. Which one of the following is a case of wrong matching?

[AIPMT PRE 2012]

(a) Somatic hybridization – Fusion of two diverse cells.
(b) Vector DNA – Site for t-RNA synthesis
(c) Micropropagation – In vitro production of plants in large numbers
(d) Callus – Unorganised mass of cells produced an tissue culture.

11. Which part would be most suitable for raising virus-free plants for micropropagation?

[AIPMT PRE 2012]

(a) Bark
(b) Vascular tissue
(c) Meristem
(d) Node

12. In plant breeding programmes, the entire collection (of plants/seeds) having all the diverse alleles for all genes in a given crop is called:

[AIPMT 2013]

(a) Selection of superior recombinants
(b) Cross–hybridisation among the selected parents
(c) Evaluation and selection of parents
(d) Germplasm collection

13. In vitro clonal propagation in plants is characterized by:

[AIPMT 2014]

(a) PCR and RAPD (b) Northern blotting
(c) Electrophoresis and HPLC (d) Microscopy

14. An alga which can be employed as food for human being is:

[AIPMT 2014]

(a) Ulothrix (b) Chlorella
(c) Spirigyra (d) Polysiphonia

15. To obtain virus – free healthy plants from a diseased one by tissue culture technique, which part/parts of the diseased plant will be taken?

[AIPMT 2014]

(a) Apical meristem only (b) Palisade parenchyma
(c) Both apical and axillary meristems (d) Epidermis only

16. A technique of micro propagation is:

[AIPMT 2015]

(a) Somatic hybridization (b) Somatic embryogenesis
(c) Protoplast fusion (d) Embryo rescue

17. Golden rice is a genetically modified crop plant where the incorporated gene is meant for biosynthesis of:

[RE-AIPMT 2015]

(a) Vitamin C (b) Omega 3
(c) Vitamin A (d) Vitamin B

18. Outbreeding is an important strategy of animal husbandry because it:

[RE-AIPMT 2015]

(a) Is useful in producing purelines of animals
(b) Is useful in overcoming inbreeding depression
(c) Exposes harmful recessive genes that re eliminated by selection
(d) Helps in accumulation of superior genes

Answer Keys

1. (d)	2. (d)	3. (d)	4. (d)	5. (c)	6. (d)	7. (d)	8. (d)	9. (d)	10. (d)
11. (a)	12. (d)	13. (c)	14. (d)	15. (d)	16. (d)	17. (d)	18. (b)	19. (a)	20. (a)
21. (b)	22. (d)	23. (d)	24. (d)	25. (b)	26. (b)	27. (c)	28. (d)	29. (a)	30. (d)
31. (d)	32. (b)	33. (a)	34. (c)	35. (b)	36. (c)	37. (d)	38. (d)	39. (a)	40. (d)
41. (a)	42. (a)	43. (b)	44. (c)	45. (d)	46. (c)	47. (c)	48. (d)	49. (d)	50. (b)
51. (b)	52. (b)	53. (d)	54. (c)	55. (c)	56. (b)	57. (a)	58. (c)	59. (d)	60. (c)
61. (c)	62. (d)	63. (c)	64. (b)	65. (d)	66. (d)	67. (c)	68. (a)	69. (c)	70. (d)
71. (a)	72. (d)	73. (b)	74. (c)	75. (c)	76. (a)	77. (d)	78. (d)	79. (d)	80. (c)
81. (a)	82. (b)	83. (d)	84. (d)	85. (a)	86. (d)	87. (a)	88. (c)	89. (c)	90. (d)
91. (d)	92. (c)	93. (c)	94. (d)	95. (a)	96. (d)	97. (c)	98. (b)	99. (a)	100. (d)
101. (c)	102. (b)	103. (a)	104. (d)	105. (d)	106. (a)	107. (b)	108. (c)	109. (c)	110. (c)
111. (b)	112. (c)	113. (c)	114. (b)						

AIPMT Previous Year Questions

1. (c)	2. (b)	3. (b)	4. (a)	5. (c)	6. (c)	7. (c)	8. (d)	9. (c)	10. (b)
11. (c)	12. (d)	13. (a)	14. (b)	15. (c)	16. (b)	17. (c)	18. (b)		

CHAPTER

32

Microbes in Human Welfare

1. Choose the correct option with regard to statement A and B.
   A: Microbes are present everywhere on earth.
   B: They cannot live in thermal vents where temperature is as high as 100°C.
   (a) Statement A is correct and B is incorrect. (b) Statement A and B are correct.
   (c) Statement A is incorrect but B is correct. (d) Statement A and B are incorrect.
2. Prions are _________ infectious agents.
   (a) Lipidic (b) Sugar containing
   (c) Proteinaceous (d) Poison containing
3. Microbes after growth on a nutritive medium form _________.
   (a) Group (b) Colonies
   (c) Species (d) Family
4. _________ is/are responsible for converting milk into curd.
   (a) Lactobacillus only (b) *Lactobacillus* and other microbes
   (c) Microbes other than lactobacillus (d) (a) or (c)
5. Choose the correct option with regard to statement A and B.
   A: Lactic Acid Bacteria (LAB) are responsible for converting milk into curd.
   B: LAB create acidic medium necessary to coagulate and fully digest the milk proteins.
   (a) Statement A and B are correct. (b) Statement A and B are incorrect.
   (c) Statement A is correct but B is incorrect. (d) Statement B is correct and A is incorrect.
6. If someone wants to make curd from milk, a small amount of curd is added to fresh milk. The small amount of curd containing millions of LAB is known as.
   (a) accelerator (b) promoter
   (c) inoculum (d) germ
7. To prevent curd from getting sour, which parameter should be essentially controlled?
   (a) Quantity of milk (b) Amount of LAB added initially
   (c) Temperature of the surrounding (d) Amount of O_2 in surrounding air
8. Which vitamin is synthesized by LAB?
   (a) Vitamin B_2 (b) Vitamin B_6
   (c) Vitamin B_5 (d) Vitamin B_{12}
9. The puffed-up dough of dosa and idli is due to _________.
   (a) Fermentation by bacteria and production of O_2.
   (b) Hydrolysis by bacteria and production of CO_2.
   (c) Fermentation by bacteria and production of CO_2.
   (d) Hydrolysis by bacteria and production of O_2.

10. Which microbe helps us in the preparation of bread?
(a) Bacteria (b) Yeast
(c) Fungi (d) Algae

11. Baker's yeast is _________.
(a) *Saccharomyces cariocanus* (b) *Saccharomyces florentinus*
(c) *Saccharomyces cerevisiae* (d) *Saccharomyces spencerorum*

12. _________ is a traditional drink of south India.
(a) Wine (b) Toddy
(c) Tequila (d) Rum

13. The traditional drink of south India is made by fermenting sap from _________ tree.
(a) eucalyptus (b) coconut
(c) palm (d) date

Figure given for questions 14 and 15.

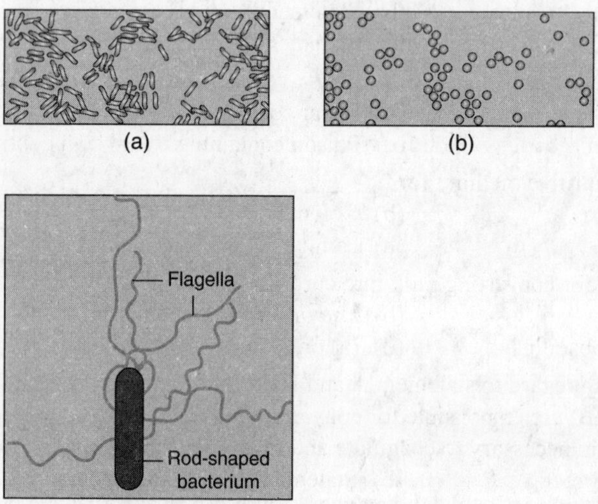

(a) (b) (c)

14. The bacteria shown in figure (a) and (b) are at which level of magnification?
(a) 150X (b) 1500X
(c) 15000X (d) 1.5 lacX

15. The rod shaped bacteria showing flagella is magnified at _________.
(a) 5×10^3 (b) 5×10^4
(c) 1.5×10^3 (d) 15×10^4

16. 'Swiss cheese' bears large holes due to the production of CO_2 by which microbe?
(a) *Lacto bacillus* (b) Sachharomyces cerevisiae
(c) *Propionibacterium sharmanii* (d) Aspergillus niger

17. Just as, Swiss cheese it to Bacteria, Roquefort cheese is to _________.
(a) algae (b) yeast
(c) bacteria (d) fungi

18. Roquefort cheese is ripened by growing a specific fungus on it which gives it a particular ________.

(a) texture (b) large holes
(c) flavour (d) color

19. Vessels for growing microbes on industrial scale are known as ________.

(a) Incubators (b) Sterilizers
(c) Fermentors (d) Microbial vessels

20. Alcoholic beverages are produced by microbial fermentation of:

(a) Malted cereals (b) Fruit juices
(c) Vegetable juices (d) Both (a) and (b)

21. Brewer's Yeast is:

(a) *Saccharomyces cariocanus* (b) *Saccharomyces florentinus*
(c) *Saccharomyces cerevisiae* (d) *Saccharomyces spencerorum*

22. ________ is the alcoholic beverage obtained without distillation.

(a) Whiskey (b) Brandy
(c) Wine (d) Rum

23. Point the odd one out.

(a) Rum (b) Beer
(c) Whiskey (d) Brandy

24. 'Antibiotics' literally means:

(a) Protecting life (b) Against life
(c) Healing life (d) Accelerating life

25. Penicillin was discovered by ________.

(a) Edward Jenner (b) Louis Pastew
(c) Alexander Fleming (d) Howard Florey

26. Penicillin was discovered by chance as the organism producing it retarded growth of ________.

(a) Lactobacilli (b) Staphylococci
(c) Streptococci (d) E. Coli

27. The name penicillin was given after the mould ________.

(a) *Penicillium notatum* (b) *Penicillium chrysogenum*
(c) *Penicillium candidum* (d) *Penicillium glaucum*

28. The full potential as an effective antibiotic in context of penicillin was studied by ________.

(a) Sutton and Boveri (b) Chain and Florey
(c) Watson and Crick (d) Edward Jenner

29. Penicillin was extensively used during which war?

(a) World War I (b) World War II
(c) Both (a) and (b) (d) Cold War

30. ________ soldiers were extensively treated with penicillin during World War II.

(a) German (b) Austrian
(c) American (d) Japanese

31. 'Gal ghotu' is a common name for which disease?

(a) Whooping cough (b) Diphtheria
(c) Plague (d) Leprosy

32. 'Kusht rog' is a common name for which disease?
(a) Dermatitis (b) Plague
(c) Leprosy (d) Whooping cough

33. Citric acid is produced by _________.
(a) *Aspergillus niger* (b) *Sachharomyces cerevisiae*
(c) *Lactobacillus* (d) *Clostridium butylicum*

34. *Acetobacter aceti* essentially produces _________.
(a) Citric acid (b) Acetic acid
(c) Butyric acid (d) Lactic acid

35. Which microbe produces butyric acid?
(a) *Sachharomyces cerevisiae* (b) *Clostridium butylicum*
(c) *Aspergillus niger* (d) *Propionibacterium sharmanii*

Figures given for questions 36 and 37.

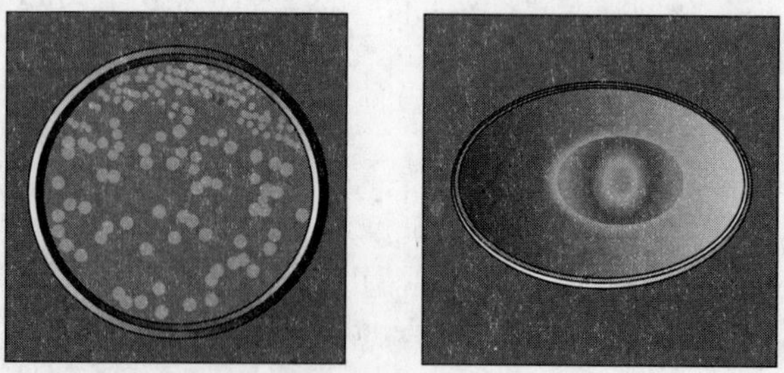

(a) (b)

36. What is depicted in figure (a)?
(a) Fungal colony (b) Algal colony
(c) Bacterial colony (d) Viral colony

37. What is depicted in figure 'b'?
(a) Fungal colony (b) Algal colony
(c) Bacterial colony (d) Viral colony

38. A bacterium which is a rich source of lactic acid is _________.
(a) *Lactobacillus* (b) *Aspergillus*
(c) *Clostridium* (d) *Sachharomyces*

39. Which enzyme produced by microbes is an important ingredient in detergent formulations?
(a) Hydrourse (b) Lipase
(c) Pectinase (d) Cleansase

40. The fruit juices available commercially are clearer than ones which are homemade. Which ingredient is added in commercially available fruit juices?
(a) Lipase and Protease (b) Pectinase and Hydrolase
(c) Pectinase and Protease (d) Hydrolase and Protease

41. Which enzyme is known as 'clot-buster'?
(a) Protease (b) Thrombokinase
(c) Streptokinase (d) Hydrolase

42. 'Clot-buster' is produced by which microbe?
(a) Staphylococcus (b) Streptococcus
(c) Penicillium (d) Aspergillus

43. The enzyme streptokinase is used medicinally to:
(a) Check growth of microbes in body fluids
(b) Remove blood clots from the blood vessels
(c) Weaken walls of blood vessels
(d) Create blood clots in blood vessels

44. Which drugs are often administered before and after organ transplant procedure?
(a) Immuno modulators (b) Immuno suppressants
(c) Vaccination (d) Anabolic steroids

45. Which drug is generally administered at the time of organ-transplant procedure?
(a) Actinomycin-D (b) Bleomycin
(c) Cyclosporin-A (d) Paclitaxel

46. Cyclosporine-A is produced by fungus _________.
(a) *Trichoderma polysporum* (b) *Penicillium notatum*
(c) *Micromonospora* (d) *Aspergillums niger*

47. Blood cholesterol lowering agents are known as _________.
(a) Steroids (b) Statins
(c) Lipolytics (d) Diuretics

48. *Monascus purpureus* is a commercial source of _________.
(a) Antibiotices (b) Statins
(c) Pectinase (d) Ethanol

49. The mechanism of action of statins is _________.
(a) allosteric inhibition of enzyme responsible for synthesis of cholesterol
(b) competitive inhibition of enzyme responsible for synthesis of cholesterol
(c) irreversible inhibition of enzyme responsible for synthesis of cholesterol
(d) None of the above

50. The major portion of waste water in cities and towns is _________.
(a) Household waste (b) Industrial waste
(c) Human excreta (d) Both (a) and (b)

51. Municipal waste water is also known as _________.
(a) Drainage (b) Sewage
(c) Spillage (d) Gutter

52. Sewage is treated in _________.
(a) STD (b) STP
(c) SPT (d) SDT

53. STP stands for:
(a) Sequential Topographical Projection (b) Standard Test Procedure
(c) Sewage Treatment Plant (d) None of the above

54. Which microbes help in sewage treatment?
(a) Autotrophic (b) Heterotrophic
(c) Symbiotic (d) Saprophytic

55. Sewage water treatment is done in how many stages?
(a) 1 (b) 3
(c) 2 (d) 4

56. Primary treatment of sewage waste involves which processes?
(a) Filtration and incubation (b) Sedimentation and decantation
(c) Filtration and sedimentation (d) Sedimentation and microbial proliferation

57. In sewage treatment plant, primary treatment involving removal of floating debris is done by:
(a) Vacuum filtration (b) Pressure filtration
(c) Sequential filtration (d) Sedimentation

58. In primary treatment of sewage water, removal of grit involves which process?
(a) Decantation (b) Picking
(c) Filtration (d) Sedimentation

59. In primary treatment of sewage water, after sedimentation, the solids that settle form ________.
(a) activated sludge (b) primary sludge
(c) secondary sludge (d) Both (a) and (c)

60. The supernatant left after sedimentation of sewage water during primary treatment is known as:
(a) Affluent (b) Flocs
(c) Sludge (d) Effluent

61. Which of the following is transferred from primary setting tank to another tank for secondary treatment?
(a) Grit (b) Sludge
(c) Effluent (d) Floc

Figures given for questions 62 – 70.

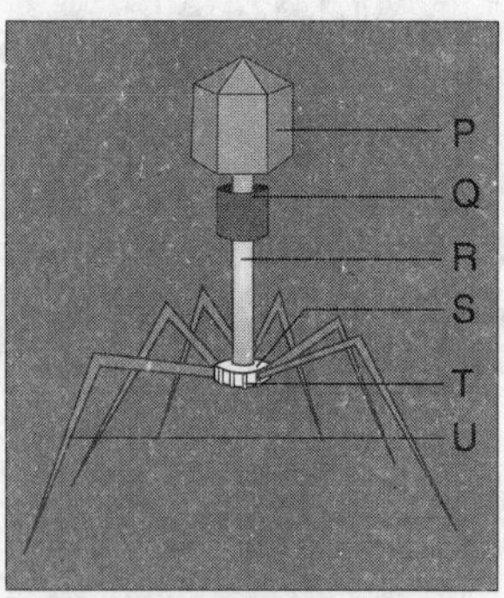

(a)

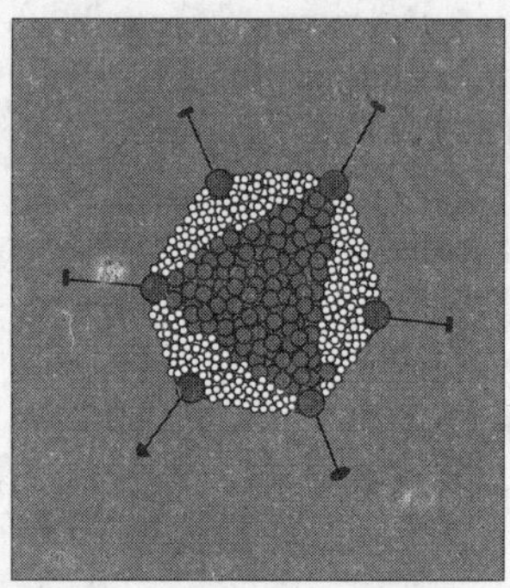
(b)

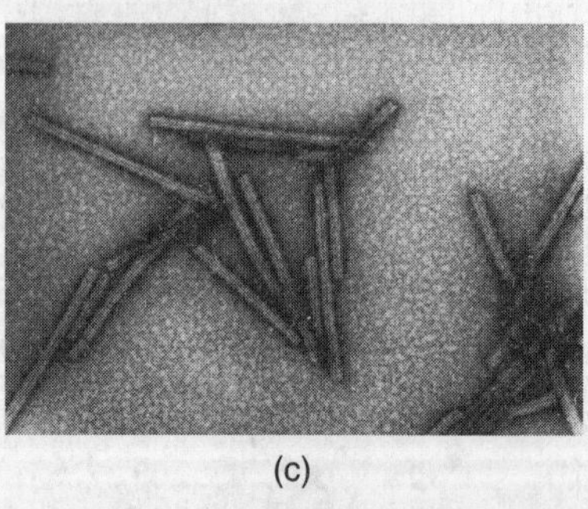
(c)

62. What does figure (a) depict?
(a) Adenovirus (b) Rhinovirus
(c) Bacteriophage (d) Tobacco mosaic Virus

63. What does 's' represent in the figure (a)?
(a) Plate (b) Head
(c) Tail (d) Prongs

64. What does 'p' indicate in the figure (a)?
(a) Plate (b) Head
(c) Collar (d) Prongs

65. What does 'r' indicate in the figure (a)?
(a) Head (b) Collar
(c) Tail (d) Plate

66. What does 'u' represent in the figure (a)?
(a) Prongs (b) Pins
(c) Plate (d) Collar

67. What does 'q' indicate in the figure (a)?
(a) Head (b) Collar
(c) Tail (d) Plate

68. What does 't' represent in the figure (a)?
(a) Collar (b) Prongs
(c) Tail (d) Pins

69. What does figure (b) depict?
(a) Adenovirus (b) Rhinovirus
(c) Bacteriophage (d) Tobacco mosaic Virus

70. Which does figure (c) depict?
(a) Fungal cells (b) Sclercids
(c) TMV (d) Bacteria

71. The secondary treatment of sewage waste is also known as _________.
(a) Chemical treatment (b) Physical treatment
(c) Biological treatment (d) Detoxification

72. Which of the following is used in secondary treatment of sewage water?
(a) Fermentation tanks (b) Digester tanks
(c) Detoxification tanks (d) Aeration tanks

73. What kind of microbes is present in 'flocs' formed during secondary treatment of sewage?
(a) Aerobic (b) Anaerobic
(c) Symbiotic (d) Aero tolerant

74. In context of secondary treatment of sewage, 'flocs' is associated with which microbes?
(a) Bacteria and algae (b) Algae and fungus
(c) Fungi and bacteria (d) Fungi and lichen

75. What is BOD?
(a) Bacterial Oxygen Demand (b) Biological Organic Debris
(c) Biochemical Organic Demand (d) Biochemical Oxygen Demand

76. The 'flocs' present in large aeration tanks causes _________ in BOD.
(a) decrease (b) increases
(c) no change (d) Either (a) or (b)

77. BOD can be defined as:
(a) Amount of CO_2 consumed if all the inorganic matter in one litre of water is oxidized by bacteria.
(b) Amount of O_2 consumed if all the organic matter in one decilitre of water is reduced by bacteria.
(c) Amount of O_2 consumed if all the organic matter in one litre of water is oxidized by bacteria.
(d) Amount of O_2 consumed if all the inorganic matter in one litre of water is oxidized by bacteria.

78. BOD is the measure of _________ in water.
(a) organic matter
(b) inorganic matter
(c) bacterial load
(d) toxicity

79. BOD _________ polluting potential of waste water.
(a) is not proportional to
(b) is directly proportional to
(c) is inversely proportional to
(d) None of the above

80. Once BOD from the sewage is reduced significantly, the 'flocs' are allowed to sediment and it is known as _________.
(a) Primary Sludge
(b) Secondary Sludge
(c) Activated Sludge
(d) Inactivated Sludge

81. Assertion (A): A small part of activated sludge is pumped back into aeration tank.
Reason (R): It serves as inoculum.
(a) A is true but R is false.
(b) A is true and R is correct explanation for A.
(c) A is false but R is true.
(d) Both A and R is false.

82. What is shown in this figure?

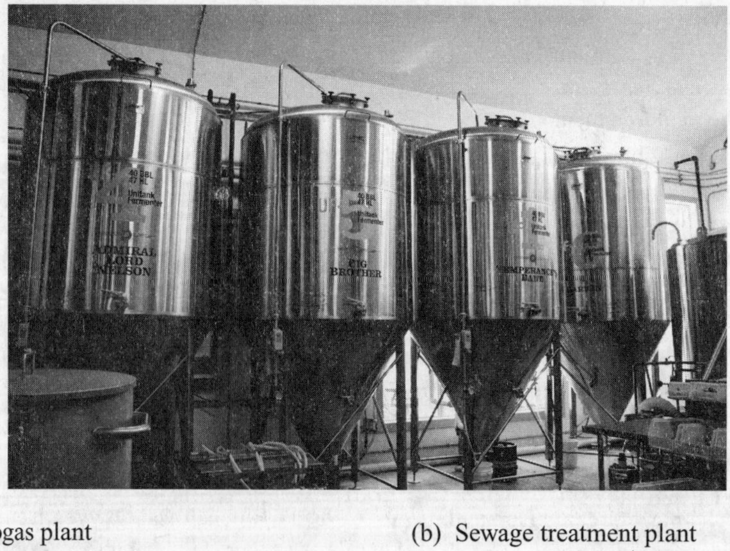

(a) Biogas plant
(b) Sewage treatment plant
(c) Fermentors
(d) Distillation apparatus

83. The remaining major part of activated sludge is pumped into large tanks called ________.
(a) Aerobic fermenters
(b) Anaerobic fermenters
(c) Aerobic Sludge digesters
(d) Anaerobic Sludge digesters

84. In an anaerobic sludge digester, anaerobically digesting bacteria digest which microbes?
(a) Fungi
(b) Bacteria
(c) Algae
(d) Both (a) and (b)

85. What is shown in the figure?

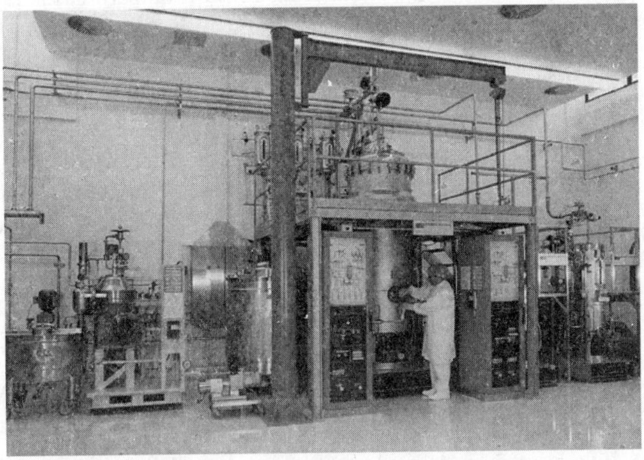

(a) Transmission electron microscope
(b) Fermentation plant
(c) Sewage treatment
(d) Large Hadron Collider

86. In an anaerobic sludge digester, during the digestion process, mixture of gases like ________ are produced.
(a) CH_4, H_2O, O_2
(b) C_2H_6, H_2S, CO_2
(c) CH_4, H_2O_2, CO_2
(d) CH_4, H_2S, CO_2

87. The gases that evolve from anaerobic sludge digester constitute ________.
(a) Natural gas
(b) Biogas
(c) Water gas
(d) None of the above

88. After secondary treatment, the effluent is released into:
(a) Digester tank
(b) Filtration Unit
(c) Water bodies
(d) Chemical treatment unit

89. Which ministry has initiated Ganga Action Plan and Yamuna Action Plan?
(a) Ministry of Chemicals and Fertilizers
(b) Ministry of Health and Family Welfare
(c) Ministry of Community Health and Diseases
(d) Ministry of Environment and Forest

90. Which gas is the main constituent of biogas?
(a) H_2S
(b) CH_4
(c) C_2H_6
(d) C_3H_8

91. The gas produced as end-product during growth and metabolism of microbes depends on:
(a) Nature of microbe and substrate
(b) Nature of digester tank and microbe
(c) Nature of microbe only
(d) Oxygen levels in the digester tank

92. Methanogens produce certain gases by growing on cellulosic material. What kind of organisms are they?

(a) Fungi (b) Algae
(c) Bacteria (d) Lichen

93. Methanogens are ________ microbes.

(a) Anaerobic (b) Aerobic
(c) Microaerophils (d) Aerotobront

94. Methanogens produces which gases amongst the following list of gases?

CH_4, O_2, CO_2, H_2O_2, H_2S, H_2

(a) CH_4, H_2O_2, H_2 (b) H_2S, H_2, CO_2
(c) CH_4, H_2, CO_2 (d) H_2S, H_2O_2, CO_2

95. The most commonly found methanogens in anaerobic sludge is ________.

(a) Ethanobacterium (b) Methanobacterium
(c) Cyanobacterium (d) Both (b) and (c)

96. The rumen of cattle harbours which bacteria?

(a) Methanogens (b) Cyanobacteria
(c) Cellulogens (d) Ethanogens

97. What is the role of bacteria present in the rumen of cattle?

(a) Production of methane (b) Regulation of digestion
(c) Breakdown of cellulose (d) Synthesis of polysaccharides

98. Gobar gas is the same as ________.

(a) Water gas (b) Biogas
(c) Natural gas (d) None of the above

99. The depth of concrete tank, a part of biogas plant, ranges from ________ to ________.

(a) 10–15 feet (b) 10–15 metre
(c) 15–20 feet (d) 15–20 metre

100. What is the input material for a biogas plant?

(a) Bio wastes (b) Slurry of dung
(c) Industrial waste (d) Both (a) and (b)

101. A ________ is placed over the slurry in biogas plant.

(a) gas holder (b) floating cover
(c) digester (d) gas filter

102. The spent slurry in a biogas plant is used as ________.

(a) pesticide (b) fertilizer
(c) insecticide (d) herbicide

103. Apart from cooking, biogas is generally used in rural areas for ________.

(a) Mechanical work (b) Lighting
(c) Chemical transformation (d) None of the above

104. Which institutes have actively participated in development of technology for biogas production?

IARI, IIT, IISC, KVIM, KVIC.

(a) IIT and KVIM (b) IISC and KVIC
(c) KVIC and IARI (d) IARI and KVIM

105. IARI stands for:
(a) Indian Aviation Research Institute
(b) Indian Aerospace Research Institute
(c) Indian Atomic Research Institute
(d) Indian Agricultural Research Institute

106. Biocontrol refers to:
(a) Indiscriminate use of microbes for human welfare
(b) Use of microbes to control plant diseases
(c) Use of microbes to control cattle diseases
(d) Both (b) and (c)

107. A beetle with 'red and black' markings is known as ________.
(a) Dragonfly
(b) Ladybird
(c) Clever Wasp
(d) Queen Ant

108. Dragonflies are useful to get rid of ________.
(a) Ladybird
(b) Aphids
(c) Mosquitoes
(d) Both (b) and (c)

109. Butterfly caterpillars can be controlled by use of the microbe ________.
(a) *Bacillus thermophilus*
(b) *Bacillus thruingiensis*
(c) *Bacillus Chemophilus*
(d) *Bacillus terminates*

110. 'Bt' is available in sachets as dried ________.
(a) spores
(b) capsules
(c) seeds
(d) Both (a) and (b)

111. The figure shows:

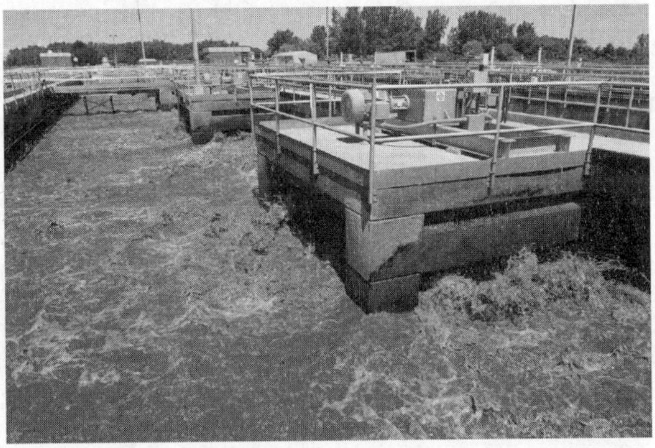

(a) Primary treatment
(b) Activated sludge
(c) Secondary treatment
(d) Flocs

112. 'Bt' spores are mixed with ________ and sprayed on vulnerable plants.
(a) only alcohol
(b) any organic solvent
(c) only water
(d) any aqueous solvent

113. Scientists have introduced ________ gene into plants to impart resistance to insect pests.
(a) Ct gene
(b) Bt gene
(c) Tt gene
(d) Mt gene

114. Which fungus is used in plants to provide control against pests?
(a) *Aspergillus* (b) *Trichoderma*
(c) *Trichophyton* (d) *Rhizopus*

115. _________ are the pathogens that attack insects and other arthropods.
(a) *Rhinovirus* (b) *Baculovirus*
(c) *Ranikhet Virus* (d) *Bean Virus*

116. Baculovirus belongs to the genus:
(a) *Retrohedro Virus* (b) *Nucleohedero-Virus*
(c) *Nucleopolyhedro Virus* (d) *Polyhedron Virus*

117. IPM stands for:
(a) Indian Pollution Management (b) Institute of Pest Management
(c) Integrated Pest Management (d) Institute of Pollution Management

118. Root nodules of leguminous plants bear which microbe?
(a) *Rhizopus* (b) *Rhino Virus*
(c) *Rhizome* (d) *Rhizobium*

119. This image is an aerial view of a _________ .

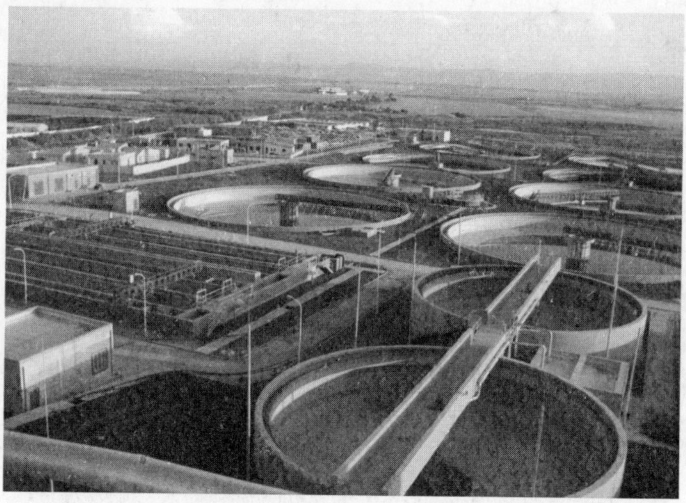

(a) Nuclear reactor (b) Sewage plant
(c) Biogas plant (d) Fermentation plant

120. _________ are free living bacteria which fix atmospheric nitrogen in soil.
(a) Azobacterium (b) Acetobacterium
(c) Azotobacter (d) Azabacterium

121. Fungi which form symbiotic associations with plants are _________.
(a) *Rhizobium* (b) *Mycorrhiza*
(c) *Azospirillum* (d) *Oscillatoria*

122. Mycorrhiza absorbs _________ from soil and passes it to the plant.
(a) K (b) P
(c) Fe (d) Mg

123. ________ bacteria fix atmospheric N_2 in aquatic and terrestrial environments.
(a) *Cyanobacteria* (b) *Azotobactor*
(c) *Methanobacteria* (d) *Mycorrhiza*

124. ________ serve as an important bio-fertilizer in paddy fields.
(a) *Cyanobacteria* (b) *Azotobactor*
(c) *Methanobacteria* (d) *Mycorrhiza*

125. Which microbe adds organic matter to the soil to increase its fertility?
(a) *Cyanobacteria* (b) *Bluegreen algae*
(c) *Rhizobium* (d) *Trichoderma*

Figure given for questions 126 – 130.

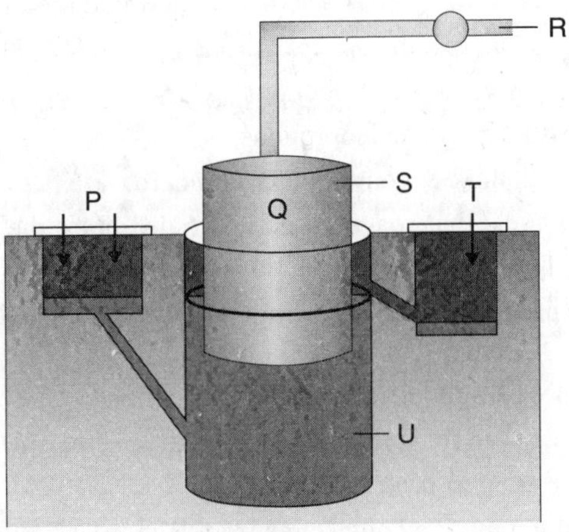

126. What does 'P' indicate in the figure?
(a) Dung and Vegetable waste (b) Water and dung
(c) Vegetable and Human excreta (d) All of the above

127. What does 'R' indicate in the figure?
(a) Effluent (b) Gas
(c) Gas holder (d) Filtration

128. What does 'S' indicate in the figure?
(a) Digester (b) Gas purifier
(c) Gas holder (d) Sludge tank

129. What does 'T' indicate in the figure?
(a) By-product collector (b) Sludge
(c) Digester (d) Gas holder

130. What does 'U' indicate in the figure?
(a) Gas holder (b) Digester
(c) Sludge (d) Waste collector

Read the ***assertion*** *and* ***reason*** *carefully to mark the correct option out of the options given below:*

(a) If both the assertion and the reason are true and the reason is a correct explanation of the assertion

(b) If both the assertion and reason are true but the reason is not a correct explanation of the assertion

(c) If the assertion is true but the reason is false

(d) If both the assertion and reason are false

131. Assertion: In paddy field, cyanobacteria serve as important biofertilizer.
Reason: Cyanobacteria can fix atmosphere nitrogen

132. Assertion: Prions are proteinaceous infectious agents.
Reason: Prions are made up of Nucleoproteins.

133. Assertion: LAB grow in milk & convert milk into curd.
Reason: LAB produce acid that coagulate and partially digest the milk protein.

134. Assertion: There are large holes present in Swiss cheese.
Reason: Large holes produce due to production of large amount of SO_2 by Propioni bacterium sharmanii.

135. Assertion: Wine & Beer are produced without distillation.
Reason: Brewer's yeast used for fermentation of malted cereals & fruit juices.

136. Assertion: Lipases are used in detergent formation.
Reason: Lipases help in removing oily stains from laundry.

137. Assertion: Bottled fruit juices bought from the market are clearer as compared to those made at home.
Reason: Bottled juices are clarified by the use of pectinases and proteases.

138. Assertion: Streptokinase is given to patient suffering from myocardial infarction.
Reason: Streptokinase act a clot -buster.

139. Assertion: Greater is BOD of waste water, more is its polluting potential.
Reason: BOD is a measure of organic matter present in water.

AIPMT PREVIOUS YEAR QUESTIONS

1. When domestic sewage mixes with river water

[AIPMT MAINS 2010]

(a) Small animals like rats will die after drinking river water
(b) The increased microbial activity releases micronutrients such as iron
(c) The increased microbial activity uses up dissolved oxygen
(d) The river water is still suitable for drinking as impurities are only about 0.1%

2. An example of endomycorrhiza is:

[AIPMT MAINS 2010]

(a) Nostoc
(b) Glomus
(c) Agaricus
(d) Rhizobium

3. Select the correct statement from the following

[AIPMT PRE 2010]

(a) Biogas is produced by the activity of aerobic bacteria on animal waste
(b) Methanobacterium is an aerobic bacterium found in rumen of cattle
(c) Biogas, commonly called gobar gas, is pure methane
(d) Activated sludge-sediment in settlement tank of sewage treatment plant is a right source of aerobic bacteria

4. A common biocontrol agent for the control of plant diseases is

[AIPMT PRE 2010]

(a) Baculovirus
(b) Bacillus thuringiensis
(c) Glomus
(d) Trichoderma

5. Which one of the following is not used in organic farming?

[AIPMT PRE 2010]

(a) Glomus
(b) Earthworm
(c) Oscillatoria
(d) Snail

6. Read the following statement having two blanks (A and B).
"A drug used for A patients is obtained from a species of the organism B
The one correct option for the two blanks is

[AIPMT MAINS 2011]

	A	B
(a)	Heart	Penicilliumm
(b)	Organ-tranplant	Trichoderma
(c)	Swine flu	Monascus
(d)	AIDS	Pseudomonas

7. Which one of the following is a wrong matching of a microbe and its industrial product, while the remaining three are correct?

[AIPMT MAINS 2011]

(a) Yeast - statins
(b) Acetobacter aceti – acetic acid
(c) Clostridium butylicum – lactic acid
(d) Aspergillus niger – citric acid

8. Which of the following is mainly produced by the activity of anaerobic bacteria on sewage?

[AIPMT PRE 2011]

(a) Propane
(b) Mustard gas
(c) Marsh gas
(d) Laughing gas

9. Which one of the following helps in absorption of phosphorus from soil by plants?

[AIPMT PRE 2011]

(a) Rhizobium
(b) Frankia
(c) Anabaena
(d) Glomus

10. Continuous addition of sugars in 'fed batch' fermentation is done to:

[AIPMT PRE 2011]

(a) Obtain antibiotics
(b) Purify enzymes
(c) Degrade sewage
(d) Produce methane

11. Secondary sewage treatment is mainly a: [AIPMT PRE 2011]

(a) Mechanical process (b) Chemical process
(c) Biological process (d) Physical process

12. Which one of the following is not a biofertilizer? [AIPMT PRE 2011]

(a) Rhizobium (b) Nostoc
(c) Mycorrhiza (d) Agrobacterium

13. The most common substrate used in distilleries for the production of ethanol is: [AIPMT PRE 2011]

(a) Soya meal (b) Ground gram
(c) Molasses (d) Corn meal

14. Ethanol is commercially produced through a particular species of [AIPMT PRE 2011]

(a) Clostridium (b) Trichoderma
(c) Aspergillus (d) Saccharomyces

15. In gobar gas, the maximum amount is that of: [AIPMT MAINS 2012]

(a) Methane (b) Propane
(c) Carbon dioxide (d) Butane

16. Read the following four statements (A-D):
(A) Colostrum is recommended for the new born because it is rich in antigen
(B) Chikengunya is caused by a Gram negative bacterium
(C) Tissue culture has proved useful in obtaining virus-free plants
(D) Beer is manufactured by distillation of fermented grape juice

[AIPMT MAINS 2012]

How many of the above statements are wrong
(a) Three (b) Four
(c) One (d) Two

17. The domestic sewage in large cities: [AIPMT MAINS 2012]

(a) Is processed by aerobic and then anaerobic bacteria in the secondary treatment in Sewage Treatment Plant (STPs)
(b) When treated in STPs does not really require the aeration step as the sewage contains adequate oxygen
(c) Has very high amounts of suspended solids and dissolved salts
(d) Has a high BOD as it contains both aerobic and anaerobic bacteria.

18. Monascus purpureus is yeast used commercially in the production of; [AIPMT PRE 2012]

(a) Ethanol
(b) Streptokinase for removing clots from the blood vessels
(c) Citric acid
(d) Blood cholesterol lowering statins

19. A patient brought to a hospital with my myocardial infarction is normally immediately given: [AIPMT PRE 2012]

(a) Penicillin (b) Streptokinase
(c) Cyclosporin-A (d) Statins

20. Which of the following microbes forms symbiotic association with plants and helps them in their nutrition? [AIPMT PRE 2012]

(a) Azotobacter (b) Aspergillus
(c) Glomus (d) Trichoderma

21. Yeast used on the production of: [AIPMT PRE 2012]

(a) Citric acid and lactic acid (b) Lipase and pectinase
(c) Bread and beer (d) Cheese and butter

22. A nitrogen-fixing microbe associated with Azolla in rice field is: [AIPMT PRE 2012]

(a) Spirulina (b) Anabaena
(c) Frankia (d) Tolypothrix

23. Which one of the following is an example of carrying out biological control of pests / diseases using microbes? [AIPMT PRE 2012]

(a) Trichoderma sp. Against certain plant pathogens
(b) Nucleopolyhedorvirus against white rust in Brassica
(c) Bt-cotton to increase cotton yield
(d) Lady bird beetal against aphids in mustard

24. A good producer of citric acid is: [AIPMT 2013]

(a) Aspergillus (b) Pseudomonas
(c) Clostridium (d) Saccharomyces

25. Which of the following are likely to be present deep sea water? [AIPMT 2013]

(a) Archaebacteria (b) Eubacteria
(c) Blue-green algae (d)Saprophytic fungi

26. During sewage treatment, biogases are produced which include: [AIPMT 2015]

(a) Methane, hydrogensulphide, carbon dioxide
(b) Methane, oxygen, hydrogensulphide
(c) Hydrogensulphide, methane, sulphur dioxide
(d) Hydrogensulphide, nitrogen, methane

27. What gases are produced in anaerobic sludge digesters? [AIPMT 2014]

(a) Methane and CO_2 only
(b) Methane, Hydrogen Sulphide and CO_2
(c) Methane, Hydrogen Sulphide and O_2
(d) Hydrogen Sulphide and CO_2

28. High value of BOD (Biochemical Oxygen Demand) indicates that : [AIPMT 2015]

(a) Water is pure
(b) Water is highly polluted
(c) Water is less polluted
(d) Consumption of organic matter in the water is higher by the microbes

29. Match the following list of microbes and their importance:

(a) sacharomyces cerevisiae	production of immunosuppressive agents
(b) monoscus purpureus	ripening of Swiss cheese
(c) Trichoderma polysporum	Commercial production of ethanol
(d) Propionibacterium sharmanii	Production of blood-cholesterol lowering agnets

[RE-AIPMT 2015]

	(a)	(b)	(c)	(d)
(a)	(iv)	(iii)	(ii)	(i)
(b)	(iv)	(ii)	(i)	(iii)
(c)	(iii)	(i)	(iv)	(ii)
(d)	(iii)	(iv)	(i)	(ii)

Answer Keys

1. (a)	2. (c)	3. (b)	4. (b)	5. (c)	6. (c)	7. (c)	8. (d)	9. (c)	10. (b)
11. (c)	12. (b)	13. (c)	14. (b)	15. (b)	16. (c)	17. (d)	18. (c)	19. (c)	20. (d)
21. (c)	22. (c)	23. (b)	24. (b)	25. (c)	26. (b)	27. (a)	28. (b)	29. (b)	30. (c)
31. (b)	32. (c)	33. (a)	34. (b)	35. (b)	36. (c)	37. (a)	38. (a)	39. (b)	40. (c)
41. (c)	42. (b)	43. (b)	44. (b)	45. (c)	46. (a)	47. (b)	48. (b)	49. (b)	50. (c)
51. (b)	52. (b)	53. (c)	54. (b)	55. (c)	56. (c)	57. (c)	58. (d)	59. (b)	60. (d)
61. (c)	62. (c)	63. (a)	64. (b)	65. (c)	66. (a)	67. (b)	68. (d)	69. (a)	70. (c)
71. (c)	72. (d)	73. (a)	74. (c)	75. (d)	76. (a)	77. (c)	78. (a)	79. (b)	80. (c)
81. (b)	82. (c)	83. (d)	84. (d)	85. (b)	86. (d)	87. (b)	88. (c)	89. (d)	90. (b)
91. (a)	92. (c)	93. (a)	94. (c)	95. (b)	96. (a)	97. (c)	98. (b)	99. (a)	100. (d)
101. (b)	102. (b)	103. (b)	104. (c)	105. (d)	106. (b)	107. (b)	108. (d)	109. (b)	110. (a)
111. (c)	112. (c)	113. (b)	114. (b)	115. (b)	116. (c)	117. (c)	118. (d)	119. (b)	120. (c)
121. (b)	122. (b)	123. (a)	124. (a)	125. (b)	126. (b)	127. (b)	128. (c)	129. (b)	130. (b)
131. (a)	132. (c)	133. (a)	134. (c)	135. (b)	136. (a)	137. (a)	138. (a)	139. (b)	

AIPMT Previous Year Questions

1. (c)	2. (b)	3. (d)	4. (d)	5. (d)	6. (b)	7. (c)	8. (c)	9. (d)	10. (b)
11. (c)	12. (d)	13. (c)	14. (d)	15. (a)	16. (a)	17. (a)	18. (b)	19. (b)	20. (c)
21. (c)	22. (b)	23. (c)	24. (a)	25. (a)	26. (a)	27. (b)	28. (b)	29. (d)	

Unit IX

Biotechnology

This unit comprises two chapters—Biotechnology: Principles and Processes and Biotechnology and its Applications. It is advised that before reading this unit, you need to go through the chapter on Molecular Basis of Inheritance. Some topics like RNA-i Mechanism, PCR Technique, Blotting technique, and Gene Therapy require in-depth knowledge. Hence, read all these topics in detail, as from this topic, 3–5 questions are asked every year in **AIPMT**. Again, diagrams are very important, so study them carefully.

CHAPTER 33

Biotechnology Principles and Processes

1. Biotechnology deals with techniques of using which of the following to produce product and processes useful to humans?
   (a) Enzyme from organism
   (b) Live organism
   (c) Vitamins
   (d) Both (a) and (b)
2. Biotechnology mainly uses
   (a) GMO
   (b) Bacteria
   (c) Virus
   (d) Animals
3. Select the process/technique included under biotechnology.
   (a) IVF (test tube baby)
   (b) Gene synthesis
   (c) Developing DNA vaccine
   (d) All of the above
4. Which of the following is true about EFB definition of biotechnology?
   (a) It includes traditional view
   (b) It includes modern molecular biotechnology
   (c) Definition is the integration of natural science and organisms, cells, parts thereof, and molecular analogues for products and services
   (d) All of the above
5. Following can be biotechnological products
   (a) Antibiotics
   (b) Vaccine
   (c) Enzymes
   (d) All of these
6. Select the false statement from the following.
   (a) Genetic engineering includes techniques to alter chemistry of genetic material (DNA and RNA).
   (b) Sexual reproduction is more advantageous than asexual reproduction.
   (c) Genetic engineering allows us to introduce desirable set of genes without the undesirable gene into the target organism.
   (d) Plasmid is autonomously replicating linear extra chromosomal DNA.
7. Multiplication of alien DNA in organism requires
   (a) ROP
   (b) ORI
   (c) Stop codon
   (d) TATA box

8. We can cut DNA with the help of
   (a) DNAase
   (b) RNAase
   (c) Knife
   (d) Restriction enzyme

9. For making GMO, the three basic steps that are required are
   (a) Identification of DNA with desirable gene
   (b) Introduction of identified DNA into the host
   (c) Maintance of introduced DNA in the host and transfer of the DNA to its progeny
   (d) All of the above

10. Who isolated antibiotic resistance gene from salmonella typhimurium in 1972?
   (a) Jacob and Monad
   (b) Stanley Cohen and Herbert Boyer
   (c) Osborn
   (d) Boliver

11. Which diagram correctly represents the cutting of both strands of DNA by EcoRI?

(a)
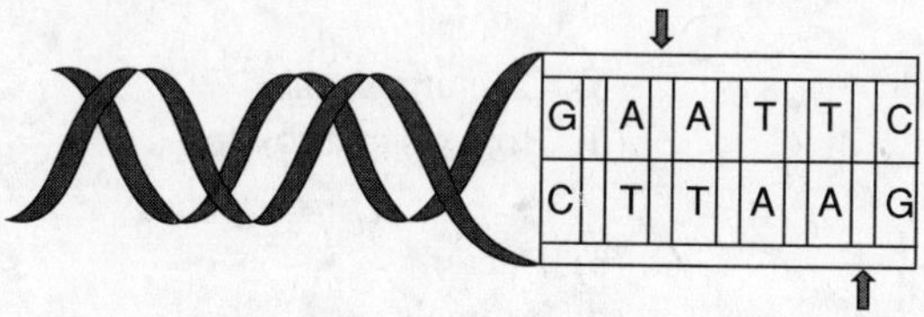

(b)
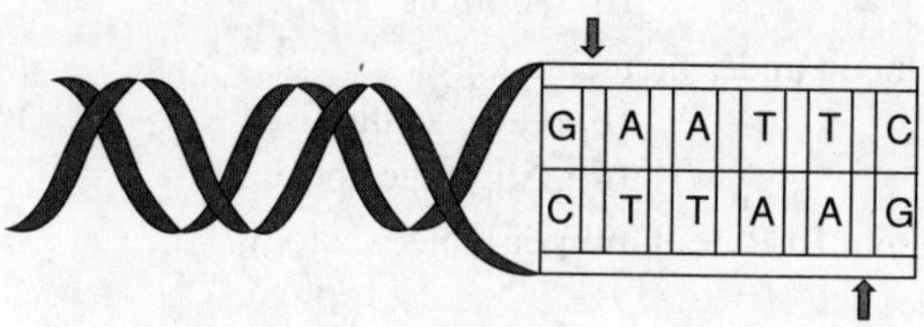

(c)
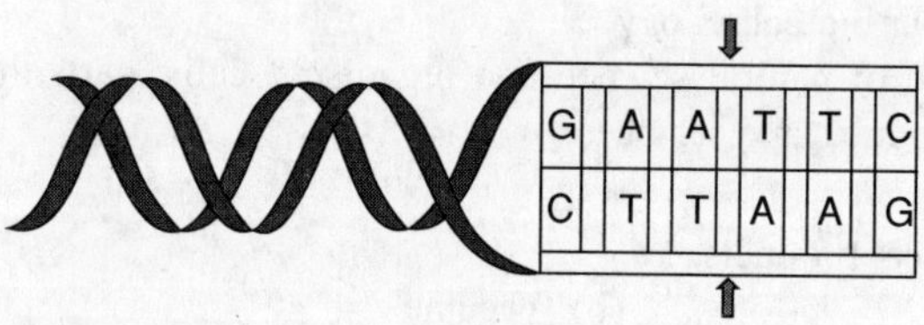

(d)
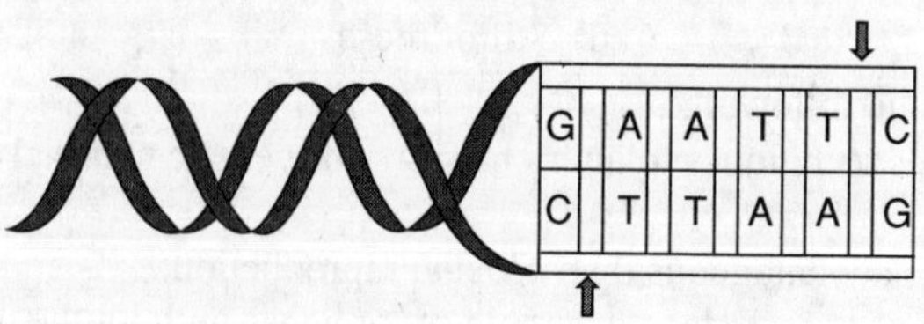

12. Hind II recognizes a specific sequence of how many base pairs?
   (a) 4
   (b) 6
   (c) 8
   (d) 10

13. The sequence recognized by restriction endonucleases
   (a) ORI
   (b) Recognition sequence
   (c) Palindrome sequence
   (d) Both (b) and (c)

14. Select the incorrect statement.
    (a) More than 900 restriction enzymes have been isolated from over 230 strains of bacteria.
    (b) In the year 1963, the two enzymes responsible for restricting the growth of bacteriophage in Escherichia coli were isolated.
    (c) Some key tools for recombinant DNA technology are restriction enzyme, polymerase enzyme, ligase, vectors and host root organisms.
    (d) EcoRI cut the DNA between bases A and T only when the sequence GAATTC is present in the DNA.
15. In 'EcoRI' R stands for
    (a) Genus
    (b) Species
    (c) Strain
    (d) Restriction enzyme
16. In 'EcoRI' 'co' stands for
    (a) Genus
    (b) Species
    (c) Strain
    (d) Restriction enzyme
17. What is 'B' in the figure?

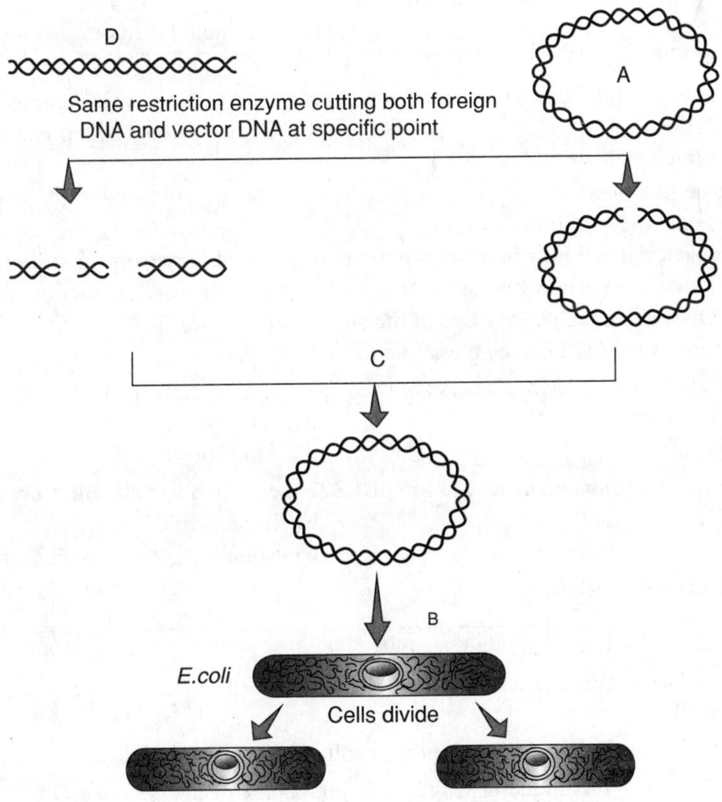

    (a) Transformation
    (b) Transduction
    (c) Conjugation
    (d) Vector DNA

18. Restriction enzyme breaks
(a) Glycosidic linkage
(b) H-bond
(c) Sugar–phosphate linkage
(d) All of the above

19. Sequence recognize by Eco RI is
(a) 5′-GAATTC-3′ 3′-CTTAAG-5′
(b) 5′-CCAATG-3′ 3′-GAATCC-5′
(c) 5′-GATACC-3′ 3′-CCTAAG-5′
(d) 5′-CATTAG-3′ 3′-GATAAC-5′

20. EcoRI cut palindrome sequence which produces overhanging stretches called sticky ends on each strand. These are named sticky because
(a) They can combine with any DNA.
(b) They form hydrogen bonds with their complementary cut counterpart.
(c) They facilitate the action of the enzyme DNA ligase.
(d) Both (b) and (c)

21. The extraction of DNA from a gel piece is known as
(a) Spooling
(b) Elution
(c) AGE
(d) Annealing

22. The fragmented DNA can be visualized by staining DNA with
(a) NaCl
(b) Ethidium bromide
(c) Ethylene bromide
(d) NaBr

23. For cloning of foreign DNA it is attached with *ori* gene of vector which control
(a) Replication
(b) Copy noumber of replicating DNA
(c) Both (a) and (b)
(d) None

24. Find the true statement.
(a) *Ori* means origin of transcription.
(b) Some bacterial cell may have copy number of plasmid vary from 15–100.
(c) Vector should have many recognition sites for commonly used restriction enzymes so that alien DNA can attach to any one of the sites easily.
(d) tetR gene in pBR322 can be cleaved by Pvu I and Pst I.

25. Following antibiotic resistance genes are used as selectable marker for E. coli
(a) Chloromphenicol
(b) Tetracycline
(c) Kanamycin
(d) All of these

26. If alien DNA in introduced using Sal I in pBR322 then transformant will grow on
(a) Ampicillin
(b) Tetracycline
(c) Both
(d) None

27. Select the incorrect matching

(a) pBR322	– E. coli cloning vector
(b) Eco R I, Cla I, Hind III	– Restriction enzyme
(c) ROP	– Protein involved in the replication of the plasmid
(d) PCR	– Technique in which multiple copies of the gene (or DNA) of interest in synthesized in vitro

28. Select the incorrect statement.
   (a) Selection of recombinants due to inactivation of antibiotic is a cumbersome procedure.
   (b) Insertional inactivation of β-galctosidase leads to colorless colonies.
   (c) Insertional inactivation of β-glactosidase leads to blue color colonies.
   (d) In insertional inactivation, the r-DNA is inserted within the coding sequence of an enzyme β-glactosidase.
29. Which vector is use to deliver gene in animal cell?
   (a) Retroviruses (b) Disarmed retroviruses
   (c) Ti-plasmid (d) E. coli
30. To make bacterium competent (Transformation with recombinant DNA) we use
   (a) Specific concentration of Ca^{2+} ion (b) Heat shock (42°C)
   (c) Both (d) None
31. By which method is rDNA directly placed in nucleus of animal cell?
   (a) Gene gun (biolistics) (b) Heat shock
   (c) $CaCl_2$ (d) Micro-injection
32. Way to introduce alien DNA into host cell includes
   (a) Disarmed pathogens (b) Biolistics or gene gun
   (c) Micro-injection (d) All of the above
33. Which method is suitable for transferring an alien DNA into a plant cell?
   (a) $CaCl_2$ (b) Biolistics or gene gun
   (c) Micro-infection (d) Heat shock

Figure given for questions 34 and 35.

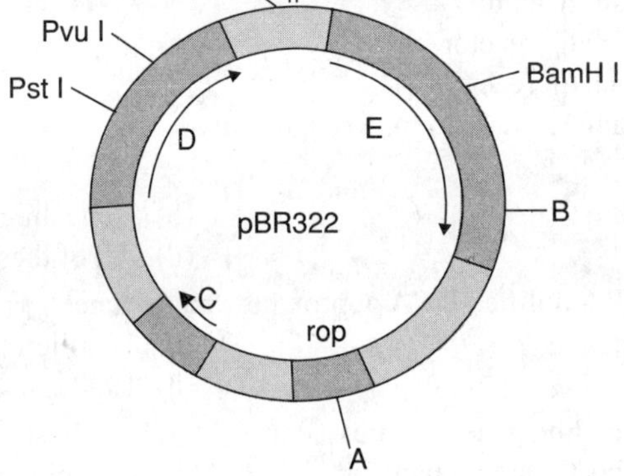

34. Restriction enzymne 'A' is
   (a) Pst I (b) PVU II
   (c) Bam HI (d) Sal I
35. 'E' is
   (a) Amp^R gene (b) tet^R gene
   (c) Chlor^R gene (d) Eco^R gene

36. Arrange the following process in the sequence used in r-DNA technology.
(1) Isolation of DNA
(2) Fragmentation of DNA by RE
(3) Isolation of desired DNA fragment
(4) Ligation of DNA fragment into vector
(5) Transferring r-DNA into host
(6) Culturing host cells in a medium at large scale
(7) Extraction of the desired product
(a) 1, 2, 3, 4, 5, 6, 7 (b) 1, 2, 3, 4, 6, 5, 7
(c) 2, 1, 3, 4, 5, 6, 7 (d) 1, 2, 3, 5, 4, 6, 7

37. In majority of organism genetic material is
(a) DNA (b) RNA
(c) m-RNA (d) Protein

38. In order to extract DNA we use the following enzyme for the following organism, which matching is correct?
(a) Plant cell–Cellulose (b) Fungus–Chitinase
(c) Bacteria–Lysozyme (d) All are correct

39. In isolation of genetic material (DNA) from nucleus, the RNA can be removed by ribonuclease and protein by protease. Purified DNA then precipitates after the addition of ________ .
(a) $CaCl_2$ (b) ether
(c) chilled ethanol (d) acetic acid

40. Which of the following is used to check progression of restriction enzyme digestion?
(a) PCR (b) ROP
(c) AGE (d) All

41. PCR stands for
(a) Polymer chain reaction
(b) Polymerase chain reactor
(c) Polymerase chain reaction
(d) Polymerisation, combination, Recognition

42. PCR includes
(a) Denaturation (b) Annealing
(c) Extension (d) All of these

43. 30 cycles of PCR amplified DNA approx how many times
(a) 1 billion times (b) 1 million times
(c) 100 times (d) 1000 times

44. If any protein encoding gene is expressed in a ________ host, it is called a ________ protein.
(a) homologus host, recombinant (b) heterologus host, recombinant
(c) heterologus host, non-recombinant (d) homologus host, non-recombinant

45. What is the maximum volume of culture that can be processed in bioreactors?
(a) 10–100 liters (b) 100–1000 liters
(c) 1–10 liters (d) 1000–1,00,000 liters

46. The host cultured in a continuous culture system where inside the used medium is drained out from one side while fresh medium is added from the other to maintain cells in their physiologically _________ phase.
    (a) lag
    (b) log
    (c) stationary
    (d) declining
47. Bioreactors have
    (a) Foam control system, temperature control system
    (b) Oxygen delivery system
    (c) pH control system
    (d) All of the above
48. Following will be done with product formed by r-DNA technology?
    (a) Product has to be formulated with suitable preservation.
    (b) Formulation has to undergo clinical trials.
    (c) Strict quality control testing is done.
    (d) All of the above
49. Which of the following DNA is undigested by restriction endonuclease in this diagram?

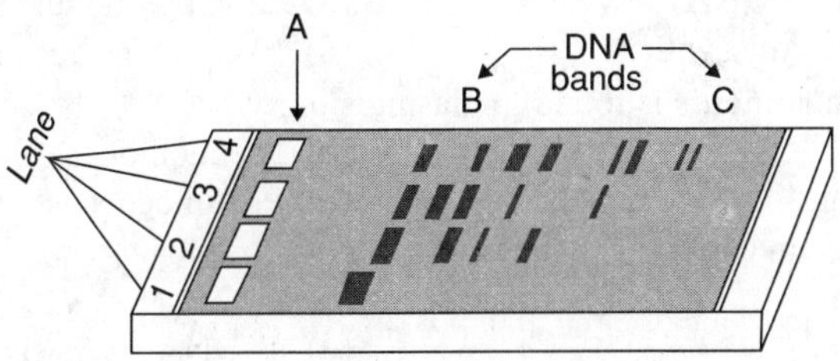

    (a) Lane 1
    (b) Lane 2
    (c) Lane 3
    (d) Lane 4
50. r-DNA is a
    (a) Chimeric DNA
    (b) Hybrid DNA-RNA
    (c) Recombinant of vector DNA and desired gene/s
    (d) Both (a) and (c)
51. Foreign DNA is also called
    (a) Vehicle DNA
    (b) Passenger DNA
    (c) r-DNA
    (d) Vector DNA
52. Plasmids are
    (a) ss-DNA
    (b) ds-DNA (linear)
    (c) ds-DNA (circular)
    (d) denatured-DNA
53. pBR322 is most extensively studied
    (a) Plasmid DNA of E. coli
    (b) Foreign gene
    (c) r-DNA
    (d) Clone
54. Restriction enzymes recognize specific
    (a) Palindromic region
    (b) Exons
    (c) Introns
    (d) None of these

55. First restriction enzyme was isolated from
(a) E. coli (b) Haemophilus influenza
(c) Pseudomonas (d) Xanthomonas

56. Restriction endonuclease is a
(a) Enzyme for transcription (b) Molecular blade
(c) Enzyme for replication (d) Enzyme for transduction

57. Restriction enzymes of E. coli are
(a) Hind.III (b) Bam H.I
(c) Eco R.I, Eco R.II (d) All of these

58. Plasmids are
(a) Extranuclear genes of bacteria (b) Endosymbiont of bacterial cells
(c) Best vector DNA (d) All of the above

59. Best cloning organism for genetic engineering and biotechnology is
(a) Agrobacterium (b) Pseudomonas
(c) E. coli (d) Lambda phage

60. Bacteriophages are used in biotechnology as
(a) Vector or vehicle DNA (b) Cloning organism
(c) Restriction enzyme synthesizers (d) None of the above

61. The ability to form tumours is found in plasmids of
(a) E. coli (b) Pseudomonas
(c) Agrobacterium (d) Pneumococcus

62. Engineered bacterium carries
(a) Plasmids (b) r-DNA
(c) c-DNA (d) ss-DNA

63. Engineered bacteria are reproduced by inserting
(a) Plasmids DNA
(b) Desired DNA (gene/s) loaded on vector DNA
(c) Vehicle DNA
(d) Phage DNA

64. Oncogenic character is seen in
(a) E. coli (b) pBR322
(c) T_i plasmids (d) R_i plasmids

65. Transgenic plants are produced by inserting desired genes in
(a) pBR-322 (b) T_i plasmids
(c) Lambda phage (d) None of these

66. Which is not a vector for r-DNA technology?
(a) Plasmids (b) Cosmids
(c) Phages (d) Mosquitoes

67. Broken ends of two DNA strands are joined by
(a) Exonuclease (b) Endonuclease
(c) DNA ligase (d) Gyrases

68. Which is a correct matching?

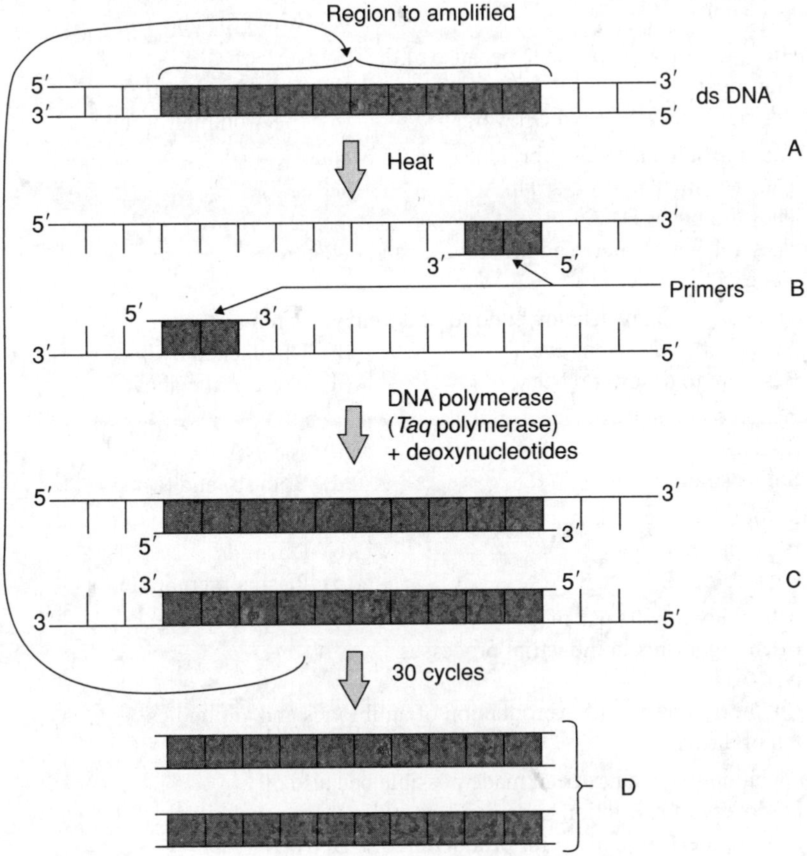

(a) Denaturation	Occurs at room temperature
(b) Annealing	DNA polymerase is required for this process
(c) Extension	Taq polymerse and deoxynucleotides are required
(d) Amplification	1 billion times in 10 cycles

69. Electrophoresis and Southern blotting techniques are used in
(a) DNA fingerprinting (b) Gene synthesis
(c) Gene cloning (d) All of the above

70. PCR technique was discovered by
(a) Hamilton Smith (b) Mullis
(c) E. Southern (d) Milstein

71. Genetic engineering means
(a) Gene manipulation (b) Tissue culture
(c) Utilization of microbes in industries (d) Somatic hybridization

72. Biotechnology helps in synthesizing
(a) New generation antibiotics (b) New vaccines
(c) MAB (d) All of the above

73. Genetic engineering is possible because of the discovery of
(a) Transduction (b) Transformation
(c) Restriction enzyme and DNA ligase (d) Electron microscopy

74. Plasmids are suitable vector for gene cloning because
(a) They are smaller circular DNA
(b) They are linear DNA
(c) They can shuttle between prokaryotes and eukaryotes
(d) None of the above

75. Bacteria possessing restriction endonuclease enzymes remain
(a) Affected by bacteriophages (b) Unattacked by bacteriophages
(c) Resistant to drugs and heat (d) None of the above

76. Restriction endonuclease cuts
(a) ds-DNA (b) ss-DNA
(c) Single strand of ds-DNA (d) Both (b) and (c)

77. Genes for antibiotic resistance are located on
(a) Bacterial genome (b) Plasmids
(c) Mesosomes (d) Plasma membrane

78. Biotechnology reveals use of
(a) Microorganisms in industrial processes
(b) r-DNA
(c) Engineered bacteria for production of antibiotics and antibodies
(d) All of the above

79. Manipulation in gene has been made possible because of
(a) Discovery of restriction endonuclease
(b) Development of method for production of r-DNA
(c) Discovery of producing desired genes
(d) All of the above

80. Tumour producing plasmid transforms
(a) Animals (b) Plants
(c) Bacteria (d) Fungi

81. The specific DNA sequence in which EcoRI cuts is
(a) GATTCG (b) GAATTC
(c) GTTCAA (d) TTCCAA

82. PCR is related to
(a) DNA cloning (b) DNA amplification
(c) DNA selective replication (d) All of the above

83. ________ is use of biology in industrial process and improvement of quality of life.
(a) Genetic engineering (b) Biotechnology
(c) Eugenics (d) Microbiology

84. T_i plasmid used in plant genetic engineering is a plasmid of
(a) Azotobacter (b) Rhizobium
(c) Agrobacterium (d) Saccharomyces

85. The below figure represents

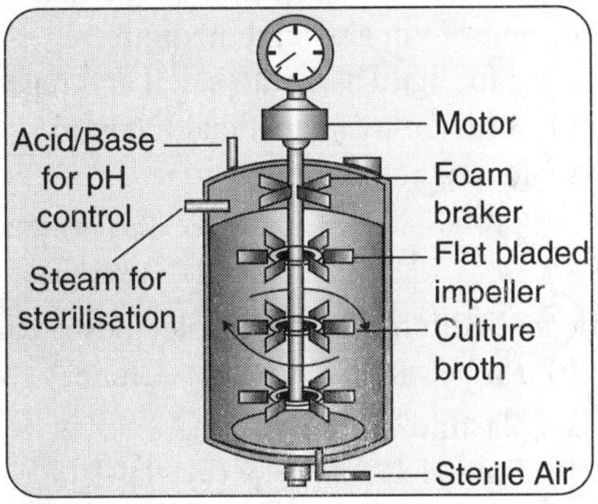

(a) Sparged stirred-tank bioreactor
(b) Simple stirred-tank bioreactor
(c) Thermo regulator
(d) Power generator

86. Plasmids are a suitable vector for gene cloning because
(a) they are small circular DNA capable of integrating with host genome.
(b) they have site for origin of replication.
(c) they can be used as a shuttle between prokaryotes and eukaryotes.
(d) they often carry antibiotic resistance genes.

87. PCR technique is best for
(a) DNA synthesis
(b) DNA amplification
(c) Protein synthesis
(d) Amino acid synthesis

88. Gel electrophoresis is used for
(a) construction of r-DNA
(b) isolation of DNA
(c) cutting of DNA
(d) separation of DNA fragments according to their size or length

89. Bacteria protect themselves from viral attack by producing
(a) exonuclease
(b) endonuclease
(c) DNA ligase
(d) gyrase

90. Restriction endonuclease
(a) cuts DNA molecule at random
(b) cuts DNA from specific palindromic site
(c) restrict DNA synthesis
(d) synthesize DNA

91. Molecular scissor is
(a) restriction endonuclease
(b) helicase
(c) urease
(d) peptidase

92. Which one of the following is commonly used in the transfer of foreign DNA to crop plants?
(a) Penicillium expansum
(b) Trichoderma harzianum
(c) Meloidogyne incognita
(d) Agrobacterium tumefaciens

93. Electroporation involves
(a) Promotion of seed germination by induced inhibition of water with electric current
(b) Making transient pores in cell membrane to facilitate entry of gene constructs
(c) Purification of saline water with the help of an artificial membrane
(d) Passage of sucrose through sieve pores by electro-osmosis

94. Transgenic plants are the ones
(a) grown in artificial medium after hybridization in the field
(b) produced by a somatic embryo in artificial medium
(c) generated by introducing foreign DNA into a cell and regenerating a plant from the cell
(d) produced after protoplast fusion in an artificial medium

95. The enzyme used in PCR technology is
(a) DNA polymerase (b) Taq polymerase
(c) Reverse transcriptase (d) Both (a) and (b)

96. DNA or RNA segment tagged with radioactive molecules is called
(a) Vector (b) Probe (c) Clone (d) Plasmid

97. Which of the following is a plasmid?
(a) pBR322 (b) Bam H-I (c) Sal-I (d) Eco R-II

98. In the PCR technology, the DNA segment is replicated over a billion times. This repeated replication is catalyzed by the enzyme
(a) DNA polymerase (b) Taq polymerase
(c) DNA dependent RNA polymerase (d) Primase

99. An antibiotic resistance gene in a vector usually helps in the selection of
(a) Competent cells (b) Transformed cells
(c) Recombinant cells (d) None of the above

100. Significance of 'heat shock' method in bacterial transformation is to facilitate
(a) binding of DNA to the cell wall
(b) uptake of DNA through membrane transport proteins
(c) uptake of DNA through transient pores in the bacterial cell wall
(d) expression of antibiotic resistance gene

101. The role of DNA ligase in the construction of a recombinant DNA molecule is
(a) Formation of phosphodiester bond between two DNA fragments
(b) Formation of hydrogen bonds between sticky ends of DNA fragments
(c) Ligation of all purine and pyrimidine bases
(d) None of the above

102. Which of the following bacteria is not a source of restriction endonuclease?
(a) Haemophilus influenzae (b) Escherichia coli
(c) Agrobacterium tumefaciens (d) Bacillius amyloli

103. Which of the following steps are catalysed by Taq polymerase in a PCR reaction?
(a) Denaturation of template DNA
(b) Annealing of primers to template DNA
(c) Extension of primer end on the template DNA
(d) All of the above

104. A bacterial cell was transformed with a recombinant DNA that was generated using a human gene. However, the transformed cells did not produce the desired protein. Reasons could be
(a) human gene may have intron which bacteria cannot process.
(b) amino acid codons for humans and bacteria are different.
(c) human protein is formed but degraded by bacteria.
(d) all of the above

105. Which of the following should be chosen for best yield if one were to produce a recombinant protein in large amounts?
(a) Laboratory flask of largest capacity
(b) A stirred-tank bioreactor without in-lets and outlets
(c) A continuous culture system
(d) Any of the above

106. Who among the following was awarded the Nobel Prize for the development of PCR technique?
(a) Herbert Boyer (b) Hargovind Khurana
(c) Kary Mullis (d) Arthur Kornberg

107. Which of the following statements does not hold true for restriction enzyme?
(a) It recognises a palindromic nucleotide sequence.
(b) It is an endonuclease.
(c) It is isolated from viruses.
(d) It produces the same kind of sticky ends in different DNA molecules.

108. The diagram represents which process?

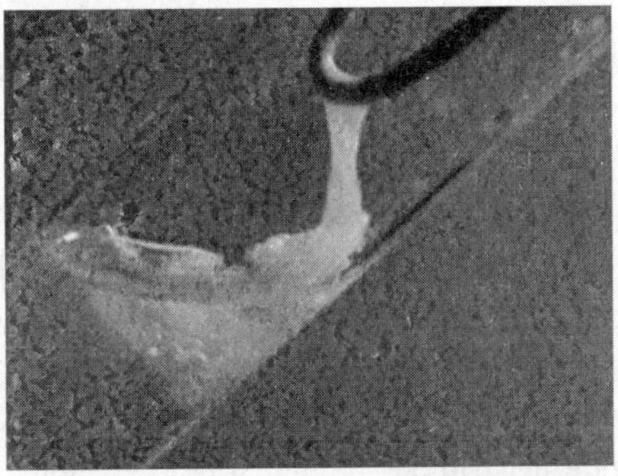

(a) PCR (b) DNA finger printing
(c) CTAB (d) DNA spooling

Read the **assertion** *and* **reason** *carefully to mark the correct option out of the options given below:*

(a) If both the assertion and the reason are true and the reason is a correct explanation of the assertion
(b) If both the assertion and reason are true but the reason is not a correct explanation of the assertion
(c) If the assertion is true but the reason is false
(d) If both the assertion and reason are false

109. **Assertion:** Biotechnology deals with techniques of using live organism or enzymes from organisms to produce products & processes useful of humans.
Reason: In vitro fertilization is a part of biotechnology.

110. Assertion: r-DNA technology is superior over hybridisation.

Reason: r-DNA technology allow us to isolate & introduce only one or a set of desirable gene without introducing undesirable genes into the target organism.

111. Assertion: Restriction endonuclease restrict the growth of bacteriophage in bacteria.

Reason: Restriction endonuclease add methyl groups to bacterial DNA.

112. Assertion: In EcoR I, the latter R is derived from the genus of bacteria.

Reason: EcoR I is the name of palindromic nucleotide sequences.

113. Assertion: In r-DNA technology restriction enzymes,those produce sticky ends are Commonly used.

Reason: Sticky ends facilitates the action of enzyme DNA ligase.

114. Assertion: Cloning vector should have selectable marker.

Reason: Selectable marker, helps in identifying and eleminating non-transformants & selectively permitting the growth of transformants.

115. Assertion: Retroviruses in animals have ability to transform normal cells into cancerous cells.

Reason: Retroviruses have ability to convert protoncogenes into oncogenes.

116. Assertion: Micro-injection technique is use to inject r-DNA directly into the nucleus of an animal cell.

Reason: Gene-gun is use to transfer r-DNA into plant cells.

117. Assertion: In case of PCR the new DNA synthesizeon template DNA, one in continuous manner & other in discontinuous manner.

Reason: PCR is an in vivo process.

118. Assertion: In bioreactors the transforming cells are maintained in their physiologically most active log / exponential phase.

Reason: This type culturing methods produces a larger biomass using to higher yields of desired protein.

AIPMT PREVIOUS YEAR QUESTIONS

1. Which one of the following is now being commercially produced by biotechnological procedures?

[AIPMT MAINS 2010]

(a) Nicotine (b) Morphine
(c) Quinine (d) Insulin

2. Which of the following are used in gene cloning?

[AIPMT MAINS 2010]

(a) Nucleosides (b) Lomasomes
(c) Mesosomes (d) Plasmids

3. In genetic engineering, a DNA segment (gene) of interest, is transferred to the host cell through a vector. Consider the following four agents (i – iv) in this regard and select the correct option about which one or more of these can be used as a vector/ vectors

(A) A Bacterium (B) Plasmid
(C) Plasmodium (D) Bacteriophage

[AIPMT MAINS 2010]

(a) (A), (B) & (D) only (b) (A) only
(c) (A) & (C) only (d) (B) & (D) only

4. Which one of the following palindromic base sequences in DNA can be easily cut at about the middle by some particular restriction enzyme?

[AIPMT PRE 2010]

(a) 5'–CGTTCG –3'
3'–ATGGTA–5'
(b) 5'-GATATG-3'
3'–CTACTA–5'
(c) 5'–GAATTC-3'
3'–CTTAAG–5'
(d) 5'–CACGTA–3'
3'–CTCAGT– 5'

5. Restriction endonucleases are enzymes which:

[AIPMT PRE 2010]

(a) Make cuts at specific positions within the DNA molecule
(b) Recognize a specific nucleotide sequence for binding of DNA ligase
(c) Restrict the action of the enzyme DNA polymerase
(d) Remove nucleotides from the ends of the DNA molecule

6. Stirred-tank bioreactors have been designed for

[AIPMT PRE 2010]

(a) Addition of preservatives of the product
(b) Purification of the product
(c) Ensuring anaerobic conditions in the culture vessel
(d*) Availability of oxygen throughout the process

7. Which one of the following techniques made it possible to genetically engineer living organisms?
[AIPMT MAINS 2011]

(a) Recombinant DNA techniques (b) X-ray diffraction
(c) Heavier isotope labelling (d) Hybridization

8. Given below is a sample of portion of DNA strand giving the base sequence on the opposite strands. What is so, special shown in it?
5'_GAATTC_3'
3'_CTTAAG_5'

[AIPMT PRE 2011]

(a) Deletion mutation (b) Start codon at the 5' end
(c) Palindromic sequence of base pairs (d) Replication completed

9. There is a restriction endonuclease called Eco RI. What does 'co' part in it stand for?
[AIPMT PRE 2011]

(a) Coelom (b) Coenzyme
(c) Coli (d) Colon

10. Agarose extracted from sea weeds finds use in

[AIPMT PRE 2011]

(a) Tissue culture (b) PCR
(c) Gel electrophoresis (d) Spectrophotometry

11. Maximum number of existing transgenic animals is of.

[AIPMT PRE 2011]

(a) Mice (b) Cow
(c) Pig (d) Fish

12. In genetic engineering, the antibiotics are used:

[AIPMT MAINS 2012]

(a) To select healthy vectors
(b) As sequences from where replication starts
(c) To keep the cultures free of infection
(d) As selectable markers

13. The figure below shows three steps (A, B, C) of Polymerase Chain Reaction (PCR). Select the option giving correct identification together with what it represents?

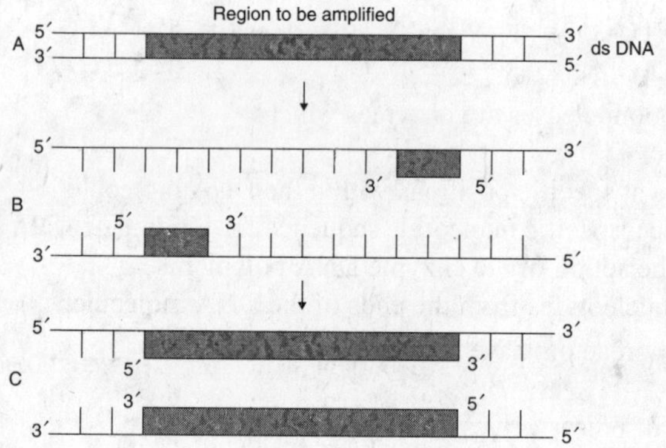

[AIPMT MAINS 2012]

Options:
(a) A: Denaturation at a temperature of about 50ºC
(b) C: Extension in the presence of heat stable DNA polymerase
(c) A: Annealing with two sets of primers
(d) B: Denaturation at a temperature of about 98ºC separating the two DNA strands

14. Which one of the following represents a palindromic sequence in DNA?

[AIPMT MAINS 2012]

(a) 5'-CCAATG-3'
3'-GAATCC-5'
(b) 5'-CATTAG-3'
3'-GATAAC-5'
(c) 5'-GATACC-3'
3'-CCTAAG-5'
(d) 5'-GAATTC-3'
3'-CTTAAG-5'

15. Biolistics (gene-gun) is suitable for:

[AIPMT MAINS 2012]

(a) Transformation of plant cells
(b) Constructing recombinant DNA by joining with vectors
(c) DNA finger printing
(d) Disarming pathogen vectors

16. The figure below is the diagrammatic representation of the E.Coli vector pBR 322. Which one of the given options correctly identifies its certain component(s)?

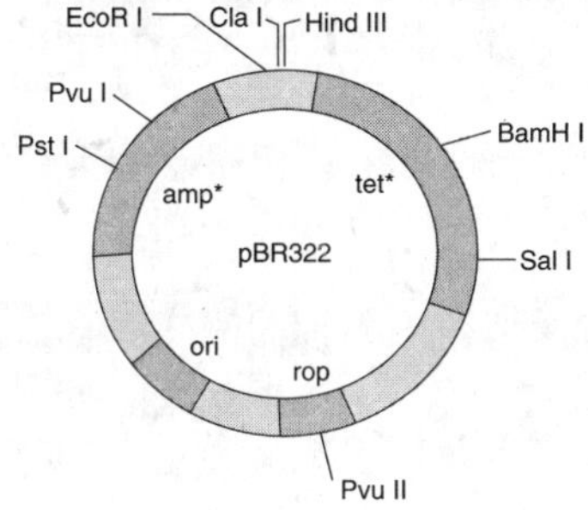

[AIPMT PRE 2012]

(a) Ori-original restriction enzyme
(b) Rop-reduced osmotic pressure
(c) Hind III, EcoRI-selectable markers
(d) amp^R, tet^R-antibiotic resistance genes

17. Which one is a true statement regarding DNA polymerase used in PCR?

[AIPMT PRE 2012]

(a) It is used to ligate introduced DNA in recipient cells
(b) It serves as a selectable marker
(c) It is isolated from a virus
(d) It remains active at high temperature

18. For transformation, micro-particles coated with DNA to be bombarded with gene gun are made up of:

[AIPMT PRE 2012]

(a) Silver or Platinum (b) Platinum or Zinc
(c) Silicon or Platinum (d) Gold or Tungsten

19. DNA fragments generated by the restriction endonucleases in a chemical reaction can be separated by:

[AIPMT 2013]

(a) Centrifugation (b) Polymerase chain reaction
(c) Electrophoresis (d) Restriction mapping

20. Which of the following is not correctly matched for the organism and its cell wall degrading enzyme?

[AIPMT 2013]

(a) Bacteria – Lysozyme (b) Plant cells – Cellulase
(c) Algae – Methylase (d) Fungi – Chitinase

21. Which vector can clone only a small fragment of DNA?

[AIPMT 2014]

(a) Bacteria artificial chromosome (b) Yeast artificial chromosome
(c) Plasmid (d) Cosmid

22. The cutting of DNA at specific locations because possible with the discovery of:

[RE-AIPMT 2015]

(a) Probes (b) Selectable markers
(c) Ligases (d) Restriction enzymes

23. The DNA molecule to which the gene of interest is integrated for cloning is called: [RE-AIPMT 2015]

(a) Vector (b) Template
(c) Carrier (d) Transformer

Answer Keys

1. (d)	2. (a)	3. (d)	4. (d)	5. (d)	6. (d)	7. (b)	8. (d)	9. (d)	10. (b)
11. (b)	12. (b)	13. (d)	14. (d)	15. (c)	16. (b)	17. (a)	18. (c)	19. (a)	20. (b)
21. (b)	22. (b)	23. (c)	24. (b)	25. (d)	26. (a)	27. (c)	28. (c)	29. (b)	30. (c)
31. (d)	32. (d)	33. (b)	34. (b)	35. (b)	36. (a)	37. (a)	38. (d)	39. (c)	40. (c)
41. (c)	42. (d)	43. (a)	44. (b)	45. (b)	46. (b)	47. (d)	48. (d)	49. (a)	50. (d)
51. (b)	52. (c)	53. (a)	54. (a)	55. (b)	56. (b)	57. (c)	58. (d)	59. (c)	60. (a)
61. (c)	62. (b)	63. (b)	64. (c)	65. (b)	66. (d)	67. (c)	68. (c)	69. (a)	70. (b)
71. (a)	72. (d)	73. (c)	74. (a)	75. (b)	76. (a)	77. (b)	78. (d)	79. (d)	80. (b)
81. (b)	82. (b)	83. (b)	84. (c)	85. (b)	86. (b)	87. (b)	88. (d)	89. (b)	90. (b)
91. (a)	92. (d)	93. (b)	94. (c)	95. (d)	96. (b)	97. (a)	98. (b)	99. (b)	100. (c)
101. (a)	102. (c)	103. (c)	104. (a)	105. (c)	106. (c)	107. (c)	108. (d)	109. (b)	110. (a)
111. (c)	112. (d)	113. (a)	114. (a)	115. (a)	116. (b)	117. (d)	118. (a)		

AIPMT Previous Year Questions

1. (d)	2. (d)	3. (d)	4. (c)	5. (a)	6. (d)	7. (a)	8. (c)	9. (c)	10. (c)
11. (a)	12. (d)	13. (b)	14. (d)	15. (a)	16. (d)	17. (d)	18. (d)	19. (c)	20. (c)
21. (c)	22. (d)	23. (a)							

CHAPTER 34

Biotechnology and Its Application

1. Transgenic plants (genetically modified or GM plants) are produced by inserting desired genes in the plasmid of
   (a) E. Coli
   (b) Pseudomonas
   (c) Bacillus subtilis
   (d) Agrobacterium
2. The applications of Biotechnology include
   (A) Therapeutics
   (B) Diagnostics
   (C) GM crops for agriculture
   (D) Processed food
   (E) Bioremediation
   (F) Waste treatment
   (G) Energy production
   (a) A, B, C, E only
   (b) C only
   (c) B, C, D, E only
   (d) All
3. Golden rice is a
   (a) Hybrid
   (b) GM plant
   (c) Transgenic plant
   (d) Both (b) and (c)
4. Which of the GMO used by biotechnology?
   (a) Microbes and fungi
   (b) Plants
   (c) Animals
   (d) All of these
5. Humulin is a
   (a) Natural insulin
   (b) Human insulin synthesized by genetically engineered E. coli
   (c) Human insulin synthesized by pancreas
   (d) Chemically synthesized insulin
6. Critical research areas of biotechnology are
   (a) Providing the best catalyst in the form of improved organism usually a microbe or pure enzyme
   (b) Creating optimal condition through engineering for a catalyst to act
   (c) Downstream processing technologies to purify the protein organic compound
   (d) All of the above
7. Salt stress, disease resistance and cold stress in plants can be introduced by
   (a) Genetic engineering
   (b) Tissue culture
   (c) Hybridoma technology
   (d) None of the above

8. Food production can be increased by
(a) Agro chemical based agriculture (b) Organic agriculture
(c) Genetically engineered based agriculture (d) All of the above

9. DNA fingerprinting was developed by
(a) Prof. Alec Jeffrey (b) Arber and Smith
(c) Barbara McClintock (d) Jacob and Monod

10. Food supply increased how many times after the Green Revolution?
(a) 2 (b) 3
(c) 4 (d) 5

11. Genetic engineering is useful for
(a) Agriculture (b) Medical research
(c) Treatment and diagnosis of diseases (d) All of the above

12. Increased yield in Green Revolution is mainly due to
(a) Use of agrochemicals (fertilizers and pesticides)
(b) Use of improved crop varieties
(c) Use of GM crops
(d) All of the above

13. DNA fingerprinting needs
(a) Suitable restriction enzyme
(b) DNA probe
(c) Facilities for gel electrophoresis and southern blotting
(d) All of the above

14. Following are the advantages of GM crops except
(a) They reduce nucliance on chemical pesticides
(b) Increase efficiency of mineral usage
(c) Enhanced nutritional value of food
(d) Post harvest losses are more

15. Bt stands for
(a) Bacterial toxin (b) Botulinum toxin
(c) Bacillus thuringiensis (d) Bacillus toxin

16. The following crops are now genetically modified by Bt-toxin gene
(A) Cotton (B) Corn
(C) Rice (D) Tomato
(E) Potato (F) Soyabean
(a) A, B and C only (b) D and E only
(c) A and F only (d) All

17. During electrophoresis, DNA fragments move towards the
(a) Anode (b) Cathode
(c) Both the poles (d) None of these

18. Some strains of Bacullus thuringiensis produce proteins that kill certain insects like
(a) Lepidopterans (b) Coleopterans
(c) Dipterans (d) All of these

19. Humulin was first marketed by
(a) Eli Lily (b) Sun pharma
(c) Nova Industry (d) May and Baker

20. Select correct matching.

(a) Lepidopterans	Tobacco bud worm, armyworm
(b) Coleopterans	Beetles and bud worm
(c) Dipterans	Flies, Mosquitoes, Spiders
(d) Aves	Lady bird, Humming bird

21. Antisense transcription is like carrying genes as much as
(a) On sense strand of DNA (b) Antisense strand of DNA
(c) On genetic RNA (d) On t-RNA

22. Bt-toxin is insecticidal because
(a) activated toxin binds to the surface of midgut epithelial cells and creates pores that causes swelling and lysis and eventually cause death of the insect.
(b) it decreases the growth of the nervous system of the insect.
(c) it makes insect unable to fly
(d) it kills insect by affecting its blood flow

23. DNA probe is used in
(a) Gel electrophoresis (b) Western blot
(c) DNA profiling technique (d) Interferon synthesis

24. Bt-crops are not affected by Bt-toxin because
(a) Toxin exist as inactive protoxin
(b) It has special antibodies against toxin
(c) Its intracellular medium is alkaline so toxin remain inactive
(d) All of the above

25. During DNA fingerprinting, DNA probes helps in
(a) Gel electrophoresis (b) Southern blotting
(c) Autoradiography (d) None of the above

26. Select the correct statement.
(a) Most Bt-toxins are insect group non-specific
(b) Bt-toxin gene is coded with the name 'CRY'
(c) Genes cry I Ac and cry II Ab form protein that control cotton bollworms
(d) CRY I Ab gene forms protein that control corn borer

27. Transfer of r-DNA through phage is done by
(a) Diffusion (b) Transformation
(c) Transduction (d) Conjugation

28. The following are all genes except
(a) cry I Ac (b) cry I Ab
(c) ROP (d) Sal I

29. Hepatitis-B vaccine is a
(a) First generation vaccine (b) Third generation vaccine
(c) Product of biotechnology (d) Both (b) and (c)

30. Protein encoded gene cry I Ab controls
(a) Cotton bollworm (b) Beetles
(c) Corn borer (d) Flies

31. Golden rice is enriched in
(a) Beta carotene (b) Lysine
(c) Vitamin C (d) Iron

32. Bt-toxin is obtained from
(a) Bacilli (b) Cocci
(c) Vibrio (d) Spirillum

33. Engineered bacteria have successfully been used for commercial production of
(a) Human insulin (b) Melstonine
(c) Thyrosine (d) Testosteron

34. A nematode _________ infects the roots of tobacco plants and causes great reduction in yield.
(a) ancylostoma (b) hookworm
(c) meloidegyne incognitia (d) wuchereria

35. The first transgenic crop plant was
(a) Cotton (b) Cereals
(c) Tobacco (d) Pea

36. RNAi process takes place in
(a) Prokaryotes (b) Unicellular eukaryotes only
(c) Multicellular eukaryote only (d) All eukaryotes

37. Which of the following cuts the DNA at a specific place?
(a) Restriction endonuclease (b) DNA ligase
(c) Exonuclease (d) Alkaline phosphatase

38. Which is true about RNA i process?
(a) Method of cellular defense
(b) It involves silencing of a specific m-RNA due to a complementary dsRNA molecule.
(c) Source of complementary RNA in this process may be infection by viruses having RNA genomes.
(d) All are correct.

39. The most commonly used bacterium in plant genetic engineering is
(a) E. coli (b) Rhizobium
(c) Klebsiella (d) Agrobacterium

40. Identify A and B in the diagram.

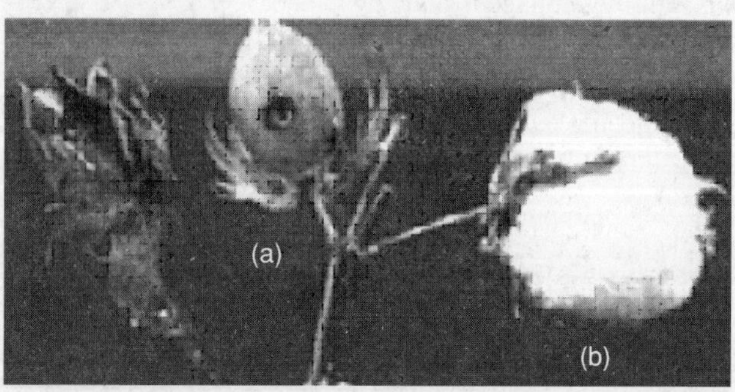

(a) A: A fully mature cotton boll, B: Destroyed by bollworms
(b) A: Destroyed by bollworms, B: Fully mature cotton boll
(c) A: Destroyed by virus, B: Immature cotton boll
(d) A: Immature normal cotton boll, B: Destroyed by virus

41. In which of the processes is both the DNA strands transcribed?
(a) PCR
(b) DNA replication
(c) RNAi
(d) Southern blotting

42. The source of Taq polymerase used in PCR technique is a
(a) Thermophilic fungus
(b) Mesophilic fungus
(c) Thermophilic bacteria
(d) Halophilic bacteria

43. Which of the following vector is used to transfer Nematode specific gene in host plant?
(a) Virus
(b) Rhizobium
(c) Agrobacterium
(d) Cosmid

44. What is true about Bt-toxin?
(a) The concerned Bacillus has antitoxins.
(b) The inactive protoxin gets converted into active form in the insect gut.
(c) Bt-protein exists as active toxin in the Bacillus.
(d) The activated toxin enters the ovary of pest to sterilize it and thus prevent its multiplication.

45. RNAi stands for
(a) RNA infection
(b) RNA induction
(c) RNA interference
(d) RNA inhibition

46. The abbreviation 'B' in Bt-toxin stands for
(a) Biotechnology
(b) Biotoxin
(c) Bacillus
(d) Toxin released by bacterium

47. Which of the following is the source of complementary strand in mRNA silencing?
(a) An infection by viruses having RNA genome
(b) Mobile genetic elements (Transposons)
(c) Both
(d) Proteins

48. Some of the characteristics of Bt-cotton are
(a) Long fibre and resistance of aphids
(b) Maximum yield, long fibre and resistance to bettle pests
(c) High yield and production of toxin protein crystal which kill dipteran pests only.
(d) High yield and resistance to bollworms

49. How many recombinant therapeutics have been approved for human use the world over?
(a) 10
(b) 20
(c) 30
(d) 90

50. Which of the following is produced by genetically engineered bacterium?
(a) Tyrosine
(b) Insulin
(c) Glycogen
(d) ADH

51. How many recombinant products are presently being marketed in India?
(a) 10
(b) 20
(c) 12
(d) 30

52. Which of the following is not used as a bioweapon?
(a) Bacillus anthracis
(b) Botulinum toxin
(c) Bacillus thuringiensis
(d) Small pox

53. The main challenge for production of insulin using rDNA technique is
(a) Production of A peptide
(b) Production of B peptide
(c) Getting insulin assembled into a mature form
(d) All of the above

54. Transgenic plants are produced by
(a) Inducing gene mutation
(b) Arresting spindle fibre formation
(c) Deleting sex chromosome
(d) Introducing foreign genes

55. Peptide A and peptide B is linked by how many disulphide linkages between their proinsulin?
(a) 1
(b) 2
(c) 3
(d) 4

56. Some of the steps involved in the production of humulin are given below. Choose the correct sequence.
(1) Purification of humulin
(2) Extraction of recombinant gene product from E. coli
(3) Culturing recombinant E. coli in bioreactors
(4) Introduction of recombinant plasmid into E. coli
(5) Synthesis of gene for human insulin artificially
(6) Insertion of human insulin gene into plasmid
(a) 2, 1, 4, 3, 5, 6
(b) 1, 3, 5, 6, 2, 4
(c) 5, 6, 4, 3, 2, 1
(d) 3, 5, 2, 1, 6, 4

57. Which American company in 1983 prepared humulin?
(a) Eli Lilly
(b) Ranbaxy
(c) Sun-pharma
(d) Glaxosmith

58. During the process of prohormone 'proinsulin' into mature insulin synthesis
(a) C-peptide is added to proinsulin
(b) C-peptide is removed from proinsulin
(c) β-peptide is added to proinsulin
(d) β-peptide is removed from proinsulin

59. Select the true statements from the following.
(1) Insulin from animal source, may develop allergy in some patients
(2) C-peptide is not present in mature insulin
(3) Recombinant therapeutics do not induce unwanted immunological response.
(4) Insulin can be administered orally to diabetic patients
(a) 1 and 3 only
(b) 1 and 2 only
(c) 3 and 4 only
(d) 1, 2, 3 only

60. Cancer is generally caused due to activation/conversion of _________ to _________ and/or inactivation of _________.
(a) oncogene, tumour suppressor gene, protooncogene
(b) tumour suppressor gene, oncogene, protooncogene
(c) proto-oncogene, oncogene, tumour-suppressor gene
(d) oncogene, protooncogene, tumour suppressor gene

61. Which of the following peptide chain is removed during maturation of pro-insulin into insulin?
(a) A-peptide
(b) B-peptide
(c) C-peptide
(d) B and C peptide

62. The Bt-toxin is not toxic to human beings because

(a) The pro Bt-toxin inactivation requires temperature above human body temperature.

(b) The Bt-toxin recognizes only insect specific target.

(c) The Bt-toxin formation from pro Bt-toxin requires pH lower than that present in the human stomach.

(d) Conversion of pro Bt-toxin to Bt-toxin takes place only in highly alkaline conditions.

63. Which part of diagram shows that insulin in our body is synthesized in immature form?

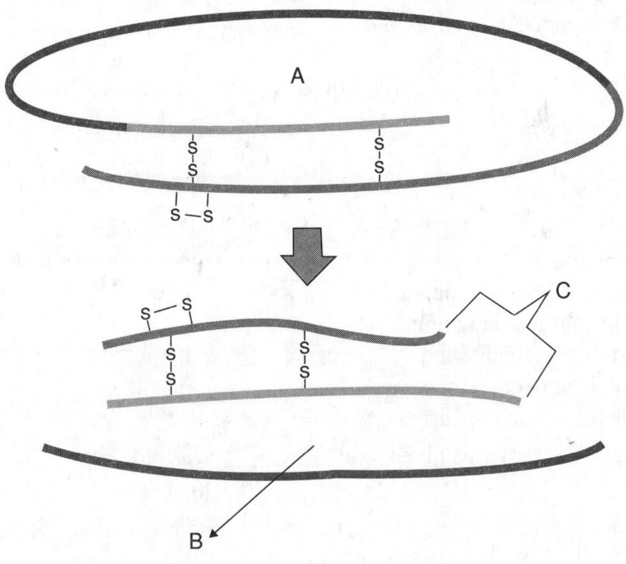

(a) A and C (b) B and C

(c) A and B (d) None of these

64. Why is insulin not administrated orally to diabetic patients?

(a) Insulin is bitter in taste.

(b) Insulin is a peptide.

(c) Insulin will lead to sudden decrease in blood sugar if given orally.

(d) Insulin leads to peptic ulcer if given orally.

65. The method of DNA fingerprinting involves the use of

(a) Restriction enzyme (b) Taq polymerase

(c) Oligonucleotide primers (d) All of the above

66. Pro-insulin contain

(a) A-peptide (b) B-peptide

(c) C-peptide (d) All of these

67. What is the source of T_i plasmid which is modified and used as a cloning vector to deliver the desired genes into plant cells?

(a) Agrobacterium tumefaciens

(b) Thermophilus aquaticus

(c) Pyrococcus furiosus

(d) Aedes aegypti

68. The first clinical gene therapy was given in
(a) 1992 (b) 1990
(c) 1995 (d) 1997

69. The thermostable enzyme 'Taq' and 'Pfu' isolated from thermophilic bacteria are
(a) RNA polymerase (b) DNA polymerase
(c) Restriction endonuclease (d) DNA ligase

70. Select the incorrect matching.
(a) ADA → Adenosine aminase
(b) ELISA → Enzyme linked inmunosorbent assay
(c) PCR → Polymers Chain Reaction
(d) PKU → Phenyl Ketonuria

71. The term 'molecular scissor' generally refers to
(a) DNA polymerase (b) RNA polymerase
(c) Restriction endonuclease (d) DNA ligase

72. ADA deficiency is due to
(a) Insertion of gene (b) Deletion of gene
(c) Duplication of gene (d) Translocation of gene

73. Permanent cure for ADA deficiency is
(a) Genetically engineered lymphocyte
(b) Bone marrow transplantation
(c) Enzyme replacement therapy
(d) ADA gene introduced in early embryonic stages

74. First clinical gene therapy was given to a ________ year old girl.
(a) 2 year (b) 6 year
(c) 4 year (d) 8 year

75. Conventional method of diagnosis involves
(a) Urine analysis (b) ELISA
(c) PCR (d) r-DNA technology

76. PCR used in detection of
(a) HIV (AIDS) (b) Cancer
(c) Genetic disorder (d) All of these

77. When a patient with defective ADA is treated, which of the following steps are performed for gene therapy?
(A) Lymphocytes are obtained from the patients.
(B) Lymphocytes are transferred to culture dishes.
(C) Lymphocytes are transected with normal ADA genes
(D) The transected cells are returned to the patients
(a) All of the above (b) Only C and D
(c) Only D (d) SCID cannot be treated

78. Which of the following is a benefit to having insulin produced by biotechnology?
(a) It is just as effective and is less expensive. (b) It can be produced in large quantity.
(c) It is non allergic. (d) All of the above

79. Which one of the following genes is defective in patients suffering from serve combined immunodeficiency syndrome (SCID)?
(a) RNAase (b) ADA
(c) Carbonic anhydrase (d) DNAase

80. A functional ADA cDNA can be introduced into cells of the patients receiving gene therapy by using vector constituted by

(a) E coli (b) Reovirus
(c) Retrovirus (d) Agrobacterium

81. Which of the following is used as probe?

(a) Single standard DNA
(b) dsDNA tagged with a radioactive molecule
(c) Single standard RNA tagged with a radioactive molecule
(d) dsRNA

82. Which gene does not appear in photographic film in autoradiography?

(a) Housekeeping gene (b) Structural gene
(c) Mutated gene (d) Transcriptionally active gene

83. Which of the following is based on antigen-antibody reaction?

(a) PCR (b) ELISA
(c) Serum analysis (d) Southern blotting

84. Which of the following can be detected in ELISA?

(a) Protein antigen (b) Glycoprotein antigen
(c) Antibodies synthesized against pathogen (d) Any of the above

85. Over 95% of all existing transgenic animals are

(a) Pig (b) Mice
(c) Sheep (d) Cow

86. Transgenic organisms are used

(a) to study disease (b) to produce biological product
(c) to test vaccine safety (d) All of the above

87. Match the columns

Column-I	Column-II
A. Emphysema	1. Test to detect antigen or antibody
B. Rosie	2. α-1 antitrypsin
C. ELISA	3. Protein-enriched milk
D. ROP	4. Codes for proteins involved in plasmid replication

(a) A-2, B-3, C-1, D-4 (b) A-1, B-3, C-4, D-2
(c) A-1, B-2, C-3, D-4 (d) A-4, B-3, C-2, D-1

88. Transgenic animals are prepared for the following disease analysis except

(a) Cancer (b) Cystic fibrosis and Alzheimer
(c) Rheumatoid arthritis (d) AIDS

89. 'Rosie' a transgenic cow known to produce a type of milk which has all the following characteristics except

(a) Protein content of 2.4 gm/litre
(b) Has human α-lactalbumin
(c) More balance diet than normal milk for babies
(d) Rich in cholesterol

90. Rosie was produced in the year
(a) 2000 (b) 1999
(c) 1997 (d) 2007

91. GMO/transgenic animal are used in testing safety of polio vaccine before they are used on human?
(a) Transgenic sheep (b) Transgenic cow
(c) Transgenic viruses (d) Transgenic mice

92. How many varieties of rice have been estimated to be present in India?
(a) 200 (b) 20,000
(c) 200,000 (d) 2,000,000

93. The use of bioresources by multinational companies and other organizations, without proper authorization from the countries and people concerned without compensatory payment, is called
(a) Bioethics (b) Biopiracy
(c) Bioterror (d) Bioweapon

94. Which variety or rice was patented by a US company even though the highest number of varieties of this rice is found in India?
(a) Sharbati Sonara (b) Co-667
(c) Basmati (d) Lerma Roja

95. The Government of India took which step to cater to the requirement of patent terms and other emergency provisions with regard to bioparacy?
(a) Biopiracy act (b) India Patents Bill
(c) RTI Act (d) Negotiable Instruments Act

96. Which Indian plants have either been patented or attempts have been made to patent them by western nations for their commercial use?
(a) Basmati rice (b) Turmeric
(c) Neem (d) All of these have been targeted.

97. Golden rice is
(a) A variety of rice grown along the yellow river in China
(b) Long stored rice having yellow colour tint
(c) A transgenic rice having gene for β-carotene
(d) Wild variety of rice with yellow coloured grains

98. In RNAi, genes are silenced using
(a) ssDNA (b) dsDNA
(c) dsRNA (d) ssRNA

99. The first clinical gene therapy was done for the treatment of
(a) AIDS
(b) Cancer
(c) Cystic fibrosis
(d) SCID (Servere Combined Immuno Deficiency resulting from deficiency of ADA)

100. ADA is an enzyme which is deficient in the genetic disorder SCID. What is the full form of ADA?
(a) Adenosine deoxyaminase (b) Adenosine deaminase
(c) Aspartate deaminase (d) Arginine dearginase

101. Silencing of a gene could be achieved through the use of
(a) Short interfering RNA (RNAi) (b) Antisense RNA
(c) By both (d) None of the above

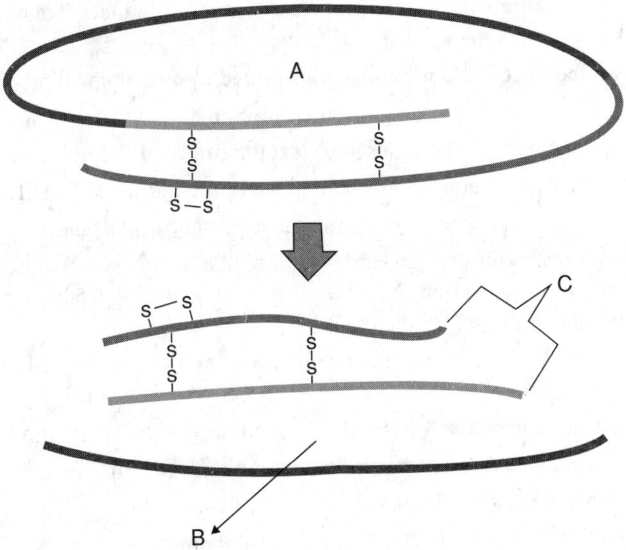

102. Identify A, B and C in the diagram.
   (a) A Proinsulin, B Free C peptide, C Insulin
   (b) A Free C peptide, B Proinsulin, C Insulin
   (c) A Insulin, B Proinsulin, C Free C peptide
   (d) A Free C peptide, B Insulin, D Proinsulin

103. Crystals of Bt-toxin produced by some bacteria do not kill the bacteria themselves because
   (a) Bacteria are resistant to the toxin.
   (b) Toxin is immature.
   (c) Toxin is inactive.
   (d) Bacteria encloses toxin in a special sac.

Read the ***assertion*** *and* ***reason*** *carefully to mark the correct option out of the options given below:*

(a) If both the assertion and the reason are true and the reason is a correct explanation of the assertion

(b) If both the assertion and reason are true but the reason is not a correct explanation of the assertion

(c) If the assertion is true but the reason is false

(d) If both the assertion and reason are false

104. **Assertion:** ELISA use to detect infection by pathogen,can be detected by the presence of antigens or by detecting the antibodies synthesized against the pathogen.
   Reason: ELISA is based on the principle of anitgen- antibody interaction.

105. **Assertion:** GEAC is genetic engineering approval committee.
   Reason: GEAC will make decisions regarding the validity of GM research.

106. **Assertion:** r-DNA therapeutic are better than similar products isolated from non-human sources.

Reason: r-DNA therapeutic do not induce unwanted immunological responses.

107. **Assertion:** ∞ - 1 – antitrypsin used to treat emphysema.

Reason: Transgenic mice are being used to test the safety of the polio vaccine.

108. **Assertion:** PCR & ELISA are techniques that serve the purpose of easily diagnosis.

Reason: For effective of a disease, early diagnosis is very important.

109. **Assertion:** Biopiracy is the team used to refer to the use of bio-resources by multinational companies and other organisations without proper authorisation from the countries and people concerned without compensatory payment.

Reason: Bioprospecting is the process of discovery and commercialisation of new products based on biological resources.

110. **Assertion:** ADA deficiency can be cured by bone marrow transplantation.

Reason: ADA deficiency can be treated by enzyme replacement therapy.

111. **Assertion:** Bt toxin do not kill Bacillus.

Reason: Bt toxin protein exist in Bacillus as inactive prototoxins.

112. **Assertion:** RNA i takes place in all eukaryotic organism as a method of cellular defence.

Reason: RNAi method involve silencing of a specific mean due to complementary dsRNA molecule that binds to and prevent translation of the m-RNA (silencing).

113. **Assertion:** Genetic modification will enhance nutritional value of food.

Reason: Vit A enriched rice is GMO.

AIPMT PREVIOUS YEAR QUESTIONS

1. Which one of the following is used as vector for cloning genes into higher organisms?

[AIPMT PRE 2010]

(a) Baculovirus
(b) Salmonella typhemurium
(c) Rhizopus nigricans
(d) Retrovirus

2. DNA or RNA segment tagged with a radioactive molecule is called

[AIPMT PRE 2010]

(a) Vector
(b) Probe
(c) Clone
(d) Plasmid

3. Genetic engineering has been successfully used for producing

[AIPMT PRE 2010]

(a) Transgenic mice for testing safety of polio vaccine before use in humans
(b) Transgenic models for studying new treatments for certain cardiac diseases
(c) Transgenic cow-Rosie which produces high fat milk for making ghee
(d) Animals like bulls for farm work as they have super power

4. Some of the characteristics of Bt cotton are [AIPMT PRE 2010]
   (a) Long fibre and resistance to aphids
   (b) Medium yield, long fibre and resistance to beetle pests
   (c) High yield and production of toxic protein crystals which kill dipteran pests
   (d) High yield and resistance to bollworms
5. Bacillus thuringiensis forms protein crystals which contain insecticidal protein. This protein [AIPMT MAINS 2011]
   (a) Binds with epithelial cells of midgut of the insect pest ultimately killing it.
   (b) Is coded by several genes including the gene cry.
   (c) Is activated by acid pH of the foregut of the insect pest.
   (d) Does not kill the carrier bacterium which is itself resistant to this toxin.
6. Silencing of mRNA has been used in producing transgenic plants resistant to [AIPMT MAINS 2011]
   (a) Bollworms (b) Nematodes
   (c) White rusts (d) Bacterial blights
7. Read the following four statements (A-D) about certain mistakes in two of them.
   (A) The first transgenic buffalo, Rosie produced milk which was human alpha-lactalbumin enriched.
   (B) Restriction enzymes are used in isolation of DNA from other macromolecules.
   (C) Downstream processing is one of the steps of rDNA technology.
   (D) Disarmed pathogen vectors are also used in transfer of rDNA into the host. [AIPMT MAINS 2011]

   Which of the two statements have mistakes?
   (a) B and C (b) C and D (c) A and C (d) A and B
8. The process of RNA interference has been used in the development of plants resistant to: [AIPMT PRE 2011]
   (a) Fungi (b) Viruses (c) Insects (d) Nematodes
9. Tobacco plants resistant to a nematode have been developed by the introduction of DNA that produced (in the host cells): [AIPMT MAINS 2012]
   (a) A particular hormone (b) An antioxidant
   (c) A toxic protein (d) Both sense and anti-sense RNA
10. Which of the following Bt crops is being grown in India by the farmers? [AIPMT 2013]
    (a) Maize (b) Cotton (c) Brinjal (d) Soybean
11. The colonies of recombinant bacteria appear white in contrast to blue colonies of non-recombinant bacteria because of: [AIPMT 2013]
    (a) Non-recombinant bacteria containing beta galactosidase
    (b) Insertional inactivation of alpha galactosidase in non-recombinant bacteria
    (c) Insertional inactivation of alpha galactosidase in recombinant bacteria
    (d) Inactivation of glycosidase enzyme in recombinant bacteria
12. Which of the following Bt crops is being grown in India by the farmers? [AIPMT 2013]
    (a) Maize (b) Cotton (c) Brinjal (d) Soybean

13. The first human hormone produced by recombinant DNA technology is [AIPMT 2014]
   (a) Insulin (b) Estrogen
   (c) Thyroxin (d) Progesterone
14. Which body of the Government of India regulates GM research and safety of introducing GM organism for public services? [AIPMT 2015]
   (a) Bio-safety committee
   (b) Indian Council of Agricultural Research
   (c) Genetic Engineering Approval Committee
   (d) Research Committee on Genetic manipulation
15. In Bt cotton the Bt toxin present in plant tissue as pro-toxin is converted into active toxin due to [AIPMT 2015]
   (a) Alkaline pH of the insect gut (b) Acidic pH of the insect gut
   (c) Action of gut micro-organisms (d) Presence of conversion factors in insect gut
16. The crops engineered for glyphosate are resistant/tolerant to: [AIPMT 2015]
   (a) Fungi (b) Bacteria (c) Insects (d) Herbicides
17. The introduction of t-DNA into plants involves: [RE-AIPMT 2015]
   (a) Altering the pH of soil, then heat-socking the plants
   (b) Exposing the plants to cold for a brief period
   (c) Allowing the plant roots to stand in water
   (d) Infection of the plant by Agrobacterium tumefaciens

Answer Keys

1. (d)	2. (d)	3. (d)	4. (d)	5. (b)	6. (d)	7. (a)	8. (d)	9. (a)	10. (b)
11. (d)	12. (a)	13. (d)	14. (d)	15. (c)	16. (d)	17. (a)	18. (d)	19. (a)	20. (a)
21. (b)	22. (a)	23. (c)	24. (a)	25. (c)	26. (c)	27. (c)	28. (d)	29. (d)	30. (c)
31. (a)	32. (a)	33. (a)	34. (c)	35. (c)	36. (d)	37. (a)	38. (d)	39. (d)	40. (b)
41. (c)	42. (c)	43. (c)	44. (b)	45. (c)	46. (c)	47. (c)	48. (d)	49. (c)	50. (b)
51. (c)	52. (c)	53. (c)	54. (d)	55. (b)	56. (c)	57. (a)	58. (b)	59. (d)	60. (c)
61. (c)	62. (d)	63. (c)	64. (b)	65. (a)	66. (d)	67. (a)	68. (b)	69. (b)	70. (a)
71. (c)	72. (b)	73. (d)	74. (c)	75. (a)	76. (d)	77. (a)	78. (d)	79. (b)	80. (c)
81. (c)	82. (c)	83. (b)	84. (d)	85. (b)	86. (d)	87. (a)	88. (d)	89. (d)	90. (c)
91. (d)	92. (c)	93. (b)	94. (c)	95. (b)	96. (d)	97. (c)	98. (c)	99. (d)	100. (b)
101. (c)	102. (a)	103. (c)	104. (a)	105. (b)	106. (a)	107. (b)	108. (b)	109. (b)	110.(b)
111. (a)	112. (b)	113. (b)							

AIPMT Previous Year Questions

1. (d)	2. (b)	3. (a)	4. (d)	5. (a)	6. (b)	7. (d)	8. (d)	9. (d)	10. (b)
11. (a)	12. (b)	13. (a)	14. (c)	15. (a)	16. (d)	17. (d)			

Unit
X

Ecology

This unit comprises four chapters—Organisms and Populations, Ecosystem, Biodiversity and Conservation and Environmental Issues. Again, diagrams and Pi-charts are very significant. In the chapter on Ecosystem, dates are very important. All graph and pyramids are also significant, and should be carefully appraised. While reading this unit, it is advisable to remember that it's nature's rule, and as we are an integral part of the nature, these rules are applicable to us. This mode of thought makes ecology a very interesting topic.

CHAPTER 35

Organisms and Populations

1. __________ is revered as the Father of Ecology in India.
   (a) Varghese Kurein
   (b) Amartya Sen
   (c) Ramdeo Misra
   (d) Hargobind Khurana
2. Ecology is a subject which studies the interactions among organisms and __________.
   (a) Amongst the organism and its chemical environment
   (b) Between the organism and its physical environment
   (c) Amongst the organism and its habitat
   (d) Between the organism and its biosphere
3. Basically, ecology is concerned with how many levels of biological organisations?
   (a) 3
   (b) 4
   (c) 5
   (d) 7
4. The levels of biological organisation in ecology are
   (a) Cell, Organism, Community, Biosphere
   (b) Organisms, Family, Communities, Biomes
   (c) Species, Populations, Communities, Biomes
   (d) Organisms, Populations, Communities, Biomes
5. Ecology at the level of an individual organism is __________.
   (a) Systemic ecology
   (b) Somatic ecology
   (c) Physiological ecology
   (d) Physical ecology
6. Which important life process is considered at organism level of ecology?
   (a) Respiration
   (b) Immunity
   (c) Reproduction
   (d) Homeostasis
7. How does seasonal variations take place on earth?
   (a) Rotation on its own axis
   (b) Rotation around sun
   (c) Rotation of moon around earth
   (d) Both (a) and (b)
8. The factors responsible for causing annual variation in the intensity and duration of temperature are __________.
   (a) Rotation of earth in solar system
   (b) Rotation of earth around sun
   (c) Tilt in axis of earth
   (d) Both (b) and (c)
9. Precipitation due to annual variation in seasons includes
   (a) Rain
   (b) Snow
   (c) Dew
   (d) Both (a) and (b)

10. Precipitation is an important factor for the formation of major biomes such as
(a) Rain forest
(b) Tundra
(c) Desert
(d) All of the above

11. **A:** Regional and local variations occur with each habitat
B: It causes formation of a wide variety of biomes
(a) A is true and B is also true
(b) A is false but B is true
(c) A is true but B is false
(d) A is false and B is also false

12. Rain-soaked forest occurs in which state of India?
(a) Assam
(b) Meghalaya
(c) Arunachal Pradesh
(d) Nagaland

13. Just as sand: desert; __________ : Polar regions
(a) Lichen
(b) Sand
(c) Perma frost
(d) Silt

14. Which part of human body is a unique habitat for hundreds of species of microbes?
(a) Mouth
(b) Urinary bladder
(c) Intestine
(d) Spleen

15. The key elements which lead to much variation in the physical and chemical conditions of different habitat are enlisted below:
Temperature, Wind, Water, Light, Soil, Humidity, UV rays.
(a) 5
(b) 6
(c) 4
(d) 3

16. A habitat of an organism constitutes __________.
(a) Abiotic components
(b) Biotic components
(c) Symbiotic compounds
(d) Both (a) and (b)

17. The organisms through natural selection have evolved __________ to optimise its survival and reproduction in its habitat.
(a) Camouflage
(b) Adaptations
(c) Specialized Physiology
(d) Higher reproduction rate

18. In tropical deserts, the temperature goes __________.
(a) > 40°C
(b) > 60°C
(c) > 50°C
(d) >70°C

19. Habitats such as thermal springs and deep-sea hydrothermal vents have average temperature exceeding __________.
(a) 100°C
(b) 150°C
(c) 80°C
(d) 1000°C

20. __________ trees cannot grow in temperate countries.
(a) Banana
(b) Mango
(c) Oranges
(d) Peaches

21. Mango cannot grow in countries like __________.
(a) Canada
(b) Germany
(c) Africa
(d) Both (a) and (b)

22. __________ are not found in Kerala forests.
(a) Snakes
(b) Snow leopards
(c) Elephants
(d) Monkeys

23. __________ fish is rarely caught beyond tropical latitudes in ocean.
(a) Salmon (b) Shark
(c) Tuna (d) Pomphret

24. The temperature of habitat affects kinetics of __________ in the body of organisms.
(a) Hormones (b) Enzymes
(c) Inflammatory mediators (d) Neurotransmitters

25. The organisms which can tolerate and thrive in a wide range of temperature are called as __________.
(a) Stenothermal (b) Homiotherm
(c) Eurythermal (d) Poikilotherm

26. The organisms which thrive in a very narrow range of temperatures are known as __________.
(a) Stenothermal (b) Poikilotherm
(c) Homiotherm (d) Eurythermal

27. The level of thermal tolerance of different species determines the extent of __________.
(a) Survival (b) Geographical distribution
(c) Morphology (d) Biodiversity

28. Life originated on earth first in
(a) Air (b) Land
(c) Water (d) All of the above

29. Special modifications with respect of __________ make it possible for an organism to survive in desert.
(a) Water (b) High temperature
(c) Sand (d) Less abundance plants

30. For aquatic organisms __________ of water becomes important.
(a) Quantity (b) Quality
(c) Conductivity (d) Specific gravity

31. The salt concentration is measured as salinity in parts per __________.
(a) Billion (b) Million
(c) Hundred (d) Thousand

32. The salinity of inland waters is __________
(a) 3 (b) 4
(c) 5 (d) 2

33. The salinity of sea water is __________
(a) > 100 (b) 30–35
(c) 60–80 (d) 10–15

34. The salinity of a hyper saline lagoon is
(a) Up to 10^3 (b) $> 10^3$
(c) Up to 10^2 (d) $> 10^2$

35. The organisms which are tolerant of a wide range of salinities are
(a) Salinotrophs (b) Euryhaline
(c) Salinosomes (d) Stenohaline

36. The organisms which are restricted to a narrow range of salinity are known as
(a) Salinosomes (b) Salinotolerants
(c) Euryhaline (d) Stenohaline

37. Fresh water animals cannot live for long in sea water because they would face problems of
(a) Vapour pressure (b) Purity
(c) Osmotic (d) Thermal change

38. **Assertion:** Photosynthesis is an essential life process of plants.
Reason: Small plants growing in forest are adapted to other process than photosynthesis because they are over-shadowed by tall canopied trees.
(a) A is true and R is also true (b) R is true and A is false
(c) A is true but R is false (d) Both A and R are false

39. For many animals, light is an important factors which regulates __________ variations.
(a) Nocturnal (b) Diurnal
(c) Urinal (d) Crepuscular

40. The activities of animals like foraging, reproductive and migratory depend on
(a) Temperature (b) Water
(c) Light (d) Air

41. Marine organisms, which live at a depth of > 500 m, receive solar energy in which form?
(a) Different rays from visible spectrum (b) UV radiations
(c) Cosmic rays (d) Infra Red radiations

42. The factors which affect percolation and water holding capacity of soil are
(a) Soil composition (b) Grain size
(c) Aggregation (d) All of the above

43. Vegetation in any area depends on
(a) pH of soil (b) Mineral composition
(c) Topography (d) All of the above

44. The __________ characteristics often determine the type of benthic animals than can thrive there
(a) Composition (b) Sediment
(c) Grain size (d) Water holding capacity

45. The internal environment of an organism is called
(a) Equilibrium (b) Organostasis
(c) Homeostasis (d) Apoptosis

46. The 'success' of mammals is due to
(a) Presence of mammary glands (b) Efficient osmoegulation
(c) Efficient thermoregulation (d) Efficient magnetoception

47. 'Shivering' during cold is beneficial for mammals. It helps to
(a) Decrease body temperature (b) Increase body temperature
(c) No change in body temperature (d) None of the above

48. Which is the most effective way to get relief from high temperature?
(a) Oil secretion increases (b) Frequent urination
(c) High water intake (d) Profuse sweating

49. Assertion: Due to changes in seasons, temperature also changes.
Reason: To cope up with this, plants can regulate internal body temperature
(a) A is true and B us also true (b) A is false but B is true
(c) A is true and B is false (d) A and B are false

50. Thousands of migratory birds from Siberia come to __________ in India.
(a) Jim Corbett National Park (b) Nal Sarovar
(c) Keolado National Park (d) Maan Sarovar

51. In case of unfavourable conditions, many lower organisms develop __________ which help them to survive.
(a) Spores (b) Buds
(c) Gametes (d) Clones

52. In higher plants __________ helps to tide over periods of stress
(a) Roots (b) Fruits
(c) Seeds (d) Stem

53. Higher plants survive stressful conditions by reducing their __________ activity.
(a) Reproductive (b) Metabolic
(c) Growth (d) Morphogenetic

54. Bears undergo a period of __________ to escape stress during winter.
(a) Hibernation (b) Aestivation
(c) Sedation (d) Metamorphosis

55. Snails and fish undergo aestivation to avoid summer related problems of heat and __________
(a) Hygroscopicity (b) Desiccation
(c) Efflorescence (d) Starvation

56. Under unfavourable conditions, many species of zooplankton which lives in small water bodies are known to enter __________
(a) Diapause (b) Metapause
(c) Neopause (d) Monopause

57. Diapause is a stage of __________
(a) Perpetual development (b) Intermittent development
(c) Suspended development (d) Sequential development

58. __________ is any attribute of an organism that enables the organism to survive and reproduce in its habitat.
(a) Mutation (b) Evolution
(c) Adaptation (d) Conformation

59. Adaption includes __________ attribute of an organism.
(a) Behavioural (b) Physiological
(c) Morphological (d) All of the above

60. Many adaptations of an organism have evolved over a long duration of evolution and are __________
(a) Genetically unstable (b) Genetically fixed
(c) Genetically disadvantageous (d) Genetically extemporaneous

61. __________ in North American deserts is capable of meeting all its water requirements through its internal biochemical process.
(a) Llama (b) Coyote
(c) Kangaroo rat (d) Weasel

62. By which biochemical process, kangaroo rat meets its water requirement?
(a) Reduction of fats (b) Oxidation of proteins
(c) Reduction of proteins (d) Oxidation of fats

63. Water molecule is a by product in which of the following process?
(a) Reduction of fats (b) Oxidation of proteins
(c) Reduction of proteins (d) Oxidation of fats

64. Desert animals have the capability of forming __________ urine.
(a) Hypotonic (b) Isosmotic
(c) Concentrated (d) Dilute

65. Select the true statement from the following options:
(a) Desert plants have thick cuticle on their body
(b) Stomata are arranged superficially
(c) Minimum loss of water through fat oxidation
(d) Special photosynthetic pathway occurs in desert plants

66. An important feature regarding CAM pathway in desert plants
(a) Enables stomata to increase the number of chloroplasts
(b) Enables stomata to remain open during any time
(c) Enables stomata to remain closed during day time
(d) Enables stomata to open during rainy weather

67. Some desert plants like __________ have no leaves.
(a) Meuhlenbeckia (b) Opuntia
(c) Nephrolepis (d) All of the above

68. Photosynthetic function in opuntia is performed by __________
(a) Roots (b) Flowers
(c) Fruits (d) Stems

69. In opuntia, leaves are reduced to __________
(a) Thorns (b) Prickles
(c) Spines (d) Buds

70. Allen's rule is with respect to __________
(a) Reptiles (b) Mammals
(c) Aves (d) Amphibia

71. Mammals from colder climates generally have __________ ears and limbs to minimize heat loss.
(a) Reduced (b) Shorter
(c) Longer (d) Wider

72. Aquatic mammals in polar seas have a thick layer of fat known as __________
(a) Blubber (b) Flubber
(c) Rubber (d) Stubber

73. A thick layer of fat under the skin in aquatic mammals essentially acts as __________
(a) Food reservoir (b) Insulator
(c) Conductor (d) Heat generator

74. Visiting a place like Manali and Mansarovar gives you an uncomfortable feeling. This is referred to as __________
(a) Motion Sickness (b) Altitude Sickness
(c) Acrophobia (d) All of the above

75. With the increase in altitude of a place __________
(a) Atmospheric pressure decreases (b) Atmospheric pressure increases
(c) Atmospheric pressure remain constant (d) Either (a) or (b)

76. The symptoms of altitude sickness are
(a) Nausea
(b) Heart palpitations
(c) Fatigue
(d) All of the above

77. How acclimatization occurs in case of altitude sickness?
(a) Decrease RBC production
(b) Increase RBC production
(c) Increase rate of breathing
(d) Both (b) and (c)

78. Which bacteria can flourish in hot springs and deep sea hydrothermal vents?
(a) Cyanobacteria
(b) Archaebacteria
(c) Actinobacteria
(d) Acidobacteria

79. Many fish thrive in Antarctic water where the temperature is __________.
(a) Always above zero
(b) Always above 4°C
(c) Always below zero
(d) Sometimes below zero

80. How much pressure is experienced by marine invertebrates and fishes living at the great depths in oceans?
(a) $<$ 100 times that of normal atmospheric pressure
(b) $<$ 100 times that of hydrostatic pressure
(c) $>$ 100 times that of hydrostatic pressure
(d) $>$ 100 times that of normal atmospheric pressure

81. Which of the following animals lack the physiological ability to deal with high temperature in their habitat?
(a) Giant frilled lizard
(b) Desert lizard
(c) Kangaroo rat
(d) Weasel

82. What adaptation desert lizard shows to deal with high temperature?
(a) Bask in sun when body temperature drops
(b) Move in shade when body temperature drops
(c) Bask in sun when ambient temperature drops.
(d) Move in shade when ambient temperature drops.

83. The main reason behind building burrows in soil by burrowing animals is __________.
(a) To escape from predators
(b) To derive nutrition parts of plants from underground
(c) The mode of evolution chose burrows as a specific habitat
(d) To hide and escape from the above-ground heat

84. Which of the following is not a population attribute?
(a) Majority of them live in groups in a well-defined geographical location
(b) Share or compete for similar resources
(c) Potentially interbreed
(d) Single individuals of any species cannot live in isolation

85. Individuals resulting from asexual reproduction are also considered __________ while performing ecological studies.
(a) Biome
(b) Ecosystem
(c) Population
(d) Species

86. As teakwood: Forest tracts, __________ : Wetland.
(a) Lotus
(b) Rats
(c) Squirrels
(d) Cormorants

87. To evolve certain desired traits, natural selection should operate at __________ level.
(a) Species (b) Biomes
(c) Population (d) Genus

88. Population ecology is a bridge between evolution and __________.
(a) Population morphology (b) Population genetics
(c) Population proteomics (d) Population variation

89. After poaching 3 lions in certain forest of Gujarat, only 15 are left in a year. Determine death rate per capita.
(a) 5.000 (b) 0.200
(c) 0.166 (d) 0.800

90. The population size of Siberian cranes at Bharatpur wetlands in any year is __________
(a) 10 (b) 100
(c) 1000 (d) 5

91. Population size in any given habitat is also known as __________
(a) Population cluster
(b) Population explosion
(c) Population abundance
(d) Population density

92. Tiger census in our national parks and tiger reserves is done by counting
(a) Tiger cubs (b) Tiger pug marks
(c) Tiger faecal pellets (d) Both (b) and (c)

93. Natality refers to
(a) No. of births in a given geographical area
(b) No. of births in a given time period
(c) No. of births under influence of given environmental factor
(d) No. of deaths in a given time period

94. A striking difference between immigration and emigration is __________
(a) Immigration considers total no. of species in a given habitat while emigration refers to a single species
(b) Emigration considers total no. of species in a given habitat while immigration refers to a single species
(c) Immigration considers total no. of dominant species in a given habitat while emigration refers to a single species
(d) Immigration considers total no. of species in a given habitat while emigration refers to a dominant single species

95. Identify the correct equation for population density at time t + 1
(a) $N = N_t + [(D + I) - (B + E)]$ (b) $N = N_t + [(B + I) - (D + E)]$
(c) $N_{t+1} = N_t + [(B + D) - (I + E)]$ (d) $N_{t+1} = N_t + [(B + I) - (D + E)]$

96. If a new habitat is just being colonized then which of the following options do you think would have a greater contribution towards population density?
(a) Mortality (b) Natality
(c) Immigration (d) Emigration

97. While developing theory of natural selection, Darwin observed that each species could realize fully its innate potential to grow in number provided in a particular habitat __________
(a) Favourable environmental conditions are prevalent
(b) Absence of natural disasters like floods and famine
(c) Availability of unlimited resources
(d) Development of mutation in certain species

98. Study the following equation in context of population growth and choose the correct option

$dN/dt = (b - d) \times N$ (i)

Substituting r in place of b – d then

$dN/dt = rN$ (ii)

Here 'r' is known as __________
(a) Extrinsic rate of natural decrease
(b) Intrinsic rate of natural decrease
(c) Intrinsic rate of natural increase
(d) Extrinsic rate of natural increase

99. The r value for Norway rat is __________
(a) 0.15 (b) 0.0015
(c) 0.015 (d) 1.5

100. The r value for flour beetle is __________
(a) 0.15 (b) 0.12
(c) 0.21 (d) 0.012

101. The r value for human population in India is __________
(a) 0.15 (b) 0.0502
(c) 0.0205 (d) 0.012

102. When N (population density) is plotted against time __________ shaped graph is obtained (using equation. (ii) as per question 99)
(a) S (b) J
(c) U (d) Inverted U

103. The integral form of equation (ii) as given in question 98 is __________
(a) $N = N_0\, e^{rN}$ (b) $N = N_0\, e^{rt}$
(c) $N_t = N_0\, e^{rN}$ (d) $N_t = N_0\, e^{rt}$

104. Any species growing exponentially under __________ resource conditions can reach massive population densities in a short time span
(a) Limited (b) Unlimited
(c) Essential (d) Non-essential

105. **Assertion (A):** A particular species in nature can achieve exponential growth
Reason (R): Availability of unlimited resources makes it possible.
(a) A is true but R is incorrect
(b) R is correct and A is incorrect
(c) Both A and R are incorrect
(d) Both A and R are correct

106. Carrying capacity K means __________
(a) Organism's capability of maximum reproduction
(b) Nature's limit for supporting maximum growth of a species
(c) Nature's limit for supporting maximum number of species
(d) Organism's capability to withstand environmental odds

107. If a population grows in a habitat with limited resources, then following phases of achievement are observed
(a) Lag → Acceleration → Deceleration → Asymptote
(b) Log → Deceleration → Acceleration → Asymptote
(c) Log → Acceleration → Deceleration → Asymptote
(d) Lag → Acceleration → Asymptote → Deceleration

108. The sigmoid curve of population growth is also known as
(a) Wagner-Nelson logistic growth (b) Lineweaver-Burk logistic growth
(c) Verhulst-Pearl logistic growth (d) Darwin's logistic growth

109. Which of the following equation correctly describes sigmoid growth curve?
(a) $dN/dt = rN\left(\frac{K-N}{r}\right)$ (b) $dN/dt = rN\left(\frac{K-N}{t}\right)$
(c) $dN/dt = N\left(\frac{K-N}{N}\right)$ (d) $dN/dt = rN\left(\frac{K-N}{K}\right)$

110. The reproductive fitness of a population in a certain habitat is also termed as ________
(a) Verhulst's fitness (b) Darwin's fitness
(c) Lamarkian fitness (d) Huxley's fitness

111. In order to achieve maximum population in a habitat, which of the following is correct?
(a) High r value (b) Low r value
(c) Independent of r value (d) Optimum r value

112. The organism breeding only once in its lifetime is ________
(a) Atlantic tuna fish (b) Indian pomphret fish
(c) Pacific salmon fish (d) Arctic whale

113. Amongst plants, select the correct option which breeds only once in lifetime.
(a) Banyan (b) Bamboo
(c) Oak (d) Pine

114. ________ is a more meaningful measure of population size.
(a) Natality (b) Mortality
(c) Biomass (d) Resources consumed

115. Pick out the essential resources for a population in a given habitat from the following Food, Water, Air, Space
(a) Food and water (b) Food and Space
(c) Air and Space (d) Water and Space

116. Nearly ________% of all insects are known to be phytophagous
(a) 25% (b) 35%
(c) 45% (d) 10%

117. Thorns are the most common morphological means of defense in
(a) Acacia (b) Cactus
(c) Calotropis (d) Both (a) and (b)

118. Which of the following weed plant produces cardiac glycosides (highly poisonous material)?
(a) Acacia (b) Cactus
(c) Calotropis (d) All

119. Which of the following substance are produced by plants as defense against grazers and browsers (count numbers)?
Nicotine, Caffeine, Quinine, Strychnine, Opium
(a) 2 (b) 3
(c) 4 (d) 5

120. In a field experiment, when all the starfish were removed from an enclosed intertidal area more than __________(A)__________ species of invertebrates become extinct within a year, because of __________(B)__________ completion.
(a) A – 10, B – Intra-specific
(b) A – 10, B – Inter-specific
(c) A – 20, B – Intra-specific
(d) A – 20, B – Inter-specific

121. Following is true about predators
(a) They keep prey population under control
(b) They may help in maintaining species diversity in a community by reducing the intensity of competition among competing prey species
(c) They are prudent in nature
(d) All of above

122. Which butterfly is highly distasteful to its predator bird because of a specific chemical present in its body?
(a) Apis mellifera (b) Viceroy
(c) Monarch (d) Apis indica

123. Who propose competitive exclusion principle?
(a) Gause (b) Robert May
(c) Darwin (d) Von Humbolt

124. Abingdon tortoise in Galapagos Islands became extinct within a decade after __________ were introduced on the island, because of the greater browsing efficiency of introduced animal.
(a) Cows (b) Buffalows
(c) Goats (d) Camels

125. A species whose distribution is restricted to a small geographical area because of the presence of a competitive superior species is found to expand its distributional range dramatically when the competing species is experimentally removed. This phenomenon is known as
(a) Competitive exclusion
(b) Competitive release
(c) Interference competition
(d) Resource partitioning

126. Who showed that five closely related species of warblers living on the same tree were able to avoid competition and co-exist due to behavioural differences in their forging activities?
(a) Connell (b) Mc Arthur
(c) Gause (d) Darwin

127. In general, which of the following appears to be more adversely affected by competition?
(a) Herbivores (b) Plants
(c) Carnivores (d) Both (a) and (b)

128. Gause's competitive exclusion principle states that
(a) Two unrelated species competing for the same resources cannot co-exist indefinitely and competitively inferior one will eliminated eventually
(b) Two closely related species competing for the same resources cannot co-exist indefinitely and competitively inferior one will eliminated eventually
(c) Two unrelated species competing for the same resources can co-exist indefinitely and can grow together
(d) Two closely related species competing for the same resources can co-exist indefinitely and can grow together

129. Connell's elegant field experiments showed that on rocky sea coasts of Scotland, the larger & competitively superior barnacle __________ dominates the intertidal area, and exclude smaller barnacle __________ from that zone
(a) Chathamalus, Balanus (b) Balanus, Balanus
(c) Chathamalus, chhathamalus (d) Balanus, Chathamalus

130. According to Darwin which competition is a potent force in organic evolution?
(a) Inter-specific (b) Intra-specific (c) Both (a) and (b) (d) None of these

131. In some shallow South American lakes, which of the following compete for the same food that is zooplanktons of lake?
(a) Visiting flamingoes (b) Resident fishes
(c) Both (a) and (b) (d) None of these

132. Find out true statement
(a) Totally unrelated species could also compete for the same resources
(b) Resources need not to be limiting for competition to occur
(c) In interference competition, feed efficiency of one species might be reduced due to the interfering and inhibitory presence of the other species, even if resources are abundant
(d) All are true

133. Which of the following are adaptations of parasite?
(a) Loss of unnecessary sense organ (b) Loss of digestive system
(c) High reproductive capacity (d) All of these

134. Liver fluke belongs to class
(a) Cestoda (b) Trematoda (c) Hirudeneria (d) Turbelleria

135. Liver fluke complete its cycle in how many intermediate hosts?
(a) 1 (b) 2
(c) 3 (d) 4

136. Human liver fluke has two intermediate hosts in its life cycle; these are
(a) Snail and Hydra (b) Crustacean and Fish
(c) Snail and Fish (d) Mosquito and Snail

137. Effect of parasite on host
(a) Reduce survival (b) Reduce growth & reproduction
(c) Reduce its population density (d) All of them

138. Malaria parasites require which vector to spread to other hosts
(a) Snail (b) Fish (c) Housefly (d) Mosquito

139. Find the correct example of Ectoparasite
(a) Lice on humans (b) Ticks on dogs
(c) Copepods on marine fishes (d) All are correct

140. Cuscata, a parasitic plant that is commonly found growing on hedge plants has lost its __________ and __________ in the course of evolution
(a) Root and Stem
(b) Leaves and Chlorophyll
(c) Root and Leaves
(d) Leaves and Stem

141. Female mosquito require our blood for
(a) Respiration
(b) Locomotion
(c) Digestion
(d) Reproduction

142. Which of the following is not parasite?
(a) Tapeworm
(b) Female anopheles mosquito
(c) Liver fluke
(d) Lice

143. Find out false statement
(a) Parasite that feeds on the external surface of the host organism are called ectoparasite
(b) The life cycle of endoparasite are more complex because of their extreme specialization
(c) Parasitism evolved in so many taxonomic groups from plants to higher vertebrates
(d) Endoparasites have greatly complex morphological and anatomical features along with high reproductive potential

144. Example of brood parasitism
(a) Cuckoo (koel) and Crow
(b) Crow and Parrot
(c) Parrot and Pigeon
(d) Koel and Parrot

145. Find out incorrect statement
(a) In brood parasitism (of Koel and Crow), the eggs of parasitic bird have evolved to resemble the host's egg in size and colour to reduce the chance of the host bird detecting the foreign eggs and ejecting them from the host
(b) Majority of parasite harming the host
(c) Many parasites have evolved to be host specific in such a way that both host and the parasite tendto co-evolve
(d) Monarch butterfly acquire chemical by feeding on a poisonous weed in its adult stage, that chemical make it high distasteful to its bird

146. Which of the following shows commensalism
(a) Sea anemone and Clown fish
(b) Lichens
(c) Lice and Human
(d) Mycorrhizae

147. Commensalism is shown by all except
(a) Orchid on mango branch
(b) Cattle egret and Grazing cattle
(c) Sea anemone and Clown fish
(d) Cuckoo (Koel) and Crow

148. Lichens are mutualistic relationship between
(a) Fungus and Photosynthetic algae
(b) Fungus and Cyanobacteria
(c) Fungus and Roots of higher plants
(d) Both (a) and (b)

149. Mycorrhizae are association between
(a) Fungus and photosynthetic algae
(b) Fungus and roots of higher plants
(c) Fungus and cyanobacteria
(d) Fig plant and wasp

150. Pseudo copulation helps in pollination in
(a) Fig plant
(b) Orchid
(c) Cuscuta
(d) Sunflower

151. Best example of co-evolution
(a) Fig trees and pollinator species of wasp
(b) Fungus and cyanobacteria
(c) Sea anemone and clown fish
(d) All of them

152. Fruit of fig species provide
(a) Egg laying site to female wasp for oviposition
(b) Developing seed as food for the developing wasp larvae
(c) Both (a) and (b)
(d) None of these

153. Select incorrect statement
(a) The mediterranean orchid ophrys employs sexual deceit to get pollinated
(b) In mycorrhazial association, fungi help the plant in the absorption of essential nutrients from the soil
(c) Pinus seeds cannot germinate and establish without the presence of mycorrhizae
(d) When resources are unlimited, the growth is usually logistic but when resources become progressively limiting, the growth pattern turns exponential

154. In Ophrys, one petal of female flower bears an uncanny resemblance to the female of the bee in which of the following aspect.
(a) Size
(b) Colour
(c) Markings
(d) All

155. Fill in the blanks A, B, C, and D respectively

Species A	Species B	Name of Interaction
+	+	Mutualism
–	–	_A_
+	–	_B_
+	–	Parasitism
+	0	_C_
–	0	_D_

(+) Beneficial (–)detrimental (0) Neutral
(a) A: Commensalism, B: Predation, C: Amensalism, D: Competition
(b) A: Predation, B: Parasitism, C: Commensalism, D: Amensalism
(c) A: Competition, B: Predation, C: Commensalism, D: Amensalism
(d) A: Competition, B: Predation, C: Amensalism, D: Commensalism

156. In which of the following interaction only one of the species benefited
(a) Mutualism
(b) Competition
(c) Parasitism and Predation
(d) Amensalism

157. Which of the natural habitat on earth that is inhabited just by a single species
(a) Hot vents
(b) Forest
(c) Polar region
(d) None

158. Following breeds many times during their lifetime except
(a) Birds
(b) Mammals
(c) Amphibians
(d) Pacific salmon fish

159. Which of the following produce large number of small sized offsprings?
(a) Oyster
(b) Pelagic fishes
(c) Mammals
(d) Both (a) and (b)

160. Populations evolve to maximize their
(a) Health fitness
(b) Body fitness
(c) Mental fitness
(d) Reproductive fitness

161. Find out correct statement

(a) Under particular set of selection progresses, organism evolve towards the most efficient reproductive strategy

(b) In amensalism, one species is farmed whereas other is benefited

(c) Some species of insects and frogs are cryptically coloured (camouflaged) to avoid being detected easily by the prey

(d) 'Biological Control' methods adopted in agricultural pest control are based on the ability of the prey to regulate predator population

162. What type of human population is represented by the adjacent pyramid?

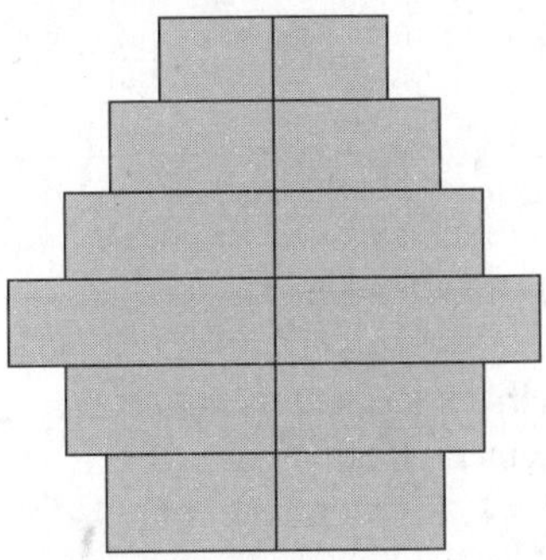

(a) Expanding population
(b) Vanishing population
(c) Stable population
(4) Declining population

163. Select correct matching for below diagram:

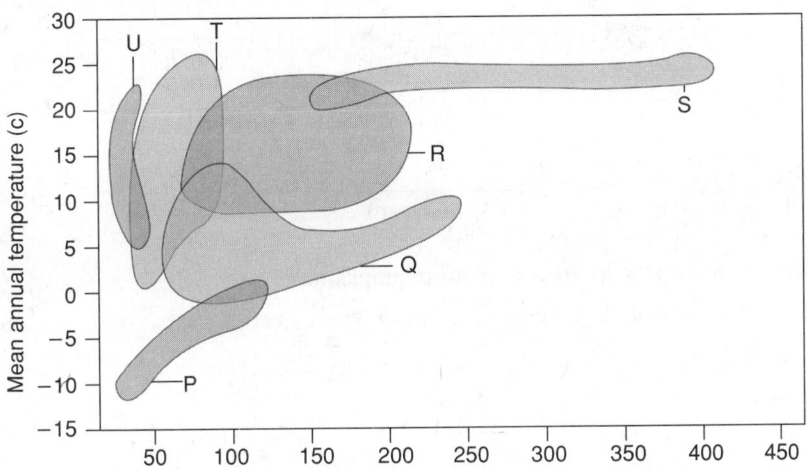

(a) P: Desert, Q: Tropical forest, R: Temperate forest, S: Coniferous forest

(b) P: Grassland, Q: Temperate forest, R: Desert, S: Arctic and Alpine tundra

(c) P: Arctic and Alpine tundra, Q: Coniferous forest, R: Temperate forest, S: Tropical forest

(d) P: Coniferous forest, Q: Grassland, R: Desert, S: Tropical forest

164. The figure given below is a diagrammatic representation of response of organisms to abiotic factors. What do (A), (B) and (C) represents respectively?

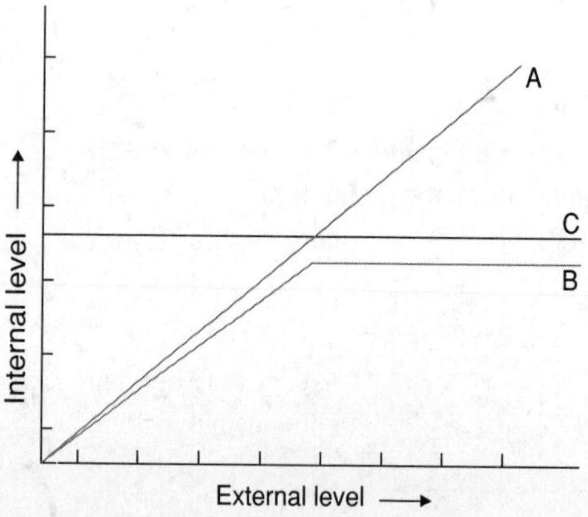

(a) A: Conformers, B: Partial regulaters C: Regulaters
(b) A: Partial regulaters, B: Conformers, C: Regulaters
(c) A: Regulaters, B: Partial regulaters, C: Conformers
(d) A: Conformers, B: Regulaters, C: Partial regulaters

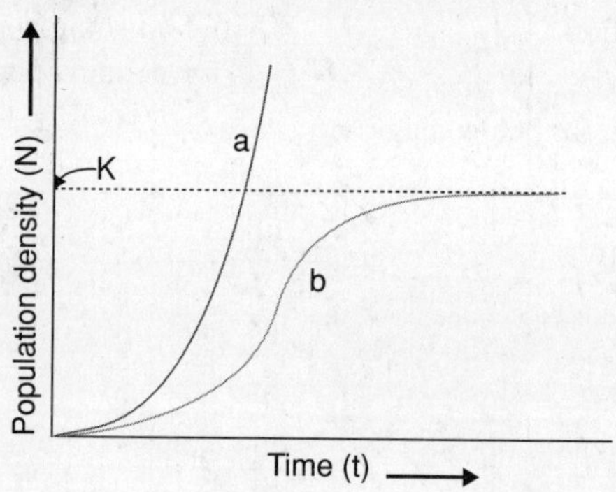

Questions 166 to 170 are based on above diagram.

165. Graph 'a' represented by formula

(a) $\frac{dN}{dt} = rN$ (b) $\frac{dN}{dt} = N$

(c) $\frac{dN}{dt} = rN\left(\frac{K-N}{K}\right)$ (d) $\frac{dN}{dt} = N\left(\frac{K-N}{K}\right)$

166. Graph 'b' represented by formula

(a) $\frac{dN}{dt} = rN$ (b) $\frac{dN}{dt} = N$

(c) $\frac{dN}{dt} = rN\left(\frac{K-N}{K}\right)$ (d) $\frac{dN}{dt} = N\left(\frac{K-N}{K}\right)$

167. What is the meaning of K?
(a) Intrinsic rate of natural reproduction
(b) Population density at time zero
(c) Carrying capacity
(d) Population density after time t

168. Plot b is known as
(a) Exponential growth curve
(b) Logistic growth curve
(c) Verhulst-Pearl Logistic growth curve
(d) Both (b) and (c)

169. Which of the growth curve is considered a more realistic one?
(a) Curve a
(b) Curve b
(c) Both (a) and (b)
(d) None of these

170. Identify the A, B, C and D in this figure.

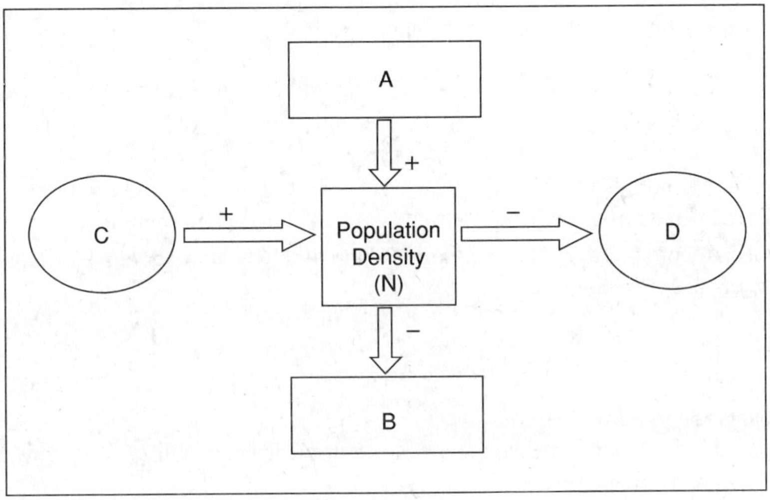

(a) A: Immigration (I), B: Emigration (E), C: Natality (B), D: Mortality (D)
(b) A: Natality (B), B: immigration (I), C: Mortality (D), D: Emigration (E)
(c) A: Mortality (D), B: Emigration (E), C: Natality (B), D: Immigration (I)
(d) A: Mortality (D), B: Natality (B), C: Emigration (E), D: Immigration (I)

171. Identify A, B and C in below figure of age pyramid for human population?

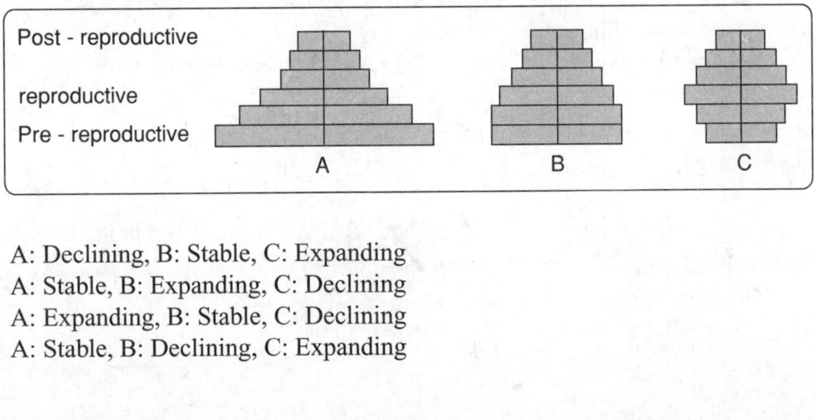

(a) A: Declining, B: Stable, C: Expanding
(b) A: Stable, B: Expanding, C: Declining
(c) A: Expanding, B: Stable, C: Declining
(d) A: Stable, B: Declining, C: Expanding

172. Biotic potential refers to
(a) Increase of population under optimum conditions.
(b) Increase of population under given conditions.
(c) Increase of population under natural conditions.
(d) Increase of population under climatic conditions.

173. A population has more young ir...viduals compared to the older individuals. What would be the status of the population after some years?
(a) It will decline
(b) It will stabilise
(c) It will increase
(d) It will first decline and then stabilise

174. What parameters are used for tiger census in our country's national parks and sanctuaries?
(a) Pug marks only
(b) Pug marks and faecal pellets
(c) Faecal pellets only
(d) Actual head counts

175. Which of the following would necessarily decrease the density of a population in a given habitat?
(a) Natality > mortality
(b) Immigration > emigration
(c) Mortality and emigration
(d) Natality and immigration

176. A protozoan reproduces by binary fission. What will be the number of protozoans in its population after six generations?
(a) 128
(b) 24
(c) 64
(d) 32

177. Diapause is
(a) Adaptation to terristerial life
(b) Stage of suspended developement seen in unfavourble conditions in many zooplankton species in lakes and ponds
(c) Method of migration from stressful habital to a more hospitable area
(d) It is a type of Symbiosis.

178. Amensalism is an association between two species where
(a) One species is harmed and other is benefitted
(b) One species is harmed and other is unaffected
(c) One species is benefitted and other is unaffected
(d) Both the species are harmed

179. Lichens are the associations of
(a) Bacteria and fungus
(b) Algae and bacterium
(c) Fungus and algae
(d) Fungus and virus

180. Which of the following is a partial root parasite?
(a) Sandal wood
(b) Mistletoe
(c) Orobanche
(d) Ganoderma

181. Which one of the following organisms reproduces sexually only once in its life time?
(a) Banana plant
(b) Mango
(c) Tomato
(d) Eucalyptus

182. Which plant is pollinated by below insect?

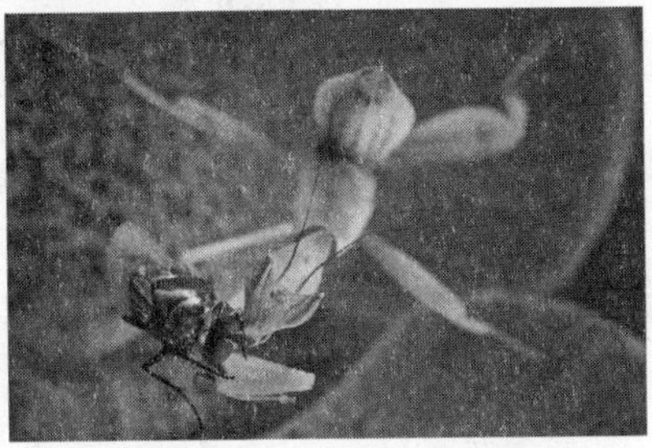

(a) Orchid flower (b) Fig flower
(c) Sunflower (d) Lotus flower

183. Below diagram represents which flower?

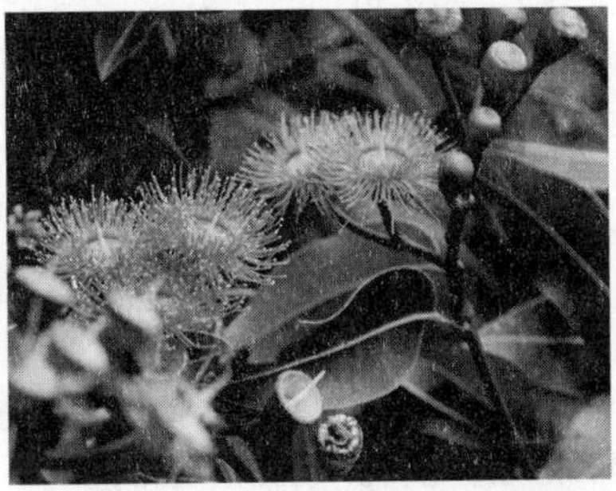

(a) Orchid flower (b) Fig flower
(c) Sunflower (d) Rose flower

184. Below diagram shows some insects laying eggs in fruit of figure. Find out insects from the following.

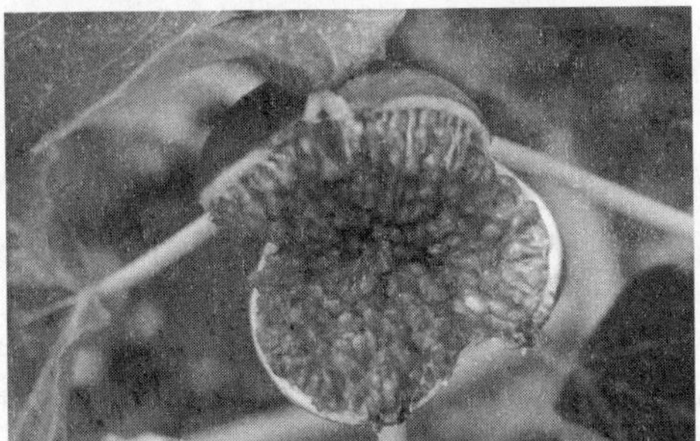

(a) Wasp (b) Female anopheles
(b) Culex (d) Honeybee

Read the ***assertion*** *and* ***reason*** *carefully to mark the correct option out of the options given below:*

(a) If both the assertion and the reason are true and the reason is a correct explanation of the assertion

(b) If both the assertion and reason are true but the reason is not a correct explanation of the assertion

(c) If the assertion is true but the reason is false

(d) If both the assertion and reason are false

185. **Assertion:** Ecology is basically concerned with four levels of biological organization organism, populations, communities and biomes.

Reason: Ecology is a subject which studies the interactions among organisms and between the organism & its physical environment.

186. **Assertion:** Temperature is the most ecologically relevant environmental factor

Reason: Temperature affects kinetics of enzyme.

187. **Assertion:** Many species of small plants (herbs & shrubs) growing in forests are adapted to photosynthesize optimally under very low light conditions.

Reason: These plants are constantly overshadowed by tall, canopied trees.

188. **Assertion:** Availability of light on land is closely linked with that of temperature.

Reason: Sun is source for both light & temperature.

189. **Assertion:** Mammals can thrive weather they live in Antarctica or in Sahara desert.

Reason: Success of mammals is largely due to their ability to maintain a constant body temperature.

190. **Assertion:** Very small animals are rarely found in Polar Regions.

Reason: Small animals have a larger surface area relative to their volume; they tend to lose body heat very fast when it is cold outside.

191. **Assertion**: Mammals from colder climates generally have shorter ears and limbs.

Reason: It is to maximize heat loss.

192. **Assertion:** Predators can help in maintaining species diversity in a community.

Reason: It is by reducing the intensity of competition among competing prey species.

193. **Assertion:** Mycorrhizae are association between fungi & roots of higher plants.

Reason: Lichens represent mutualistic relationship between fungus and photosynthetic algae or cyanobacteria.

194. **Assertion:** Parasitism and predation are considered to be negative interactions.

Reason : Parasites and predators limit the population of their host species.

AIPMT PREVIOUS YEAR QUESTIONS

1. Which one of the following is most appropriately defined?

[AIPMT MAINS 2010]

(a) Host is an organism which provides food to another organism
(b) Amensalism is a relationship in which one species is benefitted whereas the other is unaffected
(c) Predator is an organism that catches and kills other organism for food
(d) Parasite is an organism which always lives inside the body of other organism and may kill it

2. Study the four statements (1- 4) given below and select the two correct ones out of them.
(A) A lion eating a deer and a sparrow feeding on grain are ecologically similar in being consumers
(B) Predator star fish Pisaster helps in maintaining species diversity of some invertebrates
(C) Predators ultimately lead to the extinction of prey species
(D) Production of chemicals such as nicotine, strychnine by the plants are metabolic disorders
The two correct statements are

[AIPMT PRE 2010]

(a) (B) and (C) (b) (C) and (D)
(c) (A) and (D) (d) (A) and (B)

3. The figure given below is a diagrammatic representation of response of organisms to abiotic factors. What do A, B and C represent respectively?

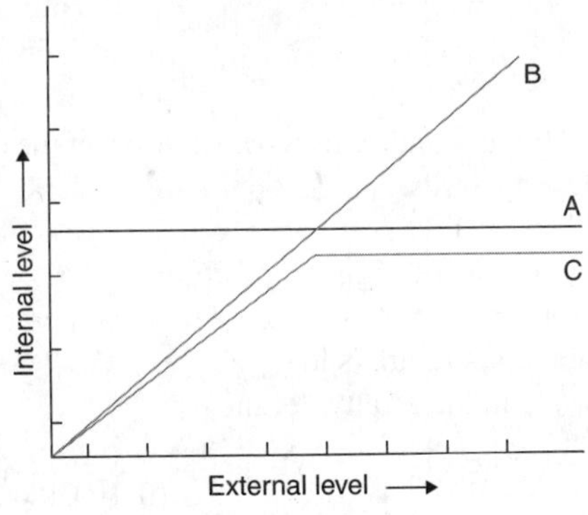

[AIPMT PRE 2010]

(a) A: Conformer, B: Regulator, C: Partial regulator
(b) A: Regulator, B: Partial, C: Conformer regulator
(c) A: Partial, B: Regulator, C: Conformer regulator
(d) A: Regulator, B: Conformer, C: Partial regulator

4. Which two of the following changes (1-4) usually tend to occur in the plain dwellers when they move to high altitudes (3,500 m or more)?
(A) Increase in red blood cell size (B) Increase in red blood cell production
(C) Increased breathing rate (D) Increase in thrombocyte count
Changes occurring are:

[AIPMT PRE 2010]

(a) (B) and (C) (b) (C) and (D)
(c) (A) and (D) (d) (A) and (B)

5. Which one of the following is one of the characteristics of a biological community? [AIPMT PRE 2010]

(a) Stratification (b) Natality
(c) Mortality (d) Sex-ratio

6. Consider the following statements (A-D) each with one or two blanks. [AIPMT MAINS 2011]

(A) Bears go into __(a)__ during winter to __(b)__ cold weather.
(B) A conical age pyramid with a broad base represents __(c)__ human population.
(C) A wasp pollinating a fig flower is an examples of __(d)__.
(D) An area with high levels of species richness is known as __(5)__.

Which one of the following options, gives the correct fill ups for the respective blank numbers from (a) to (5) in the statements?

(a) (c) stable (d) commensalism, (5) marsh
(b) (a) aestivation, (b) escape, (c) stable, (d) mutualism
(c) (c) expanding, (d) commensalism, (5) biodiversity park
(d) (a) hibernation, (b) escape, (c) Expanding (5) hot spot

7. The logistic population growth is expressed by the equation [AIPMT MAINS 2011]

(a) $dt / dN = Nr\left(\frac{K-N}{K}\right)$ (b) $dN/dt = rN\left(\frac{K-N}{K}\right)$

(c) $dN/dt = rN$ (d) $dN/dt = rN\left(\frac{N-K}{N}\right)$

8. Consider the following four conditions (A-D) and select the correct pair of them as adaptation to environment in desert lizards.

The conditions:

(A) Burrowing in soil to escape high temperature
(B) Losing heat rapidly from the body during high temperature
(C) Bask in sun when temperature is low
(D) Insulating body due to thick fatty dermis

[AIPMT PRE 2011]

(a) (A) and (C) (b) (B) and (D)
(c) (A) and (B) (d) (C) and (D)

9. What type of human population is represented by the following age pyramid?

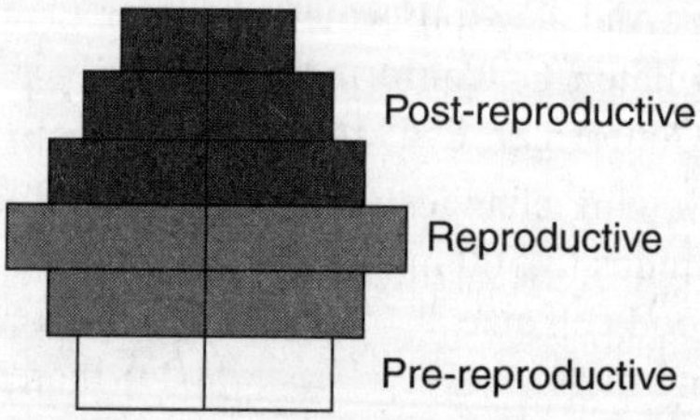

[AIPMT PRE 2011]

(a) Stable population (b) Declining population
(c) Expanding population (d) Vanishing population

10. Which one of the following is categorised as a parasite in true sense? [AIPMT PRE 2011]

(a) Human foetus developing inside the uterus draws nourishment from the mother
(b) Head louse living on the human scalp as well as laying eggs on human hair
(c) The cuckoo (koel) lays its eggs in crew's nest
(d) The female Anopheles bites and sucks blood from humans

11. Cuscuta is an example of: [AIPMT MAINS 2012]

(a) Brood parasitism (b) Predation
(c) Endoparasitism (d) Ectoparasitism

12. People who have migrated from the planes to an area adjoining Rohtang Pass about six months back: [AIPMT PRE 2012]

(a) Have more RBCs and their haemoglobin has a lower binding affinity to O_2
(b) Are not physically fit to play games like football
(c) Suffer from altitude sickness with symptoms like nausea, fatigue, etc
(d) Have the usual RBC count but then haemoglobin has very high binding affinity to O_2

13. A biologist studied the population of eats in a barn. He found that the average natality was 250, average mortality 240, immigration 20 and emigration 30. The net increase in population is: [AIPMT 2013]

(a) 10 (b) 15
(c) 05 (d) Zero

14. A sedentary sea anemone gets attached to the shell lining of hermit crab. The association is: [AIPMT 2013]

(a) Ectoparasitism (b) Symbiosis
(c) Commensalism (d) Amensalism

15. Just as a person moving from Delhi to Shimla to escape the heat for the duration of hot summer, thousands of migratory birds from Siberia and other extremely cold northern regions move to: [AIPMT 2014]

(a) Western Ghat (b) Meghalaya
(c) Corbett National Park (d) Keolado National Park

16. Leaves become modified into spines sin [AIPMT 2015]

(a) Opuntia (b) Pea
(c) Onion (d) Skin cotton

17. The following graph depicts changes in two populations (A and B) of herbivore in a grassy field. A possible reason for these changes is that :

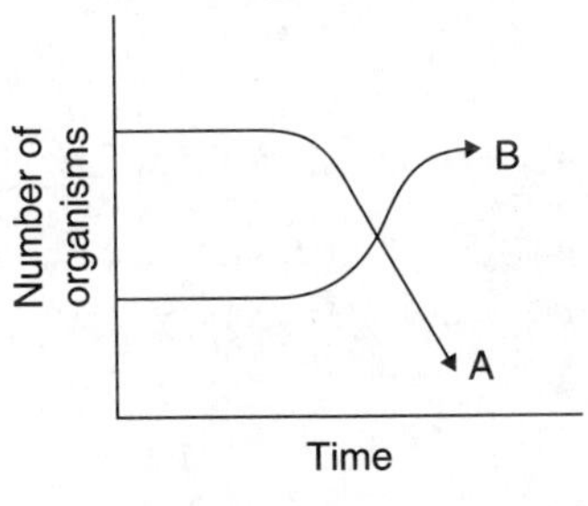

[AIPMT 2015]

(a) Both plant populations in this habitat decreased
(b) Population B compound more successfully for food than populations A.
(c) Population A produced more offspring than population B.
(d) Population A consumed the members of population B.

18. In which of the following interactions both partners are adversely affected?

[RE-AIPMT 2015]

(a) Predation
(b) Parasitism
(c) Mutualism
(d) Competition

19. An association of individuals of different species living in the same habitat and having functional interactions is:

[RE-AIPMT 2015]

(a) Biotic community
(b) Ecosystem
(c) Population
(d) Ecological niche

Answer Keys

1. (c)	2. (b)	3. (b)	4. (d)	5. (c)	6. (c)	7. (d)	8. (d)	9. (d)	10. (d)
11. (d)	12. (b)	13. (c)	14. (c)	15. (c)	16. (d)	17. (b)	18. (c)	19. (a)	20. (b)
21. (d)	22. (b)	23. (c)	24. (b)	25. (c)	26. (a)	27. (b)	28. (c)	29. (a)	30. (b)
31. (d)	32. (c)	33. (b)	34. (d)	35. (b)	36. (d)	37. (c)	38. (c)	39. (b)	40. (c)
41. (d)	42. (d)	43. (d)	44. (b)	45. (c)	46. (c)	47. (b)	48. (d)	49. (c)	50. (c)
51. (a)	52. (c)	53. (b)	54. (a)	55. (b)	56. (a)	57. (c)	58. (c)	59. (d)	60. (b)
61. (c)	62. (d)	63. (d)	64. (c)	65. (d)	66. (c)	67. (b)	68. (d)	69. (c)	70. (b)
71. (b)	72. (a)	73. (b)	74. (b)	75. (a)	76. (d)	77. (d)	78. (b)	79. (c)	80. (d)
81. (b)	82. (a)	83. (d)	84. (d)	85. (c)	86. (d)	87. (c)	88. (b)	89. (c)	90. (a)
91. (d)	92. (d)	93. (b)	94. (b)	95. (d)	96. (c)	97. (c)	98. (c)	99. (c)	100. (b)
101. (c)	102. (b)	103. (d)	104. (b)	105. (d)	106. (b)	107. (a)	108. (c)	109. (d)	110. (b)
111. (a)	112. (c)	113. (b)	114. (c)	115. (b)	116. (a)	117. (d)	118. (c)	119. (d)	120. (b)
121. (d)	122. (c)	123. (a)	124. (c)	125. (b)	126. (b)	127. (d)	128. (b)	129. (d)	130. (a)
131. (c)	132. (d)	133. (d)	134. (b)	135. (b)	136. (c)	137. (d)	138. (d)	139. (d)	140. (b)
141. (d)	142. (b)	143. (d)	144. (a)	145. (d)	146. (a)	147. (d)	148. (d)	149. (b)	150. (b)
151. (a)	152. (c)	153. (d)	154. (d)	155. (c)	156. (c)	157. (d)	158. (d)	159. (d)	160. (d)
161. (a)	162. (d)	163. (c)	164. (d)	165. (a)	166. (c)	167. (c)	168. (d)	169. (b)	170. (a)
171. (c)	172. (a)	173. (c)	174. (b)	175. (c)	176. (c)	177. (b)	178. (c)	179. (c)	180. (a)
181. (d)	182. (a)	183. (b)	184. (a)	185. (b)	186. (b)	187. (a)	188. (a)	189. (a)	190. (a)
191. (c)	192. (a)	193. (b)	194. (c)						

AIPMT Previous Year Questions

1. (c)	2. (d)	3. (d)	4. (a)	5. (a)	6. (d)	7. (b)	8. (a)	9. (b)	10. (b)
11. (d)	12. (a)	13. (d)	14. (b)	15. (d)	16. (a)	17. (b)	18. (d)	19. (a)	

CHAPTER

36

Ecosystem

1. Following are examples of terrestrial ecosystem except:
   (a) Forest
   (b) Wetland
   (c) Grassland
   (d) Desert
2. Which of these are examples of aquatic ecosystem?
   (a) Pond
   (b) River
   (c) Estuary
   (d) All
3. Which of these are examples of man-made ecosystem?
   (a) Crop field
   (b) Aquarium
   (c) Wetland
   (d) Both (a) and (b)
4. Find the incorrect statement.
   (a) Biosphere is a global ecosystem.
   (b) Transfer of energy in ecosystem explains in terms of food web and nutrient cycle.
   (c) Pond, lake and wetland are aquatic ecosystems.
   (d) Ecosystem is structural not functional unit of ecosystem.
5. Which of the following occupy top vertical strata of forest ecosystem?
   (a) Shrubs
   (b) Herbs and grasses
   (c) Tree
   (d) Phytoplankton
6. Pond is a:
   (a) Shallow fresh water body
   (b) Deep fresh water body
   (c) Shallow marine water body
   (d) Deep marine water body
7. Functional aspect of ecosystem can be explained in terms of:
   (a) Productivity
   (b) Decomposition and energy flow
   (c) Nutrient cycle
   (d) All of the above
8. At the bottom of ponds decomposers found are:
   (a) Fungi
   (b) Bacteria
   (c) Flagellates
   (d) All of these
9. Which of the following have only unidirectional flow?
   (a) Carbon
   (b) Nitrogen
   (c) Energy
   (d) Sulphur
10. The amount of biomass or organic matter produced per unit area over a period of time by plants during photosynthesis is known as:
   (a) Primary production
   (b) Secondary production
   (c) Net primary production
   (d) Net secondary production

11. Unit of primary production is:
(a) g/m^2
(b) $kcal/m^2$
(c) Both (a) and (b)
(d) None of these

12. NPP is equal to:
(a) GPP + R
(b) GPP – R
(c) GPP × R
(d) GPP ÷ R

13. Secondary productivity means:
(a) Rate of formation of organic matter by producer
(b) Rate of formation of new organic matter by consumers
(c) Rate of formation of inorganic matter by producer
(d) Rate of formation of inorganic matter by consumers

14. Primary productivity depends on which of the following factors?
(a) Environmental factor
(b) Photosynthetic capacity of plant
(c) Availability of nutrients
(d) All of the above

15. GPP means:
(a) Gross Public Partnership
(b) Gross Primary Production
(c) Gross Producer Production
(d) Gross plant production

16. Unit of productivity is:
(a) $gm^{-2}yr^{-1}$
(b) $Kcal/m^2/year$
(c) Both (a) and (b)
(d) None

17. NPP means:
(a) Available biomass for the consumption of heterotrophs
(b) Biomass produced by producers
(c) Gross primary product of respiratory losses
(d) All of the above

18. The annual net primary productivity of the whole biosphere is how much billion tons (dry weight) of organic matter?
(a) 120
(b) 170
(c) 210
(d) 150

19. Oceans occupy ________ % of the surface of earth but productivity of ocean are ________ billion tons.
(a) 70, 45
(b) 60, 55
(c) 70, 55
(d) 60, 65

20. Productivity of ocean is less because:
(a) It occupies 70% of earth's surface.
(b) Light is a major limiting factor which decreases with increase in water depth.
(c) It contains algae as a chief producer.
(d) All of the above

21. What is the percentage of primary productivity of oceans?
(a) 50%
(b) 90%
(c) 32%
(d) 70%

22. Earthworms help in:
(a) Breakdown of complex organic matter
(b) Loosening of soil
(c) Both (a) and (b)
(d) None of the above

23. Detritus contain:
   (a) Dead plant remains (leaves, bark and flower)
   (b) Dead animal remains
   (c) Fecal matter
   (d) All of the above
24. The important steps in the process of decomposition are:
   (a) Fragmentation (b) Leaching
   (c) Catabolism (d) All of these
25. Match the columns:

Column–I	Column–II
1. Fragmentation	A. Break down of detritus into smaller particles
2. Leaching	B. Precipitation of water soluble nutrients as unavailable salt
3. Catabolism	C. Degradation of detritus by bacterial and fungal enzymes

   (a) 1–A, 2–B, 3–C (b) 1–B, 2–C, 3–A
   (c) 1–C, 2–B, 3–A (d) 1–C, 2–A, 3–B
26. Which of these are true about humus?
   (a) Dark colored amorphous substance (b) Colloidal in nature
   (c) Reservoir of nutrient (d) All of the above
27. Humus is degraded by some microbes and release of inorganic nutrients occur by the process known as ________.
   (a) Fragmentation (b) Leaching
   (c) Humidification (d) Mineralization
28. Find out total number of incorrect statements from the following:
   (A) Decomposition is largely an anaerobic process.
   (B) Fragmentation, leaching and catabolism occur simultaneously on detritus.
   (C) Vertical distribution of different species occupying different level is called stratification.
   (D) Pond is a deep water body.
   (E) The rate of decomposition is controlled by chemical composition of detritus and climatic factors.
   (a) 1 (b) 2
   (c) 3 (d) 4
29. Decomposition is favoured by:
   (a) Warm and moist environment
   (b) Rich amount of nitrogen and water soluble substance like sugar in detritus
   (c) Aerobic environment
   (d) All of the above
30. Rate of decomposition process is decreased by:
   (a) Aerobic environment
   (b) Rich amount of lignin and chitin in detritus
   (c) Worm and moist environment
   (d) All of the above
31. What is the main source of energy for all ecosystems on earth?
   (a) Sun (b) Volcano
   (c) Deep sea hydro-thermal system (d) Moon

32. PAR (Photosynthetically active radiation) from incident solar radiation is:
(a) 50% (b) 30%
(c) 70% (d) 20%

33. Plant capture how much of PAR?
(a) 2–10% (b) 10–20%
(c) 50% (d) 30%

34. Which law is obeyed during energy flow in an ecosystem?
(a) First law of thermodynamics (b) Second law of thermodynamics
(c) Third law of thermodynamics (d) Both (a) and (b)

35. In a terrestrial ecosystem major producers are:
(A) Herbs (B) Woody plant
(C) Shrubs
(a) A and B only (b) A and C only
(c) A, B and C (d) B only

36. Primary producers in aquatic ecosystem are:
(a) Phytoplankton (b) Algae
(c) Higher plant (d) All of these

37. Which of these is a primary consumer?
(a) Grass (b) Goat
(c) Man (d) Tiger

38. Which of these is a common herbivores in aquatic ecosystem?
(a) Insect (b) Birds
(c) Mammals (d) Mollusc

39. Which of the following represent simple GFC (Grazing Food Chain)?
(a) Grass → Goat → Man (b) Goat → Grass → Man
(c) Detritus → Fungi → Man (d) Fungi → Detritus → Grass

40. DFC (Detritus Food Chain) begins with:
(a) Dead organic matter (b) Fungi
(c) Bacteria (d) Plant

41. Main decomposers are:
(a) Bacteria and fungus (b) Earthworm,
(c) Flagellated, Protozoans (d) Flagellated diatoms

42. Decomposers meet their energy and nutrient requirements by:
(a) Phytoplanktons (b) Zooplauktons
(c) Detritus (d) Bacteria

43. GFC is a major conduit for energy flow in:
(a) Terrestrial ecosystem (b) Aquatic ecosystem
(c) Both (a) and (b) (d) None of the above

44. Decomposers shows:
(a) Intracellular digestion (b) Extra cellular digestion
(c) Both intra and extracellular digestion (d) No digestion at all

45. Find the incorrect statement.
   (a) In terrestrial ecosystem larger fraction of energy flow occurs through DFC.
   (b) In aquatic ecosystem a major conduit for energy flow is GFC.
   (c) Detritus food chain is not at all connected with grazing food chain at any level.
   (d) Natural interconnection of food chain makes it a food web.
46. Based on the source of their nutrient or food, organisms occupy a specific place in the food chain that is known as their _________.
   (a) Hierarchy position (b) Class
   (c) Order (d) Trophic level
47. Herbivoures are:
   (a) Producers (b) Primary consumers
   (c) Secondary consumer (d) Tertiary consumers
48. Plants are:
   (a) Producers (b) Primary consumers
   (c) Secondary consumers (d) Tertiary consumers
49. Each tropic level has a certain mass of living material at a particular time called:
   (a) Standing state (b) Stranding crop
   (c) Ecological pyramid (d) GPP
50. Stranding crop is measured in terms of:
   (a) Biomass/unit area (b) Number of organism/unit area
   (c) Both (a) or (b) (d) None of the above
51. Measurement of biomass is generally done in terms of:
   (a) Fresh weight (b) Dry weight
   (c) Ash (d) Numbers of organisms
52. What does A represent in the diagram?

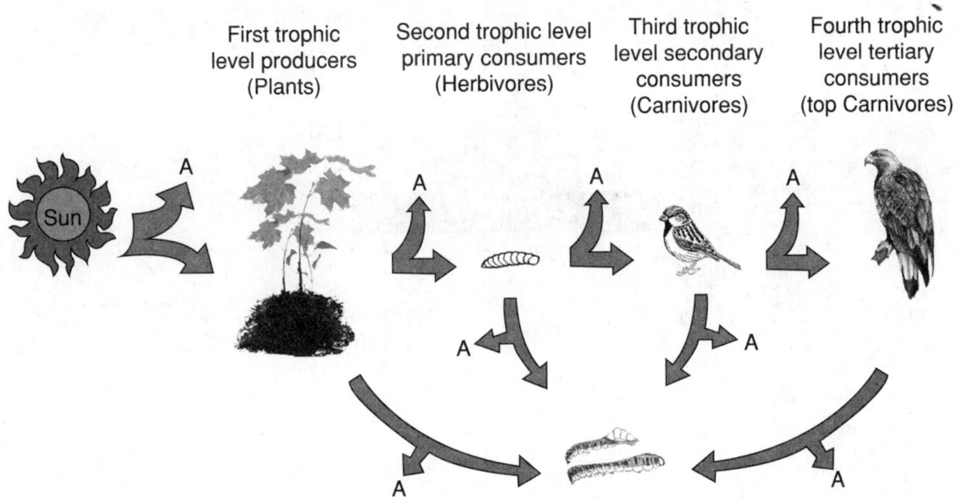

   (a) Food (b) Heat
   (c) Water (d) CO_2

53. Transfer of energy in tropic level follows:
(a) 20% law
(b) 10% law
(c) 5% law
(d) 15% law

54. A graphical representation known as ________ is required to express food or energy relationship between organisms at different trophic levels.
(a) ecological pyramid
(b) standing state
(c) ecological quadrilateral
(d) standing crop

55. Ecological pyramids are based on:
(a) Food chain
(b) Food web
(c) Energy flow
(d) All of these

56. How many ecological pyramids are usually studied?
(a) 1
(b) 2
(c) 3
(d) 4

57. Ecological pyramids are:
(a) Pyramids of number
(b) Pyramids of biomass
(c) Pyramids of energy
(d) All of the above

58. Which of following pyramid is always upright?
(a) Energy
(b) Biomass
(c) Number
(d) All

59. How much energy of sunlight is converted by primary producers into NPP in above energy pyramid?

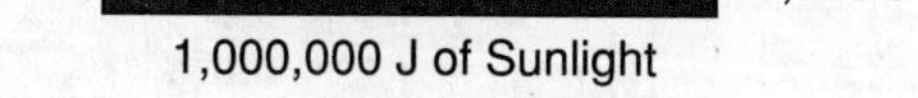

(a) 2%
(b) 10%
(c) 1%
(d) 110%

60. How many top-carnivores are supported in an above grassland ecosystem based on production of nearly 6 million plants?

Trophic level	Number of individuals
TC (Tertiary consumer)	3
SC (Secondary consumer)	3,54,000
PC (Primary consumer)	708,000
PP (Primary producer)	5,842,000

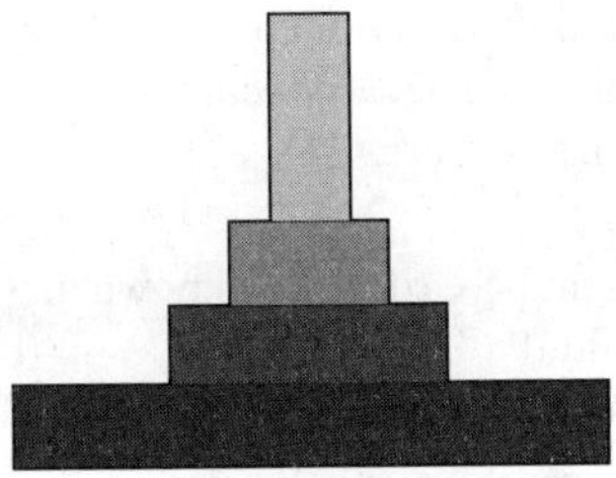

(a) 3 (b) 6
(c) 9 (d) 12

61. An inverted pyramid of biomass is seen in:
(a) Forest ecosystem (b) Grassland ecosystem
(c) Aquatic ecosystem (d) Desert

62. Find the correct statement:
(a) Trophic level represents a functional level, not a species as such.
(b) A given species never occupies more than one trophic level in the same ecosystem at the same time.
(c) In most ecosystems, producers are less in number and biomass than the herbivores.
(d) Pyramid of energy can never be upright.

63. Following are limitations of ecological pyramids:
(a) It does not take into account the same species belonging to two or more trophic levels.
(b) It assumes a simple food chain that almost does not exist in nature.
(c) Saprophytes are not given any place.
(d) All of the above

64. Which of the following may occupy more than one trophic level in the same ecosystem at the same time?
(a) Lion (b) Sparrow
(c) Snake (d) Frog

65. Which of these are true about sparrows?
(a) When it eats seeds and peas it is a primary consumer.
(b) When it eats insets and worms it is a secondary consumer.
(c) It may occupy more than one trophic level in same ecosystem at the same time.
(d) All of the above

66. Which of the following organisms have no space in ecological pyramid although they play vital role in the ecosystem?
(a) Birds (b) Snake
(c) Bacteria and fungi (d) Frog

67. Orderly and sequential changes in communities, parallel with the changes in the physical environment is known as:
(a) Ecological succession (b) Extinction
(c) Divergent evolution (d) Convergent evolution

68. The entire sequence of communities that successively change in a given area are called:
(a) Extinction (b) Evolution
(c) Succession (d) Sere

69. In the successive seral stages:
(a) There is change in diversity of species of organisms.
(b) Increase in number of species occurs.
(c) Increase in biomass occurs.
(d) All of the above

70. If succession occurs on bare rock, it is known as:
(a) Primary succession (b) Secondary succession
(c) Tertiary succession (d) Quaternary succession

71. Primary succession occurs on/in:
(a) Bare rocks (b) Newly cooled lava
(c) Newly created pond (d) All of the above

72. Secondary succession occurs in:
(a) Flooded land (b) Burned forest
(c) Abandoned farm land (d) All of the above

73. How is primary succession different from secondary succession?
(a) There is change in type of animals and plants during primary succession only.
(b) Anthropogenic disturbance can change seral stages in primary succession only.
(c) Primary succession occurs at slower rate.
(d) All of the above

74. What happened during succession?
(a) Extinction of some species (b) Increase in number of some species
(c) Change in type of decomposer species (d) All of the above

75. In secondary succession the species that invades an area depend on:
(a) Soil condition (b) Water availability
(c) Seed or propagules present (d) All of the above

76. In which succession is climax reached faster?
(a) Succession on bare rock (b) Succession on burned forest
(c) Succession on newly cooled lava (d) All of the above

77. Which is correct order of seral stages in hydrarch?
(a) Phytoplankton–submerged plant–submersed free floating plant stage–reed swamp stage–marsh-meadow stage–scrub stages–forest
(b) Scrub stages–forest–reed swamp stage–marsh-meadow stage–submersed free floating plant stage–submerged plant–phytoplankton
(c) Submerged plant–marsh-meadow stage–scrub stages–forest–phytoplankton–submersed free floating plant stage–reed swamp stage
(d) Phytoplankton–reed swamp stage–scrub stages–forest–submerged plant–submersed free floating plant stage–marsh-meadow stage

78. Which is a pioneer species in primary succession on rocks?
(a) Algae (b) Lichens
(c) Bryophyte (d) Pteridophyte

79. **A**. Lichens are pioneer species on rocks.
R. They secrete acids to dissolve rocks, helping in weathering and soil formation.
(a) A and R are both correct. (b) A and R are both incorrect.
(c) A is correct but R is incorrect. (d) R is correct but A is incorrect.

80. Find out total number of true statements from the following.
(A) Primary succession, is a very slow process, taking thousands of years for the climax to be reached.
(B) All succession whether taking place in water or land, proceeds to a similar climax community, the mesic.
(C) As succession proceeds, the number and types of animals and decomposers also change
(D) Saprophytes are not given any place in the ecological pyramids even though they play a vital role in the ecosystem.
(a) 1 (b) 2
(c) 3 (d) 4

81. The amount of nutrients such as carbon, nitrogen, phosphorus, calcium, etc., present in the soil at any given time is referred to as:
(a) Standing state (b) Standing crop
(c) Hydrarch (d) Xerarch

82. Nutrient cycling is known as:
(a) Biogeochemical cycle (b) Clavin cycle
(c) Hatch–slack pathway (d) Krebs cycle

83. Standing state:
(a) Vary according to type of ecosystem (b) Vary on seasonal basis
(c) Both (a) and (b) (d) None of the above

84. How many types of nutrient cycles are there?
(a) 1 (b) 2
(c) 3 (d) 4

85. The following elements shows gaseous type of nutrient cycles except:
(a) Carbon (b) Nitrogen
(c) Oxygen (d) Phosphorus

86. The following factors regulate the release of nutrients into the atmosphere:
(a) Soil and moisture (b) pH
(c) Temperature (d) All of these

87. Which nutrients flows through the sedimentary cycle?
(a) Sulphur (b) Phosphorus
(c) Both (a) and (b) (d) Carbon

88. What percentage of the dry weight of an organism does carbon constitute?
(a) 60% (b) 90%
(c) 49% (d) 35%

89. What percentage of global carbon does the atmosphere contain?
(a) 48% (b) 71%
(c) 1% (d) 10%

90. How much carbon is fixed approximately in biosphere annually through the process of photosynthesis?
(a) 4×10^{13} kg (b) 4×10^{10} kg
(c) 4×10^{8} kg (d) 4×10^{20} kg

91. Which of the following majorly regulates the amount of CO_2 in the atmosphere?
(a) Respiratory activities of the producers and consumers
(b) Decomposers
(c) Burning of fossil fuel
(d) Oceanic reservoir

92. Human activities mainly influence the:
(a) Carbon cycle (b) Nitrogen cycle
(c) Phosphorus cycle (d) Sulphur cycle

93. Phosphorus is a major constituent of:
(a) Biological membrane (b) Nucleic acids
(c) Cellular energy transfer system (d) All of the above

94. Following are the differences between carbon and phosphorus cycle:
(a) Carbon cycle is sedimentary whereas phosphorus cycle is gaseous.
(b) Carbon cycle is not significantly affected by human activities whereas phosphorus is significantly affected.
(c) Carbon has respiratory release but not phosphorus.
(d) All of the above

95. A chart is given to represent the phosphorus cycle in a terrestrial ecosystem. Find out what A, B, C and D represents in the flow chart.

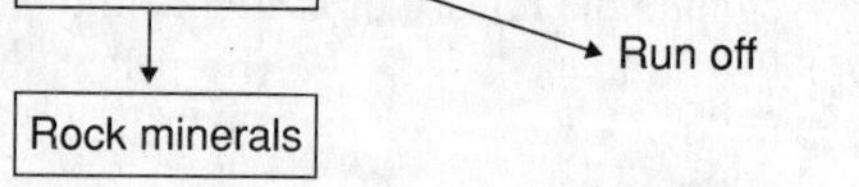

(a) A—Producers, B—Detritus, C—Soil solution, D—Litter fall
(b) A—Litter fall, B—Soil solution, C—Detritus, D—Producers
(c) A—Detritus, B—Producers, C—Litter fall, D—Soil solution
(d) A—Soil solution, B—Litter fall, C—Litter fall, D—Detritus

96. What price tag did Robert Constanza put for fundamental ecosystem services?
(a) 33 trillion US \$ (b) 22 trillion US \$
(c) 11 trillion US \$ (d) 44 trillion US \$

97. Global GNP is about:
(a) 33 trillion US \$ (b) 18 trillion US \$
(c) 12 trillion US \$ (d) 22 trillion US \$

98. Out of the total cost of various ecosystem services, the soil account for _________ %, recreation and nutrient cycling are less than _________ % and climate regulation and habitat for wildlife is about _________ % each.
(a) 50, 6, 10 (b) 50, 10, 6
(c) 50, 30, 20 (d) 20, 30, 50

99. Which one of the following has the largest population in a food chain?
(a) Producers (b) Primary consumers
(c) Secondary consumers (d) Decomposers

100. Following are ecosystem services:
(a) Purification of air and water by forest (b) Crop pollination
(c) Nutrient cycling (d) All of the above

101. Following are the two main structural features of an ecosystem:
(A) Species composition (B) Energy flow
(C) Decomposition (D) Stratification
(a) A and D only (b) B and C only
(c) A only (d) B, C and D only

102. Following are the reservoir of gaseous cycle:
(a) Atmosphere (b) Earth curst
(c) Hydrosphere (d) Both (a) and (c)

103. Which of the following nutrient cycle is the most complex?
(a) Nitrogen cycle (b) Phosphorous cycle
(c) Carbon cycle (d) Oxygen cycle

104. Biotic community is:
(a) Static
(b) Dynamic
(c) Group of population of same species in a given area
(d) All of the above

105. The stage of succession represented in the diagram is:

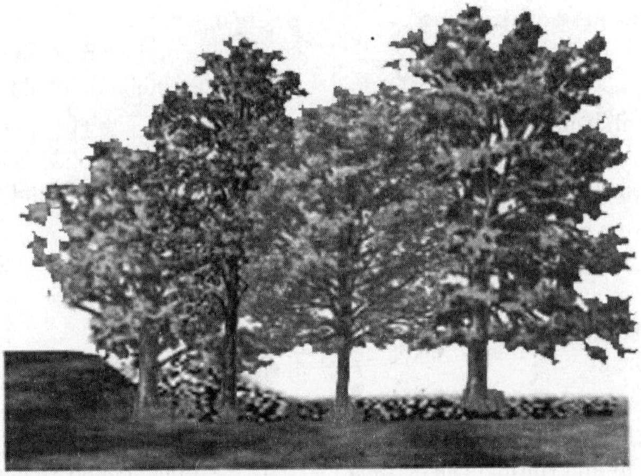

(a) Read swamp stage (b) Scrub stage
(c) Marsh-meadow stage (d) Forest stage

106. Litter is decomposed by how many organisms among the following?
Earthworm, Bacteria, Fungi, Mites
(a) 1 (b) 2
(c) 3 (d) 4

107. Following are ecosystem services except:
(a) Maintain biodiversity (b) Crop pollination
(c) Storage site for carbon (d) Flood

108. In decomposition, complex organic compounds of detritus are converted to which of the following substances by decomposers?
(a) Carbon dioxide (b) Water
(c) Inorganic nutrients (d) All of the above

109. Driving force for an ecosystem is:
(a) Primary producers (b) Secondary producers
(c) Solar radiation (d) Food chain

110. Frog, snake and eagle belong to:
(a) Three trophic levels (b) Two trophic levels
(c) Only one trophic level (d) None of these

111. Ecosystem shows:
(a) Homeostasis (b) Mineral cycling
(c) Energy flow (d) All of these

112. Diagrammatic representation of different trophic levels of an ecosystem presents:
(a) Energy flow (b) Mineral cycling
(c) Food chain and food web (d) Ecological pyramids

113. A plant eaten by a herbivorous animal which in turn is eaten by a carnivorous animal forms a:
(a) Food web (b) Food chain
(c) Food pyramid (d) Food cycle

114. Which of the following statements is correct?
(a) Producers produce energy. (b) Consumers consume energy.
(c) Decomposers decompose energy. (d) Producers transform energy.

115. Food chain operating on decaying cow dung or organic remains is referred to as:
(a) Secondary succession (b) Secondary food chain
(c) Food web (d) Detritus food chain

116. Biological equilibrium is maintained with the help of:
(a) Producers and consumers (b) Consumers and decomposers
(c) Herbivorous and carnivorous (d) Photosynthesis and respiration

117. In ecosystem, the nonliving components are:
(a) Less important than the living components
(b) Equally important as those of the living components
(c) More important than living components
(d) None of the above

118. Cycling of material in ecosystem is entirely dependent upon:
(a) Producers and Consumers (b) Primary producers and Herbivorous
(c) Herbivorous and Carnivorous (d) Producers and Decomposers

119. In a terrestrial ecosystems such as forests, maximum energy is found in which trophic level?

(a) T_1 (b) T_2
(c) T_3 (d) T_4

120. Trophic levels are formed by:

(a) Only plants (b) Only animals
(c) Only carnivores (d) Organisms linked in food chains

121. If 20 kJ energy is available at producer level, then how much energy will be transferred to the lion in the food chain: producer → deer → lion?

(a) 0.2 J (b) 0.02 J
(c) 0.002 J (d) 2 J

122. Select the correct match for the below given stages of succession.

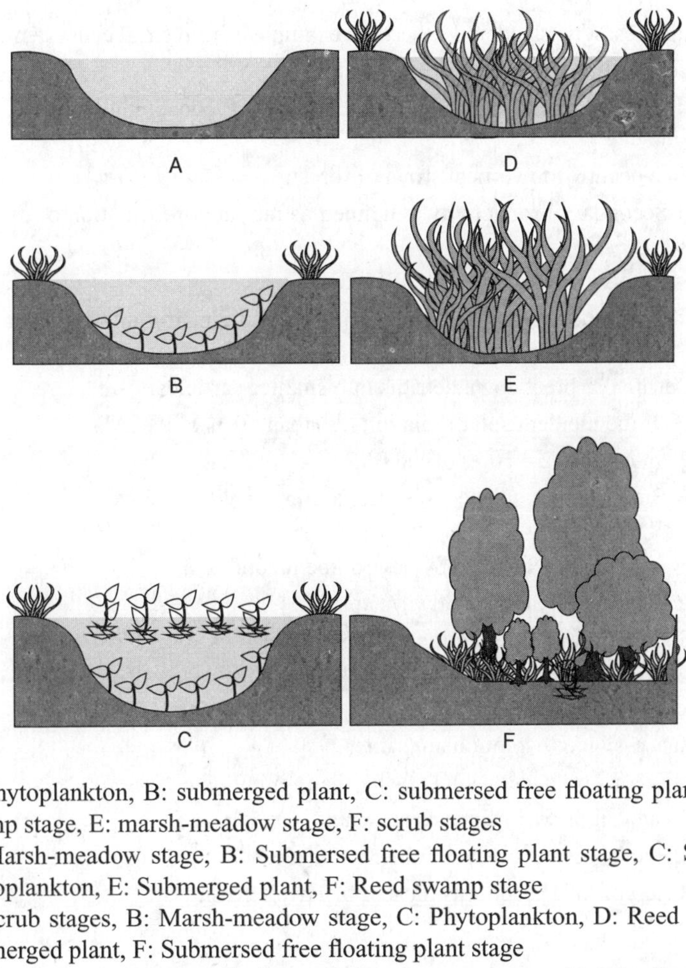

(a) A: Phytoplankton, B: submerged plant, C: submersed free floating plant stage, D: reed swamp stage, E: marsh-meadow stage, F: scrub stages
(b) A: Marsh-meadow stage, B: Submersed free floating plant stage, C: Scrub stages, D: Phytoplankton, E: Submerged plant, F: Reed swamp stage
(c) A: Scrub stages, B: Marsh-meadow stage, C: Phytoplankton, D: Reed swamp stage, E: Submerged plant, F: Submersed free floating plant stage
(d) A: Scrub stages, B: Phytoplankton, C: Reed swamp stage, D: Marsh-meadow stage, E: Submersed free floating pant stage, F: Submerged plant

*Read the **assertion** and **reason** carefully to mark the correct option out of the options given below:*

(a) If both the assertion and the reason are true and the reason is a correct explanation of the assertion

(b) If both the assertion and reason are true but the reason is not a correct explanation of the assertion

(c) If the assertion is true but the reason is false

(d) If both the assertion and reason are false

123. Assertion: Forest, grassland and desert are example of terrestrial ecosystem.
Reason: Ecosystem is functional unit of nature.

124. Assertion: Vertical distribution of different species occupying different levels is called stratification.
Reason: Tree occupy top vertical strata of forest.

125. Assertion: Secondary productivity is defined as the rate of formation of new organic matter by producers.
Reason: Secondary productivity = GPP – R.

126. Assertion: Decomposers break down complex organic matter into inorganic substances like CO_2, H_2O and nutrients.
Reason: Detritivore breakdown detritus into smaller particles.

127. Assertion: Of the incident solar radiation less than 50 % of its PAR.
Reason: Plant capture 2 – 10 % of the PAR.

128. Assertion: Biomass of a species is expressed in terms of dry weight in more accurate than fresh weight.
Reason: Fresh weight is affected by environment condition.

129. Assertion: Pyramid of energy is always upright.
Reason: Energy flow is unidirectional & some energy is always lost as heat at each step.

130. Assertion: Gradual and fairly predictable change in the species composition of a given area is called succession.
Reason: Succession & evolution are same.

131. Assertion: Secondary succession is faster than primary succession.
Reason: Some soil or sediments are presents.

132. Assertion: Phosphorus cycle is sedimentary cycle.
Reason: Reservoir of phosphorus located in earth's crust.

AIPMT PREVIOUS YEAR QUESTIONS

1. Which of the following representations shows the pyramid of numbers in a forest ecosystem?

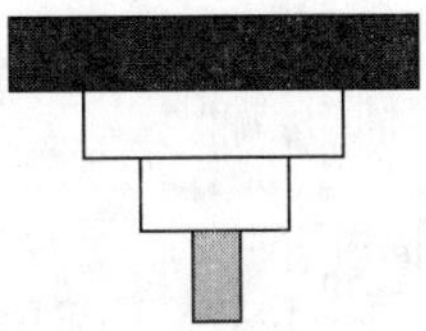
A

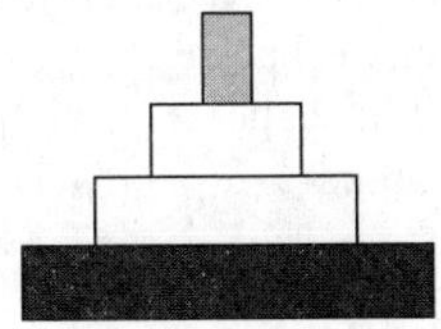
B

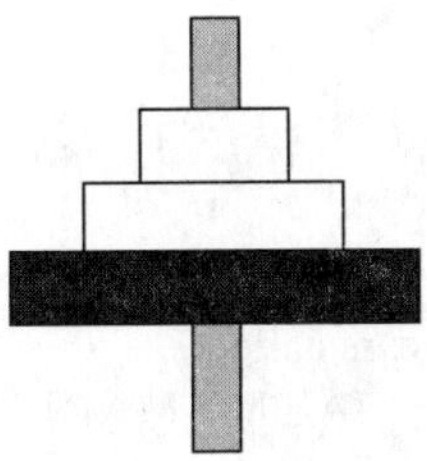
C

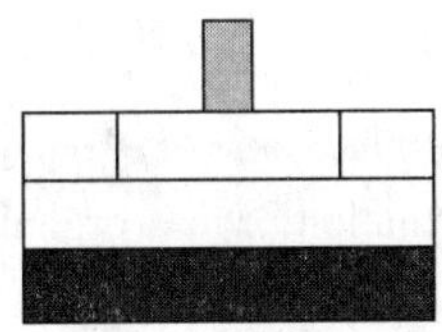
D

[AIPMT MAINS 2010]

(a) D (b) A
(c) B (d) C

2. The biomass available for consumption by the herbivores and the decomposers is called: [AIPMT PRE 2010]

(a) Net primary productivity (b) Secondary productivity
(c) Standing crop (d) Gross primary productivity

3. Which one of the following animals may occupy more than one trophic levels in the same ecosystem at the same time?

[AIPMT MAINS 2011]

(a) Sparrow (b) Lion
(c) Goat (d) Frog

4. Both hydrarch and xerarch successions lead to

[AIPMT MAINS 2011]

(a) Medium water conditions (b) Xeric conditions
(c) Highly dry conditions (d) Excessive wet conditions

5. The breakdown of detritus into smaller particles by earthworm is a process called [AIPMT MAINS 2011]

(a) Humification (b) Fragmentation
(c) Mineralisation (d) Catabolism

6. Which of the following statements is correct for secondary succession?

[AIPMT PRE 2011]

(a) It occurs on a deforested site
(b) It follows primary succession
(c) It is similar to primary succession except that it has a relatively fast pace
(d) It begins on a bare rock

7. Which one of the following statements for pyramid of energy is incorrect, whereas the remaining three are correct?

[AIPMT PRE 2011]

(a) It shows energy content of different trophic level organisms
(b) It is inverted in shape
(c) It is upright in shape
(d) Its base is broad

8. Mass of living matter at a trophic level in an area at any time is called:

[AIPMT PRE 2011]

(a) Detritus (b) Humus
(c) Standing state (d) Standing crop

9. Of the total incident solar radiation the proportion of PAR is:

[AIPMT PRE 2011]

(a) About 60% (b) Less than 50%
(c) More than 80% (d) About 70%

10. The rate of formation of new organic matter by rabbit in a grassland, is called:

[AIPMT MAINS 2012]

(a) Secondary productivity (b) Net primary productivity
(c) Gross primary productivity (d) Net productivity

11. Identify the likely organisms (a), (b), (c) and (d) in the food web shown below:

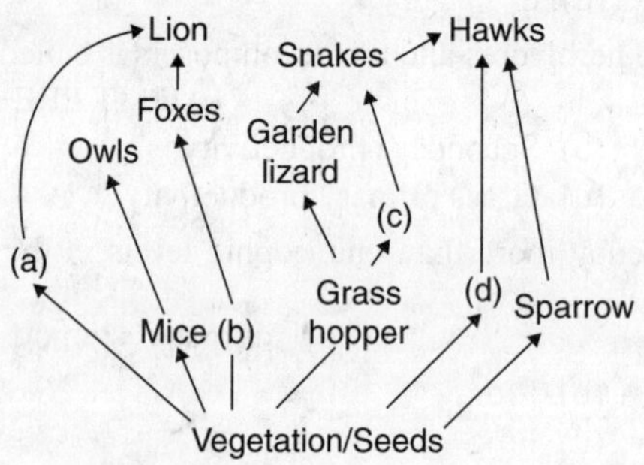

[AIPMT MAINS 2012]

Options:
(a) A: Dog, B: Squirrel, C: Bat, D: Deer
(b) A: Rat, B: Dog, C: Tortoise, D: Crow
(c) A: Squirrel, B: Cat, C: Rat, D: Pigeon
(d) A: Deer, B: Rabbit, C: Frog, D: Rat

12. The second stage of hydrosere is occupied by plants like

[AIPMT MAINS 2012]

(a) Typha (b) Salix
(c) Vallisneria (d) Azoll

13. Which one of the following is not a gaseous biogeochemical cycle in ecosystem?

[AIPMT PRE 2012]

(a) Sulphur cycle (b) Phosphorus cycle
(c) Nitrogen cycle (d) Carbon cycle

14. Identify the possible link "A" in the following feed chain:

Plant → insert → Frog → " A"→ Eagle

[AIPMT PRE 2012]

(a) Rabbit (b) Wolf
(c) Cobra (d) Parrot

15. Given below is an imaginary pyramid of numbers. What could be one of the possibilities about certain organisms at some of the different levels?

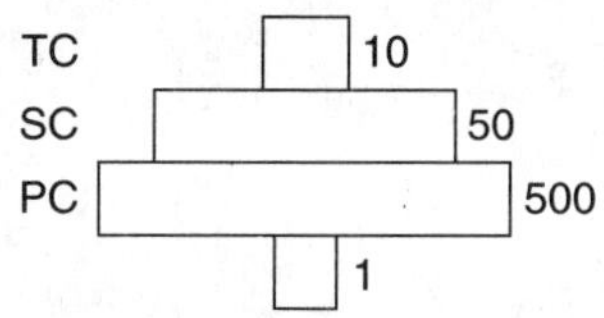

[AIPMT PRE 2012]

(a) Level PC is "insects" and level SC is "small insectivorous birds"
(b) Level PP is "phytoplanktons" in sea and "whale" on top level TC
(c) Level one PP is "pipal trees" and the level SC is "sheep"
(d) Level PC is "rats" and level SC is "cats"

16. Which one of the following is not a functional unit of an ecosystem?

[AIPMT PRE 2012]

(a) Energy flow (b) Decomposition
(c) Productivity (d) Stratification

17. The upright pyramid of number is absent in:

[AIPMT PRE 2012]

(a) Pond (b) Forest
(c) Lake (d) Grassland

18. Natural reservoir of phosphorus is:

[AIPMT 2013]

(a) Sea water (b) Animal bones
(c) Rock (d) Fossils

19. Secondary productivity is rate of formation of none organic matter by:

[AIPMT 2013]

(a) Producer (b) Parasite
(c) Consume (d) Decomposer

20. Which one of the following processes during decomposition is correctly described?

[AIPMT 2013]

(a) Fragmentation – Carried out by organisms such as earthworm
(b) Humification – Leads to the accumulation of a dark coloured substance humus which undergoes microbial action at a very fast rate
(c) Catabolism – Last step in the decomposition under fully anaerobic condition
(d) Leaching – Water soluble inorganic nutrients rise to the top layers of soil

21. Given below is a simplified model of phosphorus cycling in a terrestrial ecosystem, with four blanks (A-D). Identify the blanks.

[AIPMT 2014]

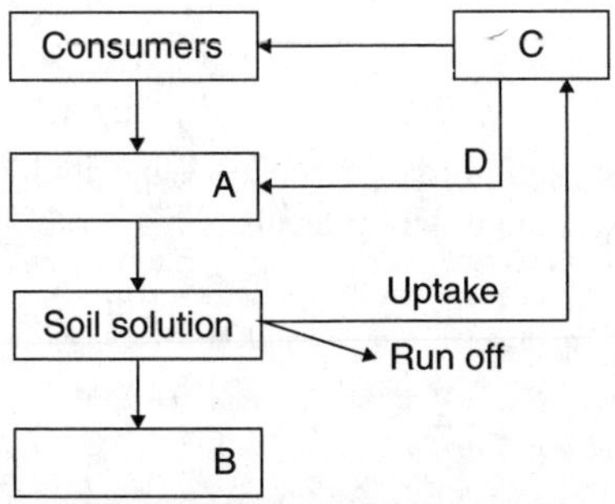

(a) A: Rock minerals, B: Detritus, C: Litter fall, D: Producers
(b) A: Litter fall, B: Producers, C: Rock minerals, D: Detritus
(c) A: Detritus, B: Rock minerals, C: Producers, D: Litter fall
(d) A: Producers, B: Litter fall, C: Rock minerals, D: Detritus

22. Match the following and select the correct option:

Column – I	Column – II
(A) Earthworm	(1) Pioneer species
(B) Succession	(2) Detritivore
(C) Ecosystem service	(3) Natality
(D) Population growth	(4) Pollination

[AIPMT 2014]

(a) A:1, B:2, C:3, D:4 (b) A:4, B:1, C:3, D:2
(c) A:3, B:2, C:4, D:1 (d) A:2, B:1, C:4, D:3

23. If 20 J of energy is trapped at producer level, then how much energy will be available to peacock as food in the following chain?

Plant $\rightarrow$ mice $\rightarrow$ snake $\rightarrow$ peacock

[AIPMT 2014]

(a) 0.02 J (b) 0.002 J
(c) 0.2 J (d) 0.0002 J

24. Secondary Succession takes place on/in

[AIPMT 2015]

(a) Bare rock (b) Degraded forest
(c) Newly created pond (d) Newly cooled lava

25. The mass of living material at a trophic level at a particular time is called

[AIPMT 2015]

(a) Gross primary productivity (b) Standing state
(c) Net primary productivity (d) Standing crop

26. In an ecosystem the rate of production of organic matter during photosynthesis is termed as:

[AIPMT 2015]

(a) Net primary productivity (b) Gross primary productivity
(c) Secondary productivity (d) Net productivity

27. During ecological succession: [RE-AIPMT 2015]

(a) The establishment of a new biotic community is very fast in its primary phase
(b) The numbers and types of animals remain constant
(c) The changes lead to a community that is in near equilibrium with the environment and is called pioneer community
(d) The gradual the predictable change in species composition occurs in a given area

28. Most animals that live in deep oceanic waters are: [RE-AIPMT 2015]

(a) Secondary consumers (b) Tertiary consumers
(c) Detritivore (d) Primary consumers

29. In which of the following both pairs have correct combination? [RE-AIPMT 2015]

(a)	Gaseous nutrient cycle	Carbon and sulphur
	Sedimentary nutrient cycle	Nitrogen and phosphorus
(b)	Gaseous nutrient cycle	Nitrogen and sulphur
	Sedimentary nutrient cycle	Carbon and phosphorus
(c)	Gaseous nutrient cycle	Sulphur and phosphorus
	Sedimentary nutrient cycle	Carbon and nitrogen
(d)	Gaseous nutrient cycle	Carbon and nitrogen
	Sedimentary nutrient cycle	Sulphur and phosphorus

Answer Keys

1. (b)	2. (d)	3. (d)	4. (d)	5. (c)	6. (a)	7. (d)	8. (d)	9. (c)	10. (a)
11. (c)	12. (b)	13. (b)	14. (d)	15. (b)	16. (c)	17. (a)	18. (b)	19. (c)	20. (b)
21. (c)	22. (c)	23. (d)	24. (d)	25. (a)	26. (d)	27. (d)	28. (b)	29. (d)	30. (b)
31. (a)	32. (a)	33. (a)	34. (d)	35. (a)	36. (d)	37. (b)	38. (d)	39. (a)	40. (a)
41. (a)	42. (c)	43. (b)	44. (b)	45. (c)	46. (d)	47. (b)	48. (a)	49. (b)	50. (c)
51. (b)	52. (b)	53. (b)	54. (a)	55. (a)	56. (c)	57. (d)	58. (a)	59. (c)	60. (a)
61. (c)	62. (a)	63. (d)	64. (b)	65. (d)	66. (c)	67. (a)	68. (d)	69. (d)	70. (a)
71. (d)	72. (d)	73. (c)	74. (d)	75. (d)	76. (b)	77. (a)	78. (b)	79. (a)	80. (d)
81. (a)	82. (a)	83. (c)	84. (b)	85. (d)	86. (d)	87. (c)	88. (c)	89. (c)	90. (a)
91. (d)	92. (a)	93. (d)	94. (c)	95. (a)	96. (a)	97. (b)	98. (b)	99. (a)	100. (d)
101. (a)	102. (d)	103. (a)	104. (b)	105. (b)	106. (d)	107. (d)	108. (d)	109. (c)	110. (a)
111. (d)	112. (d)	113. (b)	114. (d)	115. (d)	116. (d)	117. (b)	118. (d)	119. (a)	120. (d)
121. (a)	122. (a)	123. (b)	124. (b)	125. (c)	126. (b)	127. (b)	128. (a)	129. (a)	130. (c)
131. (a)	132. (a)								

AIPMT Previous Year Questions

1. (c)	2. (a)	3. (a)	4. (a)	5. (b)	6. (a)	7. (b)	8. (d)	9. (b)	10. (a)
11. (d)	12. (c)	13. (b)	14. (c)	15. (a)	16. (d)	17. (b)	18. (c)	19. (c)	20. (a)
21. (c)	22. (d)	23. (a)	24. (b)	25. (d)	26. (b)	27. (d)	28. (c)	29. (d)	

CHAPTER

37

Biodiversity and Conservation

1. Match Column-I (organism) with Column-II.

Column-I	Column-II (number of species)
1. Ants	A. 20,000
2. Orchids	B. 25,000
3. Fishes	C. 28,000
4. Beetles	D. 3,00,000

(a) 1:D, 2:C, 3:B, 4:A
(b) 1:B. 2:A, 3:C, 4:D
(c) 1:A, 2:B, 3:C, 4:D
(d) 1:A, 2:A, 3:C, 4:D

2. The term 'Biodiversity' was popularized by
(a) Robert May
(b) A. Von Humboldt
(c) Edward Wilson
(d) Paul Ehrlich

3. Identify the type/level of biodiversity from the following:
(a) Genetic
(b) Species
(c) Ecological
(d) All of these

4. Which of the following show maximum genetic diversity?
(a) Rice
(b) Mango
(c) Rauwolfia vomitoria
(d) Wheat

5. How many different varieties of mango are found in India?
(a) 50,000
(b) 5,000
(c) 2,000
(d) 1,000

6. How many genetically different strains of rice are found in India?
(a) 50,000
(b) 5,000
(c) 2,000
(d) 1,000

7. Choose correct statement from the following
(A) Western Ghats have a greater amphibian species diversity than the Eastern Ghats.
(B) Diversity exists at all levels of biological organization ranging from macromolecules within cells to biomes.
(C) Rauwolfia Vomitoria shows genetic variation in terms of potency and concentration of the reserpine produced.
(D) Norway has greater ecosystem diversity than India.
(a) A and B only
(b) B and D only
(c) A, B and C only
(d) D only

8. If the present rate of species losses continues, we will lose our biological wealth in how much time?
   (a) Less than one century (b) Less than 2 centuries
   (c) Less than 50 years (d) Next 20 years
9. Robert May places the global species diversity at about ________ million.
   (a) 2 (b) 3
   (c) 6 (d) 7
10. More than ________ % of all species recorded are animals.
    (a) 60 (b) 70
    (c) 90 (d) 10
11. Arrange following in their decreasing order of species.
    Fishes, Birds, Reptiles, Amphibian
    (a) Fishes > Birds > Reptiles > Amphibian (b) Fishes > Reptiles > Birds > Amphibian
    (c) Reptiles > Fishes > Birds > Amphibian (d) Amphibian > Fishes > Birds > Reptiles
12. Which of following have more number of species?
    (a) Fungi (b) Mosses
    (c) Angiosperm (d) Lichens
13. Which order is correct with respect to the number of species?
    (a) Fungi > Algae > Lichens > Angiosperm (b) Angiosperm > Fungi > Algae > Lichen
    (c) Fungi > Angiosperm > Algae > Lichen (d) Mosses > Ferns > Algae > Lichens
14. What does A, B, C, D, E and F represent in this figure?

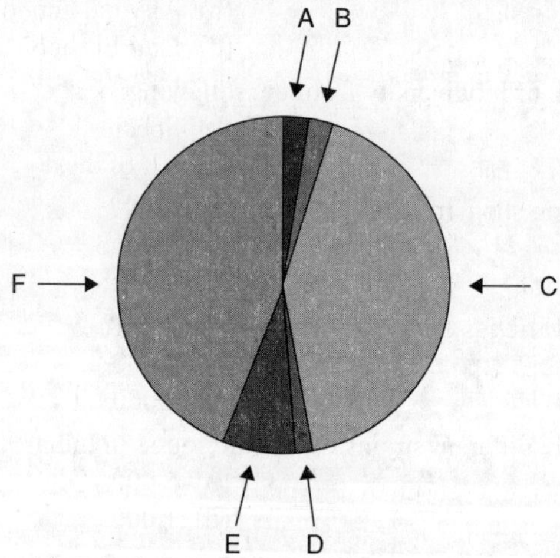

π-chart for number of species of major taxa of plants.
    (a) A: Ferns and allies, B: Mosses, C: Algae, D: Fungi, E: Lichens, F: Angiosperms
    (b) A: Fungi, B: Mosses, C: Lichens, D: Ferns and allies, E: Angiosperms, F: Algae
    (c) A: Angiosperms, B: Ferns and allies, C: Fungi, D: Lichens, E: Algae, F: Mosses
    (d) A: Mosses, B: Ferns and allies, C: Angiosperms, D: Lichens, E: Algae, F: Fungi

15. Find the false statement.
(a) The number of fungi species is more than the combined total of the species of fishes, amphibians, reptiles and mammals.
(b) Conventional taxonomic methods are not suitable for identifying microbial species.
(c) For many taxonomic groups, species inventories are more complete in temperate than in tropical countries.
(d) Insects form 70% part of all the species recorded.

16. Find the true statement.
A. If we consider biochemical or molecular criteria for micro-organisms, their diversity may run into millions.
B. There are 12 mega diversity countries in the world.
C. If we accept May's global estimates, only 32% of total species have been recorded so far.
D. Western Ghats have a greater amphibian species diversity than Eastern Ghats.
(a) A and B only
(b) D only
(c) A and D only
(d) A, B and D only

17. India has only _________ percent of the world's land area; its share of the global species diversity is an impressive _________ percent.
(a) 4.2, 1.8
(b) 2.4, 8.1
(c) 2.4, 13
(d) 4.2, 13

18. Match Column-I (Place) with Column-II (No. of bird species).

Column–I	Column –II
1. Colombia	A. 12,00
2. New York	B. 13,00
3. India	C. 14,00
4. Amazonian rain forest	D. 105

(a) A:3, B:4, C:2, D:1
(b) A:2, B:1, C:4, D:3
(c) A:2, B:4, C:3, D:1
(d) A:3, B:4, C:1, D:2

19. Find incorrect statement.
(a) India has nearly 45,000 species of plants and twice as many of animals.
(b) A forest in a tropical region like equator has 10 times as many species of vascular plants as a forest of equal area in a temperate region like the mid west of the USA.
(c) Greenland 71° N has only 56 species of birds.
(d) The diversity of plant and animals is uniform throughout the world.

20. The largely tropical Amazonian rain forest in South America has the greatest biodiversity on earth. It is home for more than _________ species of plants. _________ of fishes, _________ of birds, _________ of mammals, _________ of amphibians, _________ of reptiles and of more than _________ invertebrates.
(a) 30,000, 4000, 1200, 427, 427, 387, 1,25,000
(b) 40,000, 3000, 1200, 427, 427, 387, 1,25,000
(c) 40,000, 3000, 1300, 427, 427, 378, 1,25,000
(d) 40,000, 3000, 1200, 427, 427, 378, 1,25,000

21. What is the sum of the number of species of birds in New York 41° N and Greenland of 71° N.
(a) 112
(b) 161
(c) 170
(d) 56

22. Species richness of tropics is because of
(a) Tropics have more evolutionary time.
(b) Tropics have relatively constant environment.
(c) Tropics receive more solar energy.
(d) All of the above

23. Species–area relationship was provided by
(a) Alexander Van Humboldt (b) Robert May
(c) Paul Ehrlich (d) Edward Wilson

24. The graph formed by plotting species richness against area for a wide variety of taxa (angiosperm plants, birds, bats, fresh water fishes, etc.) turns out to be a:
(a) Parabola (b) Straight line
(c) Rectangular hyperbola (d) Any of the above

25. log S = log C + Z log A (Logarithmic formula for species–area relationship). True about this formula
(a) S = Species richness A = Area (b) Z = Regression Coefficient
(c) C = Y-intercept (d) All of the above

26. If we analyze species–area relationship among very large area like entire continents, slope of line becomes
(a) Less steeper (b) Vertical
(c) Much steeper (d) Horizontal

27. Z-value in a much steeper slope ranges between
(a) 0.6 to 1.2 (b) 0.1 to 1.2
(c) 0.01 to 0.02 (d) 0.6 to 0.12

28. For frugivorous (fruit-eating) birds and mammals in the tropical forests of different continents, the slope of species–area relationship is foud to be approx
(a) 0.6 (b) 1.3
(c) 1.15 (d) 1

29. Which is the correct formula of the graph shown below? Given:

S-species richness
A-Area
C-Y-intercept
Z-Slope of line (regression coefficient)

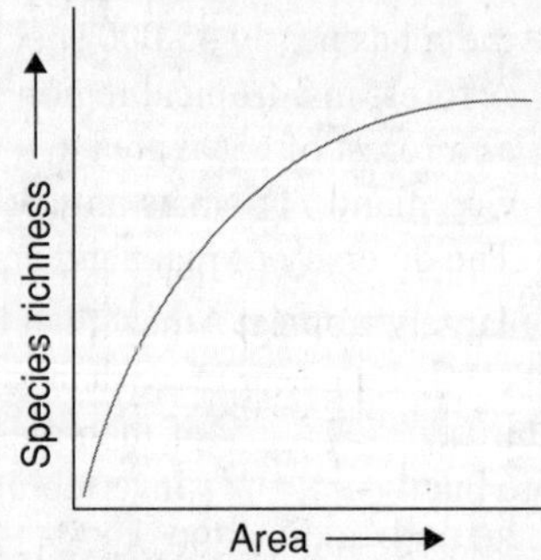

(a) $S = CA^Z$ (b) $S = CZ^A$
(c) $S = ZC^A$ (d) $Z = SC^A$

30. 'Z' value in species–area relationship lies in the rage of 0.1 to 0.2 for
(a) Plants in Britain (b) Birds in California
(c) Molluscs in New York State (d) All of the above

31. Followings are the features of a stable community
(a) Resistant or resilient to occasional disturbances (Natural or Anthropogenic)
(b) Not show much variation in productivity
(c) Resistant to invasion by alien species
(d) All of the above

32. There are two plots Plot '1' has less species and Plot '2' has more species. Which statement is true regarding the two plots?
(a) Plot '1' shows less year to year variation in total biomass.
(b) Plot '2' is less resistant to natural disturbance.
(c) Plot '1' has more productivity than plot '2'.
(d) Plot '2' has more productivity than plot '1'.

33. Rivet popper hypothesis was proposed by
(a) Robert May (b) A. Von Humboldt
(c) Paul Ehrlich (d) Edward Wilson

34. Tropical environments, unlike temperate ones, are
(a) Less seasonal (b) Relatively more constant
(c) More predictable (d) All of the above

35. Find the incorrect statement.
(a) Constant environment promote niche specialization.
(b) Key species are those which derive major ecosystem functions.
(c) Increase in diversity generally increases productivity.
(d) Increased steepness in species–area relationship curve decreases species richness in a given area.

36. The colonization of tropical Pacific Islands by humans led to extinction of more than, ________ species of native birds
(a) 2000 (b) 50
(c) 4000 (d) 3000

37. IUCN Red list (b004) documents the extinction of how many species in last 500 years?
(a) 784 (b) 874
(c) 478 (d) 487

38. Match the Column- I (Recently extinct animals) with Column-II (Places from where they are extinct).

Column-I	Column-II
A. Dodo	1. Russia
B. Quagga	2. Australia
C. Thylacine	3. Africa
D. Steller's sea cow	4. Mauritius

(a) A:1, B:2, C:3, D:4 (b) A:4, B:3, C:2, D:1
(c) A:4, B:2, C:3, D:1 (d) A:4, B:1, C:2, D:3

39. Find the false statement.

(A) In the last 20 years alone there is a disappearance of 27 species.
(B) Three species (Bali, Javan and Caspian) of tiger are included in recently extinct animals.
(C) If we apply May's estimate then there are probably more than 1,00,000 plant species in India that are yet to be discovered and described.
(D) There is more solar energy available in tropics, which contribute to higher productivity; this in turn contributes directly to greater diversity.

(a) A only (b) C, D only
(c) B, D only (d) A and C only

40. According to the IUCN Red list (2004) how many vertebrates became extinct in the last 550 years?

(a) 359 (b) 338
(c) 487 (d) 87

41. According to IUCN Red list (2004) how many invertebrates became extinct in the last 500 years?

(a) 359 (b) 338
(c) 784 (d) 87

42. Which group is most vulnerable to extinction?

(a) Fishes (b) Amphibians
(c) Reptiles (d) Birds

43. Approximately how many species face the threat of extinction?

(a) 3000 (b) 1500
(c) 15,500 (d) 70,000

44. Presently_________% of all bird species, _________% of all mammals species, _________% of all amphibian species and _________% of all gymnosperm species in the world face the threat of extinction.

(a) 23, 32, 12, 31
(b) 12, 23, 32, 31
(c) 12, 23, 31, 32
(d) 23, 12, 32, 81

45. Since the origin and diversification of life on earth how many episodes of mass extinction of species have occurred till date?

(a) 2 (b) 3
(c) 4 (d) 5

46. What is the A, B, C and D in this figure?

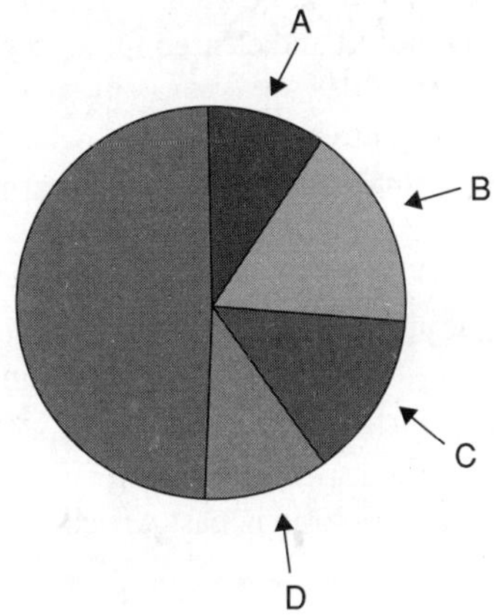

π-chart for number of species of major taxa of vertebrates

(a) A: Mammals, B: Birds, C: Reptiles, D: Amphibians
(b) A: Amphibians, B: Birds, C: Mammals, D: Reptiles
(c) A: Reptiles, B: Amphibians, C: Birds, D: mammals
(d) A: Mammals, B: Reptiles, C: Birds, D: Amphibians

47. The current rate of species extinction is how many times faster than the pre-human time?

(a) 10 to 50 times
(b) 100 to 1000 times
(c) 1000 to 10,000 times
(d) 10,000 to 1,00,000 times

48. Find the incorrect statement.

(a) 'Sixth extinction' is different from previous extinction in terms of rate of extinction.
(b) Ecologist warn that if the present trend of extinction continues, nearly 50% all species on earth might be wiped out within the next 100 years.
(c) Amphibians appear to be vulnerable to extinction.
(d) Recent extinction is completely natural.

49. Loss of biodiversity in a region may lead to

(a) Decline in plants production
(b) Lowered resistance to environmental perturbations such as draught.
(c) Increased variability in certain ecosystem processes such as plant productivity, water use, and pest and disease cycle.
(d) All of the above

50. Which of the following is major cause of loss of biodiversity?

(a) Habitat loss and fragmentation
(b) Over-exploitation
(c) Alien species invasion
(d) Co-extinction

51. Most dramatic examples of habitat loss comes from the

(a) Tropical rain forests
(b) Temperate forests
(c) Grasslands
(d) Deserts

52. Find the incorrect statement from the following.
(A) Tropic rain forests cover around 6% of earth's land surface.
(B) Amazonian rain forest is being cut and cleared for soya bean cultivation or for conversion to grasslands for raising beef cattle.
(C) Animals with migratory habits are badly affected by habitat loss and fragmentation.
(D) Mammals and birds require small territories.
(a) A and B only
(b) A and D only
(c) D only
(d) B and C only

53. Steller's sea cow and Passenger pigeon became extinct due to
(a) Alien species invasion
(b) Co-extinction
(c) Habitat loss and fragmentation
(d) Over exploitation

54. Which of these are examples of alien species invasion?
(a) Nile perch introduced in Lake Victoria in east Africa
(b) African catfish in Indian River
(c) Water hyacinth in India
(d) All of the above

55. Which of these are invasive weeds?
(a) Carrot grass (Parthenium)
(b) Gandhari (lantana)
(c) Water hyacinth (Eicchornia)
(d) All of the above

56. Co-extinction means
(a) Introduction of alien species leading to decline or extinction of indigenous species
(b) Extinction due to over exploitation
(c) Extinction due to Habitat loss
(d) Extinction due to obligatory association of plant or animal

57. Which of these is not a narrowly utilitarian argument for conserving biodiversity?
(a) Food
(b) Medicine
(c) Construction material
(d) Pollination

58. All are examples of broadly utilitarian except
(a) Pollination
(b) Oxygen
(c) Aesthetic pleasure of walking through thick woods
(d) Firewood

59. Find the incorrect statement from the following.
(a) Introduction of Nile perch in Lake Victoria in east Africa lead to extinction of more than 200 species of cichlid fish in the lake.
(b) Fast dwindling Amazon forest is estimated to produce, through photosynthesis, 20% of the total oxygen in the earth's atmosphere.
(c) More than 25% of drugs currently sold worldwide are derived from plants.
(d) Illegal introduction of American catfish Clarias gariepinus for aquaculture purpose is posing threat to indigenous cat fishes in our rivers.

60. 'We save the entire forest to save the tiger'. This approach of conservation is
(a) In situ
(b) Ex situ
(c) In vitro
(d) In vivo

61. What percentage of the earth's land area is covered by all biodiversity hotspots put together?
(a) 6% (b) 10%
(c) 2% (d) 15%

62. Following are examples of ex situ conservation except
(a) Zoological parks (b) Botanical garden
(c) Wildlife safari park (d) Biosphere reserve

63. Following are example of In situ conservation except?
(a) Biosphere reverse (b) National park
(c) Sacred groves (d) Gene-bank

64. Hotspots are characterized by
(a) Very high species richness (b) High degree of endemism
(c) Region of accelerated habitat loss (d) All of the above

65. In India, ecologically unique and biodiversity rich regions are legally protected as
(a) Biosphere reserve (b) National park
(c) Sanctuaries (d) All

66. The Earth Summit (Historic Convention on Biological Diversity) was held in
(a) Johannesburg, South Africa, 2002 (b) Rio De Janerio, 1992
(c) Kyoto, Japan (d) Montreal, Canada

67. World Summit on sustainable development was held in
(a) Johannesburg, South Africa, 2002 (b) Rio De Janerio, 1992
(c) Kyoto, Japan (d) Montreal, Canada

68. Which of these are hotspots of India?
(a) Western Ghats (b) Himalaya
(c) Indo-Burma (d) All of the above

69. Ex situ conservation include
(a) Cryopreservation of gametes (b) In vitro fertilization
(c) Tissue culture (d) All of the above

70. The reasons for biodiversity conservation are
(a) Broadly utilization (b) Narrowly utilization
(c) Ethical (d) All of the above

71. Following are broadly utilitarian except
(a) Pest control (b) Flood control
(c) Climate moderation (d) Pharmaceuticals

72. In the World Summit on sustainable development held in 2002 in Johannesburg, South Africa, how many countries pledged their commitment to achieve a significant reduction in the current rate of biodiversity loss at global, regions and local levels, by 2010?
(a) 100 (b) 180
(c) 190 (d) 200

73. Sacred groves are present in
(a) Khasi and Jaintia Hills in Meghalaya
(b) Aravalli Hills of Rajasthan
(c) Western Ghat regions of Karnataka and Maharashtra
(d) All of the above

74. How do ecologists estimate the total number of species present in the world?
(a) By counting them all
(b) By counting the number of any one species and applying this to various genus.
(c) By making statistical comparison of the temperate–tropical species richness of an exhaustively studied group of insects and extrapolating this ratio to other group of animals and plants.
(d) By calculating biomass of all the species

75. The species diversity of plants (22%) is much less than that of animals (72%), what could be the explanation to how animals achieved greater diversification?
(a) Animal are non-motile.
(b) Their movement to diverse habitats resulted in more evolutionary changes occurring in animals.
(c) Animals use carbohydrate and lipid as a source of energy
(d) Animal DNA is different from plant DNA in terms of type of nitrogen bases.

76. Which extinction is presently in progress?
(a) Fifth (b) Sixth (c) Forth (d) Third

77. Identify A, B, C and D in this figure.

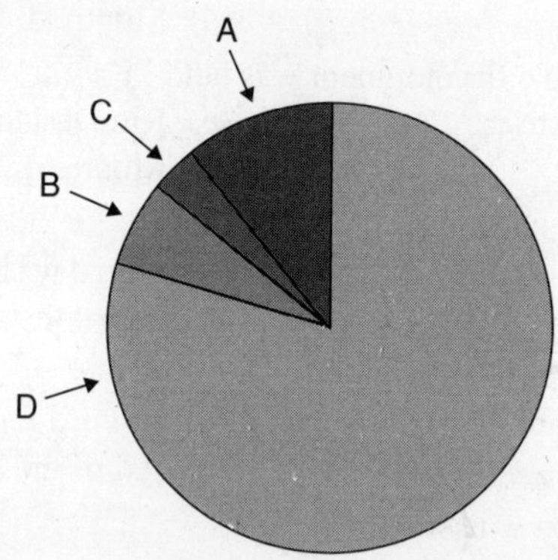

π-chart for number of species of major taxa of Invertebrates
(a) A: Insects, B: Crustaceans, C: Molluscs, D: Other animal groups
(b) A: Other animal groups, B: Molluscs, C: Crustaceans, D: Insects
(c) A: Molluscs, B: Insects, C: Other animal groups, D: Crustaceans
(d) A: Insects, B: Molluscs, C: Crustaceans, D: Other animal groups

78. Which of the following require large territories?
(a) Birds (b) Amphibians
(b) Mammals (d) Both (a) and (c)

79. Presently which of the following face maximum threat of extinction?
(a) Birds (b) Amphibians
(c) Mammals (d) Gymnosperm

80. Loss of biodiversity in a region leads to increase in variability in certain ecosystem processes like
(a) Plant productivity (b) Water use
(c) Pest and disease cycle (d) All of these

81. Gametes of threatened species can be preserved in viable and fertile condition for long periods using
(a) PCR technique (b) CTAB
(c) Cryopreservation technique (d) In situ conservation

82. At present, how many biosphere reserves does India have?
(a) 11 (b) 14 (c) 17 (d) 20

83. How many biodiversity hotspots are found in the world?
(a) 25 (b) 34 (c) 9 (d) 20

84. Hotspot is a region of
(a) Endemism (b) Accelerated habitat loss
(c) Low level of species richness (d) Both (a) and (b)

85. Following are direct benefits from biodiversity except
(a) Firewood (b) Fibre (c) Food (d) Pollination

86. Following are indirect benefits from biodiversity except?
(a) Pest control (b) Climate moderation
(c) Flood control (d) Dyes, resins and perfumes

87. Which area of M.P. (Madhya Pradesh) contain sacred groves?
(a) Sarguja (b) Chanda (c) Bastar (d) All of these

88. Find the incorrect match.

(a) Pollinator – Bees, Bumblebees, Bats and Birds
(b) Legally protected biodiversity rich region – Biosphere reserve, National park, wildlife sanctuaries, sacred groves
(c) Lung of planet – Amazonian rain forest
(d) Rivet popper hypothesis – Harvard ecologist Paul Ehrlich

89. Stellar's Sea cow became extinct from
(a) Mauritius (b) Africa (c) Russia (d) Australia

90. Strict protection of hotspots can reduce ongoing mass extinction by
(a) 20% (b) 30% (c) 40% (d) 50%

*Read the **assertion** and **reason** carefully to mark the correct option out of the options given below:*

(a) If both the assertion and the reason are true and the reason is a correct explanation of the assertion
(b) If both the assertion and reason are true but the reason is not a correct explanation of the assertion
(c) If the assertion is true but the reason is false
(d) If both the assertion and reason are false

91. Assertion: Current estimates do not give any figure for prokaryotes taxonomic.
Reason: Conventional taxonomic methods are not suitable for identifying microbial species.

92. Assertion: Tropics have greater biological diversity.
Reason: Tropics have long evolutionary time for species diversification is one of the reasons.

93. **Assertion:** Stable community must be either resistant or resilient to occasional disturbances.
Reason: Stable community not shows too much variation in productivity from year to year.

94. **Assertion:** Sixth extinction presently in progress different from the previous episode.
Reason: Difference is in the rate; current species extinction rates are estimated to be 100 to 1000 times faster than in the pre-human times.

95. **Assertion:** Bioremediation is the use of living organisms, usually prokaryotes, fungi plants, to detoxify polluted ecosystems.
Reason: Biological augmentation uses organisms to add essential materials to a degraded ecosystem.

96. **Assertion:** Steller's sea cow becomes extinct.
Reason: It is due to over exploitation by humans.

97. **Assertion:** Biodiversity hotspots are example of in situ conservation.
Reason: It is conservation of biological wealth on site.

98. **Assertion:** Ex-situ conservation is carried out in biosphere reserves, national parks and sanctuaries.
Reason: NGOs are involved in maintenance of these protected areas.

99. **Assertion:** Insects are enormously diversified.
Reason: It is because of the presence of exoskeleton made up of chitin.

100. **Assertion:** Habitat loss and fragmentaion is the most important cause driving animals and plants to extinction.
Reason: Habitat loss and fragmentaion causes alien species invasion.

AIPMT PREVIOUS YEAR QUESTIONS

1. Which one of the following is an example of ex-situ conservation?
[AIPMT PRE 2010]
(a) Wildlife sanctuary
(b) Seed bank
(c) Sacred groves
(d) National park

2. Biodiversity of a geographical region represents
[AIPMT MAINS 2011]
(a) Endangered species found in the region
(b) The diversity in the organism living in the region
(c) Genetic diversity in the dominant species of the region
(d) Species endemic to the region

3. Large woody vines are more commonly found in
[AIPMT PRE 2011]
(a) Mangroves
(b) Tropical rainforests
(c) Alpine forests
(d) Temperate-forests

4. Which one of the following shows maximum genetic diversity in India?
[AIPMT PRE 2011]
(a) Rice
(b) Maize
(c) Mango
(d) Groundnut

5. Select the correct statement about biodiversity [AIPMT MAINS 2012]
   (a) Large scale planting of Bt cotton has no adverse effect on biodiversity
   (b) Western Ghats have a very high degree of species richness and endemism
   (c) Conservation of biodiversity is just a fad pursued by the developed countries
   (d) The desert areas of Rajasthan and Gujarat have a very high level of desert animal species as well as numerous rare animals

6. Sacred groves are specially useful in: [AIPMT MAINS 2012]
   (a) Preventing soil erosion
   (b) Year-round flow of water in rivers
   (c) Conserving rare and threatened species
   (d) Generating environmental awareness

7. Which one of the following areas in India is a hotspot of biodiversity? [AIPMT PRE 2012]
   (a) Eastern Ghats
   (b) Gangetic Plain
   (c) Sunderbans
   (d) Western Ghats

8. The highest number of species in the world is represented by: [AIPMT PRE 2012]
   (a) Fungi
   (b) Mosses
   (c) Algae
   (d) Lichens

9. Which of the following is not used for ex situ plant conservation? [AIPMT 2013]
   (a) Field gene banks
   (b) Seed banks
   (c) Shifting cultivation
   (d) Botanical Gardens

10. Which of the following represent maximum number of species among global biodiversity? [AIPMT 2013]
   (a) Algae
   (b) Lichens
   (c) Fungi
   (d) Mosses and Ferns

11. An example of ex situ conservation is: [AIPMT 2014]
   (a) National Park
   (b) Seed Bank
   (c) Wildlife Sanctuary
   (d) Sacred Grove

12. A species facing extremely high risk of extinction in the immediate future is called: [AIPMT 2014]
   (a) Vulnerable
   (b) Endemic
   (c) Critically Endangered
   (d) Extinct

13. The organization which publishes the Red list of species is: [AIPMT 2014]
   (a) ICFRE
   (b) IUCN
   (c) UNEP
   (d) WWF

14. Given below is the representation of the extent of global diversity of invertebrates. What groups the four portions (A-D) represent respectively?

[AIPMT 2014]

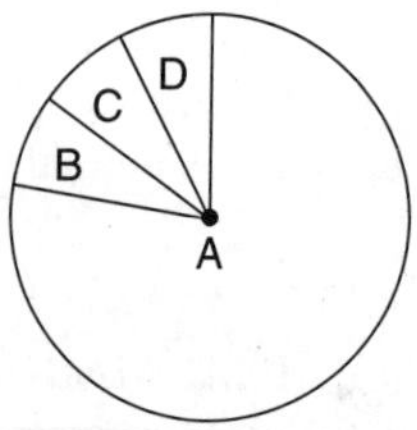

(a) A: Insects, B: Crustaceans, C: Other animal groups, D: Molluscs
(b) A: Crustaceans, B: Insects, C: Molluscs, D: Other animal groups
(c) A: Molluscs, B: Other animal groups, C: Crustaceans, D: Insects
(d) A: Insects, B: Molluscs, C: Crustaceans, D: Other animal groups

15. Vertical distribution of different species occupying different levels in a biotic community is known as:
(a) Divergence (b) Stratification
(c) Zonation (d) Pyramid

16. In which of the following both pairs have correct combination?

[AIPMT 2015]

(a) In situ conservation : National park
Ex situ conservation : Botanical Garden
(b) In situ conservation : Cryopreservation
Ex situ conservation : Wildlife Sanctuary
(c) In situ conservation : Seed Bank
Ex situ conservation : National park
(d) In situ conservation : Tissue culture
Ex situ conservation : Sacred groves

17. Which of the following characteristics is mainly responsible for diversification of insects of land?

[AIPMT 2015]

(a) Segmentation (b) Bilateral symmetry
(c) Exoskeleton (d) Eyes

18. Most animals are tree dwellers in a

[AIPMT 2015]

(a) Coniferous forest (b) Thorn woodland
(c) Temperature deciduous forest (d) Tropical rain forest

19. Cryopreservation of gametes of threatened species in viable and fertile condition can be referred to as

[AIPMT 2015]

(a) In situ conservation of biodiversity
(b) Advanced ex-situ conservation of biodiversity
(c) In situ conservation by sacred groves
(d) In situ cryo-conservation of biodiversity

20. The species confined to a particular region and not found elsewhere is termed as: [RE-AIPMT 2015]

(a) Alien (b) Endemic
(c) Rare (d) Keystone

Answer Keys

1. (d)	2. (c)	3. (d)	4. (a)	5. (d)	6. (a)	7. (c)	8. (b)	9. (d)	10. (b)
11. (a)	12. (a)	13. (c)	14. (d)	15. (d)	16. (d)	17. (b)	18. (d)	19. (d)	20. (c)
21. (b)	22. (d)	23. (a)	24. (c)	25. (d)	26. (c)	27. (a)	28. (c)	29. (a)	30. (d)
31. (d)	32. (d)	33. (c)	34. (d)	35. (d)	36. (a)	37. (a)	38. (b)	39. (c)	40. (b)
41. (a)	42. (b)	43. (c)	44. (b)	45. (d)	46. (a)	47. (b)	48. (d)	49. (d)	50. (a)
51. (a)	52. (c)	53. (d)	54. (d)	55. (d)	56. (d)	57. (d)	58. (d)	59. (d)	60. (a)
61. (c)	62. (d)	63. (d)	64. (d)	65. (d)	66. (b)	67. (a)	68. (d)	69. (d)	70. (d)
71. (d)	72. (c)	73. (d)	74. (c)	75. (b)	76. (b)	77. (b)	78. (d)	79. (b)	80. (d)
81. (c)	82. (c)	83. (b)	84. (d)	85. (d)	86. (d)	87. (d)	88. (d)	89. (c)	90. (b)
91. (a)	92. (a)	93. (b)	94. (a)	95. (b)	96. (a)	97. (a)	98. (d)	99. (a)	100. (c)

AIPMT Previous Year Questions

1. (b)	2. (b)	3. (d)	4. (a)	5. (b)	6. (a)	7. (d)	8. (a)	9. (c)	10. (c)
11. (b)	12. (c)	13. (b)	14. (d)	15. (b)	16. (a)	17. (c)	18. (d)	19. (b)	20. (b)

CHAPTER

38 Environmental Issues

1. Pollution is any undesirable change in physical, chemical or biological characteristics of:
   (a) Air
   (b) Land
   (c) Water or soil
   (d) All of the above
2. Agents which cause pollution are known as:
   (a) Mutants
   (b) Carcinogens
   (c) Pollutants
   (d) Allergens
3. In which year did Government of India pass the Environment (Protection) Act to protect and improve the quality of environment (air, water and soil)?
   (a) 1978
   (b) 1986
   (c) 1981
   (d) 1987
4. What are the effects of air pollution on plants?
   (a) Growth retardation
   (b) Decrease in yield
   (c) Premature death
   (d) All of the above
5. Which system of humans and animals are affected mostly by air pollution?
   (a) Respiratory system
   (b) Digestive system
   (c) Circulatory system
   (d) Excretory system
6. Harmful effects of air pollution depends on:
   (a) Concentration of pollutants
   (b) Duration of exposure
   (c) Type of organism
   (d) All of the above
7. The most widely used and effective device for removing particulate matter is:
   (a) Arrester
   (b) Scrubber
   (c) Electrostatic precipitator
   (d) Converters
8. Identify A, B, C and D in the diagram

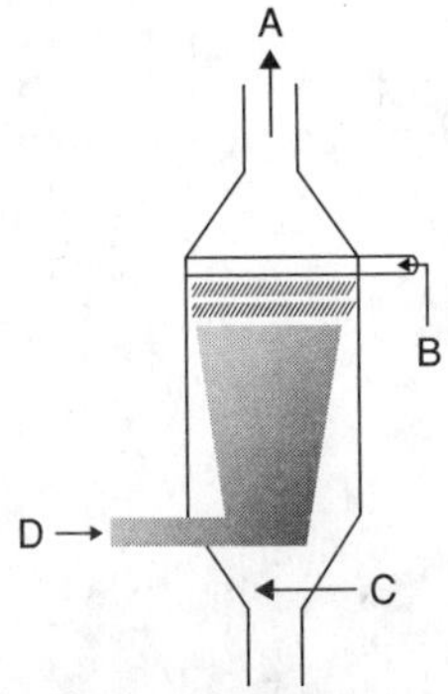

Scrubber

(a) A: Dirty air, B: Water line spray, C: Clean air, D: Particulate matter
(b) A: Clean air, B: Water line spray, C: Particulate matter, D: Dirty air
(c) A: Water line spray, B: Particulate matter, C: Clean air, D: Dirty air
(d) A: Particulate matter, B: Dirty air, C: Clean air, D: Water line spray

9. ESP removes approx ________% of particulate matter present in exhaust from a thermal power plant.
(a) 60% (b) 80%
(c) 99% (d) 85%

10. Which is incorrect about ESP (Electrostatic Precipitator)?
(a) Corona produces electrons
(b) Collecting plates are grounded, so use to attract the charged dust particle
(c) Velocity of air between the plates must be low
(d) Electrodes wires that are maintained at hundred volts produces corona.

11. Scrubber is used to remove following gas
(a) SO_2 (b) N_2
(c) O_2 (d) CO_2

12. According to CPCB which particulate size causes greatest harm to human health?
(a) 2.5 μm (b) 3.5 μm
(c) 4.5 μm (d) 5.2 μm

13. PM 2.5 or less than that in diameter in air causes:
(a) Irritation and inflammation in lungs (b) Damage to lungs
(c) Premature deaths (d) All of the above

14. ________ is a major cause of air pollution in metro cities
(a) Factory (b) Automobiles
(c) Smoking (d) Thermal power plant

15. Automobile pollution is reduced by using:
(a) Lead-free petrol or diesel (b) Catalytic converters
(c) Both (a) and (b) (d) None of the above

16. The metal used in catalytic converter in automobiles is:
(a) Platinum (b) Palladium
(c) Rhodium (d) Any of the above

17. What is/are done by catalytic converters?
(a) Unburnt hydrocarbons are converted to CO_2 and H_2O.
(b) CO in converted to CO_2.
(c) Nitric oxide is changed to N_2.
(d) All of the above

18. Motor vehicle equipped with catalytic converters should use unleaded petrol because:
(a) Lead activates the catalyst (b) Lead deactivates catalyst
(c) Lead increase fuel efficiency. (d) Lead decrease fuel efficiency.

19. Match the columns.

Column–I	Column–II
A. Air (Prevention and Control of Pollution) Act	1. 1987
B. Water (Prevention and Control of Pollution) Act	2. 1981
C. Noise added as air pollutant	3. 1974
D. Environment (Protection) Act	4. 1986

(a) A:2, B:3, C:4, D:1 (b) A:2, B:3, C:1, D:4
(c) A:4, B:3, C:2, D:1 (d) A:4, B:3, C:1, D:2

20. Noise is undesirable high level of sound and causes all of these except;
(a) Psychological disorder (b) Increased heart beat
(c) Altered breathing pattern (d) Sleepiness

21. A brief exposes of extremely high sound level, of ________ or more generated by takeoff of jet plane or rocket, may damage ear drums thus permanently impairing hearting ability.
(a) 80 dB (b) 20 dB
(c) 150 dB (d) 60 dB

22. Which of these measures can be adopted to control noise pollution?
(a) Areas around hospitals and schools should be made Horn-free zones.
(b) Use of loud-speaker should be restricted to a fixed intensity and fixed hours of the day,
(c) Occupational exposure to noise can be reduced by using cotton plugs.
(d) All of the above

23. In the 1990s Delhi ranked ________ among the 41 most polluted cities in the world.
(a) 1st (b) 2nd
(c) 3rd (d) 4th

24. CNG is better fuel than petrol or diesel because CNG:
(a) Burns efficiently (b) Cannot be siphoned off and adulterated
(c) Non-carcinogenic and non-corrosive (d) All of the above

25. According to Euro II norms, sulphur should be controlled at ________ in diesel and ________ in petrol.
(a) 350 ppm, 150 ppm (b) 50 ppm, 150 ppm
(c) 50 ppm, 50 ppm (d) 350 ppm, 50 ppm

26. Four wheelers have to follow Bharat stage IV in how many mega cities of India since April, 2010?
(a) 11 (b) 12
(c) 13 (d) 14

27. Bharat stage III is applicable to 2 and 3 wheelers throughout the country since:
(a) 2008 (b) 2009
(c) 2010 (d) 2011

28. What is the minimum percentage of impurity that makes domestic sewage unfit for human use?
(a) 0.1% (b) 1%
(c) 3% (d) 10%

29. Match the columns for the composition of waste water which contains 0.1% impurities.

Column–I	Column–II
A. Suspended solid	1. Nitrate, NH_3, sodium, calcium and phosphate
B. Colloidal material	2. Fecal matter, bacteria, cloth and paper
C. Dissolved material	3. Sand, silt and clay

(a) A:1, B:2, C:3
(b) A:3, B:2, C:1
(c) A:2, B:3, C:1
(d) A:1, B:3, C:2

30. Identify A, B and C in the figure.

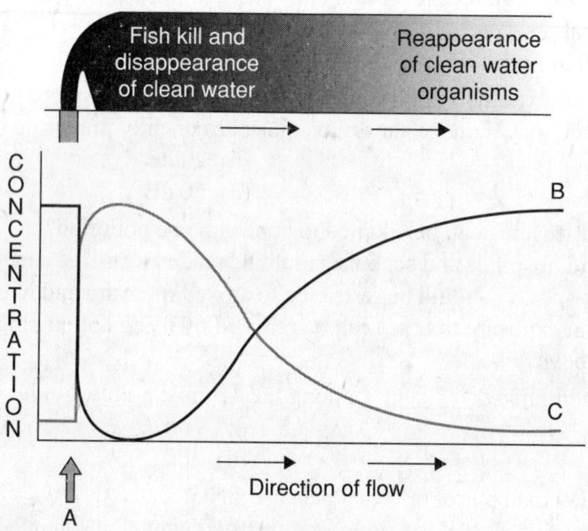

(a) A: Dissolved oxygen, B: BOD, C: Sewage discharge
(b) A: Sewage discharge, B: Dissolved oxygen, C: BOD
(c) A: BOD, B: Sewage discharge, C: Dissolved oxygen
(d) A: Dissolved oxygen, B: Sewage discharge, C: BOD

31. Which of the following is the most difficult to remove from waste water?
(a) Suspended Solids
(b) Dissolved salts
(c) Biodegradable waste matter
(d) All of the above

32. Select the incorrect matching.
(a) BOD → Biochemical Oxygen Demand
(b) JFM → Joint Forest Management
(c) DU → Degree of Unstauration
(d) FOAM → Friends of the Arcata March

33. What happens to sewage water from the point of sewage discharge?
(a) Dissolved oxygen ↓eses
(b) Mortality of fish ↑eses
(c) Biological oxygen demand ↑eses
(d) All of the above

34. World's most problematic aquatic weed is
(a) Terror of Bengal
(b) Water hyacinth
(c) *Eichhornia crassipes*
(d) All of the above

35. Water hyacinth is introduced in India for
(a) High growth rate
(b) Beautiful flowers
(c) Disease resistance gene
(d) All of the above

36. The presence of large amount of nutrients in water causes excessive growth of planktonic (free-floating) algae, called. This is called
(a) Red tide
(b) Bio-magnification
(c) Algal bloom
(d) Biofortification

37. Which of these diseases is/are caused by contaminated water?
(a) Dysentery
(b) Typhoid, jaundice
(c) Cholera
(d) All of the above

38. Heavy metal in waste water comes from:
(a) Petroleum industries
(b) Paper manufacturing industries
(c) Metal extraction industries
(d) All of the above

39. Which of the following are heavy metals (density > 5gm/cc)?
(a) Hg, Cd
(b) Cu
(c) Pb
(d) All of these

40. Increase in concentration of the toxic substances at successive trophic levels is known as:
(a) Bio-fortification
(b) Bio-war
(c) Bio-informatics
(d) Bio-magnification

41. The phenomena of biomagnification in aquatic ecosystem is well-known for the rising presence of:
(a) Hg
(b) DDT
(c) Both (a) and (b)
(d) None of these

42. If the water contains 0.003ppb of DDT then fish eating birds contain what level of DDT?
(a) 0.04 ppm
(b) 2 ppm
(c) 0.5 ppm
(d) 25 ppm

43. High concentration of DDT causes decline in:
(a) Fish population
(b) 200 plankton population
(c) Small fish population
(d) Bird population

44. Which of these is/are true about DDT?
(a) Undergo biomagnifications in aquatic ecosystem
(b) Disturb calcium metabolism in bird
(c) Causes thinning of eggshell leads to premature breaking
(d) All of the above

45. Natural aging of lake by nutrient enrichment of its water is:
(a) Bio-fortification
(b) Bio-magnification
(c) Bio-geochemical cycle
(d) Eutrophication

46. Eutrophication occurs because of:
(a) Ca and Mg
(b) Nitrogen and phosphorous
(c) Carbon and oxygen
(d) Hg and DDT

47. Natural aging of lake depends on:
(a) Climatic factors
(b) Size of lake
(c) Nutrient content of lake
(d) All of the above

48. Accelerated aging process of lake, because of pollutants from activities like effluents from the industries and homes, is known as:
(a) Cultural Eutrophication
(b) Accelerated Eutrophication
(c) Both a and b
(d) Bio-magnification

49. Which of the following is/are caused by algal bloom in a water body?
(a) Scum
(b) Unpleasant odour
(c) Robbing the water of dissolved oxygen
(d) All of the above

50. Select the correct statement from the following.
(A) Thermal wastewater eliminates or reduces the number of organisms sensitive to high temperature.
(B) In a young lake the water is cold and clear supporting little life.
(C) DDT disturbs calcium metabolism in birds, which causes thinning of eggshell and their premature breaking, eventually causing decline in bird population.
(D) Terror of Bengal grows abundantly in eutrophic water bodies.
(a) A and B only
(b) C and D only
(c) A and D only
(d) A, B, C and D all

51. Which of these facts are true with regard to wastewater treatment in the town of Arcata, California?
(a) The cleaning occurs in two stages.
(b) In the first stage conventional sedimentation, filtering and chlorine treatment are given.
(c) In the second stage biologists developed a series of six connected marshes of over 60 hectors of marshland, appropriate plant, algae, fungi and bacteria are seeded in this area, which neutralizes, absorb and assimilates the pollutants.
(d) All of the above

52. Dry composting toilet is useful in handling human excreta because this is:
(a) Practical and hygienic
(b) Efficient
(c) Cost-effective
(d) All of the above

53. 'EcoSan' toilets have been made effective in many areas of:
(a) Kerala
(b) Sri Lanka
(c) Both (a) and (b)
(d) None of these

54. Find the incorrect statement.
(a) Sanitary landfills were adopted as the substitute for open burning dumps.
(b) Seepage of chemical from landfills pollutes the underground water resources.
(c) All waste that we generate can be categorized into three types, i.e., bio-degradable, recyclable and non-biodegradable.
(d) Open dumps inhibit breeding of rats and flies.

55. Select the correct statement.
(A) Use of incinerator is crucial to disposal of hospital waste.
(B) Recycling is the only solution for the treatment of e-waste.
(C) Fish-eating birds containing 2ppm DDT become agents of biomagnifications.
(D) Polybend, is a fine powder of bitumen
(a) A and B only
(b) B and C only
(c) C and D only
(d) A, B and C only

56. Road laid by polyblend with bitumen have all of the following properties except:
(a) More water repellant
(b) Increase road life by factor of three
(c) Less bleeding in summer
(d) Increase cost of road laying

57. Who prepared polyblend?
(a) Ahmed Khan
(b) Ramesh Chand Dagar
(c) Amrita Devi
(d) Sunderlal Bahuguna

58. Who created Haryana Kisan Welfare Club?
(a) Ahmed Khan (b) Ramesh Chand Dagar
(c) Amrita Devi (d) Sunderlal Bahuguna

59. Integrated organic farming is a ________ and ________ procedure.
(a) non-cyclical, zero waste (b) cyclical, zero waste
(c) non-cyclical, wasteful (d) cyclical, wasteful

60. Accidental leakage in nuclear plants occurred in:
(a) Three mile island (b) Chernobyl
(c) Bhopal (d) Both (a) and (b)

61. Problem with use of nuclear energy is:
(a) Accidental leakage (b) Safe disposal of radioactive waste
(c) Both (a) and (b) (d) None of these

62. Which of these is/are true with regard to nuclear radiation coming from nuclear waste?
(a) It causes mutation at very high rate (b) High dose of radiation is lethal
(c) Low doses causes diseases like cancer (d) All of the above

63. How deep should nuclear waste after sufficient pre-treatment be buried (in shielded containers) within the rocks below the earth's surface?
(a) 100 m (b) 200 m
(c) 300 m (d) 500 m

64. Without greenhouse effect the average temperature at surface of Earth would have been ________.
(a) –0°C (b) 15°C
(c) –18°C (d) 6°C

65. Earth's present average temperature is:
(a) 0°C (b) 15°C
(c) –18°C (d) 6°C

66. What part of the incoming solar radiation actually comes through and falls on Earth's surface heating it?
(a) 1/4 (b) 1/2
(c) 1/3 (d) 2/3

67. Which gas contributes the maximum to the greenhouse effect?
(a) CH_4 (b) CO_2
(c) CFCs (d) N_2O

68. What is the contribution of methane gas to the total global warming?
(a) 60% (b) 20%
(c) 14% (d) 6%

69. During the past century, the temperature of earth has increased by ________.
(a) 0.6°C (b) 5°C
(c) 6°C (d) 1°C

70. Greenhouse gases absorb ________ radiation from the earth and emit it again towards the earth. The cycle continues till the earth's surface has no____________ radiation to emit.
(a) long wave (infrared), long wave (b) short wave (uv), long wave
(c) long wave (infrared), short wave (uv) (d) short wave (uv), short wave (uv)

71. Rise in temperature is leading to deleterious changes in the environment and resulting is odd climatic change such as:
(a) Ozone depletion (b) Greenhouse effect
(c) Water logging (d) El Nino effect

72. We can control global warming by the following means except:
(a) Cut down use of fossil fuel (b) Slow down growth of human population
(c) Improving efficiency of energy uses (d) Deforestation

73. Thickness of ozone is measured in terms of:
(a) BOD (b) D.O.
(c) DU (d) ROP

74. Bad ozone is formed in:
(a) Stratosphere (b) Ionosphere
(c) Troposphere (d) Lithosphere

75. Which of the following biomolecule absorbs UV radiation?
(a) DNA (b) Protein
(c) Both a and b (d) Carbohydrates

76. Good ozone is found in:
(a) Stratosphere (b) Ionosphere
(c) Troposphere (d) Lithosphere

77. Ozone degradation is done by:
(a) DDT (b) CFCs
(c) CH_4 (d) CO_2

78. In stratosphere, UV rays act on CFCs (Chlorofluoro Carbons) and release which atom leading to ozone depletion?
(a) 'F' atoms (b) 'Cl' atoms
(c) 'H' atoms (d) 'C' atoms

79. Which of these is incorrect about ozone depletion?
(a) CFCs releases 'Cl' atom causes degradation of O_3.
(b) 'Cl' atoms acts as catalyst.
(c) 'Cl' atom is not consumed in the reaction.
(d) It is minimum over Antarctica region

80. Antarctic region has a large area of thinned ozone layer, commonly known as:
(a) Dobson unit (b) Ozone hole
(c) Black hole (d) All of the above

81. UV-B radiation causes:
(a) Damage to DNA (b) Aging of skin
(c) Skin cancer (d) All of the above

82. In human eye, cornea absorbs UV- B radiation, and a high dose of UV-B causes inflammation of cornea, known as:
(a) Night blindness (b) Xerophthalmia
(c) Epicanthus (d) Snow-blindness

83. Which international treaty was signed at Montreal (Canada) in 1987 (effective in 1989) to control the emission of ozone depleting substances?
(a) Kyoto Protocol (b) Earth Summit
(c) Montreal Protocol (d) All of the above

84. Ozone hole over Antarctica develops each year between:
(a) Late August and early October (b) Late February and early April
(c) Late December and early February (d) Late October and early December

85. In which year did Government of India introduce the concept of Joint Forest Management (JFM)?
(a) 1974 (b) 1980
(c) 1990 (d) 1970

86. 'Chipko movement' was started by which community?
(a) Bishnois (b) Garhwal
(c) Sahiwal (d) Jain

87. How many daughters of Amrita Devi were cut down along with trees?
(a) 1 (b) 2
(c) 3 (d) 4

88. Government of India has recently instituted which award for individuals or communities from rural areas that have shown extra-ordinary courage and dedication in protecting wildlife?
(a) Padam Bhushan
(b) Chipko Award
(c) Baharat Ratna
(d) Amrita Devi Bishnoi Wildlife Protection Award

89. According to an estimate, almost ________ percent forests have been lost in the tropics, compared to only ________ percent in the temperate region.
(a) 40, 10 (b) 60, 20
(c) 40, 1 (d) 20, 1

90. National Forest Policy (1988) of India has recommended ________ percent forest cover for the plains and ________ percent for the hills.
(a) 60, 40 (b) 33, 67
(c) 40, 60 (d) 67, 33

91. By the end of 20th century India lost how much forest cover?
(a) 30% (b) 19.4%
(c) 33% (d) 10.6

92. Jhum cultivation (slash and burn agriculture) is found in which part of India?
(a) North- eastern state (b) Western state
(c) Southern state (d) Desert state

93. Which of these statements is/are true about slash and burn agriculture?
(a) Farmers cut down trees of the forest and burn the plant remains.
(b) Ash is used as fertilizer.
(c) Land is used for farming or cattle grazing.
(d) All of the above

94. Deforestation causes all of these except:
(a) Soil erosion and loss of biodiversity (b) Desertification
(c) Increase CO_2, conc. in atmosphere (d) Undisturbed hydrological cycle

95. Which of these statements is/are true about reforestation?
(a) It is process of restoring forest. (b) It may occur naturally.
(c) It can be sped up by planting trees. (d) All of the above

96. Soil erosion occurs because of:
(a) Over-cultivation (b) Unrestricted grazing
(c) Deforestation and poor irrigation practice (d) All of the above

97. Problems which came with Green Revolution are:
(a) Water logging (b) Increased soil salinity
(c) Both (a) and (b) (d) None of these

98. Irrigation without proper drainage leads to:
(a) Decrease soil salinity (b) Water logging
(c) Increased yield of crop (d) Increased aeration in soil

99. Desertification is a major problem nowadays, mainly due to:
(a) Over grazing (b) Over-cultivation
(c) Increased urbanization (d) Water logging

100. Match the columns.

Column–I	Column–II
A. DU	1. Dobson unit
B. CFCs	2. Chloro fluoro carbons
C. BOD	3. Biological oxygen demand
D. PIL	4. Public Interest Litigation
E. CNG	5. Compressed natural gas

(a) A:1, B:3, C:2, D:4, E:5 (b) A:4, B:3, C:2, D:1, E:5
(c) A:1, B:2, C:3, D:4, E:5 (d) A:1, B:2, C:4, D:3, E:5

101. Select the incorrect match.
(a) El Nino effect—odd climatic changes
(b) Radioactive leakage—Three Mile Island
(c) Biomagnification—Hg and DDT
(d) Haryana Kisan Welfare Club—Ahmed Khan

102. Which among these is the most common source of pollution of water bodies?
(a) Waste from thermal power plant (b) Effluents from chemical factories
(c) Hospital waste (d) Domestic sewage

103. Air pollution primarily result from:
(a) Deforestation (b) Forestation
(c) Burning of fossil fuel (d) Eutrophication

104. Identify A, B, C and D in this figure.

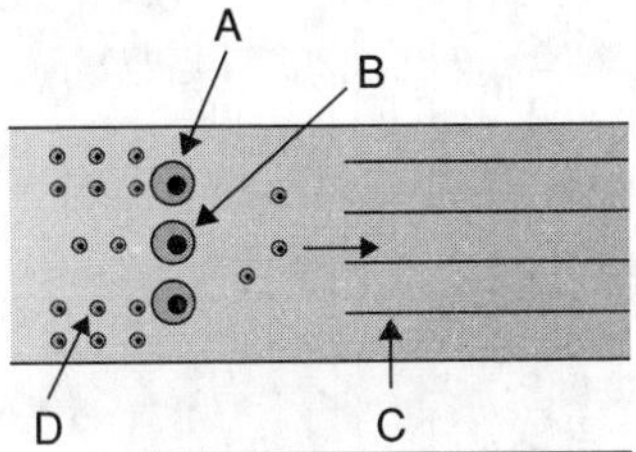

Electrostatic precipitator

(a) A: Discharge corona, B: Negatively charged wire, C: Collection plate grounded, D: Dust particles
(b) A: Dust particles, B: Discharge corona, C: Negatively charged wire, D: Collection plate grounded
(c) A: Negatively charged wire, B: Discharge corona, C: Collection plate grounded, D: Dust particles
(d) A: Collection plate grounded, B: Dust particles, C: Negatively charge wire, D: Discharge corona

105. What is the relative contribution (A, B, C, D) of various greenhouse gases according to pi-chart?

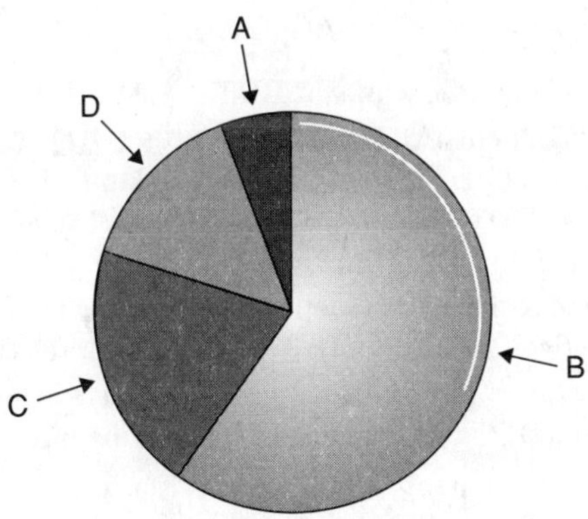

(a) A: N_2O (6%), B: Carbon dioxide (60%), Methane (25%), D: CFCs (14%)
(b) A: Methane (25%), B: CFCs (14%), C: N_2O (6%), D: Carbon dioxide (60%)
(c) A: Carbon dioxide (6%), B: N_2O (6%), C: Methane (25%), D: CFCs (14%)
(d) A: CFCs (14%), B: Carbon dioxide (60%), C: Methane (25%), D: N_2O (6%)

106. What is the concentration of DDT in stages A, B, C, D and E in the figure?

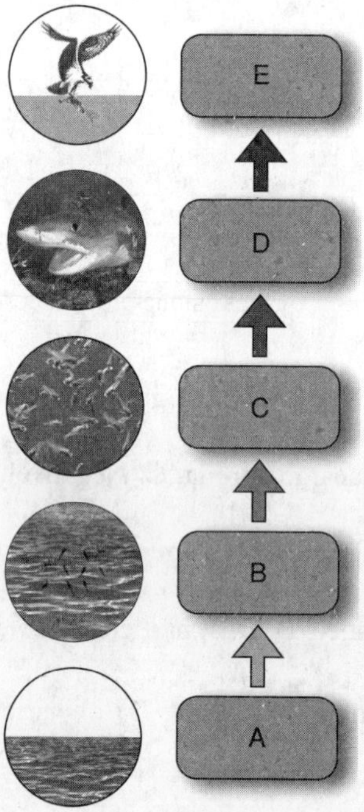

Diagram showing of biomagnifications of DDT

(a) A: Water (DDT 0.003 ppm), B: Fish-eating birds (DDT 25 ppm), C: Small fish (DDT 0.5 ppm), D: Large fish (DDT 2 ppm), E: Zooplankton (DDT 0.04 ppm)
(b) A: Fish-eating birds (DDT 25 ppm), B: Large fish (DDT 2 ppm), C: Small fish (DDT 0.5 ppm), D: Zooplankton (DDT 0.04 ppm), E: Water (DDT 0.003 ppb)
(c) A: Water (DDT 0.003 ppb), B: Zooplankton (DDT 0.04 ppm), C: Small fish (DDT 0.5 ppm), D: Large fish (DDT 2 ppm), E: Fish-eating birds (DDT 25 ppm)
(d) A: Small fish (DDT 0.5 ppm), B: Large fish (DDT 2 ppm), C: Zooplankton (DDT 0.04 ppm), D: Water (DDT 0.003 ppm), E: Fish-eating birds (DDT 25 ppm)

*Read the **assertion** and **reason** carefully to mark the correct option out of the options given below:*

(a) If both the assertion and the reason are true and the reason is a correct explanation of the assertion
(b) If both the assertion and reason are true but the reason is not a correct explanation of the assertion
(c) If the assertion is true but the reason is false
(d) If both the assertion and reason are false

107. **Assertion:** Noise is undesirable high level of sound.
Reason: Noise causes psychological and physiological disorder in humans.

108. **Assertion:** CNG is better fuel than dieses.
Reason: CNG burns most efficiently and cheaper than petrol.

109. **Assertion:** Presence of large amounts of nutrients in waters also causes excessive growth of planktonic (free-floating) algae, called algal bloom.
Reason: Algal bloom imparts a distinct colour to the water bodies.

110. **Assertion:** Water hyacinth is an aquatic weed.
Reason: They grow abundantly in eutrophic water bodies.

111. **Assertion:** DDT & Hg undergo biological magnification.
Reason: Hg & DDT are not metabolised & excreted by body of organism,

112. **Assertion:** Sanitary landfills in also not a good method for disposal of solid waste.
Reason: These landfills causes pollution of underground water resources due to seepage of chemicals.

113. **Assertion:** Nuclear energy in non-polluting way for generating electricity.
Reason: Nuclear waste is not all dangerous for organism.

114. **Assertion:** UV rays are highly injurious to living organism.
Reason: DNAs proteins of living organism preferentially absorb UV rays, and its high energy breaks the chemical bonds within these molecules.

115. **Assertion:** Large area of thinned ozone layer particularly marked over the Antarctic region is known as ozone hole.
Reason: CFCs causes ozone depletion.

116. **Assertion:** Deforestation may causes desertification.
Reason: It causes, loss of biodiversity, disturb hydrological cycle, causes soil erosion, may lead to desertification, in extreme cases.

AIPMT PREVIOUS YEAR QUESTIONS

1. A renewable exhaustible natural resource is

[AIPMT PRE 2010]

(a) Coal (b) Petroleum
(c) Minerals (d) Forest

2. dB is a standard abbreviation used for the quantitative expression of

[AIPMT PRE 2010]

(a) The density of bacteria in a medium (b) A particular pollutant
(c) The dominant Bacillus in a culture (d) A certain pesticide

3. The two gases making highest relative contribution to the greenhouse gases are

[AIPMT PRE 2010]

(a) CO_2 and CH_4 (b) CH_4 and NO_2
(c) CFCs and N_2O (d) CO_2 and N_2O

4. "Good ozone" is found in the:

[AIPMT MAINS 2011]

(a) Mesosphere (b) Troposphere
(c) Stratosphere (d) Ionosphere

5. Which one of the following pairs of gases are the major-cause of 'Green house effect'?

[AIPMT PRE 2011]

(a) CO_2 and CO (b) CFCs and SO_2
(c) CO_2 and N_2O (d) CO_2 and O_3

6. Which one of the following expanded forms of the following acronyms is correct?

[AIPMT PRE 2011]

(a) UNEP United Nations Environmental Policy
(b) EPA Environmental Pollution Agency
(c) IVCN International Union for Conservation of Nature and Natural Resources
(d) IPCC International Penal for Climahange

7. Which one of the following statements is wrong in case Bhopal gas tragedy?

[AIPMT PRE 2011]

(a) Thousands of human beings died
(b) Radioactive fallout engulfed Bhopal
(c) It took place in the night of December 2/3, 1984
(d) Methyl isocyariate gas leakage took place

8. Eutrophication is often seen in:

[AIPMT PRE 2011]

(a) Fresh water lakes (b) Ocean
(c) Mountains (d) Deserts

9. In an area where DDT had been used extensively the population of birds declined significantly because:

[AIPMT PRE 2012]

(a) Birds stopped laying eggs
(b) Earthworms in the area got eradicated
(c) Cobras were feeding exclusively on birds
(d) Many of the birds eggs laid, did not hatch

10. Which one of the following is a wrong statement?

[AIPMT PRE 2012]

(a) Most of the forests have been lost in tropical areas
(b) Ozone in upper part of atmosphere is harmful to animals
(c) Greenhouse effect is a natural phenomenon
(d) Eutrophication is a natural phenomenon in freshwater bodies

11. Measuring Biochemical Oxygen Demand (BOD) is a method used for:

[AIPMT PRE 2012]

(a) Estimating the amount of organic matter in sewage water
(b) Working out the efficiency of oil driven automobile engines.
(c) Measuring the activity of Saccharomyces cerevisae in producing curd on a commercial scale.
(d) Working out the efficiency of R.B.Cs. about their capacity to carry oxygen.

12. Kyoto Protocol was endorsed at:

[AIPMT 2013]

(a) CoP-3 (b) CoP-5
(c) CoP-6 (d) CoP-4

13. Global warming can be controlled by:

[AIPMT 2013]

(a) Reducing deforestation, cutting down use of fossil fuel
(b) Reducing reforestation, increasing the use of fossil fuel
(c) Increasing deforestation, slowing down the growth of human population
(d) Increasing deforestation, reducing efficiency of energy usage.

14. The Air Prevention and Control of Pollution Act came into force in:

[AIPMT 2013]

(a) 1975 (b) 1981
(c) 1985 (d) 1990

15. The zone of atmosphere in which the ozone layer is present is called:

[AIPMT 2014]

(a) Ionosphere (b) Mesosphere
(c) Stratosphere (d) Troposphere

16. A scrubber in the exhaust of a chemical industrial plant removes:

[AIPMT 2014]

(a) Gases like sulphur dioxide
(b) Particulate matter of the size 5 micrometer or above
(c) Gases like ozone and methane
(d) Particulate matter of the size 2.5 micrometer or less

17. Rachel Carson's famous book "Silent Spring" is related to :

[AIPMT 2015]

(a) Pesticide pollution (b) Noise Pollution
(c) Population explosion (d) Ecosystem management

18. Which of the following is not one of the prime health risks associated with greater UV radiation through the atmosphere due to depletion of stratospheric ozone?

[AIPMT 2015]

(a) Increased skin caner (b) Reduced Immune System
(c) Damage to eyes (d) Increased liver cancer

19. The UN conference of Parties on climate change in the year 2011 was held in :

[AIPMT 2015]

(a) Poland (b) South Africa
(c) Peru (d) Qatar

20. The UN conference of Parties on climate change in the year 2012 was held at:

[RE-AIPMT 2015]

(a) Doha (b) Lima
(c) Warsaw (d) Durban

21. Acid rain is caused by increase in the atmospheric concentration of:

[RE-AIPMT 2015]

(a) SO_3 and CO (b) CO_2 and CO
(c) O_3 and dust (d) SO_2 and NO_2

22. Increase in concentration of the toxicant at successive trophic levels is known as: [RE-AIPMT 2015]

(a) Biodeterioration
(b) Biotransformation
(c) Biogeochemical cycling
(d) Biomagnification

23. Which of the following are most suitable indicators of SO_2 pollution in the environment? [RE-AIPMT 2015]

(a) Conifers
(b) Algae
(c) Fungi
(d) Lichens

24. Eutrophication of water bodies leading to killing of fishes is mainly due to non-availability of: [RE-AIPMT 2015]

(a) Light
(b) Essential minerals
(c) Oxygen
(d) Food

Answer Keys

1. (d)	2. (c)	3. (b)	4. (d)	5. (a)	6. (d)	7. (c)	8. (b)	9. (c)	10. (d)
11. (a)	12. (a)	13. (d)	14. (b)	15. (c)	16. (d)	17. (d)	18. (b)	19. (b)	20. (d)
21. (c)	22. (d)	23. (d)	24. (d)	25. (a)	26. (c)	27. (c)	28. (a)	29. (b)	30. (b)
31. (b)	32. (c)	33. (d)	34. (d)	35. (b)	36. (c)	37. (d)	38. (d)	39. (d)	40. (d)
41. (c)	42. (d)	43. (d)	44. (d)	45. (d)	46. (b)	47. (d)	48. (c)	49. (d)	50. (d)
51. (d)	52. (d)	53. (c)	54. (d)	55. (a)	56. (d)	57. (a)	58. (a)	59. (b)	60. (d)
61. (c)	62. (d)	63. (d)	64. (c)	65. (b)	66. (b)	67. (b)	68. (b)	69. (a)	70. (a)
71. (d)	72. (d)	73. (c)	74. (c)	75. (c)	76. (a)	77. (b)	78. (b)	79. (d)	80. (b)
81. (d)	82. (d)	83. (c)	84. (a)	85. (b)	86. (b)	87. (c)	88. (d)	89. (c)	90. (b)
91. (d)	92. (a)	93. (d)	94. (d)	95. (d)	96. (d)	97. (c)	98. (b)	99. (c)	100. (c)
101. (d)	102. (d)	103. (c)	104. (a)	105. (a)	106. (c)	107. (b)	108. (a)	109. (b)	110. (a)
111. (a)	112. (a)	113. (d)	114. (a)	115. (b)	116. (a)				

AIPMT Previous Year Questions

1. (d)	2. (b)	3. (a)	4. (c)	5. (c)	6. (c)	7. (b)	8. (b)	9. (d)	10. (b)
11. (a)	12. (a)	13. (a)	14. (b)	15. (c)	16. (a)	17. (a)	18. (d)	19. (b)	20. (a)
21. (d)	22. (d)	23. (d)	24. (c)						

Mock Test-I

1. How many pair of gill slits are present in class from which Hagfish belongs
(a) 3–15 (b) 4–15 (c) 5–15 (d) 6–15

2. How much % of angiosperm pollen grains sheds at 2-celled stage?
(a) >40 (b) >50 (c) >60 (d) >70

3. During a period of 1960 to 2000, wheat production increased from 11 million tonnes to 75 million tonnes, while rice production went up from 35 million tones to __________ million tones.
(a) 79.5 (b) 89.5 (c) 99.5 (d) 69.5

4. What is the typical size of bacteria?
(a) 1–2 μm (b) 2–3 μm (c) 3–4 μm (d) 0.1–1.0 μm

5. How many metameric segments present in earthworm?
(a) 100–200 (b) 100–150 (c) 120–150 (d) 100–120

6. If 4 individuals in a laboratory population of 40 fruit flies died during specified time interval, say a week, the death rate in the population during that period is __________ individuals per fruit fly per weeks
(a) 0.01 (b) 0.10 (c) 1.0 (d) 10.0

7. Plant capture only __________ percent of the PAR
(a) 10–15 (b) 2–10 (c) 2–20 (d) >20

8. How many restriction sites are present in *E. Coli.* cloning vector pBR322?
(a) 6 (b) 7 (c) 8 (d) 9

9. Yeast poison themselves to death when the concentration of alcohol reaches about _______ percent during fermentation.
(a) 10 (b) 13 (c) 25 (d) 20

10. Xylem formed by how many different kinds of elements?
(a) 1 (b) 3 (c) 4 (d) 5

11. A mere __________ per cent impurities make domestic sewage unfit for human use.
(a) 0.001 (b) 0.1 (c) 1.0 (d) 10.0

12. Any mineral ion concentration in the tissue that reduces the dry weight of tissue by about __________ per cent is considered to be toxic.
(a) 20 (b) 10 (c) 5 (d) 30

13. In malaria, the rupture of RBCs is associated with release of a toxic substance, haemozoin, which is responsible for the chill and high fever recurring every __________ days.
(a) 1– 2 (b) 4–5 (c) 3–4 (d) 5–6

14. It has been calculated that a 250 kg of cow produces 200 gm of proteins per day. In the same period, 250 gm of a micro-organism like Methylophilus methylotropus, because of its high rate of biomass production and growth, can be expected to produce __________ tonnes of protein.
(a) 10 (b) 20 (c) 25 (d) 35

15. Of the total incident solar radiation, the proportion of PAR is
(a) About 70% (b) About 60%
(c) Less than 50% (d) More than 80%

16. Nearly all of the essential nutrients and __________ percent of electrolytes and water are absorbed by PCT.
(a) 30–40 (b) 99 (c) 70–80 (d) 25

17. Robert made more conservative and scientifically estimate the global species diversity at about __________ million.
(a) 4 (b) 1.5 (c) 20–50 (d) 7

18. National Forest Policy (1988) of India has recommended __________ per cent forest cover for the plains and ________ per cent for the hills.
(a) 33, 67 (b) 67, 33 (c) 40, 60 (d) 60, 40

19. ABO blood group is controlled by the gene I.
The gene I has how many types of alleles?
(a) 1 (b) 2 (c) 3 (d) 4

20. The recent record of __________ years old viable seed is of the date palm, Phoenix dactylifera discovered during archaeological excavation at King Herod's palace near the dead sea.
(a) 1000 (b) 2000 (c) 3000 (d) 500

21. In the human beings, the membrane of the erythrocyte has approximately ________ percent protein.
(a) 42 (b) 52 (c) 62 (d) 40

22. Nitrogenase requires how many molecules of ATP for each molecule of NH_3 produced?
(a) 8 (b) 4 (c) 16 (d) 2

23. Penicillin was extensively used to treat American soldiers wounded in World War II. Fleming, Chain and Florey were awarded the Nobel Prize in which year?
(a) 1945 (b) 1935
(c) 1955 (d) 1940

24. There are lymphoid tissues located within the lining of the major tract (respiratory, digestive and urogenital tracts) called mucosal associated lymphoid tissue (MALT). It constitutes how much percent of lymphoid tissue in human body?
(a) 30 (b) 40
(c) 50 (d) 60

25. A typical angiosperm embryo sac, at maturity, though ________ nucleated is ________ celled
(a) 8, 7 (b) 7, 8
(c) 6, 8 (d) 8, 8

26. Blood normally contain how many (in lacs) platelets per mm?
(a) 1–1.5 (b) 1.5–3.5
(c) 2.0–2.5 (d) 2.0

27. Amount of residual volume (RV) in ml is
(a) 1100–1200 (b) 1000–1100
(c) 2500–3000 (d) 500

28. In given diagram, rod shaped Tobacco Mosaic Virus (TMV) magnified about

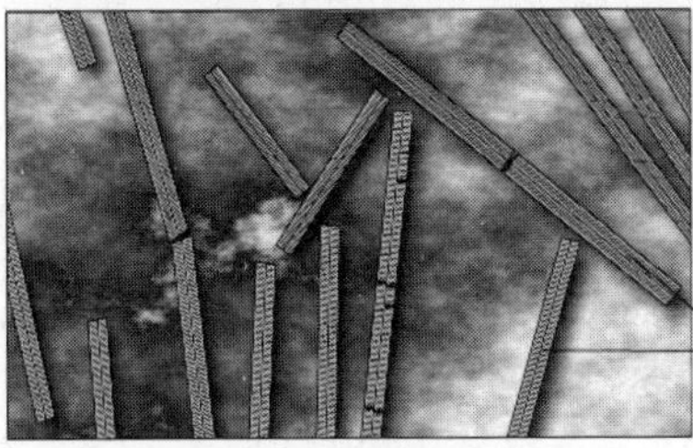

(a) 1000X (b) 1500X
(c) 50,000X (d) 1,00,000–1,50,000X

29. Which of the following is the number of chromosomes present in gamete of rat?
(a) 12 (b) 21 (c) 19 (d) 24

30. How many parathyroid glands are present in humans?
(a) 1 (b) 2 (c) 3 (d) 4

31. Some interesting aspects of about earth's biodiversity are based on the currently available species inventories. More than __________ percent of all the species recorded are animals.
(a) 50 (b) 60 (c) 70 (d) 90

32. How many stamens are present in a flower of Indigofera?
(a) 5 (b)10 (c) 9 (d) 4

33. Mitochondria is sausage shaped or cylindrical having a diameter of ______.
(a) 0.2–1.0 μm (b) 1.0–2.0 μm
(c) 0.01–0.1 μm (d) 0.001–.01 μm

34. How many pairs of gills are present in osteicthyes?
(a) 1 (2) 2 (c) 3 (d) 4

35. The largely tropical Amazonian rain forest in south America has greatest biodiversity on earth. It is home to more than 40,000 species of plants, 3000 of fishes, 1,300 of birds, __________ of mammals, __________ of amphibians, 378 of reptiles and of more than 1,25,000 invertebrates.
(a) 427,327 (b) 427,427
(c) 472,372 (d) 274,273

36. The biogas plant consists of a concrete tank (__________ feet deep) in which bio-waste are collected and slurry of dung is fed.
(a) 1–2 (b) 10–15 (c) 30–40 (d) 40–60

37. Plasma is a straw coloured, viscous fluid constituting nearly 55% of the blood. 90–92 % of plasma is water and proteins contribute __________ % of it.
(a) 3–4 (b) 6–8 (c) 10–15 (d) 10–12

38. How many molecules of NADH $+H^+$ formed from one molecule of pyruvic acid inside mitochondria?
(a) 2 (b) 4 (c) 8 (d) 16

39. How many carbon atoms are present in Arachidonic acid excluding the carboxyl carbon?
(a) 19 (b) 20
(c) 18 (d) 17

40. In plant cells, the vacuole can occupy up to __________ % of the volume of the cell.
(a) 20 (b) 60 (c) 90 (d) 100

41. Adrenal cortex cab be histologically divide in to how many layers?
(a) 1 (b) 2 (c) 3 (d) 4

42. How many genes are present in chromosomes X and chromosome Y, respectively?
(a) 2968,213 (b) 2896,231 (c) 2869,312 (d) 2968,231

43. Macronutrients are generally present in the plant tissues in large amounts (in excess of __________ m mole Kg^{-1} of the dry weight)
(a) 5 (b) 10 (c) 15 (d) 20

44. What is the life span of Crocodile in years?
(a) 10 (b) 20 (c) 60 (d) 30

45. How much temperature is provided to cells and recombinant DNA during heat shock?
(a) 22°C (b) 32°C (c) 42°C (d) 72°C

46. How much % of CO_2 is carried in a dissolved state through plasma?
(a) 70 (b) 7 (c) 20–25 (d) 3

47. Stomatal apparatus is made of how many components?
(a) 1 (b) 3 (c) 4 (d) 5

48. Administration of progestogens or progestogen-estrogen combination or IUDs within __________ hours(max) of coitus have found to be very effective emergency contraceptives as they could be used to avoid possible pregnancy due to rape or causal unprotected intercourse.
(a) 24 (b) 36 (c) 72 (d) 84

49. How many chitinous teeth are present in gizzard of cockroach?
(a) 3 (b) 6 (c) 8 (d) 10

50. Every 100 ml of blood can deliver around how many ml of oxygen to tissue under normal physiological condition?
(a) 4 (b) 5 (c) 14 (d) 20

51. The number of chromosomes in meiocyte of rice
(a) 1 (b) 24 (c) 16 (d) 32

52. The number of chromosome in meiocyte of dog
(a) 34 (b) 20 (c) 78 (d) 380

53. The size of each ovary in cm (length)
(a) 2–4 (b) 4–6 (c) 6–8 (d) 8–10

54. At puberty, total number of primary follicle present in human female body
(a) 60,000–80,000 (b) 1,20,000–1,60,000
(c) 30,000–40,000 (d) 15,000–20,000

55. Menopause generally occur at which age
(a) 45 (b) 50 (c) 55 (d) 40

56. In which year Miller do his experiment for chemical evolution of life and Watson and Crick propose d double stranded model of DNA?
(a) 1926 (b) 1869 (c) 1953 (d) 1952

57. In which year 1st transgenic cow, Rosie, is produced (protein content of milk is 2.4 gm/lt)?
(a) 1997 (b) 1995 (c) 1999 (d) 1993

58. In which year, Whittaker proposed a five kingdom classification?
(a) 1935 (b) 1969 (c) 1839 (d) 1972

59. In which year, Ribosome was first observed by George Palade?
(a) 1926 (b) 1869 (c) 1953 (d) 1952

60. How much filtrate is reabsorbed by renal tubules?
(a) 70–80 (b) 90 (c) 99 (d) 95

61. In which year, T.O. Diener discovered viroids?
(a) 1971 (b) 1961 (c) 1981 (d) 1991

62. In Dictyota, how many flagella are present?
(a) 2 (b) 4 (c) 6 (d) 8

63. How many external rows of ciliated comb plates present on the body of ctenophores?
(a) 4 (b) 6 (c) 8 (d) 10

64. Heart of crocodile posses how many chambers?
(a) 1 (b) 2 (c) 3 (d) 4

65. How many carpels are present in flower of sem?
(a) 1 (b) 2 (c) 3 (d) 4

66. How many petals are present in one flower of Makoi?
(a) 4 (b) 5 (c) 3 (d) 6

67. Keel in a pea flower is formed by how many petals?
(a) 1 (b) 2 (c) 3 (d) 5

68. Head of Cockroach is formed by fusion of how many segments?
(a) 2 (b) 6 (c) 4 (d) 8

69. How many eggs are present in each Oothecae of Cockroach?
(a) 14–16 (b) 12–14 (c) 10–12 (d) 8–10

70. Hind limb of frog has how digits
(a) 3 (b) 4 (c) 5 (d) 6

71. What is the size of Ribosomes?
(a) 15–20 nm (b) 10–15 nm (c) 20–25 nm (d) 5–10 nm

72. How many nucleus present in human RBC?
(a) 1 (b) 2 (c) 3 (d) 0

73. Percentage wt. of carbon in human body is
(a) 65 (b) 18.5 (c) 0.5 (d) 3.3

74. How many carbons are present in serine?
(a) 3 (b) 2 (c) 4 (d) 5

75. Cell cycle of yeast is about
(a) 60 min (b) 90 min (c) 30 min (d) 20 min

76. Saturation point of CO_2 for C_4-plant is (in μ/L)
(a) 360 (b) 450 (c) 120 (d) 200

77. How many ATP are produced when $16H^+$ ion passed through F-unit of F_0–F_1 particle?
(a) 16 (b) 8 (c) 4 (d) 2

78. At which thoracic vertebra, trachea is divided into 1^0 bronchi-
(a) 6th (b) 5th (c) 4th (d) 7th

79. How much % of Plasma is water?
(a) 95–97 (b) 90–92 (c) 80–85 (d) 75–80

80. Hipopocampus has how many chamber in heart?
(a) 3 (b) 2 (c) 4 (d) 1

81. GFR is (in m/minute)
(a) 120 (b) 125 (c) 130 (d) 180

82. What is the molarity of outer part of inner medulla in Kidney (in m 0% mol/litre)?
(a) 1200 (b) 600 (c) 900 (d) 300

83. Cranial bones are __________ in number.
(a) 6 (b) 8 (c) 4 (d) 10

84. Coxal bone is formed by fusion of how many bones?
(a) 3 (b) 6 (c) 4 (d) 2

85. The ventral portion of the mid brain consists of how many round swelling (lobes)?
(a) 2 (b) 4 (c) 0 (d) 3

86. The wall of eye ball is made up of how many layers?
(a) 1 (b) 2 (c) 3 (d) 4

87. Find out the total number of secondary messenger from the following?
ATP, AMP, IP_3, Ca^{2+}
(a) 1 (b) 2 (c) 3 (d) 4

88. Each eye of cockroach is consisting of about how many ommatidia?
(a) 1000 (b) 2000 (c) 4000 (d) 3000

89. How many genes are present in a human cell?
(a) 20,000 (b) 30,000 (c) 50,000 (d) 80,000

90. How many genes are present in 1st chromosome of human?
(a) 2968 (b) 2986 (c) 231 (d) 132

Answer Keys

1. (d)	2. (c)	3. (b)	4. (a)	5. (d)	6. (b)	7. (b)	8. (c)	9. (b)	10. (c)
11. (b)	12. (b)	13. (c)	14. (c)	15. (c)	16. (c)	17. (d)	18. (a)	19. (c)	20. (b)
21. (b)	22. (a)	23. (a)	24. (c)	25. (a)	26. (b)	27. (a)	28. (d)	29. (b)	30. (d)
31. (c)	32. (b)	33. (a)	34. (d)	35. (b)	36. (b)	37. (b)	38. (b)	39. (a)	40. (c)
41. (c)	42. (d)	43. (b)	44. (c)	45. (c)	46. (b)	47. (b)	48. (c)	49. (b)	50. (b)
51. (b)	52. (c)	53. (a)	54. (b)	55. (b)	56. (c)	57. (a)	58. (b)	59. (c)	60. (c)
61. (a)	62. (a)	63. (c)	64. (d)	65. (a)	66. (b)	67. (b)	68. (b)	69. (a)	70. (c)
71. (a)	72. (d)	73. (b)	74. (a)	75. (b)	76. (a)	77. (b)	78. (b)	79. (b)	80. (b)
81. (b)	82. (c)	83. (b)	84. (a)	85. (c)	86. (c)	87. (c)	88. (b)	89. (b)	90. (a)

Mock Test-2

1. Specialised procedure to form an embryo in the laboratory in which a sperm is directly injected in to the ovum is
   (a) ZIFT (b) GIFT
   (c) ICSI (d) AI
2. Which one of the following structures between two adjacent cells is an effective transport pathway?
   (a) Plasmodesmata (b) Plastoquinones
   (c) Endoplasmic reticulum (d) Plasmalemma
3. Multicellular loose tissue organisation found in
   (a) Protista (b) Fungi
   (c) Archaea (d) Monera
4. Which of the following plants can express Bt genes: **Cotton, corn, rice, tomato, potato, soyabean, brinjal**. Find total numbers from the following
   (a) 3 (b) 4
   (c) 5 (d) 7
5. Ovary is one chambered but it become two chambered due to the formation of false septum in
   (a) mustard (b) dianthus
   (c) merigold (d) sunflower
6. Which of the following are free living nitrogen fixer in soil
   (a) Rhizobium (b) Alnus
   (c) Frankia (d) Nostoc
7. Leydig cells are found in
   (a) ovaries and secrete progesterone
   (b) adrenal cortex and secrete adrenalin
   (c) seminiferous tubules and provide nutrition to germ cells
   (d) seminiferous tubules and secrete androgens
8. Which one of the following cannot be explained on the basis of Mendel's Law of Dominance?
   (a) The discrete unit controlling a particular character is called a factor
   (b) Out of one pair of factors one is dominant, and the other recessive
   (c) Alleles do not show any blending and both the characters recover as such in F_2 generation
   (d) Factors occur in pairs
9. Apomictic embryos in Citrus arise from
   (a) synergids (b) maternal sporophytic tissue in ovule
   (c) antipodal cells (d) diploid egg

10. One example of animals having a single opening to the outside that serves both mouth as well as anus is
(a) Octopus (b) Asterias
(c) Ascidia (d) Dugesia

11. Select the correct statement from the ones given below
(a) Barbiturates when given to criminals make them tell the truth
(b) Morphine is often given to persons who have under gone surgery as a pain killer
(c) Chewing tobacco lowers blood pressure and heart rate
(d) Cocaine is given to patients after surgery as it stimulates recovery

12. Select correct statement from the following
A: Wheezing sound is produced in asthma
B: Emphysema is chronic disorder and one of its major cause is cigarette smoking
C: Pneumotaxic cetre present in medulla
(a) A and B (b) A and C
(c) B and C (d) A, B and C

13. Phloem of gymnosperm contain
(a) sieve tubes (b) albuminous cells
(c) companion cells (d) tracheids

14. Many fungi belong to the following genera causes ringworm
(a) Microsporum (b) Trichophyton
(c) Epidermophyton (d) All

15. Which one of the following is not a micronutrient?
(a) Molybdenum (b) Calcium
(c) Zinc (d) Boron

16. Membrane-bound organelles are absent in
(a) Saccharomyces (b) Nostoc
(c) Cladophora (d) Plasmodium

17. At puberty how many primary follicles found in female body
(a) 60,000–80,000 (b) 20,000–40,000
(c) 1,20,000–1,60,000 (d) 30,000–60,000

18. Select the correct statement from the following
(a) Biogas is produced by the activity of aerobic bacteria on animal waste
(b) Methanobacterium is an anerobic bacterium found in rumen of cattle
(c) Biogas, commonly called gobar gas, is pure ethane
(d) Activated sludge-sediment in settlement tanks of sewage treatment plant is a right source of aerobic bacteria

19. Select the two statements out of the four (1–4) given below about lac operon.
(1) Glucose or galactose may bind with the repressor and inactivate it
(2) In the presence of lactose, the repressor binds with the operator region
(3) The y-gene codes for permease
(4) This was elucidated by Francois Jacob and Jacques Monod
The correct statements are
(a) (2) and (3) (b) (1) and (3)
(c) (3) and (4) (d) (1) and (2)

20. Keel is characteristic of the flowers of
(a) gulmohur (b) cassia
(c) calotropis (d) pea

21. The kind of epithelium which forms the inner walls of alveoli is
(a) cuboidal epithelium (b) columnar epithelium
(c) ciliated columnar epithelium (d) squamous epithelium

22. Which one of the following has its own DNA?
(a) Chloroplast (b) Dictyosome
(c) Lysosome (d) Peroxisome

23. Transfer of pollen grains from the anther to the stigma of same flower of the same plant is called
(a) xenogamy (b) geitonogamy
(c) karyogamy (d) autogamy

24. The genotype of a plant showing the dominant phenotype can be determined by
(a) test cross (b) dihybrid cross
(c) pedigree analysis (d) back cross

25. PGA as the first CO_2 fixation product was discovered in photosynthesis of
(a) pteridophyte (b) gymnosperm
(c) angiosperm (d) alga

26. Study the four statements (1–4) given below and select the two correct ones out of them.
(1) A lion eating a deer and a sparrow feeding on grain are ecologically similar in being consumers
(2) Predator star fish Pisaster helps in maintaining species diversity of some invertebrates
(3) Predators ultimately lead to the extinction of prey species
(4) Production of chemicals such as nicotine, strychnine by the plants are metabolic disorders
The two correct statements are
(a) (2) and (3) (b) (3) and (4)
(c) (1) and (4) (d) (1) and (2)

27. Seminal plasma in human males is rich in
(a) fructose and calcium (b) glucose and calcium
(c) DNA and testosterone (d) ribose and potassium

28. ABO blood groups in humans are controlled by the gene I. It has three alleles-I^A, I^B and i. Since there are three different alleles, six different genotypes are possible. How many phenotypes can occur?
(a) Three (b) One
(c) Four (d) Two

29. Which variety of wheat has high protein content?
(a) Himgiri (b) P 1542
(c) Sonalika (d) Atlas 66

30. True about Nucleopolyhedrovirus (biocontrol agent)
(a) species-non specific
(b) narrow spectrum
(c) harmful to non target insect also
(d) has negative impact on plant, mammals, birds

31. Widal test is used for the diagnosis of
(a) Malaria (b) AIDS
(c) Plague (d) Typhoid

32. Injury to adrenal medulla is likely to affect the secretion of which one of the following?
(a) Aldosterone
(b) Both androstenedione and dehydroepiandrosterone
(c) Adrenalin
(d) Cortisol

33. High uric acid be the cause of
(a) tetany (b) anaemia
(c) angina pectoris (d) gout

34. Which one of the following pairs is incorrectly matched?
(a) Thyroid follicles-T_3 and T_4 (secretion)
(b) Somatostatin-Alpha cells (source)
(c) Corpus luteum-Relaxin (secretion)
(d) Insulin-Diabetes mellitus (disease)

35. Select the correct statement from the ones given below with respect to dihybrid cross.
(a) Tightly linked genes on the same chromosome show higher recombinations
(b) Genes far apart on the same chromosome show very few recombinations
(c) Genes loosely linked on the same chromosome show similar recombinations as the tightly linked ones
(d) Tightly linked genes on the same chromosome show very few recombinations

36. Which one of the following statements in regard to the excretion by the human kidneys is correct?
(a) Descending limb of Loop of Henle is impermeable to water
(b) Distal convoluted tubule is incapable of reabsorbing HCO_3
(c) Nearly 99 per cent of the glomerular filtrate is reabsorbed by the renal tubules
(d) Ascending limb of loop of Henle is impermeable to electrolytes

37. The vomit centre situated at
(a) hypothalamus (b) pons
(c) cerebellum (d) medulla

38. The full form of GFC
(a) glucose fructose carrier (b) Grazing food chain
(c) grafted food crop (d) gross food capacity

39. Which of the following disease is related to circulatory system (find total no)
Hypertension, CAD, angina, uremia, osteoporosis, tetany, gout
(a) 2 (b) 3
(c) 1 (d) 5

40. Ovary is inferior in the flowers of
(a) peach (b) plum
(c) mustard (d) guava

41. Which one of the following is used as vector for cloning genes into higher plants?
(a) Baculovirus (b) Agrobacterium tumifaciens
(c) Rhizopus nigricans (d) Retrovirus

42. Select incorrect matching
(a) GCA-Ala (b) GUU-Val
(c) AAU-Asn (d) UCC-Leu

43. Which one of the following is an example of in situ conservation?
(a) botanical garden (b) Seed bank
(c) Sacred groves (d) zoological park

44. Which one of the following restriction enzyme can cut Tet ^{R} site of pBR322
(a) Pvu I, Pst I (b) BamH I, Sal I
(c) Pvu II (d) EcoR I

45. Which one of the following statements is correct with respect to Cancer?
(a) The cancer cell have the full ability of contact inhibition
(b) Metastasis is shown by Benign tumors
(c) The cancer causing agents are known as oncogens
(d) c–onc or proto oncogenes when activated can cause cancer

46. Which of the following is used to initiate flowering and synchronising fruit–set in pineapples
(a) gibberellin (b) phytochrome
(c) ethylene (d) auxin

47. The figure given below is a diagrammatic representation of response of organisms to abiotic factors. What do A, Band C represent respectively?

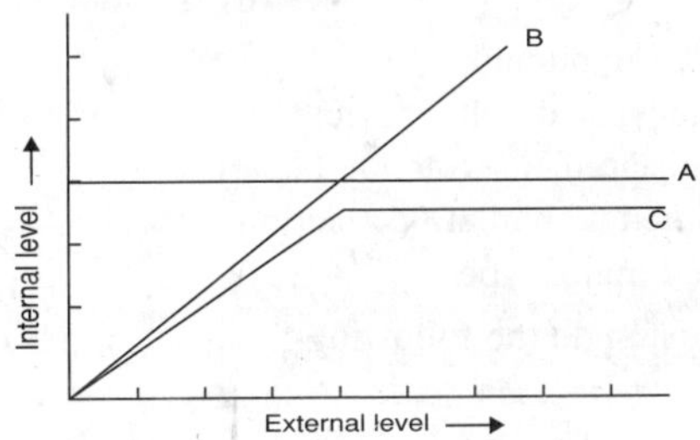

A	B	C
(a) conformer	regulator	partial regulator
(b) regulator	partial regulator	conformer
(c) partial regulator	regulator	conformer
(d) regulator	conformer	partial regulator

48. Find the total number of algae belongs to class phaeophyceae from the following
Volvox, **ectocarpus**, gelidium, **dictyota**, ficus, **laminaria**, porphyra, chara, gracilaria, cladophora
(a) 3 (b) 4
(c) 2 (d) 5

49. The technical term used for the androecium in a flower of Pea (Pisum sativum) is
(a) monadelphous (b) diadelphous
(c) polyandrous (d) polyadelphous

50. Potato spindle tuber disease is caused by
(a) virus (b) viriods
(c) fungi (d) bacteria

51. The permissible use of the technique amniocentesis is for
(a) detecting sex of the unborn foetus
(b) artificial insemination
(c) transfer, of embryo into the uterus of a surrogate mother
(d) detecting any genetic abnormality

52. During mitosis ER and nucleolus begin to disappear at
(a) late prophase (b) early metaphase
(c) late metaphase (d) early prophase

53. The free-living, anaerobic nitrogen-fixer is
(a) Beijerinckia (b) Rhodospirillum
(c) Rhizobium (d) Azotobacter

54. DNA or RNA segment tagged with a radioactive molecule is called
(a) vector (b) probe
(c) clone (d) plasmid

55. Darwin's finches are a good example of
(a) industrial melanism (b) connecting link
(c) divergent evolution (d) convergent evolution

56. The length of fallopian tube is
(a) 5–6 cm (b) 10–12 cm
(c) 14–16 cm (d) 2–4 cm

57. What is false about WBCs in humans?
(a) Netrophils and monocytes are phagocytes
(b) Basophiles secrete histamine, serotonin, heparin
(c) Eosinophiles associated with allergic reaction
(d) Lymphocytes are of 4 major type

58. Which stages of cell division do the following figures A and B represent respectively?

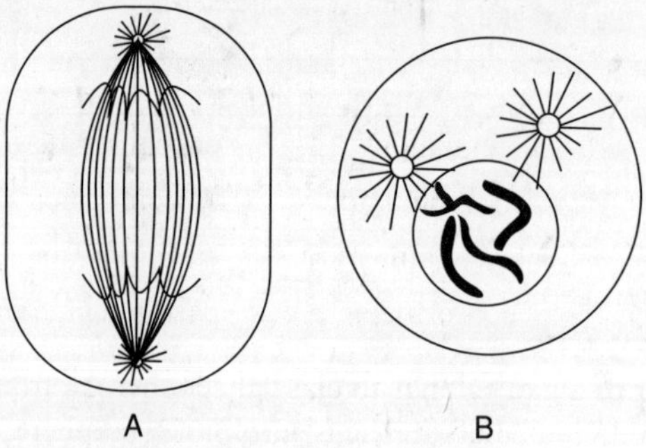

A		B
(a) Metaphase	-	Telophase
(b) Telophase	-	Metaphase
(c) Late anaphase	-	Prophase
(d) Prophase	-	Anaphase

59. Which of the following are inclusion bodies
(a) Phosphate granules (b) Glycogen granules
(c) Gas vacuoles (d) all

60. The common nitrogen-fixer in paddy fields is
(a) Rhizobium (b) Azospirillum
(c) Oscillatoria (d) Frankia

61. The principal nitrogenous excretory compound in humans is synthesised
(a) in kidneys but eliminated mostly through liver
(b) in kidneys as well as eliminated by kidneys
(c) in liver and also eliminated by the same through bile
(d) in the liver, but eliminated mostly through kidneys

62. Carrier ions like Na^+ facilitate the absorption of substance like
(a) amino acids and glucose (b) glucose and fatty acids
(c) fatty acids and glycerol (d) fructose and Some amino acids

63. Which one of the following symbols and its representation, used' in human pedigree analysis is correct?
(a) 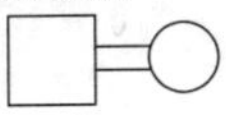 = Mating between relatives (b)  = Unaffected male
(c) 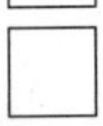 = Unaffected female (d)  = Male affected

64. Which two of the following changes (1–4) usually tend to occur in the plain dwellers when they move to high altitudes (3,500 m or more)?
(1) Increase in red blood cell size
(2) Increase in red blood cell production
(3) Decreasing breathing rate
(4) Decreasing the binding affinity of hemoglobin
(a) (2) and (3) (b) (3) and (4)
(c) (2) and (4) (d) (1) and (2)

65. Aldosterone helps in maintenance of
(a) electrolyte (b) body fluid volume
(c) blood pressure (d) All

66. If for some reason our goblet cells are non functional, this will adversely affect
(a) production of rennin
(b) secretion of cerumen
(c) maturation of sperms
(d) smooth movement of food down the intestine

67. The loose sheath of glycocalyx known as
(a) capsule (b) cell wall
(c) slime layer (d) mesosome

68. Which one of the following statements about all the four of Physalia, obelia, ctenoplana and sea fan is correct?
(a) all are tribloblastic
(b) digestion is both intra cellular and extra cellular
(c) all posses cnidoblast
(d) All are bilaterally symmetrical

69. The first movements of the foetus and appearance of hair on its head are usually observed during which month of pregnancy?
(a) Fourth month (b) Fifth month
(c) Sixth month (d) Third month

70. Select the total number from the following which have one ovule in an ovary?
wheat, watermelon, papaya, paddy, mango, orchid
(a) 2 (b) 3
(c) 1 (d) 4

71. Which one of the following kinds of animals are triploblastic acoelomate?
(a) Taenia (b) torpedo
(c) tusk chell (d) trygon

72. Select incorrect matching?
(a) Petromyzon – 6–15 pairs of gill slits (b) Labeo – 4 pair of gill slits
(c) Spiracles in cockroach – 10 pairs (d) Gizzard of cockroach – 8 chitinous teeth

73. Intra Uterine Devices (IUDs) from the following are
(a) Cu T (b) Cu 7
(c) Multiload 375 (d) All

74. Copper centres are present in which complex
(a) complex I (b) complex II
(c) complex III (d) complex IV

75. Restriction endonucleases are enzymes which
(a) make cuts at specific positions within the DNA molecule
(b) recognize a specific nucleotide sequence for binding of DNA ligase
(c) restrict the action of the enzyme DNA polymerase
(d) remove nucleotides from the ends of the DNA molecule

76. Which one of the following is not a lateral meristem?
(a) Intrafascicular cambium (b) Interfascicular cambium
(c) Phellogen (d) Intercalary meristem

77. In India, the Air (prevention and control of pollution) Act came into force in
(a) 1981 (b) 1978
(c) 1918 (d) 1997

78. Which of the following is not a function of gibberellins
(a) Delay senescence
(b) improve shape of apple
(c) increase length of grapes stalks
(d) speed down the malting process in brewing industry

79. C_4-plants are more efficient in photosynthesis than C_3-plants due to
(a) higher leaf area
(b) presence of larger number of chloroplasts in the leaf cells
(c) presence of thin cuticle
(d) lower rate of photorespiration

80. Algae have cell wall made up of
(a) cellulose, galactans and mannans (b) hemicellulose, pectins and proteins
(c) pectins, cellulose and proteins (d) cellulose, hemicellulose and pectins

81. Some hyperthermophilic organisms that grow in highly acidic (pH 2) habitats belong to the two groups called
(a) eubacteria and archaea (b) cyanobacteria and diatoms
(c) protists and mosses (d) liverworts and yeasts

82. Genetic engineering has been successfully used for producing
(a) transgenic mice for testing safety of polio vaccine before use in humans
(b) transgenic models for studying new treatments for certain cardiac diseases
(c) transgenic cow-Rosie which produces high fat milk for making ghee
(d) animals like bulls for farm work as they have super power

83. Some of the characteristics of Bt cotton are
(a) long fibre and resistance to aphids
(b) medium yield, long fibre and resistance to beetle pests
(c) high yield and production of toxic protein crystals which kill dipteran pests
(d) high yield and resistance to bollworms

84. Spring wood differs from autumn wood in
(a) having high density (b) having dark colour
(c) having less xylary element (d) having vessel with wider lumen

85. Satellite DNA is useful tool in
(a) organ transplantation (b) Sex determination
(c) forensic science (d) genetic engineering

86. The second maturation division of the mammalian ovum occurs
(a) shortly after ovulation before the ovum makes entry into the Fallopian tube
(b) until after the ovum has been penetrated by a sperm
(c) until the nucleus of the sperm has fused with that of the ovum
(d) in the Graafian follicle following the first maturation division

87. Which one of the following does not follow the central dogma of molecular biology?
(a) Pea (b) Mucor
(c) Chlamydomonas (d) TMV

88. Mark the odd one.
(a) Endometrium (b) Corpus luteum
(c) Acrosome (d) Graafian follicle

89. Identify the true statements –
I. Abstinence from drugs of dependence causes withdrawal symptoms but not craving.
II. Chikungunya is confirmed by Widal test.
III. Rheumatoid arthritis which affects many people in our society is an auto-immune disease.
IV. AIDS was first reported in 1981 and is caused by a member of a group of viruses called restroviruses
V. Benign tumors are normally considered with metastasis.
VI. Most powerful stimulant is cocaine.
(a) I, II, V (b) I, III, IV, VI
(c) III, V, VI (d) III, IV, V

90. Wind pollinated flowers are
(a) small, brightly coloured, producing large number of pollen grains
(b) small, producing large number of dry pollen grains
(c) large, producing abundant nectar and pollen
(d) small, producing nectar and dry pollen

Answer Keys

1. (c)	2. (a)	3. (b)	4. (d)	5. (a)	6. (d)	7. (d)	8. (c)	9. (b)	10. (d)
11. (b)	12. (a)	13. (b)	14. (d)	15. (b)	16. (b)	17. (c)	18. (b)	19. (c)	20. (d)
21. (d)	22. (a)	23. (d)	24. (a)	25. (d)	26. (d)	27. (a)	28. (c)	29. (d)	30. (b)
31. (d)	32. (c)	33. (d)	34. (b)	35. (d)	36. (c)	37. (d)	38. (b)	39. (b)	40. (d)
41. (b)	42. (d)	43. (c)	44. (b)	45. (d)	46. (c)	47. (a)	48. (a)	49. (b)	50. (b)
51. (d)	52. (a)	53. (b)	54. (b)	55. (c)	56. (b)	57. (d)	58. (c)	59. (d)	60. (c)
61. (d)	62. (d)	63. (a)	64. (c)	65. (d)	66. (d)	67. (c)	68. (b)	69. (b)	70. (b)
71. (a)	72. (d)	73. (d)	74. (d)	75. (a)	76. (d)	77. (a)	78. (d)	79. (d)	80. (a)
81. (a)	82. (a)	83. (c)	84. (d)	85. (c)	86. (b)	87. (d)	88. (c)	89. (b)	90. (b)

Mock Test-3

1. The most important factor which determined the increase in human population in India during the 20th century is
   (a) Natality
   (b) Mortality
   (c) Immigration
   (d) Emigration
2. Vascular bundles in monocotyledons are considered closed because
   (a) Xylem is surrounded all around by phloem
   (b) There are no vessels with perforations
   (c) A bundle sheath surrounds each bundle
   (d) There is no secondary growth
3. When there are two haploid nuclei per cell in some fungi before the formation of diploid, this stage is called
   (a) diplotene
   (b) diplophase
   (c) dikaryophase
   (d) dikaryote
4. In blood group typing in human, if an allele contributed by one parent is I^A and an allele contributed by the other parent is i, the resulting blood group of the offspring will be
   (a) A
   (b) B
   (c) AB
   (d) O
5. A population growing in a habitat with limited resources shows four phases of growth in the following sequence
   (a) Acceleration - Deceleration-Lag phase - Asymptote
   (b) Asymptote - Acceleration - Deceleration - Lag phase
   (c) Lag phase - Acceleration - Deceleration - Asymptote
   (d) Acceleration - Lag phase - Deceleration - Asymptote
6. Necrosis in crops is due to the deficiency of
   (a) Ca, K, S and Mo
   (b) N, K, S and Mo
   (c) N, S, Fe and Zn
   (d) Mg, S, Mn and Ca
7. Presence of bundle sheath is a characteristics of
   (a) Xerophytic plants
   (b) Members of grass family
   (c) C_4 plants
   (d) C_3 plants
8. Which one of the following would not lead to formation of clones?
   (a) Double fertilization
   (b) Apomixis
   (c) Vegetative reproduction
   (d) Tissue culture
9. The variation/difference in the offsprings of a species from their parents constitutes an important component of
   (a) genetics
   (b) speciation
   (c) species fixation
   (d) heredity

10. If two pea plants having red (dominant) coloured flowers with unknown genotypes are crossed, 75% of the flowers are red and 25% are white. The genotypic constitution of the parents having red coloured flowers will be
(a) both homozygous
(b) one homozygous and other heterozygous
(c) both heterozygous
(d) both hemizygous

11. If the total amount of adenine and thymine in a double-stranded DNA is 60%, the amount of guanine in this DNA will be
(a) 15%
(b) 20%
(c) 30%
(d) 40%

12. The protein products of the following Bt toxin genes cry I Ac and cry II Ab are responsible for controlling
(a) bollworm
(b) roundworm
(c) moth
(d) fruit fly

13. In a flowering plant, the pollen tube first arrives in
(a) egg
(b) an antipodal cell
(c) a synergid
(d) central cell

14. A peculiar odour that prevails in marshy areas and cow-sheds is on account of a gas produced by
(a) mycoplasma
(b) archaebacteria
(c) slime moulds
(d) cyanobacteria

15. A germplasm collection is a
(a) Collection of specimens of all the species of an area in a herbarium or botanical garden
(b) Collection of modern varieties of a crop
(c) Collection of plants or seeds having diverse alleles of all genes in a crop
(d) Collection of seeds or pollen of rare and threatened species of a group or area

16. Walter Sutton is famous for his contribution to
(a) Genetic engineering
(b) Totipotency
(c) Quantitative genetics
(d) Chromosomal theory of inheritance

17. The reaction, Amino acid + ATP $\rightarrow$ Aminoacyl AMP + P-P depicts
(a) Amino acid assimilation
(b) Amino acid transformation
(c) Amino acid activation
(d) Amino acid translocation

18. The problem of blindness in poor countries can be taken care of by using the following
(a) golden rice
(b) transgenic tomato
(c) transgenic maize
(d) Bt brinjal

19. The transcription of any gene is the indication of its
(a) induction
(b) activity
(c) stimulation
(d) hypersensitivity

20. In C_4-plants, the bundle sheath cells
(a) have thin walls to facilitate gaseous exchange
(b) have large intercellular spaces
(c) are rich in PEP carboxylase
(d) have a high density of chloroplasts

21. In root nodules of legumes, leghaemoglobin is important because it
    (a) transports oxygen to the root nodule
    (b) acts as an oxygen scavenger
    (c) provides energy to the nitrogen fixing bacterium
    (d) acts as a catalyst in transamination
22. Darwin judged the fitness of an individual by
    (a) ability to defend itself
    (b) strategy to obtain food
    (c) number of offsprings
    (d) dominance over other individuals
23. Which of the following statements is wrong?
    (a) Pollen grains remain viable for several months because their outer covering is made of sporopollenin.
    (b) No enzyme can degrade sporopollenin.
    (c) Pollen grains are well represented in fossil strata due to sporopollenin.
    (d) Pollen wall has cavities containing proteins.
24. In plant biotechnology, PEG is used in
    (a) protoplast isolation
    (b) cell culture preparation
    (c) protoplast fusion
    (d) hardening
25. Analogous structures are
    (a) anatomically different but performing similar functions
    (b) anatomically similar but performing different functions
    (c) anatomically similar and functioning similarly
    (d) anatomically different and functioning differently
26. A polygenic trait is controlled by 3 genes: A, B and C. In a cross AaBbCc × AaBbCc, the phenotypic ratio of the offsprings was observed as 1:6:x:20:x:6:1. What is the possible value of x?
    (a) 3
    (b) 9
    (c) 15
    (d) 25
27. A transgenic rice (golden rice) has been developed for increased content of
    (a) vitamin A
    (b) vitamin B_1
    (c) vitamin C
    (d) vitamin D
28. When the conditions are dry, a grass leaf curls inward to minimize water loss due to presence of
    (a) thick cuticle
    (b) large xylem cavities
    (c) parallel venation
    (d) bulliform cells
29. The chromosome constitution $2n - 2$ of an organism represents
    (a) monosomic
    (b) nullisomic
    (c) haploid
    (d) trisomic
30. Meristem culture is practised in horticulture to get
    (a) somaclonal variation
    (b) haploids
    (c) virus-free plants
    (d) slow-growing callus
31. Tendril in cucurbita & Thorn in Bougainvillea are example of
    (a) convergent evolution
    (b) radiation
    (c) divergent evolution
    (d) co-evolution
32. Haemoglobin is
    (a) an oxygen carrier in human blood
    (b) a protein used as food supplement
    (c) an oxygen scavenger in root nodules
    (d) a plant protein with high lysine content

33. Stomatal opening is affected by
(a) Nitrogen concentration, carbon dioxide concentration and light
(b) carbon dioxide concentration, temperature and light
(c) nitrogen concentration, light and temperature
(d) carbon dioxide concentration, nitrogen concentration and temperature

34. Taxonomic hierarchy refers to
(a) step-wise arrangement of all categories for classification of plants and animals
(b) a group of senior taxonomists, who decide the nomenclature of plants and animals
(c) a list of botanists or zoologists, who have worked on taxonomy of a species or group
(d) classification of a species based on fossil record

35. Which of the following get accumulated in the vacuoles of guard cells during stomatal opening?
(a) Water, calcium and magnesium
(b) Starch, potassium and chloride ions
(c) Malate, sodium and potassium ions
(d) Malate, potassium and chloride ions

36. Which of the following is the most accepted theory for movement of water through plants?
(a) Cohesion-tension-transpiration pull theory
(b) Capillarity
(c) Passive transport
(d) Root pressure

37. Scutellum in a caryopsis represents
(a) outermost layer of endosperm
(b) a sheath that protects the radical
(c) the place where the seed is attached to raphe
(d) a cotyledon

38. In an annual ring, the light coloured part is known as
(a) early wood
(b) late wood
(c) heartwood
(d) sapwood

39. Natural cytokinins are synthesised in tissue that are
(a) senescent
(b) dividing rapidly
(c) storing food material
(d) differentiating

40. Resemblance of one organism to another for protection and hiding is
(a) mimicry
(b) predation
(c) adaptation
(d) camouflage

41. The rough endoplasmic reticulum (RER) in the cells are because of the presence of
(a) mitochondria associated with ER
(b) ribosomes on the surface of ER
(c) volutin granules on the surface of ER
(d) sulphur granules on the surface of ER

42. Elaioplasts store
(a) starch
(b) proteins
(c) fats
(d) essential amino acids

43. Aggregates of lymphoid tissue present in the distal portion of the small intestine are known as
(a) villi
(b) Peyer's patches
(c) rugae
(d) choroid plexus

44. Mendel's principle of segregation means that the gametes always receive
(a) one pair of alleles
(b) one quarter of the genes
(c) one of the paired alleles
(d) any pair of alleles

45. Which of the following vitamins help in absorption of calcium ion from intestine
(a) Vitamin A
(b) Vitamin D
(c) Vitamin C
(d) Vitamin B

46. Somatostatin
(a) stimulates glucagon release while inhibits insulin release
(b) stimulates release of insulin and glucagon
(c) inhibits release of insulin and glucagon
(d) inhibits glucagon release while stimulates insulin release

47. Starch graine in pea plant shows
(a) Complete Dominance
(b) Incomplete Dominance
(c) Co-Dominance
(d) Epistasis

48. ELISA assay
(a) uses complement mediated cell lysis
(b) uses a radiolabelled second antibody
(c) involves addition of substrate which is converted into coloured end product
(d) requires red blood cells

49. 'Complete competitors cannot coexist' is true for
(a) character displacement
(b) competitive exclusion
(c) primary succession
(d) Secondary succession

50. mRNA directs the building of proteins through a sequence of
(a) introns
(b) codons
(c) exons
(d) anticodons

51. Foramen ovale
(a) connects the two atria in the foetal heart
(b) is a condition in which the heart valves do not completely close
(c) is a shallow depression in the interventricular septum
(d) is a connection between the pulmonary trunk and the aorta in the foetus

52. Which of the following is a Gram negative bacterium?
(a) Escherichia coli
(b) Bacillus subtilis
(c) Streptomyces coelicolor
(d) Ampycolatopsis orientalis

53. What is meant by the term 'Darwin fitness'?
(a) The ability to survive and reproduce
(b) High aggressiveness
(c) Healthy appearance
(d) Physical strength

54. Absence of one sex chromosome causes
(a) Turner's syndrome
(b) Klinefelter's syndrome
(c) Down's syndrome
(d) Tay-Sach's syndrome

55. Comparing small and large cells, which statement is correct?
(a) Small cells have a small surface area per volume ratio
(b) Exchange rate of nutrients is fast with large cells
(c) Small cells have a large surface area per volume ratio
(d) Exchange rate of nutrients is slow with small cells

56. The number of autosomes in human primary spermatocyte is
(a) 46 (b) 44
(c) 23 (d) 22

57. The most abundant molecule in cell is
(a) Water (b) Carbohydrate
(c) Lipid (d) Protein

58. How many chromosomes will the cell have at G_1, after S and after M-phase respectively, if it has 14 chromosomes at interphase?
(a) 14, 14, 7 (b) 14, 14, 14
(c) 7, 7, 7 (d) 7, 14, 14

59. The Golgi apparatus
(a) is found only in animals (b) is found in prokaryotes
(c) is a site of rapid ATP production (d) modifies and packages proteins

60. Glycolysis
(a) takes place in the mitochondria
(b) produces no ATP
(c) has no connection with electron transport chain
(d) reduces two molecules of NAD^+ for every glucose molecule processed

61. Total number of all species of organisms in a given region is known as the region's
(a) biota (b) flora
(c) fauna (d) diversity

62. The arthropod exoskeleton is composed of
(a) Globulin
(b) Chitin
(c) several kinds of proteins
(d) single complex protein called arthropodin

63. C-DNA is
(a) Copy DNA (b) Conjugated DNA
(c) Chimeric DNA (d) Complex DNA

64. Maltose gives rise to two molecules of ________ on hydrolysis
(a) fructose (b) lactose
(c) glucose (d) sucrose

65. Sigmoid growth curve is represented by
(a) $dN/dt = rN$ (b) $dN/dt = rN\,(1 - N/K)$
(c) $Nt = No + B + I - D - E$ (d) $dN/dt = 1 - N/K$

66. Beadle and Tatum showed that each kind of mutant bread mould they studied lacked a specific enzyme. Their experiments demonstrated that
(a) cells need specific enzymes in order to function
(b) genes are made of DNA
(c) genes carry information for making proteins
(d) Enzymes are required to repair damaged DNA information

67. DNA has equal number of adenine and thymine residues (A = T) and equal number of guanine and cytosine (G = C). These relationships are known as
(a) Chargaff's rule (b) Coulomb's law
(c) Le-Chatelier's principle (d) Van't Hoff plot

68. 'Balancing selection' promotes
(a) homozygotes (b) heterozygotes
(c) polyploids (d) recessive traits

69. Vomiting centre is located in the
(a) medulla oblongata (b) stomach and sometimes in duodenum
(c) GI tract (d) hypothalamus

70. How many bio-geographical regions are present in India?
(a) 3 (b) 4
(c) 7 (d) 10

71. Which of the following organs in earthworm neutralizes humic acid present in humus?
(a) Typhlosole (b) Calciferous glands
(c) Intestinal caecum (d) Gizzard

72. Fertilized eggs of *P. americana* are encased in
(a) ootheca (b) cocoon
(c) genital chamber (d) phallomere

73. Insufficient quantities of antidiuretic hormone in blood lead to
(a) diabetes mellitus (b) glycosuria
(c) diabetes insipidus (d) uremia

74. Sphincter of Oddi guards
(a) hepato-pancreatic duct (b) common bile duct
(c) pancreatic duct (d) cystic duct

75. Graveyard for RBCs is
(a) liver (b) spleen
(c) kidney (d) lymph glands

76. Blood cells involved in inflammatory reactions are
(a) basophils (b) neutrophils
(c) eosinophils (d) monocytes

77. To obtain a standard ECG, a patient is connected to the machine with three electrodes
(a) one to each wrist and to the left ankle
(b) one to each ankle and to the left wrist
(c) one to each wrist and to the left chest region
(d) one to each ankle and to the left chest region

78. The clavicle articulates with ________ of scapula.
(a) acromion process (b) glenoid cavity
(c) acetabulum cavity (d) ball and socket joint

79. The age of pyramid with broad base indicates
(a) high percentage of young individuals (b) low percentage of young individuals
(c) high percentage of old individuals (d) low percentage of old individuals

80. Thymosin hormone is secreted by
(a) thyroid gland (b) parathyroid gland
(c) thymus gland (d) hypothalamus gland

81. Which of the following groups is absolutely essential functional component of the ecosystem?
(a) Producers (b) Producers and herbivores
(c) Producers and detritivores (d) Detritivores

82. Phagocytosis and pinocytosis are collectively termed as
(a) endocytosis (b) suspension feeding
(c) omnivores (d) mucous trap

83. PCR proceeds in three distinct steps governed by temperature. They are in order of
(a) denaturation, annealing, synthesis (b) synthesis, annealing, denaturation
(c) annealing, synthesis, denaturation (d) denaturation, synthesis, annealing

84. Corpus luteum releases
(a) oestrogen (b) progesterone
(c) oestrogen and progesterone (d) androgen

85. Which of the following organs is devoid of glands?
(a) uterus (b) vagina
(c) vulva (d) oviduct

86. Primary spermatocyte differs from spermatogonium in
(a) number of chromosomes (b) size and volume
(c) DNA content (d) size of chromosomes

87. In human, cleavage divisions are
(a) slow and synchronous (b) fast and synchronous
(c) slow and asynchronous (d) fast and asynchronous

88. The basic unit of study in Ecology is
(a) population (b) organism
(c) community (d) species

89. Which of the following is example of ex-situ conservation?
(a) Botanical garden (b) Sacred groves
(c) Wild life safari park (d) Both (a) and (c)

90. How many species of birds are there in Greenland?
(a) 1400 (b) 105
(c) 1300 (d) 56

Answer Keys

1. (a)	2. (d)	3. (c)	4. (a)	5. (c)	6. (a)	7. (c)	8. (a)	9. (a)	10. (c)
11. (b)	12. (c)	13. (c)	14. (b)	15. (c)	16. (d)	17. (c)	18. (a)	19. (b)	20. (d)
21. (b)	22. (c)	23. (d)	24. (c)	25. (a)	26. (c)	27. (a)	28. (d)	29. (b)	30. (c)
31. (c)	32. (a)	33. (b)	34. (a)	35. (d)	36. (a)	37. (d)	38. (a)	39. (b)	40. (a)
41. (b)	42. (c)	43. (b)	44. (c)	45. (b)	46. (c)	47. (b)	48. (c)	49. (b)	50. (b)
51. (a)	52. (a)	53. (a)	54. (a)	55. (c)	56. (b)	57. (a)	58. (b)	59. (d)	60. (d)
61. (a)	62. (b)	63. (a)	64. (c)	65. (b)	66. (c)	67. (a)	68. (a)	69. (a)	70. (d)
71. (b)	72. (a)	73. (c)	74. (a)	75. (b)	76. (a)	77. (a)	78. (a)	79. (a)	80. (c)
81. (c)	82. (a)	83. (a)	84. (b)	85. (d)	86. (b)	87. (a)	88. (b)	89. (d)	90. (d)

Sample Paper-I

1. Which of the following event occurs during G_1-phase?
   (a) DNA replication
   (b) Growth and normal function of cell
   (c) Mutation
   (d) Fertilization
2. The stage during which, cell decides to get specialized
   (a) S-phase
   (b) M-phase
   (c) G_1-phase
   (d) G_2-phase
3. In which of the following wavelength, photo system–I is inactive?
   (a) 780 nm
   (b) 680 nm
   (c) 690 nm
   (d) 550 nm
4. ADH deficiency causes
   (a) diabetes insipidus
   (b) goitre
   (c) tetany
   (d) acromegaly
5. Law of limiting factor of photosynthesis was proposed by
   (a) von Mayer
   (b) Arnon
   (c) F F Blackmann
   (d) Hill
6. Opening of stomata is not affected by
   (a) N_2
   (b) K^+ ions
   (c) Starch
   (d) None of these
7. The IV cranial nerve is
   (a) oculomotor
   (b) trochlear
   (c) olfactory
   (d) facial
8. Subunits of 80S ribosome are
   (a) 40S
   (b) 60S
   (c) Both (a) and (b)
   (d) None of these
9. The stored food in animals is called
   (a) cellulose
   (b) starch
   (c) glucose
   (d) glycogen
10. The cellular respiration first takes place in the
    (a) cytoplasm
    (b) Golgi bodies
    (c) ER
    (d) lysosomes
11. Which of the following substrate is used in the formation of alcohol?
    (a) Sucrose
    (b) Glucose
    (c) Galactose
    (d) Fructose
12. Rubisco stands for
    (a) Ribulose bisphosphate carboxylase oxygenase
    (b) Ribulose phosphate carboxylase oxygenase

(c) Ribulose phosphate carboxylic oxygenase
(d) None of the above

13. Net gain of ATP molecules per hexose during aerobic respiration is
(a) 12 (b) 18
(c) 36 (d) 30

14. The term "hot dilute soup" was used by
(a) Haldane (b) von Helmont
(c) Redi (d) LouisPasteur

15. Which of the following classification is based on some morphological characters?
(a) Artificial (b) Natural
(c) Phylogenetic (d) Both (b) and (c)

16. Sweet potato and potato are examples of
(a) Homologous structure (b) Analogous structure
(c) Both (a) and (b) (d) None of the above

17. 'Systema Naturae' was written by
(a) Hutchinson (b) Lamarck
(c) Linnaeus (d) Bentham and Hooker

18. In the origin of life, microspheres are most primitive protobiont, which have a membrane of
(a) lipid and proteins (b) lipid
(c) carbohydrates (d) fats

19. Rabies is caused by
(a) Virus (b) Bacteria
(c) Protozoa (d) All of these

20. Tuberculosis is caused by
(a) *Vibrio cholerae* (b) *Mycobacterium*
(c) *Salmonella typhi* (d) None of these

21. Which of the following provides nutrition to sperm?
(a) Leydig cells (b) Scrotum
(c) Sertoli cells (d) Epididymis

22. Oral contraceptive pills function by
(a) Fertilization (b) Inhibiting ovulation
(c) Reproduction (d) None of the above

23. *Sphagnum* belongs to
(a) Bryophyta (b) Pteridophyta
(c) Gymnosperm (d) Angiosperm

24. Fungi differs from slime moulds by lacking of
(a) Flagellated spores (b) Ascospores
(c) basidiospores (d) zygospores

25. Fungi are classified on the basis of
(a) Sexual reproduction (b) Asexual reproduction
(c) Vegetative reproduction (d) None of the above

26. Which one of the following does not belong to kingdom–Monera?
(a) Mycoplasma (b) Archaebacteria
(c) Slime mould (d) Eubacteria

27. Which one of the following is not a plastid?
(a) Mitoplast (b) Chromoplast
(c) Chloroplast (d) Leucoplast

28. In retroviruses, RNA dependent DNA polymerase synthesizes
(a) RNA–DNA (b) DNA
(c) RNA (d) None of these

29. What will happen, when glucose is administered orally?
(a) Excretion (b) Digestion
(c) Circulation (d) Respiration

30. Agrose is a gel, which is used to separate
(a) carbohydrate (b) fats
(c) Both (a) and (b) (d) protein

31. The process of reverse transcription was discovered by
(a) Temin and Baltimore (b) Watson and Crick
(c) Alfred Hershey (d) None of the above

32. Which one of the following animal has pseudocoelome?
(a) Cockroach (b) *Ancylostoma*
(c) Aurelia (d) *Fasiola*

33. The process of joining of amino acids is called
(a) Transcription (b) Translation
(c) Conjugation (d) None of these

34. The infective stage of *Plasmodium vivax* is
(a) sporozoite (b) gametocyte
(c) trophozoite (d) cryptozoite

35. Which of the following is obtained from genetic engineering?
(a) Haemoglobin (b) Glucose
(c) Golden rice (d) None of these

36. Which of the following is a test cross?
(a) Ww × ww (b) WW × ww
(c) Ww × Ww (d) ww × ww

37. One gene–one enzyme hypothesis was propounded by
(a) Beadle and Tatum (b) Louis Pasteur
(c) J B S Haldane (d) None of the above

38. The glenoid cavity is associated with
(a) scapula (b) humerus
(c) Both (a) and (b) (d) None of these

39. The nerve fibre in its resting stage is
(a) More- permeable to K^+ (b) Semi-permeable to K^+
(c) Less permeable to K^+ (d) All of the above

40. Genes when close together on a chromosome are known as
(a) Linkage (b) Mutation
(c) Translation (d) Transcription

41. In human beings, 45 chromosomes/single X/XO abnormality causes
(a) Down's syndrome (b) Klinefelter's syndrome
(c) Turner's syndrome (d) Edward's syndrome

42. An evolutionary process, giving rise to new species adapting to new habitats and ways of life is called
(a) adaptive radiation (b) adaptation
(c) convergent evolution (d) microevolution

43. The chromosomal arrangement results in
(a) euploidy (b) aneuploidy
(c) duplication (d) polyploidy

44. One of these is associated with terminator codon?
(a) AGG (b) UAA
(c) UUA (d) AUG

45. The inherent maximum capacity of an organism to reproduce or increase in number is called as
(a) biotic potential (b) ecosystem
(c) population (d) ecology

46. Which of the following is best suited for co-dominance?
(a) Both are recessive (b) Both are dominance
(c) One is recessive (d) One is dominance

47. The substance which is metal ion for the normal functioning of enzyme is called
(a) cofactor (b) coenzyme
(c) holoenzyme (d) None of these

48. Scala Naturae was written by
(a) Linnaeus (b) Darwin
(c) Aristotle (d) Whittaker

49. The gene which masks the effect of another gene is called
(a) Epistasis (b) Lethal gene
(c) Multiple allele (d) Complementary gene

50. In a DNA molecule, the adenine is 15%. What will be the percentage of guanine in this DNA?
(a) 15% (b) 35%
(c) 70% (d) 30%

51. Which one is used in the production of insulin by genetic engineering?
(a) *Eschereria coli* (b) *Mycobacterium*
(c) Both (a) and (b) (d) None of these

52. The synthesis of complex molecules from simple molecules was proved by
(a) Arrhenius (b) Pasteur
(c) Stanley Miller (d) Redi

53. Which is not correct according to Chargaff's rule?
(a) $A+T=C+G$ (b) $A+G=C+T$
(c) $\frac{A+G}{C+T}=1$ (d) None of these

54. Which of the following cells are associated with identification of colours in bright light?
(a) Rod cells (b) Cone cells
(c) Both (a) and (b) (d) None of these

55. Which of the following defines Hardey Weinberg's law?
(a) $p^2+2pq+q^2=1$ (b) $p^2+2pq+q^2=1$
(c) $p^2+2pq+q^2=0$ (d) $q^2+p^2+2pq=0$

56. Photochemical smog pollution does not contain
(a) ozone (b) nitrogen dioxide
(c) carbon dioxide (d) PAN

57. Decrease in the calcium level in blood is caused by
(a) prolactin (b) calcitonin
(c) adrenocorticotropin (d) oxytocin

58. The ozone layer is found in
(a) troposphere (b) mesosphere
(c) stratosphere (d) atmosphere

59. The pectoral fins get enlarged in
(a) *Exocoetus* (b) *Scoliodon*
(c) *Hippocampus* (d) *Coccosteus*

60. What is a keystone species?
(a) A species which adds upto only a small proportion of the total biomass of a community, yet has a huge impact on the community's organization and survival.
(b) A common species that has plenty of biomass, yet has a fairly low impact on the community's organization.
(c) A rare species that has minimal impact on the biomass and on other species in the community.
(d) A dominant species that constitutes a large proportion of the biomass and which affects many other species.

61. Which one of the following plant functions as symbiotic nitrogen fixing plant?
(a) *Azolla* (b) *Cycas*
(c) Moss (d) *Marchantia*

62. Bowman's glands are found in
(a) olfactory epithelium (b) external auditory canal
(c) cortical nephrons only (d) juxta medullary nephrons

63. An important evidence in favour of organic evolution is the occurrence
(a) Homologous and vestigial organs (b) Analogous and vestigial organs
(c) Homologous organs only (d) Homologous and analogous organs

64. Eutrophication is the result of
(a) Bryophyte (b) Algae and aquatic plants
(c) Gymnosperm (d) Pteridophyte

65. Which one of the following is non-biodegradable?
(a) Sewage (b) DDT
(c) Live stock waste (d) Market garbage

66. ADH controls water permeability of
(a) Distal convoluted tubule (b) Proximal convoluted tubule
(c) Bowman's capsule (d) All of the above

67. The cause of decline in the population of reptiles and birds is
(a) DDT (b) bio-fertilizer
(c) bio-insecticides (d) biodegradable

68. Which one of the following shows detritus food chain?
(a) Organic waste → Bacteria → Mollusc (b) Grass → Insects → Snakes
(c) Plankton → Small fishes → Large fishes (d) All of the above

69. Which of the following enzyme helps in digesting protein in stomach?
(a) Trypsin (b) Pepsin
(c) Ptyalin (d) Rennin

70. The Leydig cells secrete
(a) estrogen (b) testosterone
(c) progesterone (d) cortisol

71. Which one of the following is not a bio-fertilizer?
(a) *Bacillus thuringiensis* (b) *Azotobacter*
(c) *Azolla* (d) *Clostridium*

72. In India hot spot area is found in
(a) Western Himalaya (b) Tropical Andes
(c) Madagascar (d) Mesoamerica

73. The thalloid body of a slime mould (Myxomycetes) is known as
(a) Protonema (b) Plasmodium
(c) Fruiting body (d) Mycelium

74. A normal woman whose father was a colour blind person is married to a normal man. Her sons would likely to be
(a) 75% colour-blind (b) 50% colour-blind
(c) All normal (d) All colour-blind

75. Which of the following is not a function of liver?
(a) Production of bile (b) Production of insulin
(c) Glycogen storage (d) Detoxification

76. The vital capacity of human lung is equal to
(a) 500 mL (b) 4600 mL
(c) 5800 mL (d) 2300 mL

77. Wavelength of visible light/PAR is
(a) 200-400 nm (b) 700-900 nm
(c) 400-700 nm (d) 100-200 nm

78. DNA can be formed by
(a) transaminase (b) lyases
(c) RNA dependent DNA polymerase (d) All of the above

79. A cell active in protein synthesis will rich in
(a) ribosomes (b) Golgi bodies
(c) mitochondria (d) lysosomes

80. The RNA primer is used in
(a) Translation (b) Replication
(c) Conjugation (d) Transformation

81. Which part is edible in Jack fruit.
(a) Bracts (b) Seeds
(c) Perianth (d) All of these

82. Bands generally used for plant karyotyping.
(a) Q and C band (b) Q and R band
(c) G and C band (d) N and C band

83. Example of non competitive inhibition
(a) G-6-P /Hexokinase (b) Sulpha drugs and /P- amino benzoic acid.
(c) Cytochrome oxidase/Cyanide (d) All of these

84. Example of inhibitory gene from below options
(a) Fruit shape in Squash
(b) Coat color in mouse.
(c) Fruit color in squash
(d) Feather color in Fowls

85. Failure of chloride ion transport mechanism is seen in
(a) PKU
(b) Cystic fibrosis
(c) Huntigton's disease
(d) Sickle cell anemia

86. Match the column

Antibiotic	Effect
A. Tetracycline	(i) Inhibits translocation of m RNA along ribosome
B. Chloramphenicol	(ii) Inhibit interaction between tRNA and m-RNA
C. Erythromycin	(iii) Inhibit binding amino-acyl tRNA to ribosome
D. Neomycin	(iv) Inhibit peptidyl transferase

(a) A – i, B – ii, C – iii, D – iv
(b) A – iii, B – iv, C – i, D – ii
(c) A – ii, B – iii, C – iii, D – i
(d) A – iv, B – i, C – ii, D – iii

87. Which of the foolowoing products now a days prepared by recombinant DNA
(a) Erythropoietin
(b) Interferons
(c) Interleukins
(d) All of these

88. In which plant terminal leaflets are modified into curved hooks for helping the plant in climbing
(a) Argemone
(b) Opuntia
(c) Bignonia unguis-cati
(d) Ficus

89. Part edible in cutard Apple is
(a) Mesocarp
(b) Pericarp
(c) Placental hairs
(d) Fleshy thalamus

90.

G ↓ G A T C C
C C T A G ↑ G

Above diagram represent recognition site for
(a) Sca I
(b) Sma I
(c) EcoRI
(d) BamH I

Answer Keys

1. (b)	2. (c)	3. (a)	4. (a)	5. (c)	6. (a)	7. (b)	8. (c)	9. (d)	10. (a)
11. (a)	12. (a)	13. (c)	14. (a)	15. (a)	16. (b)	17. (c)	18. (a)	19. (a)	20. (b)
21. (c)	22. (b)	23. (a)	24. (a)	25. (a)	26. (c)	27. (a)	28. (a)	29. (d)	30. (d)
31. (a)	32. (b)	33. (b)	34. (a)	35. (c)	36. (a)	37. (a)	38. (c)	39. (a)	40. (a)
41. (c)	42. (a)	43. (b)	44. (b)	45. (a)	46. (b)	47. (a)	48. (c)	49. (a)	50. (b)
51. (a)	52. (c)	53. (a)	54. (b)	55. (a)	56. (c)	57. (b)	58. (c)	59. (a)	60. (a)
61. (a)	62. (a)	63. (a)	64. (b)	65. (b)	66. (a)	67. (a)	68. (a)	69. (b)	70. (b)
71. (a)	72. (a)	73. (b)	74. (b)	75. (b)	76. (b)	77. (c)	78. (c)	79. (a)	80. (b)
81. (d)	82. (d)	83. (c)	84. (d)	85. (b)	86. (b)	87. (d)	88. (c)	89. (b)	90. (b)

Sample Paper-II

1. An example for symbiotic bacteria
   (a) *Erwinia amylovora*
   (b) *Rhizobium leguminosarum*
   (c) *Xanthomonas campestris*
   (d) *Agrobacterium tumefaciens*
2. In which plant, the fruit is a drupe, seed coat is thin, embryo is inconspicuous and endosperm is edible?
   (a) Groundnut
   (b) Wheat
   (c) Apple
   (d) Coconut
3. Somaclonal variation appears in plants:
   (a) Growing in polluted soil or water
   (b) Exposed to gamma rays
   (c) Raised in tissue culture
   (d) Transformed by recombinant DNA technology
4. In a monoecious plant:
   (a) Male and female sex organs are on different individuals
   (b) Male and female gametes are of two morphologically distinct types
   (c) Male and female sex organs are on the same individual
   (d) All the stamens are fused to form one unit
5. Which one of the following are intracellular obligate parasites?
   (a) Bacteria
   (b) Viruses
   (c) Slime moulds
   (d) Blue-green algae
6. Pineapple fruit develops from:
   (a) Unilocular polycarpellary flower
   (b) Multipistillate syncarpus flower
   (c) Multilocular monocarpellary flower
   (d) A cluster of compactly born flowers on an axis
7. A sewage treatment process in which a part of decomposer bacteria present in the waste is recycled into the starting of the process is called:
   (a) Cyclic treatment
   (b) Activated sludge treatment
   (c) Primary treatment
   (d) Tertiary treatment
8. Which of following mineral-nutrients plays an important role in biological nitrogen fixation?
   (a) Zinc
   (b) Iron
   (c) Molybdenum
   (d) Magnesium
9. Which of the following is true?
   (a) Vessels are unicellular and with narrow lumen
   (b) Vessels are multicellular and with wide lumen
   (c) Tracheids are unicellular and with wide lumen
   (d) Tracheids are multicellular and with narrow lumen

10. In C_4 plants, the bundle sheath cells:
(a) Have thin walls to facilitate gaseous exchange
(b) Have large intercellular spaces
(c) Are rich in PEP carboxylase
(d) Have a high density of chloroplasts

11. Potato spindle tuber disease is caused by:
(a) A nematode (b) A virus
(c) A bacterium (d) A viroid

12. In which of the following, all listed genera belong to the same class of algae?
(a) Chara, Fucus, Polysiphonia
(b) Volvox, Spirogyra, Chlamydomonas
(c) Porphyra, Ectocarpus, Ulothrix
(d) Sargassum, Laminaria, Gracillaria

13. In root nodules of legumes, leg-haemoglobin is important because:
(a) It transports oxygen to the root nodule
(b) It acts as an oxygen scavenger
(c) It provides energy to the nitrogen fixing bacterium
(d) It acts as a catalyst in transamination

14. Darwin judged the fitness of an individual by:
(a) Ability to defend itself (b) Strategy to obtain food
(c) Number of offsprings (d) Dominance over other individuals

15. Etiolation in plants is caused when:
(a) They are grown in dark (b) They have mineral deficiency
(c) They are grown in intense light (d) They are grown in blue light

16. Calorie is the unit of:
(a) Sound (b) Temperature
(c) Light (d) Heat

17. In an annual ring, the light coloured part is known as:
(a) Early wood (b) Late wood
(c) Heartwood (d) Sapwood

18. The chief component of the middle lamella in plant cell is:
(a) Potassium (b) Calcium
(c) Magnesium (d) Phosphorus

19. Tonoplast is a membrane surrounding the:
(a) Cytoplasm (b) Vacuole
(c) Nucleus (d) Mitochondria

20. Polyploidy can be produced artificially by:
(a) Colchicine (b) Inbreeding
(c) Line breeding (d) Self pollination

21. Recombination is involved in the process of:
(a) Cytokinesis (b) Spindle formation
(c) Crossing over (d) Chromosome duplication

22. A fibrous root system is excellent for:
(a) Food storage (b) Nitrogen fixation
(c) Absorbing water from deeper layer of soil (d) Providing good anchorage for the plant

23. If a primary root continues to grow, the type of root system will be known as:
(a) Secondary (b) Fibrous
(c) Tap (d) Stilt

24. A horizontal underground stem is a:
(a) Corm (b) Phylloclade
(c) Rhizome (d) Rhizoid

25. If global warming continues, the organism which may face more severe threat is:
(a) Cow (b) Banana
(c) Snow leopard (d) Dolphin

26. One advantage of cleistogamy is:
(a) It leads to greater genetic diversity
(b) Seed dispersal is more efficient and widespread
(c) Seed set is not dependent on pollinators
(d) Each visit of a pollinator results in transfer of hundreds of pollen grains

27. Jute fibres are obtained from the:
(a) Secondary phloem (b) Pith
(c) Xylem (d) Endodermis

28. A chromosome in which the centromere is situated close to its end so that one arm is very short and the other very long is:
(a) Acrocentric (b) Metacentric
(c) Sub-metacentric (d) Telocentric

29. Resin and turpentine are products of:
(a) Teak (b) Oak
(c) Eucalyptus (d) Pine

30. An inexhaustible non-conventional universal source of energy is:
(a) Wind energy (b) Solar energy
(c) Hydrothermal energy (d) Tidal energy

31. Which one of the following periods is largely associated with extinction of dinosaurs and the increase in flowering plants and reptiles?
(a) Jurassic (b) Triassic
(c) Cretaceous (d) Permian

32. Which type of water is used by the plants?
(a) Gravitational water (b) Capillary water
(c) Hygroscopic water (d) Bound water

33. Electroporation involves:
(a) Promotion of seed germination by induced imbibition of water with electric current
(b) Making transient pores in cell membrane to facilitate entry of gene constructs
(c) Purification of saline water with the help of an artificial membrane
(d) Passage of sucrose through sieve pores by electro-osmosis

34. One of the following acts as secondary pollutant:
(a) Br_2 (b) Cl_2
(c) NO_2 (d) HNO_3

35. Cuticle is absent in:
(a) Mesophytes (b) Young roots
(c) Mature stems (d) Leaves

36. The least porous soil among the following is a:
(a) Loamy soil (b) Silty soil
(c) Clayey soil (d) Peaty soil

37. In higher plants, the shape of the chloroplast is:
(a) Discoid (b) Cup-shaped
(c) Girdle-shaped (d) Reticulate

38. Which of the following statements is false?
(a) TMV has a double-stranded RNA molecule
(b) Most plant viruses are RNA viruses
(c) The bacteriophage has a double-stranded DNA molecule
(d) Most animal viruses are DNA viruses

39. A kingdom common to unicellular animals and plants is:
(a) Monera (b) Plantae
(c) Fungi (d) Protista

40. Which of the following is a rootless aquatic plant, in which a portion of the leaf forms a tiny sac for trapping insects?
(a) Nepenthes (b) Drosera
(c) Utricularia (d) Dionaea

41. Enzymes that catalyse inter-conversion of optical, geometrical or positional isomers are:
(a) Ligases (b) Lyases
(c) Hydrolases (d) Isomerases

42. According to abiogenesis life originate from:
(a) Non-living (b) Pre-existing life
(c) Chemicals (d) Extra-terrestrial matter

43. External fertilization occurs in majority of:
(a) Algae (b) Fungi
(c) Liverworts (d) Mosses

44. The final stable community in ecological succession is:
(a) Pioneers (b) Sere
(c) Climax (d) carnivores

45. Which of the following combinations of characters is true for slime moulds?
(a) Parasitic, plasmodium with true walls, spores dispersed by air currents
(b) Saprophytic, plasmodium without walls, spores dispersed by water
(c) Parasitic, plasmodium without walls, spores dispersed by water
(d) Saprophytic, plasmodium without walls, spores dispersed by air currents

46. Which is an organic compound found in most cells?
(a) Glucose (b) Water
(c) Sodium chloride (d) Oxygen

47. Taxonomic hierarchy refers to:
(a) Stepwise arrangement of all categories for classification of plants and animals
(b) A group of senior taxonomists who decide the nomenclature of plants and animals
(c) A list of botanists or zoologists who have worked on taxonomy of a species or group
(d) Classification of a species based on fossil record

48. Reproductive isolation between segments of a single population is termed:
(a) Sympatry (b) Allopatry
(c) Population divergence (d) Disruptive divergence

49. Steroid hormones easily pass through the plasma membrane by simple diffusion because they:
(a) Are water soluble (b) Contain carbon and hydrogen
(c) Enter through pores (d) Are lipid soluble

50. Industrial melanism is an example of:
(a) Defensive adaptation of skin against UV radiations
(b) Drug resistance
(c) Protective resemblance with the surrounding
(d) Darkening of skin due to industries

51. The larva of *Bombyx mori* is known as:
(a) Nymph (b) Trochophore
(c) Cocoon (d) Caterpillar

52. Which of the following is a viviparous fish?
(a) Exocoetus (b) Gambusia
(c) Clarias (d) Labeo

53. The cutaneous plexus and the papillary plexus consist of:
(a) A network of nerves to provide dermal sensation
(b) A network of arteries to provide derma supply
(c) Specialized cells for cutaneous sensations
(d) Gland cells that release cutaneous secretions

54. The function of vagus nerve innervating the heart is to:
(a) Initiate the heart beat (b) Reduce the heart beat
(c) Accelerate the heart beat (d) Maintain constant heart beat

55. The size of pupil is controlled by the:
(a) Ciliary muscles (b) Suspensory ligaments
(c) Cornea (d) Iris muscles

56. Largest single mass of lymphatic tissue in the body is:
(a) Lung (b) Spleen
(c) Liver (d) Kidney

57. HIV is classified as a retrovirus because its genetic information is carried in:
(a) DNA instead of RNA (b) DNA
(c) RNA instead of DNA (d) Protein coat

58. Vomiting centre is located in the:
(a) Stomach and sometimes in duodenum (b) Gastro-intestinal tract
(c) Hypothalamus (d) Medulla oblongata

59. Sickle cell anaemia is:
(a) Autosomal dominant inheritance (b) X-linked recessive inheritance
(c) Autosomal recessive inheritance (d) X-linked dominant inheritance

60. Skeletal muscles are controlled by:
(a) Sympathetic nerves (b) Parasympathetic nerves
(c) Somatic nerves (d) Autonomic nerves

61. Niche is defined as the:
(a) Position of species in a community in relation to other species
(b) Place where organism lives
(c) Place where organism lives and performs its duty
(d) Place where population perform their duties

62. Erythropoiesis starts in:
(a) Kidney
(b) Liver
(c) Spleen
(d) Red bone marrow

63. In an aquatic ecosystem, the trophic level equivalent to cows in grasslands is:
(a) Phytoplankton
(b) Zooplankton
(c) Nekton
(d) Benthos

64. Oxidative phosphorylation refers to:
(a) Anaerobic production of ATP
(b) The citric acid cycle production of ATP
(c) Production of ATP by chemiosmosis
(d) Alcoholic fermentation

65. Down's syndrome is due to:
(a) Linkage
(b) Sex-linked inheritance
(c) Crossing over
(d) Non-disjunction of chromosome

66. All flat worms differ from all round worms in having:
(a) Triploblastic body
(b) Solid mesoderm
(c) Bilateral symmetry
(d) Metamorphosis in the life history

67. Deserts, grasslands, forests and tundra are the examples of:
(a) Biomes
(b) Biogeographical regions
(c) Ecosystems
(d) Biospheres

68. Which of the following is a free living nitrogen fixing bacterium present in the soil?
(a) *Nitrosomonas*
(b) *Rhizobium*
(c) *Azotobacter*
(d) *Pseudomonas*

69. Aedes aegypti is a vector for:
(a) Both dengue and yellow fever
(b) Dengue fever
(c) Yellow fever
(d) Japanese encephalitis

70. Inadequate protein intake leads to kwashiorkor. The subsequent edema is most closely related to inadequate synthesis of which protein?
(a) Gamma globulin
(b) Glucagon
(c) Insulin
(d) Albumin

71. The "lock and key" model of enzyme action illustrates that a particular enzyme molecule:
(a) May be destroyed and resynthesised several times
(b) Interacts with a specific type of substrate molecule
(c) Reacts at identical rates under all conditions
(d) Forms a permanent enzyme-substrate complex

72. If the pituitary gland of an adult rat is surgically removed, which of the following endocrine glands will be less affected?
(a) Adrenal cortex
(b) Adrenal Medulla
(c) Thyroid
(d) Gonads

73. If one litre of water is introduced in human blood, then:
(a) BMR increases
(b) RBC collapses and urine production increases
(c) RBC collapses and urine production decreases
(d) BMR decreases

74. Beadle and Tatum showed that each kind of mutant bread mould they studied lacked a specific enzyme. Their experiments demonstrated that:
(a) Cells needs specific enzymes in order to function
(b) Genes are made of DNA
(c) Enzymes are required to repair damage
(d) Genes carry information for making proteins

75. mRNA directs the building of proteins through a sequence of:
(a) Exons (b) Introns
(c) Codons (d) Anticodons

76. Carbon dioxide is called green-house gas because it is:
(a) Used in green-house to increase plant growth
(b) Transparent to heat but traps sunlight
(c) Transparent to sunlight but traps heat
(d) Transparent to both sunlight and heat

77. The hormone that increases the blood calcium level and decreases its excretion by kidney is:
(a) Parathormone (b) Calcitonin
(c) Thyroxine (d) Insulin

78. Signaling between cells usually results in the activation of protein:
(a) Lipases (b) Kinases
(c) Proteases (d) Nucleases

79. Estrogen and testosterone are steroid hormones, and are most likely bind to:
(a) Membrane ions channels
(b) Enzyme-linked membrane receptors
(c) G-protein linked membrane receptors
(d) Cytoplasmic receptors

80. Which of the following is unique to mitosis and not a part of meiosis?
(a) Homologous chromosomes behave independently
(b) Chromatids are separated during anaphase
(c) Homologous chromosomes pair and form bivalents
(d) Homologous chromosomes crossover

81. Transplant between different species is
(a) Isograft (b) Allograft
(c) Xenograft (d) None of these

82. The UN conference of Parties on climate change in the year 2016 was held at
(a) Warsow (b) Lima
(c) Marrakech (d) Paris

83. Uses of organisms to add essential materials to a degraded ecosystem
(a) Bio-deterioration (b) Bio-augmentation
(c) Bio-transformation (d) Bio-magnification

84. ABA can be bioassayed by
(a) Triple pea test
(b) Root inhibition test
(c) Inhibition of α- amylase synthesis in barley endosperm test
(d) Tobacco pith culture

85. Polytene chromosome first reported by
(a) Kollar (b) Balbiani
(c) Flemming (d) Ruckert

86. What happens when sperm enters in secondary oocyte in humans
(a) Breaking of MPF (b) Turning of APC
(c) Both of above (d) None of the above

87. The science of ageing is referred as
(a) Anthropology (b) Chronology
(c) Gerontology (d) Ctetology

88. The extent of which ion accumulation in guard cells determines the size of the stomatal opening
(a) sodium ion (b) Potassium ion
(c) Chloride ion (d) Calcium ion

89. Nodule formation in leguminous plant believed to be occur due to
(i) Cytokinin produced by invading bacteria
(ii) Auxin produced by plant cell.
(iii) Auxin produced by invading bacteria
(iv) Cytokinin produced by plant cell.
(a) (i) and (ii) only (b) (i) and (iii) only
(c) (iii) and (iv) only (d) (ii) and (iv) only

90. Hydroxypyruvate in C-2 cycle formed in which cell orgenelle
(a) Chloroplast (b) Mitochondria
(c) Peroxisome (d) Vacoule

Answer Keys

1. (b)	2. (d)	3. (c)	4. (c)	5. (b)	6. (d)	7. (b)	8. (c)	9. (b)	10. (d)
11. (d)	12. (b)	13. (b)	14. (c)	15. (a)	16. (d)	17. (a)	18. (b)	19. (b)	20. (a)
21. (c)	22. (d)	23. (c)	24. (c)	25. (c)	26. (c)	27. (a)	28. (a)	29. (d)	30. (b)
31. (c)	32. (b)	33. (b)	34. (d)	35. (b)	36. (c)	37. (a)	38. (a)	39. (d)	40. (c)
41. (d)	42. (a)	43. (a)	44. (c)	45. (d)	46. (a)	47. (a)	48. (a)	49. (d)	50. (c)
51. (d)	52. (b)	53. (a)	54. (b)	55. (d)	56. (b)	57. (c)	58. (d)	59. (c)	60. (c)
61. (c)	62. (b)	63. (b)	64. (c)	65. (d)	66. (b)	67. (a)	68. (c)	69. (a)	70. (d)
71. (b)	72. (b)	73. (b)	74. (d)	75. (c)	76. (c)	77. (a)	78. (b)	79. (d)	80. (a)
81. (c)	82. (c)	83. (b)	84. (c)	85. (b)	86. (c)	87. (c)	88. (b)	89. (a)	90. (c)

Sample Paper-III

1. How many genes are found in Drosophila Melanogaster?
(a) 30,000 (b) 18,000
(c) 13,000 (d) 4,000

2. Which enzyme is responsible for degrading cell wall?
(a) Hexokinase (b) Amylase
(c) Glukcokinase (d) Cellulase

3. Enzyme found functional in lysosome is:
(a) Acid phosphatase (b) Basic phosphatase
(c) Oxido reductase (d) Liases

4. Action of lysozyme is:
(a) Physiological (b) Anatomical
(c) Morphological (d) None of these

5. Which is not phagocytic?
(a) Monocyte (b) Lymphocyte
(c) Mast-cell (d) Neutrophil

6. Which part of brain control intellectual ability?
(a) Frontal lobe (b) Parietal lobe
(c) Temporal lobe (d) Occipital lobe

7. The correct sequence of meanings of brain from outside to inside is:
(a) Duramater → arachnoid → piamater (b) Arachnoid → duramater → piamater
(c) Piamater → duramater → arachnoid (d) Duramater → piamater → arachnoid

8. The sequence of ear ossicles from outside to inside is:
(a) Malleus → Incus → Stapes (b) Incus → Stapes → Malleus
(c) Stapes → Incus → Malleus (d) Malleus → Stapes → Incus

9. Which of the following is balancing organ?
(a) Organ of Corti (b) Cochlea
(c) Vestibular region (d) All of these

10. Glenoid cavity is found in:
(a) Pelvic girdle (b) Pectoral girdle
(c) Sternum (d) Humerus

11. Vital capacity of lung is:
(a) TV + IRV + ERV (b) TV + IRV + RV
(c) TV + ERV (d) IRV + ERV

12. During normal respiration without any effort the volume of air inspired or expired is called:
(a) Tidal volume (b) Reserve volume
(c) Residual volume (d) None of these

13. Synaptic vesicle is found in:
    (a) Pre synaptic neuron (b) Post synaptic neuron
    (c) Synaptic cleft (d) None of the above
14. 3-PGA is first stable product in
    (a) carbon-reduction cycle (b) OAA
    (c) Malic acid (d) PEP
15. Fat storing granules are:
    (a) Elaioplast (b) Amyloplast
    (c) Aleuroplast (d) None of these
16. Sub units in prokaryotic ribosomes are:
    (a) 60S – 40S (b) 50S – 30S
    (c) 40S – 30S (d) 50S – 20S
17. Adaptive radiation is for:
    (a) Dissimilar character for adoption from common ancestor
    (b) Similar characters for adoption from common ancestor
    (c) Dissimilar character for adoption from different ancestor
    (d) Similar characters for adoption from different ancestor
18. Competition of species leads to:
    (a) Extinction (b) Mutation
    (c) Greater number of niches are formed (d) Symbiosis
19. Large unit of land having different types of plants and animals:
    (a) Uniform vegetation (b) Biome
    (c) Ecosystem (d) Niche
20. Pepsinogen is secreted by:
    (a) Chief cell (b) Oxyntic cell
    (c) Mast cell (d) Parietal cell
21. Haematuria means:
    (a) RBC in the urine (b) WBC in the urine
    (c) Both (a) and (b) (d) None of the above
22. Which of the following is both osmoregulator as well as nitrogenous product?
    (a) NH_3 (b) Urea
    (c) Uric acid (d) All of these
23. Phylogenetic system was given by:
    (a) Engler and Prantl (b) Pliny
    (c) John Ray (d) R.H. Whittaker
24. Coacervates are:
    (a) Protobionts having polysaccharide + protein + H_2O
    (b) Protein aggregate
    (c) Protein and lipid aggregates
    (d) None of the above
25. Bt toxin obtained from:
    (a) Prokaryotes (b) Eukaryotes
    (c) Both (a) and (b) (d) None of these

26. Which is correct?
(a) Slime moulds are haploid
(b) Protozoan lack cell wall
(c) Dinoflagellates are immotile
(d) Pellicle is absent in *Euglena*

27. Zygospore is:
(a) Give rise to zoospores on meiosis
(b) Equivalent to Ascus, *Brasilia*
(c) Dormant stage
(d) Give raise to asexual spore

28. Which disaccharide has different linkage?
(a) Maltose
(b) Starch
(c) Sucrose
(d) Lactose

29. Corpus luteum secretes
(a) Progesterone and estrogen
(b) LH
(c) Only progesterone
(d) Progesterone and LH

30. Testosterone is secreted by
(a) Leydig cell
(b) Sertoli cell
(c) Spermatogenic cell
(d) All of the above

31. Hypothyroidism causes
(a) Myxodema
(b) Cretinism
(c) Both (a) and (b)
(d) Exopthalmic goiter

32. Which of the following controls the function of Sertoli cell?
(a) FSH
(b) Estrogen
(c) ACTH
(d) Testosterone

33. Fertilization of sperm and ova takes place in:
(a) Ampulla of oviduct
(b) Isthmus of oviduct
(c) Fimbrae of oviduct
(d) None of the above

34. Rr/rr progeny: Red (dominant) flowered heterozygous crossed with white flower:
(a) 350 $\rightarrow$ red: 350 $\rightarrow$ white
(b) 450 $\rightarrow$ red: 250 $\rightarrow$ white
(c) 380 $\rightarrow$ red: 320 $\rightarrow$ white
(d) None of the above

35. Linkage group in *E. coli* is/are:
(a) 4
(b) 2
(c) 1
(d) 5

36. Which of the following first suggest the conservative model of DNA replication?
(a) Cairns
(b) Meselson and Stahl
(c) Watson and Crick
(d) Taylor

37. Lactic acid is formed in:
(a) Fermentation
(b) Glycolysis
(c) HMP pathways
(d) None of these

38. Red list in India completed by:
(a) Botanical survey of India
(b) Zoological survey of India
(c) Geological survey of India
(d) None of the above

39. National Botanical Institute is situated at:
(a) Lucknow
(b) Kolkata
(c) Mumbai
(d) Chennai

40. Penicillin was used in:
(a) I world war
(b) II world war
(c) Both (a) and (b)
(d) None of these

41. Blindness prevented by use of which crop in poor country?
(a) Golden rice (b) Wheat
(c) Gram (d) Pea

42. Movement of H_2O through cell wall is:
(a) Apoplast (b) Symplast
(c) Tonoplast (d) None of these

43. In which of the following animals Hb is found dissolved in plasma?
(a) Earthworm (b) Cockroach
(c) Sepia (d) Planaria

44. RAAS secrets which of the following hormone?
(a) Mineralo corticoids (b) Gluco corticoids
(c) Both (a) and (b) (d) None of these

45. Bones become fragile in:
(a) Osteoporosis (b) Gout
(c) Arthritis (d) None of these

46. During repolarization of nerve:
(a) K^+ gate closed and Na^+ gate open
(b) Na^+ channels are closed K^+ channels are open
(c) Both gates remain open
(d) Both K^+ and Na^+ gates are closed

47. Zn, Mo, Fe, Cu are:
(a) Trace element (b) Non-essential
(c) Macro nutrient (d) None of these

48. Depict the correct site of hormone:
(a) α-glucagons, β-insulin, δ-somatostatin
(b) α-insulin, β-glucagons, δ-somatostatin
(c) δ-insulin, α-somatostatin, β-glucagons
(d) α-somatostatin, β-insulin, δ-glucagons

49. Insulin receptors are:
(a) Extrinsic protein (b) Intrinsic protein
(c) G-protein (d) Trimeric protein

50. Mode of feeding in free living protozoan is:
(a) Holozoic (b) Saprozoic
(c) Both (a) and (b) (d) None of these

51. Protein deficiency leads to:
(a) Kwashiorkar (b) Marasmus
(c) Cretinism (d) Both (a) & (b)

52. Chloride shift in respond to:
(a) HCO_3^- (b) K^+
(c) H^+ (d) Na^+

53. Double fertilization involves:
(a) Syngamy + triple fusion (b) Double fertilization
(c) Development of antipodal cells (d) None of the above

54. Late blight of potato is caused by:
(a) *Phytophothora infestans* (b) *Xanthomonas oryzae*
(c) *Puccinia graminis* (d) TMV

55. Tendril of Cucurbita and thorns of *Bougainvillea* are:
(a) Homologous organ (b) Analogous organ
(c) Vestigial organ (d) None of these

56. O_2 dissociation curve is:
(a) Sigmoid curve (b) Parabolic
(c) Hyperbolic (d) Straight line

57. IAA is derived from or which of the following is involved in the synthesis of a plant hormone IAA and Vasoconstricter Serotonin?
(a) Tryptophan (b) Tyrosine
(c) Phenylalamine (d) None of these

58. Transverse binary fission is found in:
(a) *Paramecium* (b) *Amoeba*
(c) *Hydra* (d) *Euglena*

59. Capacitation of sperm occurs in:
(a) Female genetical tract (b) Vas deferens
(c) Vas efferens (d) Vagina

60. Phytoplankton's are found in which of the following zone?
(a) Limnetic zone (b) Profundal zone
(c) Littoral (d) Aphotic zone

61. Estuaries are considered of nutrient and trap:
(a) River (b) Pond
(c) Lake (d) Ocean

62. Green algae contains:
(a) Chlorophyll (a) and (b) (b) Starch
(c) Carotenoid (d) All of the above

63. Branch of biology dealing with study of organism in outer space is:
(a) Exobiology (b) Ethology
(c) Euphenics (d) Ethnology

64. Each immunoglobin has two heavy chains and two light chains; the antigen binding is present in:
(a) Variable region of heavy chain
(b) Variable region of both heavy and light chain
(c) Variable region of light chain
(d) Constant region of both light and heavy chain

65. Extension of plasma membrane in prokaryotic cell is:
(a) Mesosome (b) Hapnoid
(c) Ribosome (d) None of these

66. Central dogma of genetic information modified by the discovery of:
(a) Reverse transcriptase (b) DNA polymerase
(c) RNA polymerase (d) Ligase

67. Incorrect character of brown algae is:
(a) Chl a and b present
(b) They remain attached
(c) Chl a and c present
(d) Presence of fucoxanthin

68. Digestive enzymes are:
(a) Hydrolases
(b) Oxido reductases
(c) Transferases
(d) Lyases

69. Protein found in eye lens is:
(a) Crystalline
(b) Collagen
(c) Opsin
(d) Rhodopsin

70. Which cell secretes antibody?
(a) Lymphocytes
(b) Monocytes
(c) Eosinophil
(d) Neutrophil

71. Turner syndrome is:
(a) XO
(b) XXY
(c) XXX
(d) XYY

72. Operon concept was proposed by:
(a) Jacob and Monod
(b) David Baltimore
(c) Allec Jaffery
(d) None of the above

73. Blood clotting vitamin is:
(a) Vitamin-K
(b) Vitamin-A
(c) Vitamin-B_{12}
(d) Vitamin-B_6

74. Expand ELISA:
(a) Enzyme linked immunosorbent assay
(b) Enzyme linked ion sorbent assay
(c) Enzyme linked inductive assay
(d) None of the above

75. Internodes elongation is due to:
(a) Gibberellin
(b) Auxin
(c) Cytokinin
(d) Abscisic acid

76. Apical dominance is due to:
(a) Auxin
(b) Cytokinin
(c) Ethylene
(d) Gibberellin

77. Gibberellin causes:
(a) Apical dominance
(b) Flowering
(c) Internodal growth
(d) Wilting

78. If non-limiting condition are provided then, which happens?
(a) Natality increase and mortality decreases
(b) Morality decrease
(c) Natality increases
(d) Motality increases

79. Mother 'B' homozygous, father 'A' unknown ∴ possible blood group in progeny is:
(a) AB and B possible
(b) AB and A possible
(c) A + B possible
(d) O possible

80. In flagella membrane which enzyme catalyses ATP activity?
(a) Cytoplasmic dyenin
(b) Dyenin
(c) Kinesis
(d) Myosin

81. Amphivasal vascular bundles are found in
(a) Fern
(b) Cucurbita
(c) Dracaena
(d) Luffa cylindrica

82. Certain endodermal cell which are present opposite to the xylem bundle remain thin walled, these cells are
(a) Bulliform cells
(b) Passage cells
(c) Companion cells
(d) Subsidiary cells

83. Example of holocrine gland is
(a) Pancrease
(b) Mammary gland
(c) Salivary gland
(d) Sebaceous gland

84. Haversian system is found in
(a) Bone
(b) Blood
(c) Cartilage
(d) Muscles

85. Who firmly establish Germ theory of disease
(a) Darwin
(b) A.Weismann
(c) L. Pasteur
(d) Cuvier

86. Who introduce term homologus
(a) Darwin
(b) Lamarck
(c) Cuvier
(d) Richard owen

87. de Vries proposed mutation theory on the basis of his observation on the wild variety of which plant
(a) Pisum Sativum
(b) Lathyrus odoratus
(c) Oenothera lamarckiana
(d) Solanum tuberosum

88. Phenetics is
(a) Cytotaxonomy
(b) Chemotaxonomy
(c) Numerical taxonomy
(d) Classification

89. Most well known natural system of classification of angiosperm was proposed by
(a) Bentham and Hooker
(b) Aristotle
(c) Schleiden and Schwann
(d) Beadle and Tatum

90. Which of the following is known as Dead man's finger
(a) Potorion
(b) Euplectella
(c) Chalina
(d) Euspongia

Answer Keys

1. (c)	2. (b)	3. (a)	4. (a)	5. (b)	6. (a)	7. (a)	8. (a)	9. (c)	10. (b)
11. (a)	12. (a)	13. (a)	14. (a)	15. (a)	16. (b)	17. (a)	18. (a)	19. (b)	20. (a)
21. (a)	22. (b)	23. (a)	24. (a)	25. (a)	26. (b)	27. (c)	28. (c)	29. (a)	30. (a)
31. (c)	32. (a)	33. (a)	34. (a)	35. (c)	36. (b)	37. (a)	38. (a)	39. (a)	40. (b)
41. (a)	42. (a)	43. (a)	44. (a)	45. (a)	46. (b)	47. (a)	48. (a)	49. (a)	50. (a)
51. (d)	52. (a)	53. (a)	54. (a)	55. (a)	56. (a)	57. (a)	58. (a)	59. (a)	60. (c)
61. (a)	62. (d)	63. (a)	64. (b)	65. (a)	66. (a)	67. (a)	68. (a)	69. (a)	70. (a)
71. (a)	72. (a)	73. (a)	74. (a)	75. (a)	76. (a)	77. (c)	78. (a)	79. (a)	80. (b)
81. (c)	82. (b)	83. (d)	84. (a)	85. (c)	86. (d)	87. (c)	88. (c)	89. (a)	90. (c)